a Lange medical book

Current Procedures: Surgery

Rebecca M. Minter, MD
Associate Professor
Department of Surgery
University of Michigan
Ann Arbor

Gerard M. Doherty, MD
NW Thompson Professor of Surgery
Department of Surgery
University of Michigan
Ann Arbor

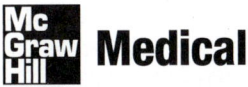

New York Chicago San Francisco Lisbon London Madrid
Mexico City Milan New Delhi San Juan Seoul Singapore Sydney Toronto

The McGraw·Hill Companies

Current Procedures: Surgery

Copyright © 2010 by The McGraw-Hill Companies, Inc. All rights reserved. Printed in the United States of America. Except as permitted under the United States Copyright Act of 1976, no part of this publication may be reproduced or distributed in any form or by any means, or stored in a database or retrieval system, without the prior written permission of the publisher.

1 2 34 5 6 7 8 9 0   WDQ/WDQ   14 13 12 11 10

ISBN 978-0-07-145316-5
MHID 0-07-145316-4
ISSN 2153-5396

Notice

Medicine is an ever-changing science. As new research and clinical experience broaden our knowledge, changes in treatment and drug therapy are required. The authors and the publisher of this work have checked with sources believed to be reliable in their efforts to provide information that is complete and generally in accord with the standards accepted at the time of publication. However, in view of the possibility of human error or changes in medical sciences, neither the authors nor the publisher nor any other party who has been involved in the preparation or publication of this work warrants that the information contained herein is in every respect accurate or complete, and they disclaim all responsibility for any errors or omissions or for the results obtained from use of the information contained in this work. Readers are encouraged to confirm the information contained herein with other sources. For example and in particular, readers are advised to check the product information sheet included in the package of each drug they plan to administer to be certain that the information contained in this work is accurate and that changes have not been made in the recommended dose or in the contraindications for administration. This recommendation is of particular importance in connection with new or infrequently used drugs.

This book was set in Minion by Glyph International.
The editors were Marsha Gelber and Harriet Lebowitz.
The production supervisor was Catherine Saggese.
Project management was provided by Somya Rustagi at Glyph International.
The illustration manager was Armen Ovsepyan.
The designer was Alan Barnett.
The illustrators were Susan Gilbert, CMI, and Peggy Firth.
Worldcolor Dubuque was the printer and binder.
Cover photo: Laurent

This book is printed on acid-free paper.

Cataloging-in Publication data for this title are on file at the Library of Congress.

McGraw-Hill books are available at special quantity discounts to use as premiums and sales promotions, or for use in corporate training programs. To contact a representative, please e-mail us at bulksales@mcgraw-hill.com.

International Edition ISBN 978-0-07-110455-5; MHID 0-07-110455-0.
Copyright © 2011. Exclusive rights by The McGraw-Hill Companies, Inc., for manufacture and export. This book cannot be re-exported from the country to which it is consigned by McGraw-Hill. The International Edition is not available in North America.

CONTENTS

Authors v

Preface ix

1 Thyroidectomy and Neck Dissection 1
   Amit K. Mathur, MD, and Gerard M. Doherty, MD

2 Parathyroidectomy 8
   Sean C. Kumer, MD, PhD and Gerard M. Doherty, MD

3 Adrenalectomy 14
   Awori J. Hayanga, MD, MPH, and Paul G. Gauger, MD

4 Surgery of the Endocrine Pancreas 22
   Brian D. Saunders, MD, and Gerard M. Doherty, MD

5 Transhiatal Esophagectomy 29
   Jennifer F. Waljee, MD, MPH, MSc, and Mark B. Orringer, MD

6 Operative Management of Gastric Lesions 42
   Erika L. Newman, MD, and Michael W. Mulholland, MD, PhD

7 Surgery of the Hiatus 57
   C. J. Lee, MD, and Jonathan F. Finks, MD

8 Emergency Operations for Peptic Ulcer Disease 67
   Susan Tsai, MD, and Michael W. Mulholland, MD, PhD

9 Surgical Therapies for Morbid Obesity 75
   John B. Ammori, MD, and Jonathan F. Finks, MD

10 Enteral Access 81
   Kerianne H. Quanstrum, MD, and Richard E. Burney, MD

11 Laparoscopic Cholecystectomy 89
   Kevin Tri Nguyen, MD, PhD, and John D. Birkmeyer, MD

12 Management of Complex Biliary Stone Disease 97
   Richard V. Ha, MD, and Charles E. Binkley, MD

13 Management of Bile Duct Injuries and
   Biliary Strictures 106
   Amit K. Mathur, MD, and James A. Knol, MD

14 Hepatectomy 115
   Theodore H. Welling, III, MD

15 Pancreaticoduodenectomy 121
   Nicholas H. Osborne, MD, and Lisa M. Colletti, MD

16 Distal Pancreatectomy 131
   K. Barrett Deatrick, MD, and Gerard M. Doherty, MD

17 Operative Management of Chronic
   Pancreatitis 137
   Jules Lin, MD, and Diane M. Simeone, MD

18 Splenectomy 145
   Brett A. Almond, MD, PhD, and Kathleen M. Diehl, MD

19 Small Bowel Resection 149
   Junewai L. Reoma, MD, and Daniel B. Hinshaw, MD

20 Appendectomy 156
   Chandu Vemuri, MD, and Jonathan F. Finks, MD

21 Loop Colostomy, End Ileostomy,
   and Loop Ileostomy 161
   Bedabrata Sarkar, MD, and Lisa M. Colletti, MD

22 Operative Management of Inflammatory
   Bowel Disease 167
   Jennifer Cannon, MD, and Emina H. Huang, MD

23 Colectomy 180
   Barry L. Rosenberg, MD, MBA, and Arden M. Morris, MD, MPH

24 Operative Management of Rectal Tumors 192
   David G. Heidt, MD, and Emina H. Huang, MD

25 Operative Management of Rectal Prolapse 203
   Brian S. Knipp, MD, and Richard E. Burney, MD

26 Benign Anorectal Procedures 210
   Erica N. Proctor, MD, and Emily V.A. Finlayson, MD

27 Operative Management of Breast Cancer 217
   Dawn M. Coleman, MD, and Kathleen M. Diehl, MD

28 Operative Management of Melanoma 229
   Amir A. Ghaferi, MD, and Michael S. Sabel, MD

29 Operative Management of Soft Tissue Sarcoma 238
   Dan G. Blazer, III, MD, and Alfred E. Chang, MD

30 Renal Transplantation 242
   Constance M. Mobley, MD, PhD, and Shawn J. Pelletier, MD

31 Pancreas Transplantation 252
   Raymond J. Lynch, MD, and Randall S. Sung, MD

32 Liver Transplantation 261
Derek A. DuBay, MD, and Randall S. Sung, MD

33 Vascular Access for Dialysis 270
Frank C. Vandy, MD, and Peter K. Henke, MD

34 Management of Infrarenal Abdominal Aortic
Aneurysm 279
Michael S. Shillingford, MD, Loay S. Kabbani, MD,
and Gilbert R. Upchurch, Jr, MD

35 Carotid Endarterectomy. 286
Christopher Longo, MD, and Ramon Berguer, MD, PhD

36 Operative Management of Aortoiliac Occlusive
Disease 292
Gorav Ailawadi, MD

37 Surgical Revascularization of Infrainguinal
Arterial Occlusive Disease 300
Loay S. Kabbani, MD, and Peter K. Henke, MD

38 Management of Lower Extremity
Venous Insufficiency 309
K. Barrett Deatrick, MD, and Thomas W. Wakefield, MD

39 Below- and Above-the-Knee Amputation. 315
Jeffrey H. Kozlow, MD, Andrew M. Zwyghuizen, MD,
and Thomas W. Wakefield, MD

40 Inguinal Hernia Repair 324
Timothy L. Frankel, MD, and Richard E. Burney, MD

41 Ventral Hernia Repair 331
Kristoffer B. Sugg, MD, Edwin Y. Chang, MD,
and Michael G. Franz, MD

42 Wound Closure Techniques 338
Brent M. Egeland, MD, and Paul S. Cederna, MD

43 Central Venous Access. 347
Laura A. Monson, MD, and Melissa E. Brunsvold, MD

44 Tube Thoracostomy. 355
Peter Sassalos, MD, and Melissa E. Brunsvold, MD

45 Tracheostomy and Emergency
Cricothyroidotomy 360
Michael L. Bernstein, MD, PhD, and Stewart C.
Wang, MD, PhD

46 Operative Management of Pyloric Stenosis:
Pyloromyotomy 366
Benjamin Levi, MD, and George B. Mychaliska, MD

47 Pediatric Vascular Access 371
Kimberly McCrudden Erickson, MD

48 Pediatric Inguinal Hernia. 378
Kimberly McCrudden Erickson, MD

Index 383

AUTHORS

Gorav Ailawadi, MD
Assistant Professor of Surgery
University of Virginia Health System

Brett A. Almond, MD, PhD
Fellow, Vascular Surgery and Endovascular Therapy
University of Florida

John B. Ammori, MD
Fellow, Surgical Oncology
Memorial Sloan-Kettering Cancer Center

Ramon Berguer, MD, PhD
Frankel Professor of Vascular Surgery
University of Michigan Health System

Michael Bernstein, MD, PhD
Assistant Professor of Surgery
Saint Louis University

John D. Birkmeyer, MD
George D. Zuidema Professor of Surgery
University of Michigan Health System

Charles E. Binkley, MD
Attending Surgeon
Hepatobliary and Pancreatic Surgery
Kaiser Permanente Medical Center, San Francisco

Dan G. Blazer, III, MD
Assistant Professor of Surgery
Duke University Medical Center

Melissa E. Brunsvold, MD
Assistant Professor of Surgery
University of Michigan Health System

Richard E. Burney, MD
Professor of Surgery
University of Michigan Health System

Jennifer Cannon, MD
Fellow in Endocrine Surgery
University of Miami, Jackson Memorial Hospital

Paul S. Cederna, MD
Associate Professor of Surgery
University of Michigan Health System

Alfred E. Chang, MD
Hugh Cabot Professor of Surgery
University of Michigan Health System

Edwin Y. Chang, MD
Spokane Plastic Surgeons

Dawn M. Coleman, MD
Resident in General Surgery
University of Michigan Health System

Lisa M. Colletti, MD
C. Gardner Child Professor of Surgery
University of Michigan Health System

K. Barrett Deatrick, MD
Resident in General Surgery
University of Michigan Health System

Kathleen M. Diehl, MD
Associate Professor of Surgery
University of Michigan Health System

Derek A. DuBay, MD
Assistant Professor of Surgery
Liver Transplant and Hepatobiliary Surgery
University of Alabama at Birmingham

Brent M. Egeland, MD
Resident in Plastic Surgery
University of Michigan Health System

Kimberly McCrudden Erickson, MD
Assistant Professor of Surgery
University of Michigan Health System

Jonathan F. Finks, MD
Assistant Professor of Surgery
University of Michigan Health System

Emily V.A. Finlayson, MD
Assistant Professor in Residence
University of California, San Francisco

Timothy L. Frankel, MD
Resident in General Surgery
University of Michigan Health System

Michael G. Franz, MD
Associate Professor of Surgery
University of Michigan Health System

Paul G. Gauger, MD
William J. Fry Professor of Surgery
University of Michigan Health System

Amir A. Ghaferi, MD
Resident in General Surgery
University of Michigan Health System

Richard V. Ha, MD
Fellow in Cardiothoracic Surgery
UCLA Medical Center

Awori J. Hayanga, MD, MPH
Resident in General Surgery
University of Michigan Health System

David G. Heidt, MD
Transplant Fellow
University of Michigan Health System

Peter K. Henke, MD
Professor of Surgery
University of Michigan Health System

Daniel B. Hinshaw, MD
Professor of Surgery
University of Michigan Health System

Emina H. Huang, MD
Associate Professor of Surgery
General Surgery/GI, Oncologic and Endocrine Surgery
University of Florida

Loay S. Kabbani, MD
Consultant Vascular Surgeon
Al Assad University Hospital
Damascus, Syria

Brian S. Knipp, MD
Resident in General Surgery
University of Michigan Health System

James A. Knol, MD
Associate Professor of Surgery
University of Michigan Health System

Jeffrey H. Kozlow, MD
Resident in Plastic Surgery
University of Michigan Health System

Sean C. Kumer, MD, PhD
Fellow, Division of Transplant Surgery
University of Virginia Health System

C.J. Lee, MD
Resident in General Surgery
University of Michigan Health System

Benjamin Levi, MD
Resident in Plastic Surgery
University of Michigan Health System

Jules Lin, MD
Assistant Professor of Thoracic Surgery
University of Michigan Health System

Christopher R. Longo, MD
Carolina Vascular Surgery and Diagnostics

Raymond J. Lynch, MD
Resident in General Surgery
University of Michigan Health System

Amit K. Mathur, MD
Resident in General Surgery
University of Michigan Health System

Constance M. Mobley, MD, PhD
Resident in General Surgery
University of Michigan Health System

Laura A. Monson, MD
Resident in Plastic Surgery
University of Michigan Health System

Arden M. Morris, MD, MPH
Associate Professor of Surgery
University of Michigan Health System

Michael W. Mulholland, MD, PhD
Frederick A. Coller Distinguished Professor
Chair, Department of Surgery
University of Michigan Health System

George B. Mychaliska, MD
Assistant Professor of Surgery
University of Michigan Health System

Erika Adams Newman, MD
Fellow, Pediatric Surgery
The University of Chicago Comer Children's Hospital

Kevin Tri Nguyen, MD, PhD
Hepatopancreaticobiliary Fellow
University of Pittsburgh

Mark B. Orringer, MD
John Alexander Distinguished Professor of Thoracic Surgery
University of Michigan Health System

Nicholas H. Osborne, MD
Resident in General Surgery
University of Michigan Health System

Shawn J. Pelletier, MD
Assistant Professor of Surgery
University of Michigan Health System

Erica N. Proctor, MD
Resident in General Surgery
University of Michigan Health System

Kerianne H. Quanstrum, MD
Resident in General Surgery
University of Michigan Health System

Junewai L. Reoma, MD
Resident in General Surgery
University of Michigan Health System

Barry L. Rosenberg, MD, MBA
Project Leader
Boston Consulting Group

Michael S. Sabel, MD
Associate Professor of Surgery
University of Michigan Health System

Bedabrata Sarkar, MD
Resident in General Surgery
University of Michigan Health System

Peter Sassalos, MD
Resident in General Surgery
University of Michigan Health System

Brian D. Saunders, MD
Assistant Professor of Surgery
Penn State Milton S. Hershey Medical Center

Michael S. Shillingford, MD
Cardiothoracic Surgery Fellow
University of Florida

Diane M. Simeone, MD
Greenfield Professor in Surgery and Molecular
And Integrative Physiology
University of Michigan Health System

Kristoffer Sugg, MD
Resident in Plastic Surgery
University of Michigan Health System

Randall S. Sung, MD
Associate Professor of Surgery
University of Michigan Health System

Susan Tsai, MD
Fellow, Surgical Oncology
Johns Hopkins University

Gilbert R. Upchurch, Jr, MD
Leland Ira Doan Research Professor of Vascular Surgery
University of Michigan Health System

Frank C. Vandy, MD
Resident in Vascular Surgery
University of Michigan Health System

Chandu Vemuri, MD
Resident in General Surgery
University of Michigan Health System

Thomas W. Wakefield, MD
S. Martin Lindenauer Collegiate Professor of Vascular Surgery
University of Michigan Health System

Jennifer Waljee, MD, MPH, MSc
Resident in Plastic Surgery
University of Michigan Health System

Stewart C. Wang, MD, PhD
Professor and Director of Burn Surgery
University of Michigan Health System

Theodore H. Welling, III, MD
Assistant Professor of Surgery
University of Michigan Health System

Andrew M. Zwyghuizen, MD
Resident in Plastic Surgery
University of Michigan Health System

PREFACE

Current Surgical Procedures is a new book intended to provide straightforward, modern guidance to common procedures performed during general surgery training. Directed at a mid-level surgery resident, the information should be equally useful to medical students, physicians assistants, higher level residents and other staff who benefit from an accessible resource to outline the key features and steps of these operations. Preparation by the faculty and house staff of the University of Michigan ensures the compilation of expert approaches to these procedures.

Outstanding Features

- All new drawings illustrate the current methods for these procedures.
- Templated presentation of the material simplifies rapid review.
- Inclusion of expected benefits, potential risks, preoperative preparation and contraindications provides a foundation for obtaining thorough informed consent prior to the procedure.
- Step-by-step presentation of key procedure steps.
- Coverage of postoperative management, potential complications, and clinical pearls complete a concise resource for timely review.

Acknowledgments

As the editors, we would like to acknowledge our tremendous good fortune to work in an outstanding Department of Surgery led by Dr. Michael Mulholland, and to be surrounded by a truly expert group of peers among both the faculty and the house staff. Their personal attention to the project has infused the text with the views of proficient practitioners that make this work special. We are particularly grateful for the patient and professional staff from McGraw-Hill including Marsha Loeb Gelber, Harriet Lebowitz, and Armen Ovsepyan, who have made great contributions to the text in both time and concentration, and allowed us to ensure an accurate, high-quality edition. The various artists who have worked to present our concepts as understandable drawings have our admiration both for their talent, and for their determination to translate our ideas into pictures. We appreciate the careful attention and good humor of Mary Kay Anderson who has provided the staff support of this work in Ann Arbor. Finally, to our families, we appreciate your indulgence of our attention to our work.

Rebecca M. Minter, MD
Gerard M. Doherty, MD
Ann Arbor, Michigan
June 2010

CHAPTER 1

Thyroidectomy and Neck Dissection

Amit K. Mathur, MD, and Gerard M. Doherty, MD

INDICATIONS

Thyroid Lobectomy
- Unilateral toxic nodule.
- Solitary adenoma or cyst.

Total Thyroidectomy
- Thyroid carcinoma.
- Graves' disease.
- Hashimoto thyroiditis.
- Multinodular goiter.
- Substernal goiter.

Neck Dissection
- Locally advanced head and neck carcinoma demonstrated by presence of nodal disease clinically, by preoperative imaging, or by sentinel node biopsy.

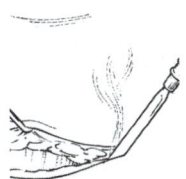 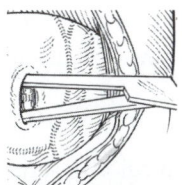 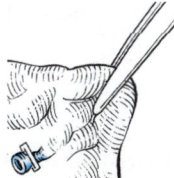
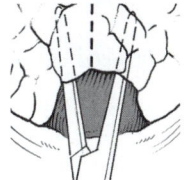 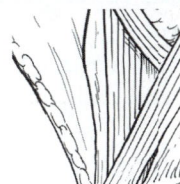 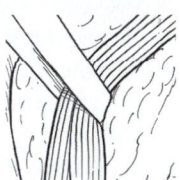
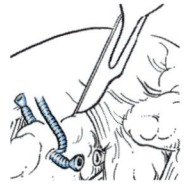 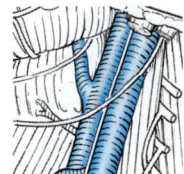 

CONTRAINDICATIONS
- Few contraindications exist for thyroidectomy or neck dissection.

Absolute (Neck Dissection)
- Randomly scattered dermal metastases precluding a full-thickness dissection.
- Intracranial extension of tumor from the neck.
- Tumor fixation to the skull base or the cervical spine.

Relative (Neck Dissection)
- Tumor fixation to the internal carotid artery.
- Locally advanced disease in the root of the neck.
- Periosteal invasion of the skull base.

INFORMED CONSENT

Thyroid Surgery

A. Expected Benefits
- Curative resection for actual or potential malignancy.
- Relief of symptoms caused by toxic or large multinodular goiters.
- Relief of symptoms resulting from benign thyroid disease.

B. Potential Risks
- Bleeding that may cause airway compression and require reoperation.
- Recurrent laryngeal nerve paresis or transection causing hoarseness (temporary or permanent).
- Hypocalcemia requiring oral calcium or vitamin D.
- Scarring.
- Infection.
- Need for additional medical or surgical treatment.

Modified Radical Neck Dissection

A. Expected Benefits
- Clearance of primary tumor and locally advanced carcinoma from the neck at all nodal levels.

B. Potential Risks
- Damage to vital adjacent structures, including spinal accessory nerve, sternocleidomastoid (SCM) muscle, internal jugular vein, and vagus nerve.
- Lymphatic leak from thoracic duct trauma.

EQUIPMENT
- No special equipment is required.
- A self-retaining retractor may be used to assist in the dissection.
- A handheld recurrent laryngeal nerve stimulator is often employed.
- A harmonic scalpel may also be used to aid in the dissection.

PATIENT PREPARATION
- Nothing by mouth the evening before surgery.
- Preoperative antibiotics if needed for valvular pathology, artificial heart valves, artificial joints, etc.
- Consultation with an anesthesiologist if necessary based on airway examination or comorbid disease, or both.
- Surgeon-directed ultrasound to identify thyroid lesion, size of thyroid, location of surrounding structures, etc.
- Additional preoperative imaging and studies to demonstrate presence of lesion and potential metastatic disease in malignancy.
- Anesthesiology consultation (see later discussion).

PATIENT POSITIONING
- The patient should be supine.
- Airway management is of particular concern. Preoperative anesthesiology consultation should alleviate positioning concerns while ensuring proper airway safety during the procedure.
- A towel roll can be placed beneath the shoulder blades to facilitate neck extension.
- Arms may be tucked.

PROCEDURE

Thyroid Procedures
- **Figure 1–1:** A curvilinear incision is made in the neck a fingerbreadth below the cricoid cartilage and approximately 2 fingerbreadths above the sternal notch.
  - Additionally, a suitable skin crease in the lower neck may be used for the incision location.
  - The subcutaneous tissue and the platysma may be divided with cautery.
  - Skin flaps are made superiorly and inferiorly above the level of the anterior jugular veins.
- **Figure 1–2:** Access to the deeper neck is made by dividing the strap muscles in the midline between the anterior jugular veins.
  - A plane is established between the sternohyoid and the sternothyroid muscles from medial to lateral.
  - A plane is established between the sternothyroid and the thyroid gland sharply.
  - The middle thyroid vein is divided.

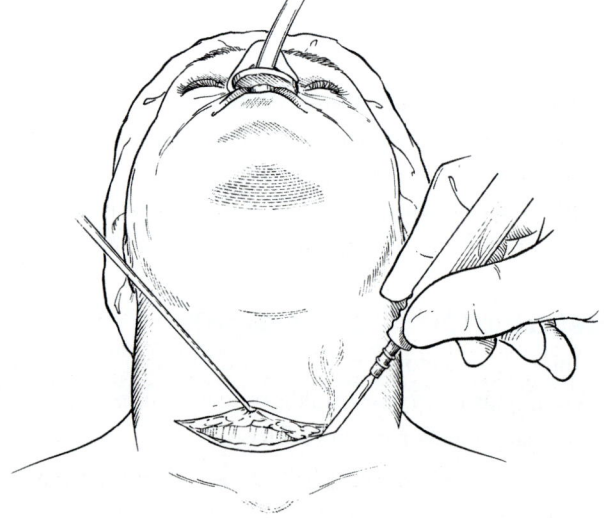

Figure 1–1

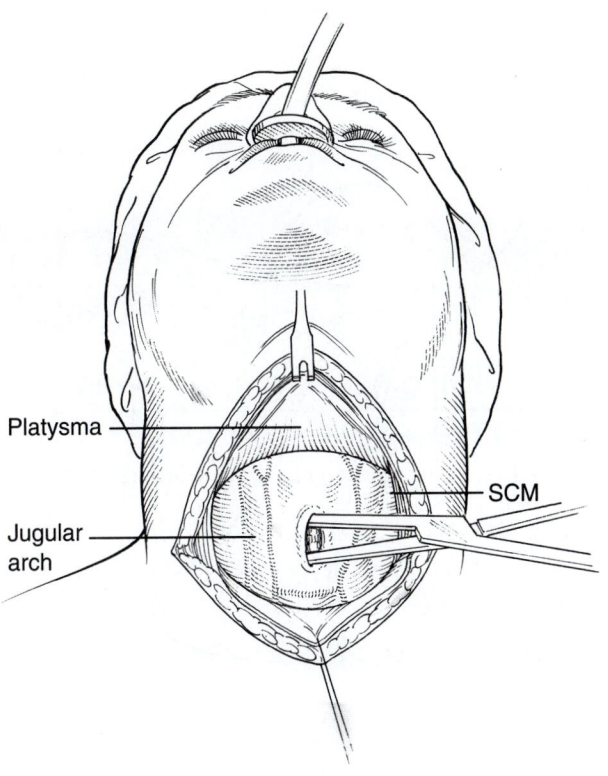

Figure 1-2

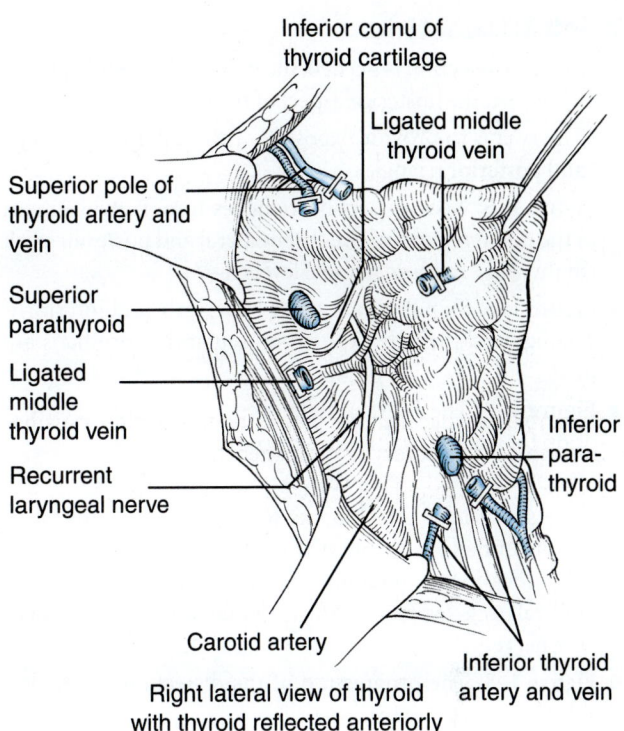

Right lateral view of thyroid with thyroid reflected anteriorly

Figure 1-3

- **Figure 1–3:** The gland is mobilized anteriorly to expose the recurrent laryngeal nerve. The superior pole attachments may be divided to assist in this mobilization.
  - The cricothyroid space is entered along the medial aspect of the lobe to mobilize the superior pole of the thyroid lobe.
  - The superior lobe attachments are divided close to the gland to avoid injury to the superior laryngeal nerve branches.
  - The superior parathyroid gland is identified posterior to the recurrent laryngeal nerve.
  - The recurrent laryngeal nerve and its course are identified and verified by the nerve stimulator.
  - The inferior parathyroid is identified anterior to the nerve. The inferior pole attachments are then divided.
  - The final attachments near the nerve and the ligament of Berry are identified and divided meticulously without traction or direct pressure on the recurrent laryngeal nerve. Use of cautery around the nerve and while dissecting with the thyroid retracted anteriorly should be avoided.
- **Figure 1–4:** The thyroid is then dissected from its attachments on the trachea and divided at the isthmus for a lobectomy.

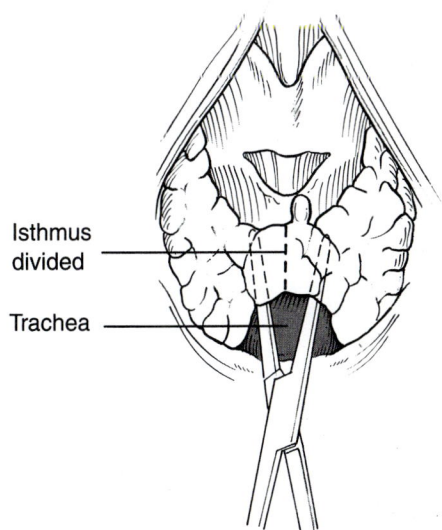

Figure 1-4

Neck Dissection

- If a neck dissection is needed, the incision is extended laterally toward the posterior aspect of the neck.
  - The goal is to provide exposure of the anterolateral neck and posterior triangles.
- **Figure 1–5:** Neck dissection removes tumor involvement in the nodal regions of the anterolateral and posterior neck (in thyroid carcinoma, nodal levels II–V).
- **Figure 1–6:** Skin flaps are made superiorly and inferiorly. The figure shows the exposed musculature once flaps are made.
- **Figure 1–7:** The SCM muscle is encircled with a Penrose drain for traction to provide exposure.
  - We prefer to initiate the dissection in the posterior triangle.
  - The specimen's attachments to the trapezius are taken down initially with blunt dissection, especially prior to identification of the spinal accessory nerve. In a modified radical neck dissection, efforts should be made to preserve the nerve.
- **Figure 1–8:** The progression of the dissection on the left side (SCM not shown).
  - The specimen is dissected from lateral to medial with attention to the underlying structures. Efforts should be made to preserve the internal jugular vein. If the vein cannot be separated from the surrounding grossly positive nodal tissue, it is included in the specimen.
  - The specimen is dissected from inferior to superior (from levels IV–II).
  - The specimen is removed en bloc, marked, and prepared for pathologic examination.

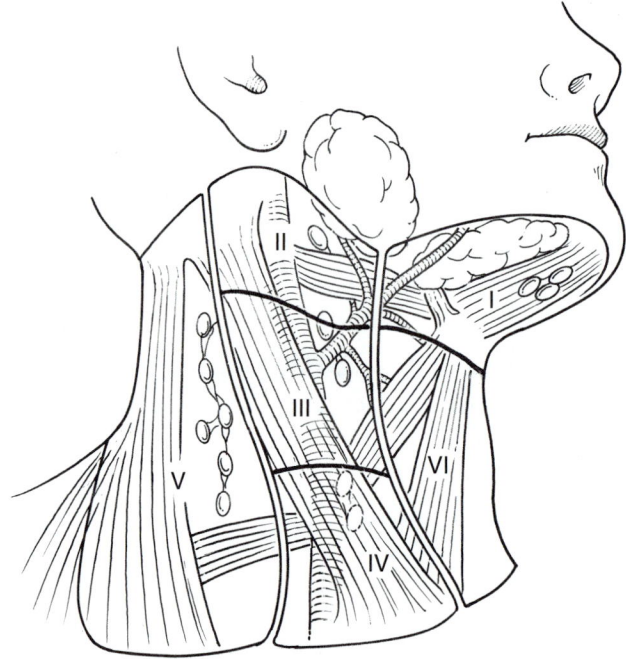

Figure 1–5

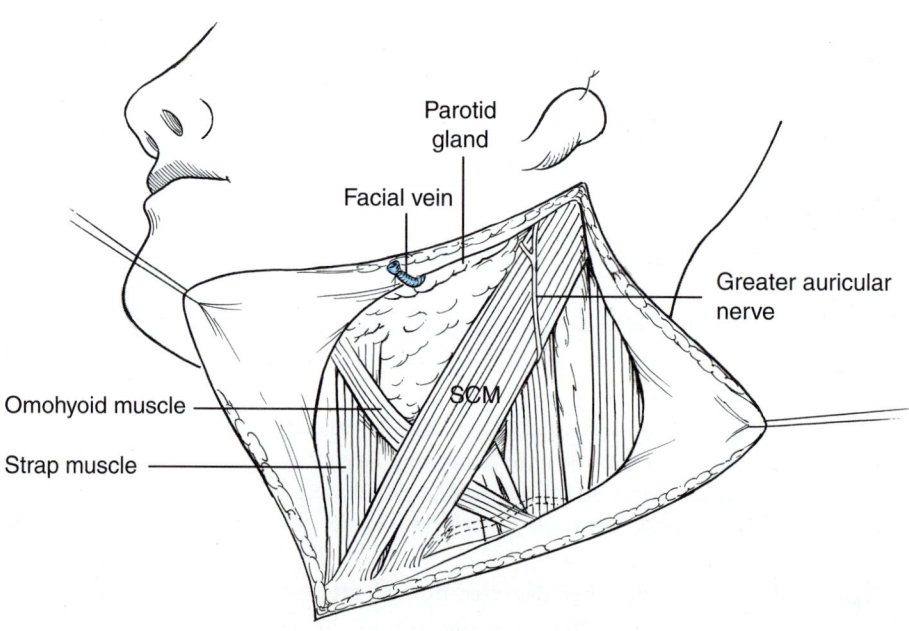

Figure 1–6

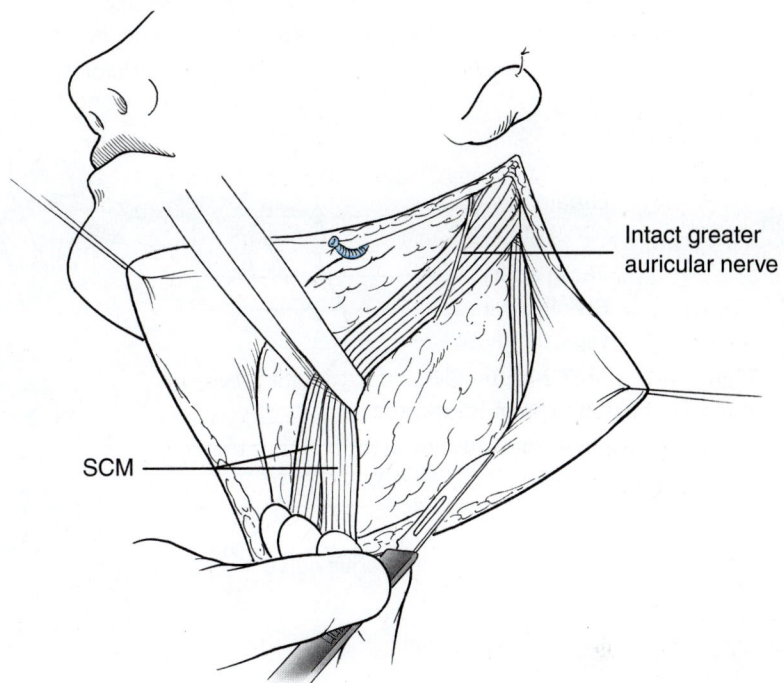

Figure 1-7

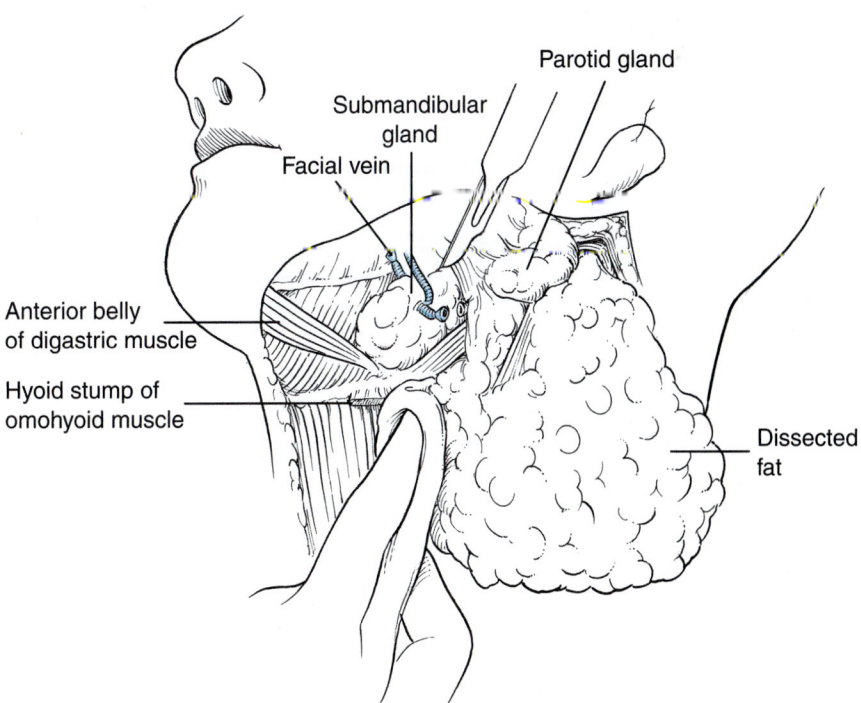

Figure 1-8

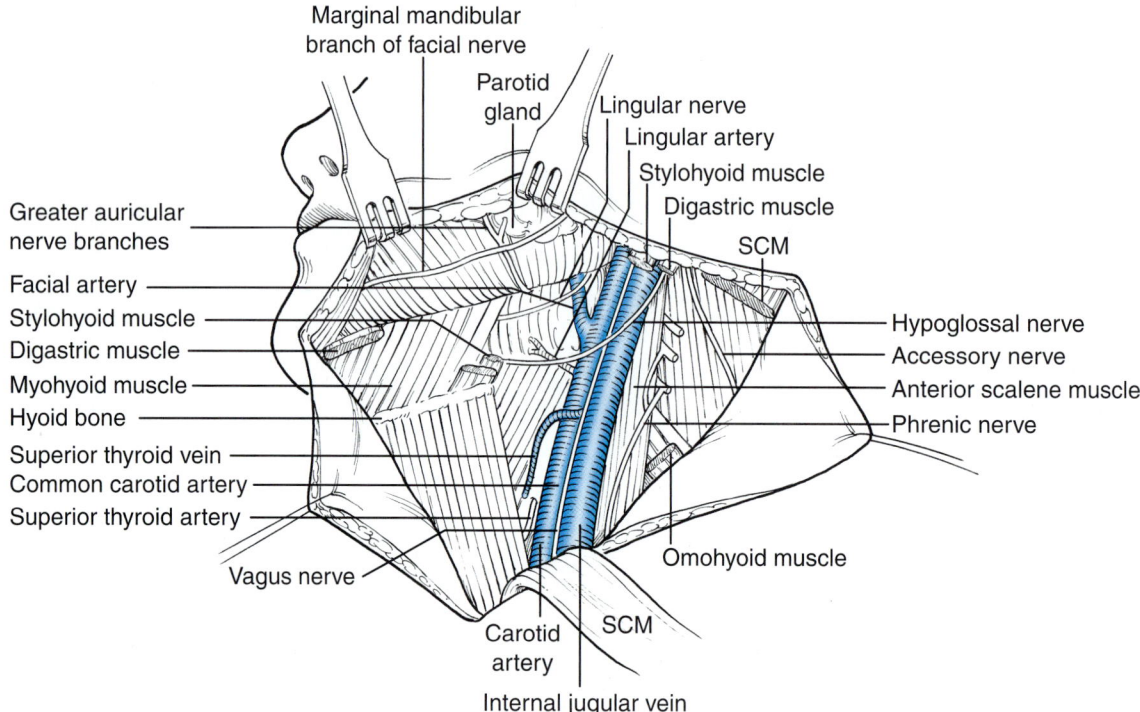

Figure 1-9

- **Figure 1–9:** As the dissection is completed, the wound is inspected for hemostasis.
  - A drain is placed through a separate stab incision in the anterolateral neck.
  - The platysma and subcutaneous tissue is reapproximated using absorbable suture, and the incision is closed with a monofilament absorbable suture or tissue glue.

POSTOPERATIVE CARE

- For benign thyroid disease, thyroid hormone replacement is initiated if total thyroidectomy has been performed.
- For malignant disease, thyroid hormone replacement is deferred until after postoperative radioactive iodine scan.
- Postoperative calcium levels are monitored and calcium replacement is given empirically.
- Pain control should be initiated with intravenous agents initially; once swallowing is adequate, the patient can be transitioned to oral narcotics.
- Diet should be advanced progressively.
- Drains should be inspected for lymphatic leak, and patients instructed on drain care.
- Drains should be removed once output decreases to 30 mL or less per day.

POTENTIAL COMPLICATIONS

- Nerve injury: spinal accessory nerve; recurrent laryngeal nerve injury (if central neck dissection is included in the procedure); brachial plexus.
- Vascular injury: internal jugular vein; carotid artery causing neck hematoma, which could potentially progress to airway compromise.
- Thoracic duct injury leading to lymphatic leak, possibly requiring operative intervention and thoracic duct ligation.
- Tracheal injury.
- Esophageal injury.
- Local disease recurrence.

PEARLS AND TIPS

- Perform neck dissection with careful attention to the underlying neurovascular structures while maintaining the goal of a complete oncologic resection.

REFERENCES

Doherty GM. Complications of Thyroid and Parathyroid Surgery. In: Mulholland MW, Doherty GM, eds. *Complications in Surgery.* Philadelphia, PA: Lippincott Williams & Wilkins; 2006:575–593.

Gauger PG. Thyroid Gland. In: Mulholland MW, Lillemoe KD, Doherty GM, et al, eds. *Greenfield's Surgery: Scientific Principles & Practice,* 4th ed. Philadelphia, PA: Lippincott Williams & Wilkins; 2006:1310–1334.

CHAPTER 2

Parathyroidectomy

Sean C. Kumer, MD, PhD, and Gerard M. Doherty, MD

INDICATIONS

Symptomatic
- Fractures (especially vertebral compression fractures).
- Nephrolithiasis.
- Severe neuromuscular weakness.
- Easy fatigability.
- Loss of stamina.
- Sleep disturbance.
- Depression.
- Memory loss.
- Pancreatitis.
- History of an episode of life-threatening hypercalcemia.
- Carcinoma.

Asymptomatic
- Markedly elevated serum calcium (> 1.0 mg/dL above normal).
- Markedly elevated 24-hour urinary calcium excretion (> 400 mg).
- Abnormal serum creatinine.
- Reduced bone mineral density (T-score < −2.5).
- Age younger than 50 years.
- Carcinoma.

CONTRAINDICATIONS
- Pregnancy (first trimester).
- Multiple comorbidities precluding safe intervention.
- Idiopathic hypercalcemia.

INFORMED CONSENT

Expected Benefits
- Treatment of symptomatic hypercalcemia.
- Prevention of deleterious effects secondary to chronic parathyroid hormone elevation and hypercalcemia.

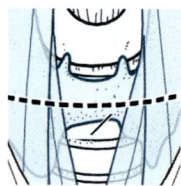
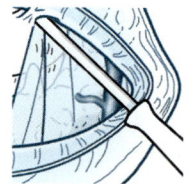
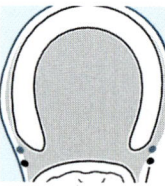
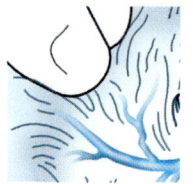
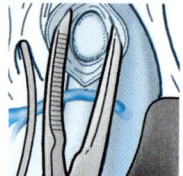
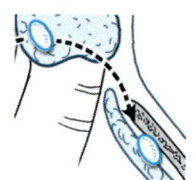

Potential Risks

- Bleeding requiring reoperation.
- Weakness of the voice or hoarseness (temporary or permanent).
- Need for oral calcium/vitamin D supplements (short or long term).
- Visible neck scar.
- Neck swelling beneath incision.
- Infection.
- Failure of operation to correct hypercalcemia or recurrence of hypercalcemia.
- Need for additional tests or procedures.

EQUIPMENT

- Intraoperative parathyroid hormone (PTH) monitoring capability with access and equipment for blood sampling (peripheral or central).
- Bipolar cautery, harmonic scalpel, LigaSure, or surgical ties can be safely used for hemostatic control.

PATIENT PREPARATION

- Nothing by mouth the evening before surgery.
- No preoperative antibiotics are necessary before surgery, except when the patient has other indications (eg, cardiac valvulopathy or orthopedic hardware).
- Anesthesiology consultation as needed.

PATIENT POSITIONING

- The patient should be supine with his or her legs slightly reclined and the head and shoulders raised (lawn chair position).
- A towel roll or other small bump is placed beneath the shoulder blades to allow for neck extension and exposure.

PROCEDURE

- Local or general anesthesia may be used.
- **Figure 2–1:** An incision is made transversely approximately 1 cm below the level of the cricoid cartilage and measuring 3–5 cm in length.

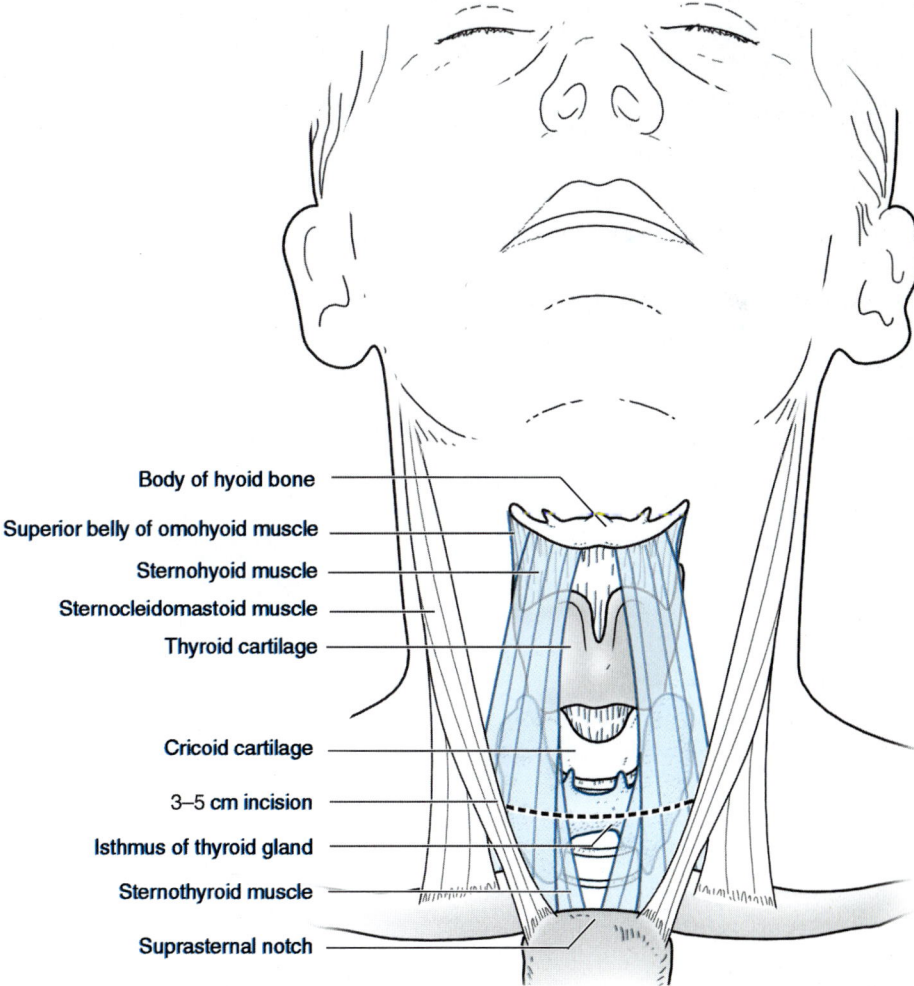

Figure 2–1

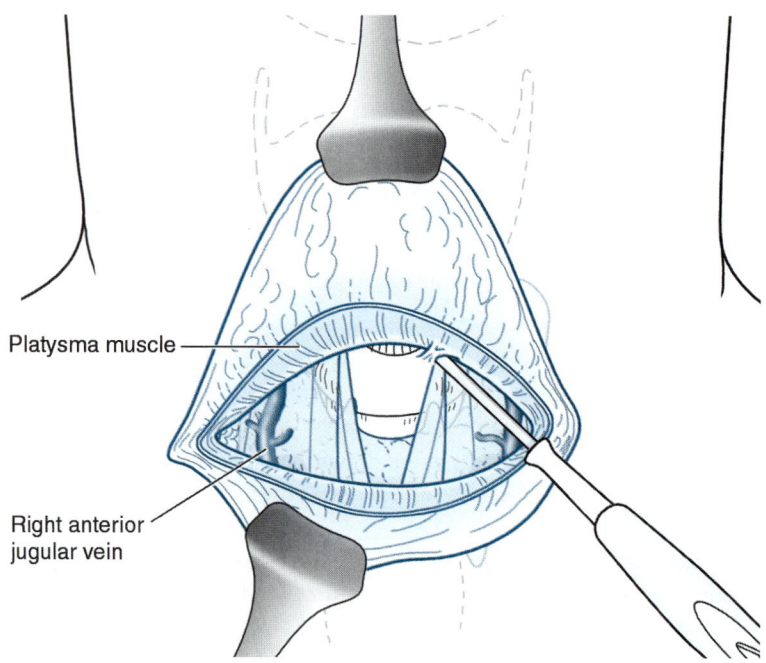

Figure 2–2

- **Figure 2–2:** This incision is carried through the level of the platysma with electrocautery.
  - Subplatysmal flaps are fashioned superiorly, laterally, and inferiorly with a combination of electrocautery and blunt dissection.
  - The strap muscles and associated fascia are entered through the midline taking care to avoid injuring the anterior jugular veins.
- **Figure 2–3:** Dissection proceeds to include all of the soft tissue associated with the thyroid down to the prevertebral fascia.

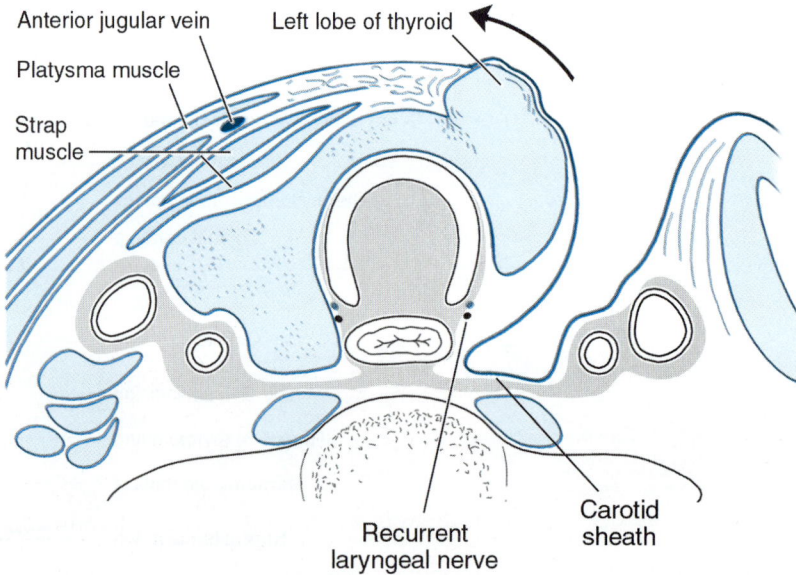

Figure 2–3

- The thyroid is retracted medially by the assistant; the carotid sheath is bluntly dissected on the medial aspect so it can be retracted laterally, allowing adequate exposure to identify the recurrent laryngeal nerve, which usually courses superiorly in the tracheoesophageal groove.
- Occasionally, the middle thyroid vein must be ligated and divided.
- At this point in the operation, a baseline PTH level is drawn and promptly placed on ice.
- **Figure 2–4:** The parathyroid glands are dissected free from the surrounding tissue, taking care to avoid disrupting their vascular supply.
  - An additional PTH level may be drawn before excision (by surgeon's choice) and PTH levels are also monitored 5, 10, and 15 minutes following excision.
  - The inferior parathyroid glands are usually more anterior than the upper glands; however, their location is more variable.

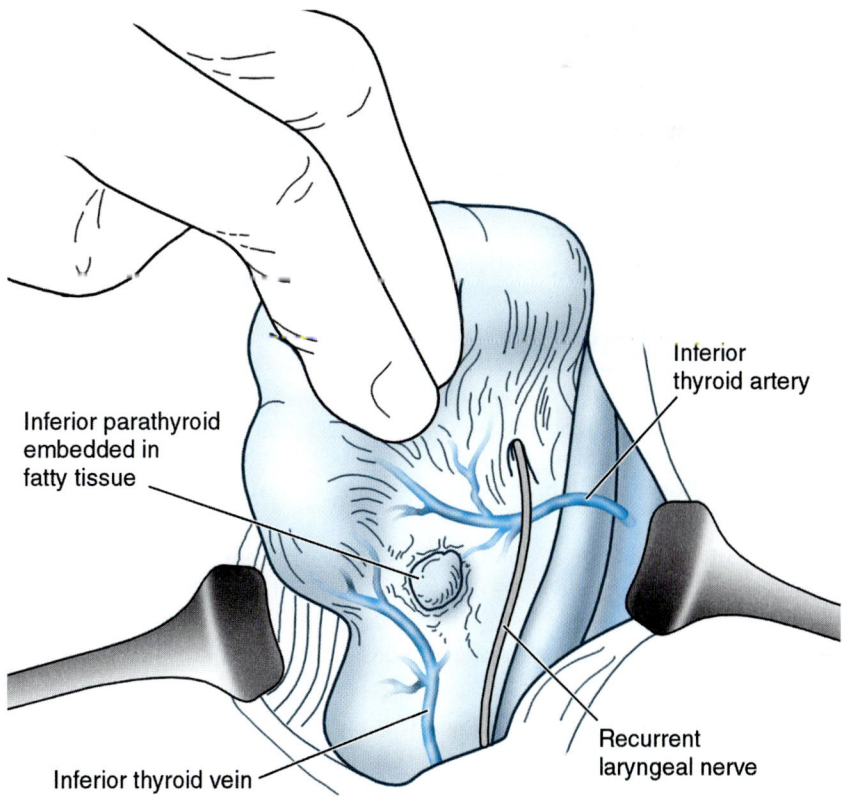

Figure 2–4

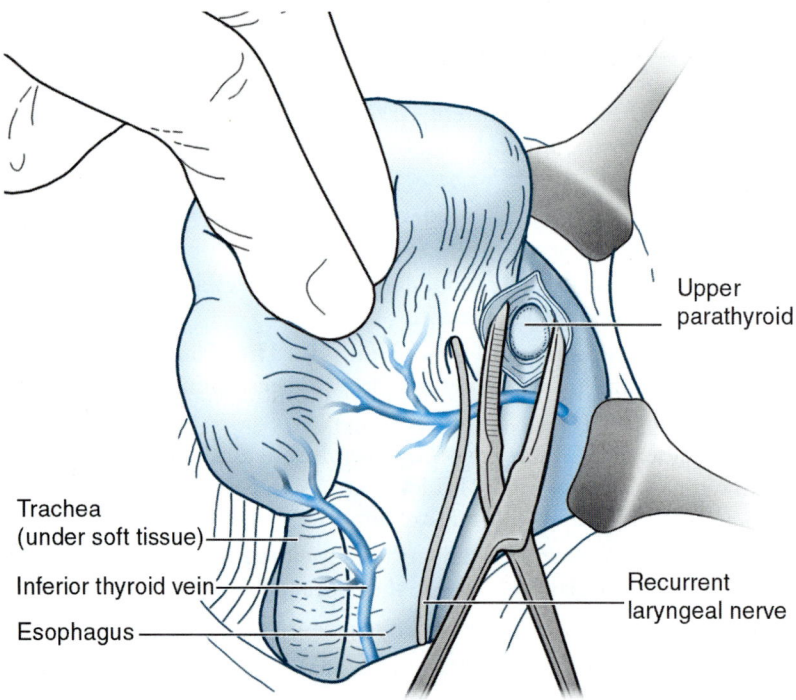

Figure 2–5

- **Figure 2–5:** The superior parathyroid glands are dissected free from surrounding tissue and removed for pathologic diagnosis. The upper glands are mostly located on the posterior surface of the thyroid at its upper two thirds.
- **Figure 2–6:** Superior parathyroid glands are less variable in location; however, they may migrate upward or downward into the posterior mediastinum.
  - Inferior parathyroid glands may migrate into the thymus, as well as the anterior or posterior mediastinum.

POSTOPERATIVE CARE

- Although uncomplicated adenoma resection may often be performed as an outpatient procedure, patients who undergo the procedure as inpatients should be admitted for overnight observation and discharged the following morning.
- In the early postoperative period, patients receive calcium carbonate, 1250 mg orally three times daily; or OsCal 500, 1 tablet orally three times daily (1 tablet OsCal 500 = 1 g $CaCO_3$ = 400 mg elemental Ca or 20 mEq Ca), which can generally be reduced within 2 weeks.
- Acetaminophen or ibuprofen, as needed, is prescribed for pain related to the procedure, and occasionally opioid agents are needed for a short time postoperatively.

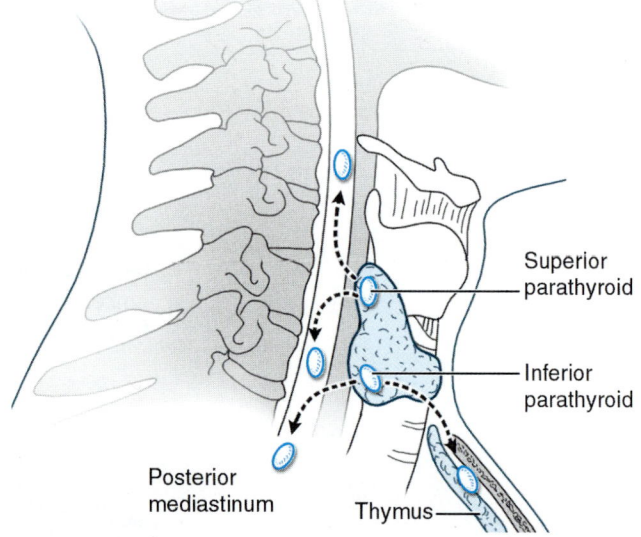

Figure 2–6

POTENTIAL COMPLICATIONS

- Neck hematoma.
  - May be self-limited if the airway is not compromised.
  - When the airway is compromised, there should be no hesitation in reopening the neck incision, including the strap musculature.
- Hypoparathyroidism and hypocalcemia.
  - Typically present as perioral paresthesias, which may progress to more serious conditions, such as cardiac arrhythmias.
  - Treatment includes oral calcium carbonate, intravenous calcium gluconate, and possibly vitamin D.
- Nerve injury: external branch of the superior laryngeal nerve.
  - Supplies motor innervation to the inferior constrictor muscles of the larynx.
  - Located near the superior pole vessels of the thyroid before entering the cricopharyngeal muscle at its superolateral aspect.
  - Damage will affect high-pitched singing or yelling.
- Nerve injury: sympathetic chain/stellate ganglion.
  - Located posterior to the thyroid.
  - Damage will produce ipsilateral miosis, ptosis, and anhidrosis (Horner syndrome).
- Nerve injury: recurrent laryngeal nerve.
  - Courses inferiorly to superiorly within the bilateral tracheoesophageal grooves and inserts at the inferior border of the cricopharyngeal muscles.
  - Damage causes ipsilateral paralysis to the vocal cord and may also affect the swallowing mechanism.
- Thoracic duct injury, which may cause collection of chyle at the site of injury.
- Tracheal injury.
- Esophageal injury.
- Persistent or recurrent hyperparathyroidism.

PEARLS AND TIPS

- Preoperative imaging (technetium sestamibi or cervical ultrasound) allows for directed operative intervention.
- Dissection should proceed anteriorly, then laterally along the posterior surface of the sternothyroid muscle.
- The dissection should continue to free the carotid medially and include all of the soft tissue down to the prevertebral fascia.
- This ensures that the parathyroid glands are included in the dissection field and prevents the surgeon from missing a potential normal or abnormal gland.
- Successful removal of the symptomatic parathyroid gland is demonstrated when intraoperative PTH monitoring shows a decrease of 50% of the preoperative PTH level and return of PTH levels to the normal range (< 70 pg/mL).

REFERENCES

Doherty GM. Complications of Thyroid and Parathyroid Surgery. In: Mulholland MW, Doherty GM, eds. *Complications in Surgery*. Philadelphia, PA: Lippincott Williams & Wilkins; 2006:575–593.

Doherty GM. Parathyroid Glands. In: Mulholland MW, Lillemoe KD, Doherty GM, et al, eds. *Greenfield's Surgery: Scientific Principles & Practice,* 4th ed. Philadelphia, PA: Lippincott Williams & Wilkins; 2006:1310–1334.

Doherty GM, Moley JF. Conventional Exploration for Hyperparathyroidism. In: Van Heerden JA, Farley DR, eds. *Operative Techniques in General Surgery*. Philadelphia, PA: WB Saunders; 1999:4–17.

CHAPTER 3

Adrenalectomy

Awori J. Hayanga, MD, MPH, and Paul G. Gauger, MD

INDICATIONS

General Indications
- Clinically or biochemically apparent adrenal hormonal hyperfunction.
- Possible or certain malignant adrenal mass.
- Adrenal mass of uncertain significance.

Specific Conditions and Disease States
- Primary hyperaldosteronism.
  - Unilateral cortical adenoma causing Conn's syndrome.
  - Bilateral hyperplasia with unilateral dominance (established by adrenal vein sampling).
- Hypercortisolism.
  - Unilateral cortical adenoma.
  - Refractory Cushing's syndrome (from Cushing's disease, primary adrenal hyperplasia, or ectopic adrenocorticotropic hormone [ACTH] syndrome).
- Pheochromocytoma.
- Unilateral cortical adenoma causing virilization.
- Myelolipoma (in selected situations).
- Adrenal cyst (if refractory or symptomatic).
- Adrenocortical carcinoma.
- Incidentaloma with indeterminate or concerning imaging characteristics.
- Adrenal metastases of other primary cancers (in selected situations).

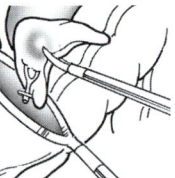 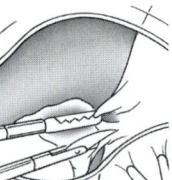 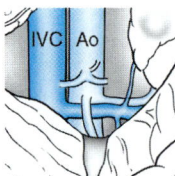
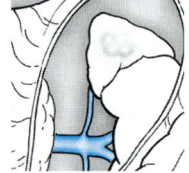 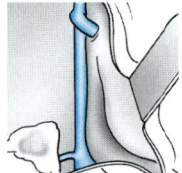 

CONTRAINDICATIONS

Laparoscopic Adrenalectomy
A. Absolute
- Adrenocortical carcinoma (certain or likely).
- Refractory coagulopathy.
- Comorbidities precluding safe general anesthesia.

B. Relative
- Previous ipsilateral partial adrenal resection.
- Previous extensive upper abdominal or retroperitoneal surgery.
- Very large adrenal tumors (> 6–8 cm).
- Suboptimal medical preparation for pheochromocytoma resection.

Open Adrenalectomy
A. Absolute
- Refractory coagulopathy.
- Comorbidities precluding safe general anesthesia.

B. Relative
- Suboptimal medical preparation for pheochromocytoma resection.

INFORMED CONSENT
Expected Benefits
- Resolution of clinical symptoms related to adrenal hypersecretory function.
- Treatment of primary or metastatic adrenal malignancies.
- Treatment of symptomatic benign adrenal masses.

Potential Risks
- For laparoscopic procedure, risk of conversion to an open procedure.
- Bleeding requiring reoperation.
- Glucocorticoid insufficiency (most commonly following preoperative hypercortisolism, bilateral adrenalectomy, or previous contralateral adrenalectomy).
- Recurrence of tumor.
- Scarring.
- Infection.
- Failure of operation to correct hypertension or adrenal hyperfunction.
- Need for additional tests or procedures.

EQUIPMENT
Laparoscopic Adrenalectomy
- Standard laparoscopic and open instrument trays.
- Surgical energy device such as harmonic scalpel or LigaSure.

Open Adrenalectomy
- Major exploratory laparotomy instrument tray.
- Retraction system such as Bookwalter or Thompson retractor.
- Surgical energy device such as harmonic scalpel or LigaSure.

PATIENT PREPARATION
General Preparation
- Nothing by mouth before surgery.
- No preoperative antibiotics are necessary before surgery except when the patient has other indications (eg, cardiac valvulopathy, orthopedic hardware).
- Anesthesiology consultation as needed.
- Invasive blood pressure monitoring if required for pheochromocytoma or other medical condition.
- Deep vein thrombosis (DVT) prophylaxis (for laparoscopic cases this should include sequential compression devices).

Disease-Specific Preparation
- Preoperative control of hypertension for patients with pheochromocytoma.
  - α-Adrenergic blockade is achieved using phenoxybenzamine, 10 mg orally three times daily, titrated upward until mild orthostatic symptoms occur.
  - Requires 7–10 days minimum preparation.
  - Phenoxybenzamine should be continued until the morning of the procedure and given with a sip of water.
  - If necessary, β-adrenergic blockade is added after α blockade is established to treat tachycardia and prevent unopposed α blockade.
- Stress-dose steroids administered to patients having adrenalectomy for hypercortisolism (benign or malignant causes) due to suppression of hypothalamic-pituitary-adrenal axis involving the contralateral adrenal gland.
  - Preoperatively, hydrocortisone, 100 mg, is given intravenously.
  - Postoperatively, suprapyhsiologic doses are weaned to physiologic replacement doses of oral steroids.

PATIENT POSITIONING
Laparoscopic Adrenalectomy
- General anesthesia is induced with the patient supine.
- An orogastric tube and a Foley catheter are placed.
- The patient is placed in the lateral decubitus position with the ipsilateral side up.
- The table is gently flexed to widen the angle between the costal margin and iliac wing.
- An axillary roll is placed and a beanbag used to hold the patient in position.
- Arms, head, and legs are appropriately padded and not abducted beyond 90 degrees.

Open Adrenalectomy

- A nasogastric tube and a Foley catheter are placed.
- The patient is placed supine with his or her arms resting on arm boards and with legs padded.

PROCEDURE

Laparoscopic Left Adrenalectomy: Figure 3–1

- A small skin incision is made to the left and superior to the umbilicus for open port placement.
- The abdomen is entered in layers under direct vision. A securing suture is placed in the external fascial layer. Alternatively, an optical port may be used.
- The Hasson port is then placed and the abdomen insufflated to 13 cm H_2O pressure.
- With the 30-degree camera in the abdomen, placement of the other two working ports is established approximately 2 fingerbreadths inferior to the subcostal margin and triangulated with the camera port.
- These ports may be 5 mm or 10 mm depending on surgeon preference and available instrumentation.
- The splenic flexure of the colon may require minor inferior mobilization by division of the lienosplenic ligament.
- The ultrasonic dissector is then used to divide the lateral peritoneal attachments of the spleen and lienophrenic ligament, often until the fundus of the stomach comes into view.
- As the spleen is reflected medially, the tail of the pancreas is mobilized with it. The splenic vein and splenic artery may be seen.
- If the adrenal gland and adrenal tumor are difficult to locate, laparoscopic ultrasonography may be helpful.
- Direct grasping of the tumor must be avoided, and grasping of the normal adrenal tissue must be very judicious and gentle.
- A plane medial to the adrenal gland and lateral to the aorta is bluntly developed.
- The superior pedicle (inferior phrenic vessels) is dissected and divided with clips or using the ultrasonic dissector.
- The central adrenal vein is dissected as it drains to the left renal vein. It is divided between double clips or with an endoscopic stapler.
- The inferior and lateral attachments of the adrenal gland are divided with the ultrasonic dissector to mobilize the gland out of the suprarenal fossa. Often this exposes the capsule of the superior renal pole.
- Once liberated, the adrenal gland is placed in a specimen retrieval bag and withdrawn from the abdomen using the original Hasson port site.

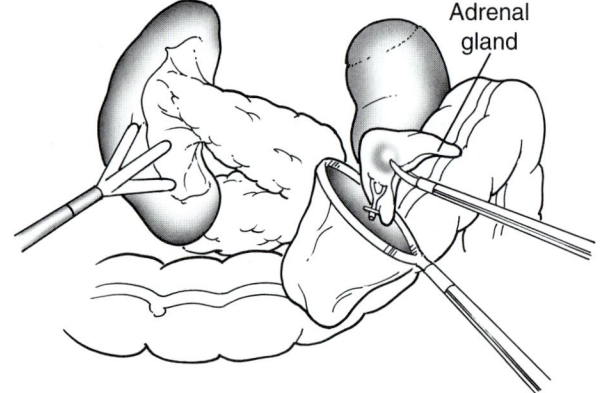

Figure 3–1

- While insufflation is maintained, the suprarenal fossa is inspected for hemostasis. The abdomen is then irrigated using saline.
- If 10-mm port sites are used, they are closed using a Carter-Thomason device.
- Local anesthetic is infiltrated into the muscle and skin of all port sites.
- The Hasson port site is closed with fascial sutures.
- The skin is then closed using absorbable monofilament suture and dressed with occlusive dressings.

Laparoscopic Right Adrenalectomy: Figure 3-2

- A small skin incision is made to the right and superior to the umbilicus for open port placement.
- The abdomen is entered in layers under direct vision. A securing suture is placed in the external fascial layer.
- The Hasson port is then placed and the abdomen insufflated to 13 cm H_2O pressure.
- With the 30-degree camera in the abdomen, placement of the other two working ports is established approximately 2 fingerbreadths inferior to the subcostal margin and triangulated with the camera port.
- These ports may be 5 mm or 10 mm depending on surgeon preference and available instrumentation.
- The lateral attachments of the liver to the diaphragm (triangular ligament) are divided with the ultrasonic dissector.
- Once the right lobe of the liver is substantially mobilized and can be retracted medially nearly 90 degrees off the horizontal view, a separate medial port is placed to accommodate a laparoscopic retractor for the liver. Port size is determined by the instrument used.
- The peritoneum overlying the medial aspect of the adrenal gland is opened from inferior to superior using the ultrasonic dissector.
- Direct grasping of the tumor must be avoided, and grasping of the normal adrenal tissue must be very judicious and gentle.
- A plane medial to the adrenal gland and posterolateral to the vena cava is bluntly developed.
- The central adrenal vein is circumferentially mobilized as it drains to the vena cava. It is divided between double clips or with an endoscopic stapler.
- The superior pedicle (inferior phrenic vessels) is dissected and divided with clips or the ultrasonic dissector.
- The inferior and lateral attachments of the adrenal are divided with the ultrasonic dissector to mobilize the gland out of the suprarenal fossa. Often this exposes the capsule of the superior renal pole.

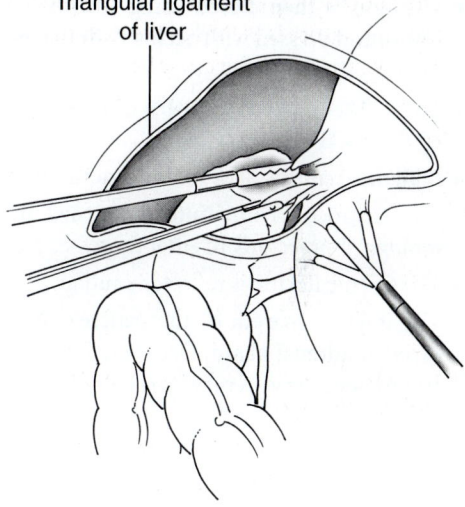

Figure 3-2

- Once liberated, the adrenal gland is placed in a specimen retrieval bag and withdrawn from the abdomen using the original Hasson port site.
- While insufflation is maintained, the suprarenal fossa is inspected for hemostasis. The abdomen is then irrigated using saline.
- If 10-mm port sites are used, they are closed using a Carter-Thomason device.
- Local anesthetic is infiltrated into the muscle and skin of all port sites.
- The Hasson port site is closed with fascial sutures.
- The skin is then closed using absorbable monofilament suture and dressed with occlusive dressings.

Open Anterior Adrenalectomy–Left: Figures 3-3 and 3-4

- A bilateral subcostal or midline incision is made.
- The gastrocolic omentum is opened or the omentum mobilized superiorly to enter the lesser sac.
- The splenic flexure is reflected caudad.
- The inferior margin of the pancreas is mobilized to the exposed adrenal gland. Occasionally, division of the inferior mesenteric vein may be required.

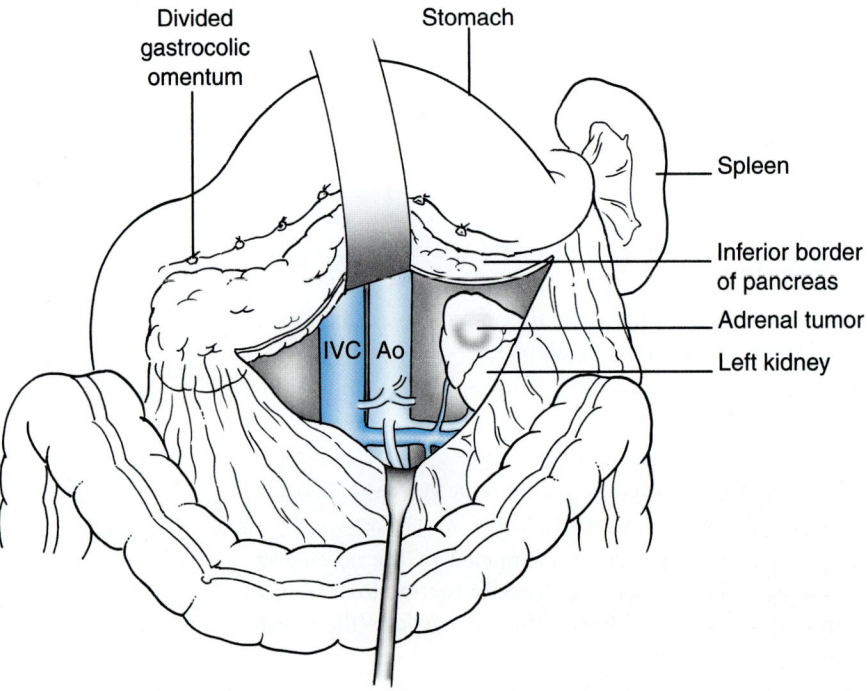

Figure 3-3

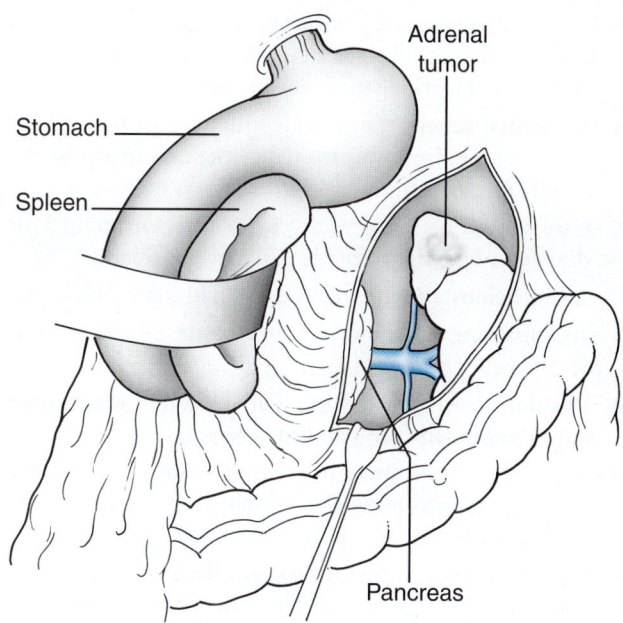

Figure 3–4

- The tail of the pancreas is gently retracted upward to expose the anterior surface of the adrenal gland (see Figure 3–3).
- The superior vascular pedicle (inferior phrenic vessels) is divided to allow caudad retraction of the tumor.
- The central adrenal vein is dissected and divided at the inferior and medial aspect of the adrenal gland as it drains to the left renal vein.
- The remaining soft tissue attachments are divided to complete the adrenalectomy.
- For large tumors, the infrapancreatic approach described earlier, and shown in Figure 3–3, may not provide adequate exposure. In that case, medial mobilization of the pancreas and spleen may be required (see Figure 3–4).
- For adrenocortical cancers, en bloc splenectomy, distal pancreatectomy, or nephrectomy may be necessary.

Open Anterior Adrenalectomy–Right: Figure 3–5

- A bilateral subcostal or midline incision is made.
- The hepatic flexure of the colon is mobilized as necessary.
- A partial Kocher maneuver is performed as necessary to expose the infrahepatic vena cava.
- The right lobe of the liver is mobilized by dividing the triangular ligament and then retracting it medially to expose the adrenal gland.
- The lateral and inferior margins of the adrenal gland are mobilized.

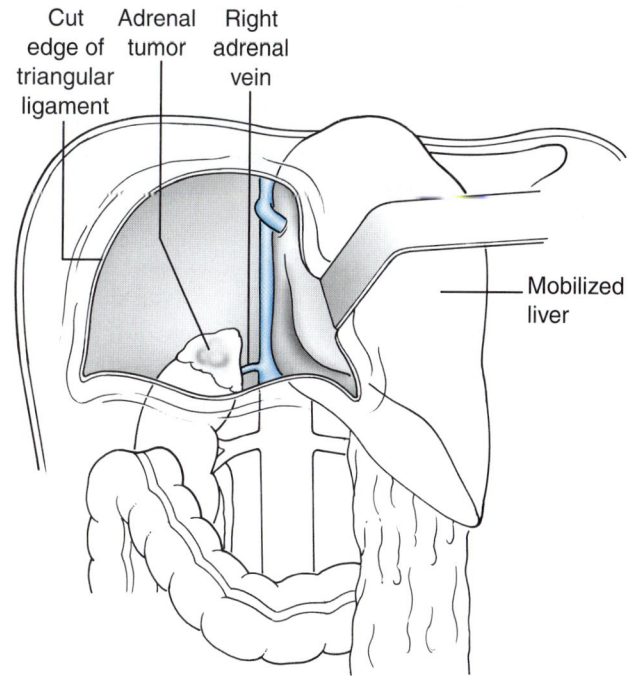

Figure 3–5

- The superior vascular pedicle (inferior phrenic vessels) is divided and controlled. Hemostatic clips may be useful as exposure and working space are limited.
- The medial superior and medial margins of the adrenal gland are mobilized away from the vena cava to expose the central adrenal vein.
  - Care should be taken as accessory veins or anomalous drainage of the right hepatic vein may be present.
  - Again, hemostatic clips may be useful to control bleeding.
- The remaining soft tissue attachments are divided to complete the adrenalectomy.
- Capsular breach and tumor spill should be assiduously avoided during the preceding maneuvers.
- Large or invasive tumors will require more extensive vena caval control, including the suprahepatic vena cava and infrahepatic vena cava superior to the renal veins.
- If adrenalectomy is performed for a large adrenocortical cancer, en bloc resection of the right hepatic lobe, right kidney, or even a portion of the vena cava may be required.

POSTOPERATIVE CARE

- Incentive spirometry should be used to prevent atelectasis and postoperative pneumonia.
- Laparoscopic procedures often require less fluid replacement than do open procedures.
- Postoperative DVT prophylaxis should be maintained until the patient is ambulatory.
  - Ambulation should be encouraged as early as possible.
  - Following laparoscopic procedures, subcutaneous heparin prophylaxis is appropriate if no concerns exist about ongoing bleeding.
- Early resumption of regular diet should be possible.
- The Foley catheter may be discontinued once hemodynamics, urinary output, and electrolytes are stable and within the normal range.

Patients with Hyperaldosteronism

- Potassium supplementation should be stopped immediately postoperatively.
- Antihypertensives should be weaned.
- Electrolytes, including potassium, should be checked the morning after surgery.

Patients with Pheochromocytoma

- Patients should be monitored for signs of postoperative hypotension resulting from vascular relaxation.
  - Significant intravenous fluid resuscitation or pressors may be required, although this is less of a problem following adequate α blockade.
- α Blockade may be discontinued immediately postoperatively and β blockade weaned, except in cases of residual metastatic pheochromocytoma.
- Monitoring for hypoglycemia includes measurement of serum glucose every 4 hours for the first 24 hours postoperatively.

Patients with Preoperative Hypercortisolism

- Following bilateral adrenalectomy or adrenalectomy for Cushing's syndrome, hydrocortisone should be available at the bedside.
- Patients should be monitored for hypotension, decreased urine output, gastrointestinal abnormalities, hyponatremia, hyperkalemia, hypoglycemia, and fever.
- Treatment should be immediate, with fluid resuscitation followed by administration of parenteral steroids, typically 100 mg of intravenous hydrocortisone given every 8 hours.
  - This dose possesses sufficient mineralocorticoid activity to preclude the need for fludrocortisone.
  - Fludrocortisone may be necessary in the event of bilateral adrenalectomy and consequent lifelong adrenal insufficiency.

Patients with Uncertain Suppression Status

- The ACTH stimulation test may be performed to test the adrenal hypothalamo-pituitary axis (HPA).
  - Baseline serum cortisol is measured.
  - Intramuscular ACTH, 250 mcg, is then administered, and serum cortisol rechecked 30 and 60 minutes later.
  - An increase of 7 mcg/dL from baseline, or an absolute baseline of 20 mcg/dL of serum cortisol, suggests a functional HPA for most patients.
  - Results lower than these values warrant steroid replacement.

POTENTIAL COMPLICATIONS

- Bleeding.
- Glucocorticoid insufficiency.
- Pneumothorax.
- Vascular injuries.
- Hypertension.
- Hypotension.
- Wound infection.
- Pneumonia.
- Splenic injury.
- Hepatic injury.
- Pancreatic injury and resultant pancreatitis.

- Incisional hernia.
- Ileus.
- Subphrenic abscess.
- Nelson's syndrome (more specifically related to bilateral adrenalectomy).
- Mineralocorticoid insufficiency (more specifically related to bilateral adrenalectomy).

PEARLS AND TIPS

- Ensure careful patient selection and matching of operative approach to patient factors and disease factors.
- Mobilization of the liver (for right adrenalectomy) and of the pancreas and spleen (for left adrenalectomy) during laparoscopic adrenalectomy always needs to be developed more than might be expected to improve exposure of the adrenal gland.
- Avoid direct grasping of the adrenal gland early in laparoscopic adrenalectomy because bleeding will occur. Grasping is less traumatic after the gland has been devascularized.
- If the central adrenal vein is broader than can be safely secured with an endoclip, use an endoscopic linear stapler/cutter (eg, Endo-GIA).

REFERENCES

Findling JW, Raff H. Cushing's syndrome: important issues in diagnosis and management. *J Clin Endocrinol Metab.* 2006;91:3746–3753.

Gauger PG. Complications of Adrenal Surgery. In: Mulholland MW, Doherty GM, eds. *Complications in Surgery.* Philadelphia, PA: Lippincott Williams & Wilkins; 2006:559–574.

Gawande A, Moore FD. Laparoscopic Adrenalectomy. In: Zinner MJ, Ashley SW, eds. *Maingot's Abdominal Operations,* 11th ed. New York: McGraw-Hill; 2007:1205–1216.

Mishra AK, Agarwal A, Gupta S, et al. Outcome of adrenalectomy for Cushing's syndrome: experience from a tertiary care center. *World J Surg.* 2007;31:1425–1432.

Woodrum DT, Gauger PG. Benign and Malignant Tumors of the Adrenal Gland. In: Sabel M, Sondak VK, Sussman JJ, eds. *Essentials of Surgical Oncology: Surgical Foundations.* Philadelphia, PA: Mosby/Elsevier; 2006:197.

CHAPTER 4

Surgery of the Endocrine Pancreas

Brian D. Saunders, MD, and Gerard M. Doherty, MD

INDICATIONS

- Tumors may be functional (ie, a clinical syndrome of excessive levels of such hormones as insulin, gastrin, VIP, somatostatin, and glucagon) or nonfunctional (ie, normal serum marker levels [excluding pancreatic polypeptide, chromogranin A]).
- Tumors may be sporadic or a manifestation of an inherited endocrinopathy (multiple endocrine neoplasia type 1 [MEN-1], von Hippel-Lindau [VHL]).
- Nonfunctional tumors demonstrable via radiologic examination should be resected.
- All functional tumors should be resected.
- Sinistral portal hypertension.

CONTRAINDICATIONS

- Inoperable, metastatic disease.
- Small (< 1 cm), nonfunctional tumors in patients with an inherited endocrinopathy.
- Functional tumors with a medically controlled syndrome in patients with an inherited endocrinopathy who have undergone previous pancreatic resection.
- Pregnancy (first trimester).
- Multiple comorbidities precluding safe surgical intervention.

INFORMED CONSENT

- For major pancreatic resections, morbidity is roughly 10–12% and mortality is 1–2%.

Expected Benefits

- Treatment of pancreatic hypersecretory syndromes in patients with functional tumors.
- Treatment of potentially malignant neuroendocrine tumors.

Potential Risks

- Bleeding, possibly requiring blood product transfusion.
- Surgical site infection.

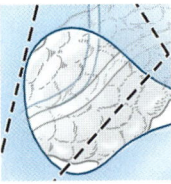
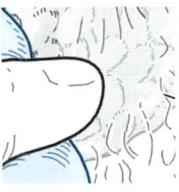
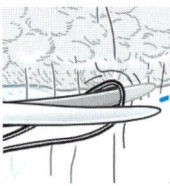
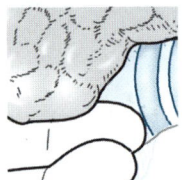
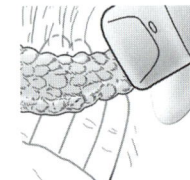
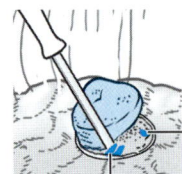
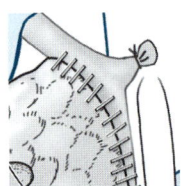

- Pancreatic fistula.
- Biliary fistula.
- Gastric outlet obstruction or delayed gastric emptying.
- Overwhelming post-splenectomy sepsis.
- Incisional hernia.
- Glucose intolerance or diabetes.
- Pancreatic exocrine insufficiency or malabsorption.

EQUIPMENT

- Intraoperative ultrasound with a high-resolution 7.5–10 MHz probe should be available for primary tumor localization or identification of hepatic metastatic disease.

PATIENT PREPARATION

- Medical control of hormone excess (eg, with proton pump inhibitors or somatostatin analogue therapy) to the degree possible.
- Any patient who is to undergo splenectomy should receive the pneumococcal, *Haemophilus influenzae* B, and meningococcal vaccines preoperatively.
- Nothing by mouth the evening before surgery.
- Preoperative antibiotics.
- Both mechanical and pharmacologic deep venous thrombosis prophylaxis should be given.
- Anesthesiology consultation as needed.

PATIENT POSITIONING

- The patient should be supine, preferably with the arms extended.

PROCEDURE

- **Figure 4–1**: For patients with documented hypergastrinemia, the primary tumor will almost always lie in the gastrinoma triangle (bounded by the confluence of the cystic and common hepatic ducts, the second and third portion of the duodenum, and the confluence of the neck and body of the pancreas).
- A vertical, upper midline incision or a subcostal incision is used.
  - The former is preferred for patients with a relatively acutely angled costal margin.
  - The latter incision can either be predominantly left sided for a distal pancreatectomy or bilateral in the case of a pancreaticoduodenectomy.
- Inspection of the abdomen for metastatic disease includes visualization and palpation of the liver, peritoneal surfaces, mesentery, omentum, and, in women, the ovaries.

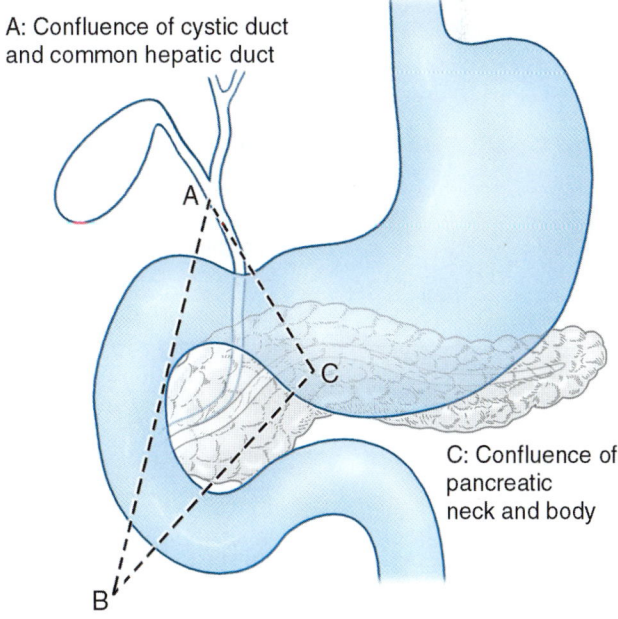

A: Confluence of cystic duct and common hepatic duct

C: Confluence of pancreatic neck and body

B: Junction of second and third portion of duodenum

Figure 4–1

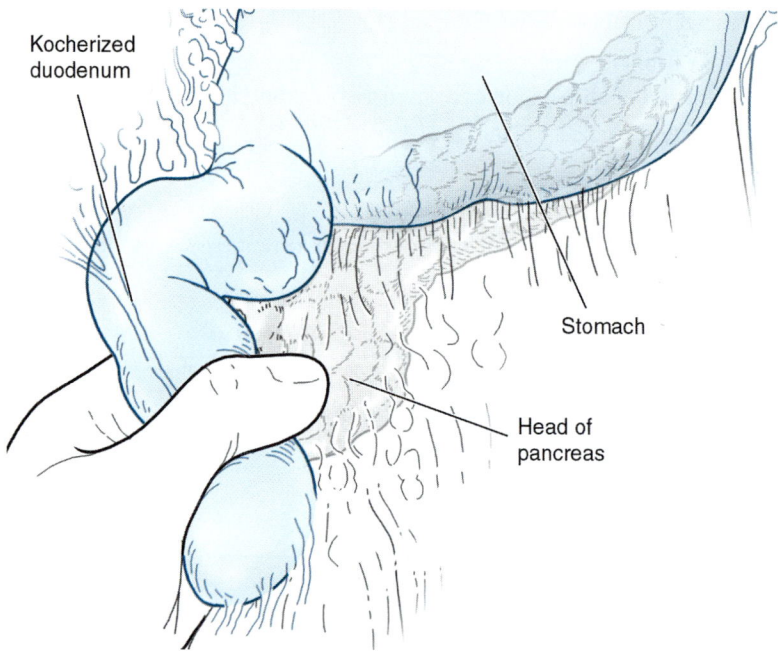

Figure 4–2

- **Figure 4–2:** The entire pancreas is mobilized for localization of the tumor.
  - This step begins with a mobilization of the pancreatic head via release of the duodenum from its lateral abdominal wall and retroperitoneal attachments (Kocher maneuver).
  - This should be continued toward the patient's left side until the aorta is encountered.
- **Figure 4–3:** The body and tail of the pancreas is exposed via entry through the lesser sac.

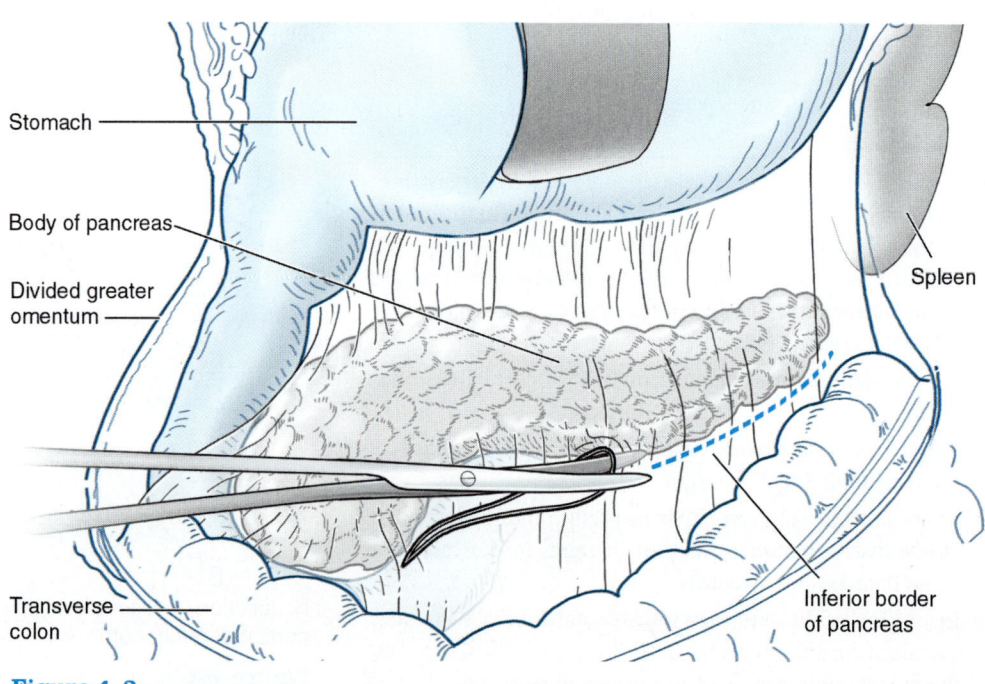

Figure 4–3

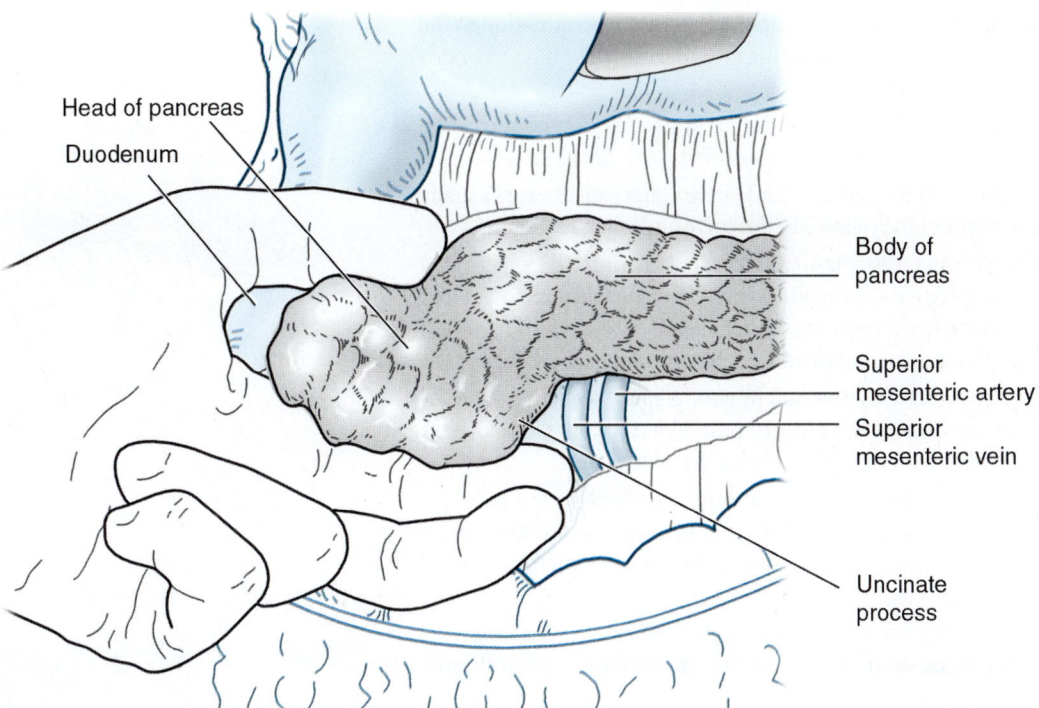

Figure 4–4A

- The gastrocolic ligament is opened, taking care not to enter the transverse mesocolon or injure the middle colic vessels.
- The retroperitoneum at the inferior border of the pancreas is opened with electrocautery or scissors.
- The superior mesenteric vein (SMV) can be identified at this stage by following the middle colic vein to its insertion into the SMV.
- **Figure 4–4A, B:** The avascular attachments of the pancreas to the posterior wall of the pancreas are divided, and the retroperitoneum overlying the superior edge of the pancreas is opened.
  - The lateral peritoneal reflection of the spleen is divided.
  - This allows for bimanual palpation of the entire length of the pancreas.
- Great care should be taken when a pancreatic neoplasm has resulted in splenic vein occlusion, leading to sinistral portal hypertension, because there may be many perilous collateral vessels in the area of dissection. In this scenario, early ligation and division of the splenic artery may reduce flow in the collateral vessels.

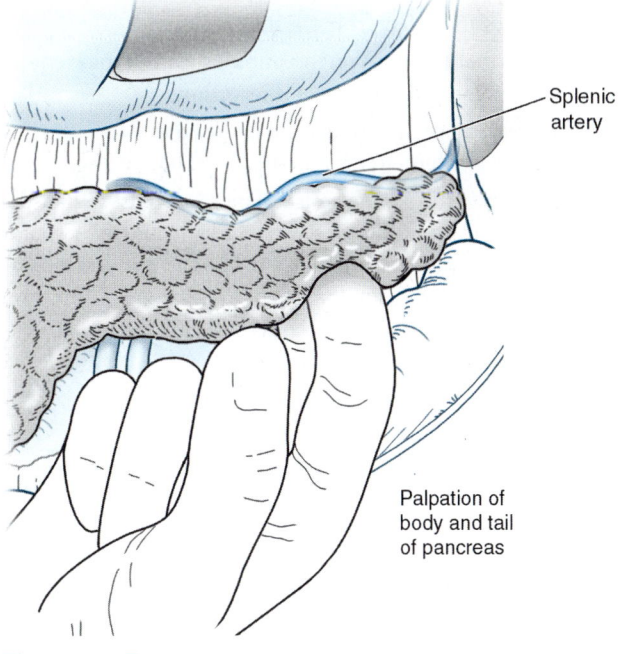

Figure 4–4B

- **Figure 4–5A-C:** A thorough ultrasound examination of the entire pancreas allows for identification of all neuroendocrine tumors.
  - The main pancreatic duct and its spatial relationship to the tumor can also be identified.
  - Endocrine tumors and their metastases are usually hypoechoic relative to the surrounding parenchyma.
  - An operative plan can then be formulated, which may involve pancreaticoduodenectomy, distal pancreatectomy and splenectomy, tumor enucleation, or a combination of enucleation and formal anatomic pancreatic resection.
- The operative approach in familial pancreatic neuroendocrine tumors should attempt to resect all gross disease while preserving normal pancreatic function.
- **Figure 4–6A-C:** Benign tumors anywhere in the pancreas can be enucleated with sharp dissection around the capsule of the tumor, with care taken to avoid a pancreatic ductal injury.
  - Cautery on the surface of the pancreas should be used with caution to prevent the transmission of a thermal injury to the pancreatic duct.
  - Closed suction drains should be left in place near the site of an enucleation or an anatomic resection to detect and control a possible pancreatic fluid leak.
- **Figure 4–7:** In patients with hypergastrinemia, routine digital exploration of the duodenum for a submucosal tumor is recommended.
  - This is accomplished with a longitudinal duodenotomy in the free wall of the second portion of the duodenum.
  - Tumors may be as small as a few millimeters; these can be resected by a full-thickness duodenal wall resection, and closure of the defect from the inside.
  - Tumors that encroach on the ampulla of Vater may require pancreaticoduodenectomy for resection.
  - The free wall of the duodenum is closed in two layers in a transverse fashion to prevent duodenal narrowing.
  - Also shown in this figure is a pancreas transected at the level of the superior mesenteric vessels and two tumor enucleation sites in the pancreatic head. (This is the operation described and popularized by Dr. Norman Thompson as initial treatment of MEN-1–related pancreatic neuroendocrine disease.)

POSTOPERATIVE CARE

- Routine postoperative admission to an ICU is not mandatory. Rather, ICU observation (usually one night) is guided by intraoperative blood loss as well as preexisting cardiac and pulmonary comorbidities the patient may have.
- Nasogastric tube decompression is continued postoperatively; the length of time the tube remains in place is guided by the volume of output.

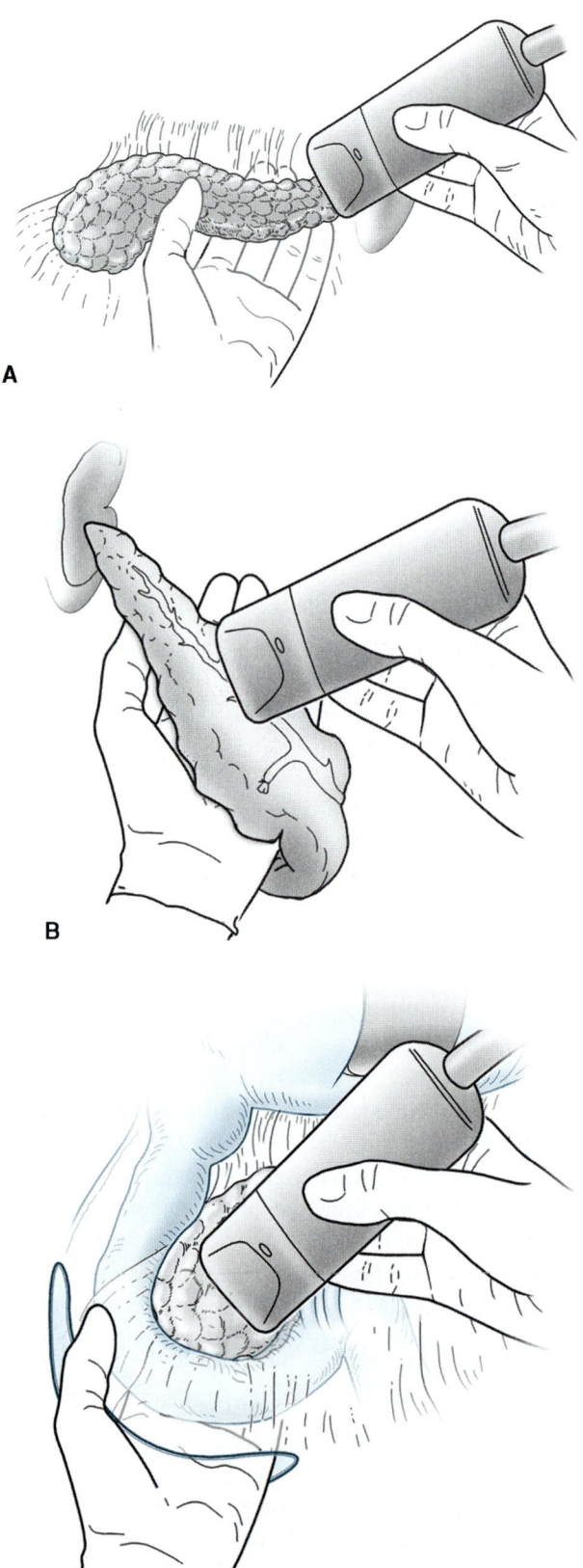

Figure 4–5 A–C

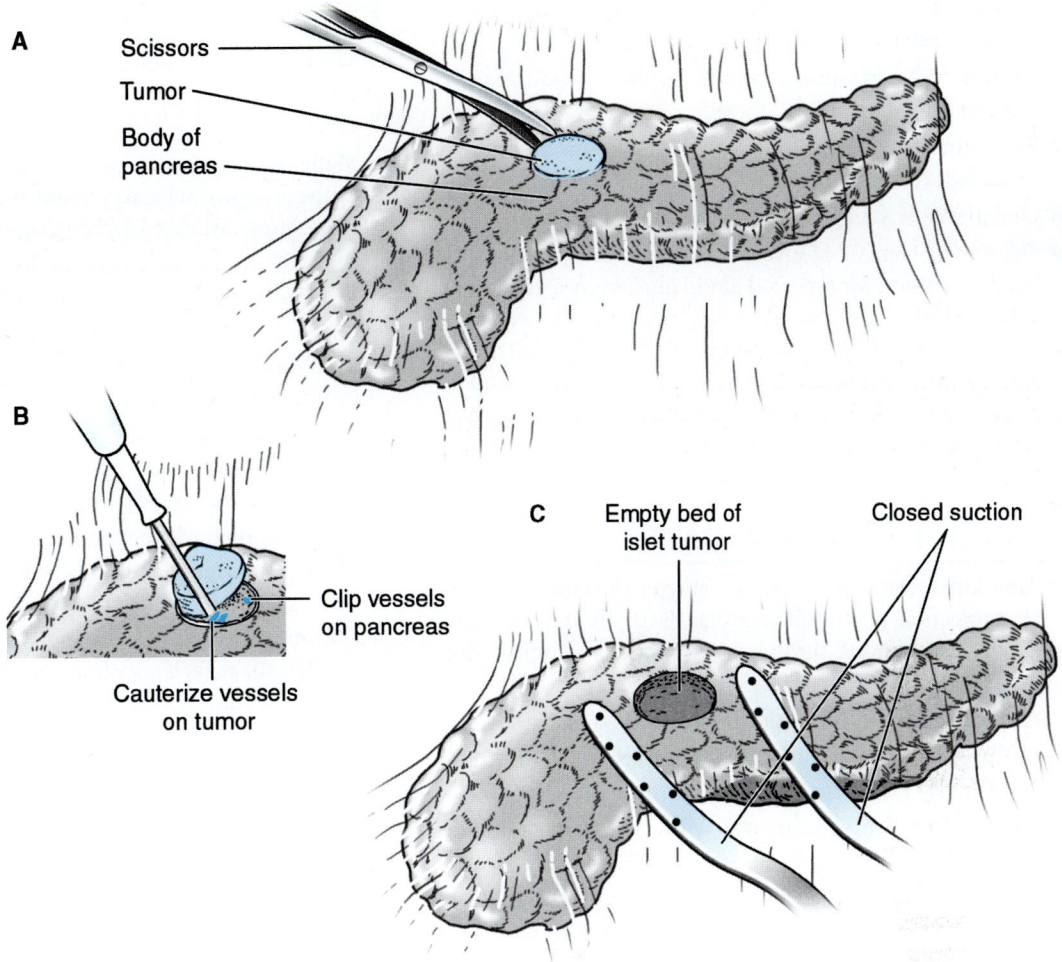

Figure 4–6 A–C

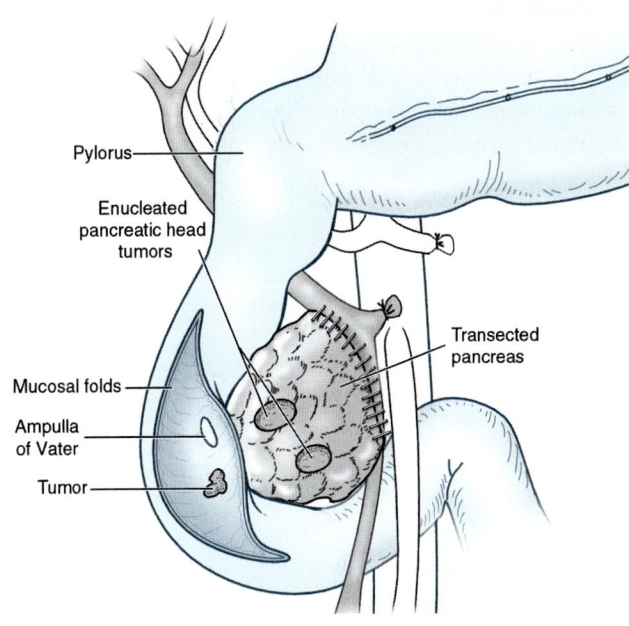

Figure 4–7

- Patient-controlled intravenous or epidural analgesia is routinely used.
- Urinary catheterization continues while an epidural pain catheter is in place.
- Early ambulation and physical therapy consultation, if indicated.
- Oral diet is slowly introduced once ileus is fully resolved.
- Strict management of glycemic control, with continuous insulin infusion for repeated blood glucose measurements > 140 mg/dL.
- Closed suction drain output is tested for amylase and lipase content prior to removal.
- Routine use of octreotide therapy to reduce the pancreatic fistula rate is not supported by published evidence.

POTENTIAL COMPLICATIONS

- After laparotomy: intravenous catheter infection, urinary tract infection, pneumonia, cardiac dysrhythmias and ischemia, deep venous thrombosis, superficial surgical site infection, fascial dehiscence.
- Pancreatic leakage and fistula occur in 5–8% of cases.
  - Leakage or fistula is confirmed by amylase and lipase-rich drainage in closed suction drain output.
  - Nontoxic patients are treated with maintenance of the drain.
  - Patients with fevers, tachycardia, acidosis, or leukocytosis should undergo abdominal and pelvic CT scan to evaluate for abscess or inadequately controlled fistula.
  - Inadequately controlled fistula can usually be managed with an additional percutaneous drain, replacement of lost fluid and electrolytes, adequate nutrition, and consideration of octreotide therapy for high-output fistulas.
- Postoperative hemorrhage, most commonly resulting from a bleeding short gastric vessel or a gastroduodenal or pancreaticoduodenal pseudoaneurysm.
- Delayed gastric emptying.

PEARLS AND TIPS

- Most clinically recognized pancreatic endocrine neoplasms are functional, producing clinically recognizable syndromes.
- Malignant pancreatic endocrine neoplasms are determined by the presence of local invasion and lymph node or hepatic metastases, not based on histologic examination.
- The initial imaging technique for a pancreatic endocrine neoplasm is a high-quality spiral CT scan.
- Endoscopic ultrasonography is particularly useful for localization of tumors in patients with gastrinoma and insulinoma.
- The characteristic severe dermatitis (necrolytic migratory erythema) associated with a glucagonoma is effectively treated with octreotide.
- Nonfunctional islet cell tumors of the pancreas, although often quite large at diagnosis, tend to grow slowly and have a more indolent course than pancreatic ductal cancer.
- Chromogranin A and pancreatic polypeptide are useful markers for surveillance following resection of a pancreatic endocrine tumor.

REFERENCES

Lairmore TC. Complications in Endocrine Pancreatic Surgery. In: Mulholland MW, Doherty GM, eds. *Complications in Surgery*. Philadelphia, PA: Lippincott Williams & Wilkins; 2006:594–602.

Lowney J, Doherty GM. Surgery for Endocrine Tumors of the Pancreas. In: Doherty GM, Skogseid B, eds. *Surgical Endocrinology*. Philadelphia, PA: Lippincott Williams & Wilkins; 2001:381–392.

Riall TS, Yeo CJ. Neoplasms of the Endocrine Pancreas. In: Mulholland MW, Lillemoe KD, Doherty GM, et al, eds. *Greenfield's Surgery, Scientific Principles & Practice*. Philadelphia, PA: Lippincott Williams & Wilkins; 2006:880–891.

Thompson NW. Pancreatic Surgery for Endocrine Tumors. In: Clark OH, Duh QY, Kebebew E, eds. *Textbook of Endocrine Surgery*. Philadelphia, PA: Elsevier Saunders; 2005:737–744.

[CHAPTER 5]

Transhiatal Esophagectomy

Jennifer F. Waljee, MD, MPH, MSc, and Mark B. Orringer, MD

INDICATIONS

- Resectable esophageal carcinoma.
- Barrett esophagus with high-grade dysplasia.
- Carcinoma of the cardia or proximal stomach.
- Achalasia.
- Advanced disease (mega-esophagus).
- Failed esophagomyotomy.
- Benign (undilatable) stricture.
- Recurrent hiatal hernia or reflux esophagitis following multiple hiatal hernia repairs.

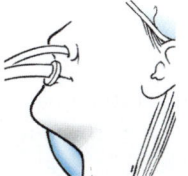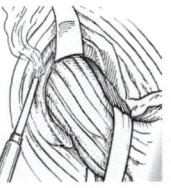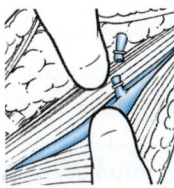
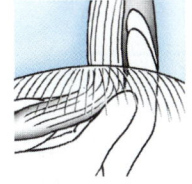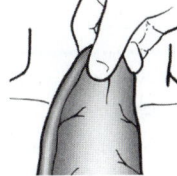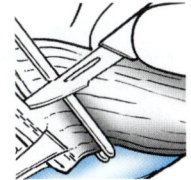
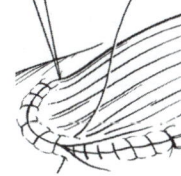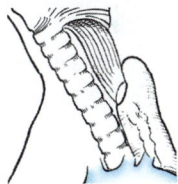

CONTRAINDICATIONS

Absolute

- Biopsy-proven distant metastatic (stage IV) esophageal cancer.
- Tracheobronchial invasion by upper or mid-third tumors visualized on bronchoscopy.
- Aortic invasion demonstrated on MRI, CT scan, or endoscopic ultrasound (EUS).

Relative

- Cardiopulmonary comorbidities.
- Previous esophageal surgery causing excessive mediastinal adhesions.
- Previous radiation therapy (more than 6–12 months prior) causing mediastinal and esophageal radiation fibrosis.

INFORMED CONSENT

- In our series of patients, overall mortality is 1%, and more than 70% of patients experience no postoperative complications.

Expected Benefits
- Resection of the intrathoracic esophagus and accessible associated adenopathy for definitive therapy or local management of disease, while restoring normal swallowing and digestive function as much as possible.

Potential Risks
- Cervical esophagogastric anastomotic leak (5–10%).
- Cervical dysphagia or esophageal stricture requiring early postoperative dilation (50–60%).
- Postvagotomy dumping symptoms (25–50%).
- Recurrent laryngeal nerve injury ($< 5\%$).
- Chylothorax ($< 2\%$).
- Mediastinal hemorrhage ($< 1\%$).
- Membranous tracheal injury ($< 1\%$).
- Gastric tip necrosis ($< 1\%$).
- Surgical site infections and systemic complications common to any major operation (eg, pneumonia, venous thromboembolism, and cardiovascular events).

EQUIPMENT
- A table-mounted "upper hand" retractor facilitates exposure of the operative field.
- Endoscope for preoperative visualization of the esophageal abnormality and to ensure an adequate normal proximal margin.
- 14-inch right-angle clamps.
- Extra-long 16-inch electrocauterizing device.
- Gastrointestinal anastomosis (GIA) stapler

PATIENT PREPARATION

Preoperative Planning
- Thorough preoperative staging evaluation is essential before performing transhiatal esophagectomy for malignancy.
  - Esophagoscopy and biopsy, to establish the location of the tumor and histology.
  - CT scanning, to demonstrate the local extent of the tumor and presence of distant metastatic disease.
  - EUS, to define the depth of tumor invasion within the esophageal wall and surrounding tissues. EUS can also identify dissemination of tumor into regional lymph nodes and can be combined with fine-needle aspiration for confirmation of malignancy.
  - Positron emission tomography has recently become a standard part of the staging evaluation and determines occult distant metastatic disease.

- For patients with a history of gastric disease or previous gastric surgery, or patients with esophagogastric junction tumors that may necessitate resection of a major portion of the stomach, a barium enema should be performed to assess the colon as an alternate conduit if the stomach is not suitable.
- Maximizing the patient's preoperative cardiopulmonary status is paramount to successful recovery.
- Patients should abstain from cigarette smoking and alcohol use for a minimum of 3 weeks before the operation.
- Patients should use an incentive spirometer on a regular basis (10 deep breaths three times daily), and walk at least 1–3 miles per day.
- For patients with severe dysphagia, weight loss, or dehydration, liquid supplementation by either oral or nasogastric routes should be considered.
- Placement of percutaneous gastrostomy and jejunostomy tubes should be avoided for preoperative feeding as they increase the risk of surgical site infection, risk injuring the right gastroepiploic artery, and complicate subsequent mobilization of the stomach at the time of operation.
- Patients who may require colonic interposition should receive a preoperative bowel preparation.

Anesthetic Management
- Continuous radial intra-arterial blood pressure monitoring.
- Two large-bore peripheral intravenous catheters.
- Epidural catheter for postoperative analgesia.
- Standard endotracheal tube.
- Foley catheter.

PATIENT POSITIONING
- After induction of general anesthesia, flexible endoscopy is performed by the operating surgeon to verify the exact location of the mass or abnormality and to ensure that there is an adequate normal length of proximal esophagus above for construction of a cervical esophagogastric anastomosis.
- Following completion of endoscopy, a 16 French nasogastric tube is placed to evacuate air from the stomach.
- **Figure 5–1:** The patient should be supine with a folded blanket under the shoulders to provide adequate neck extension.
  - The head is turned to the right and supported on a padded head ring.
  - The skin of the neck, chest, and abdomen is prepared and draped from the angle of the mandible superiorly to the pubis inferiorly, and from both midaxillary lines anteriorly.
  - Both arms are padded and tucked at the patient's side following the placement of arterial and venous access lines.

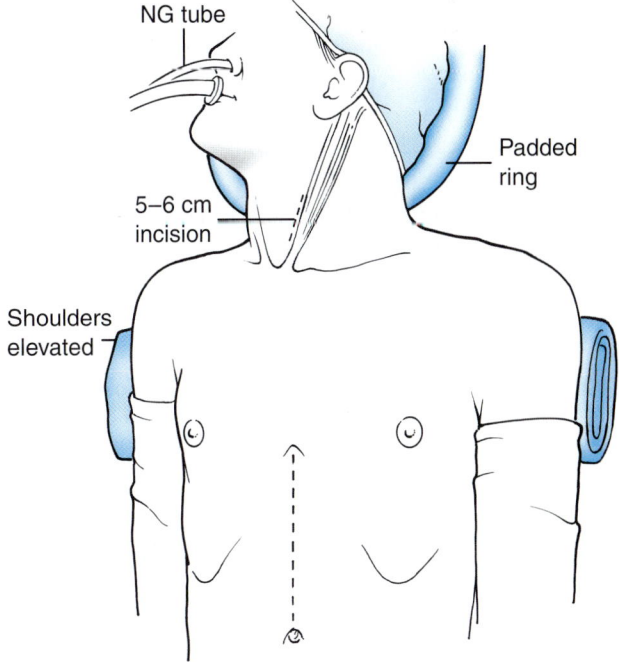

Figure 5–1

PROCEDURE

Overview

- Transhiatal esophagectomy is widely used for the resection of both benign and malignant esophageal disease.
- In experienced hands, it is a safe and well-tolerated alternative to transthoracic esophagectomy, and it avoids the morbidity of mediastinitis resulting from an intrathoracic anastomotic leak.
- Using this approach, the thoracic esophagus is resected through a widened diaphragmatic hiatus and a cervical incision.
- Alimentary continuity is restored with a gastric conduit anastomosed to the remaining cervical esophagus above the level of the clavicles.

Abdominal Phase

- The abdomen is entered through a midline supraumbilical incision (see Figure 5–1).
- Exploration of the abdomen is performed to confirm that the stomach is an appropriate conduit and is not extensively replaced by tumor nor contracted from prior surgery or caustic ingestion.
- Mobilization of the stomach.
  - Following exploration, the triangular ligament of the liver is divided using electrocautery.
  - A self-retaining, upper hand, table-mounted retractor is used to facilitate exposure, and the left lobe of the liver is padded and retracted to the right with a liver blade.
  - The greater curvature of the stomach is visualized, and the course of the right gastroepiploic artery is identified.
  - Beginning at the midpoint of the greater curvature of the stomach, the greater omentum is separated from the stomach to the level of the pylorus between right-angled clamps, using 2-0 silk ties for hemostasis.
  - Care is taken to apply the clamps 1–2 cm below the right gastroepiploic artery to avoid injury to this vessel.
  - Attention is then directed to the superior aspect of the greater curvature of the stomach. The left gastroepiploic artery and short gastric vessels are identified and divided between right-angled clamps using 2-0 silk ties for hemostasis.
  - To prevent gastric necrosis, it is important to avoid ligation of these vessels too close to the stomach.
  - Additionally, the surgeon must take care to avoid injury to the spleen during this portion of the dissection.
- **Figure 5–2:** Mobilization of the lower esophagus.
  - Following the division of these vessels, attention is turned to the diaphragmatic hiatus.
  - The peritoneum overlying the esophageal hiatus is incised, and the esophagus is encircled with a 1-inch Penrose drain.

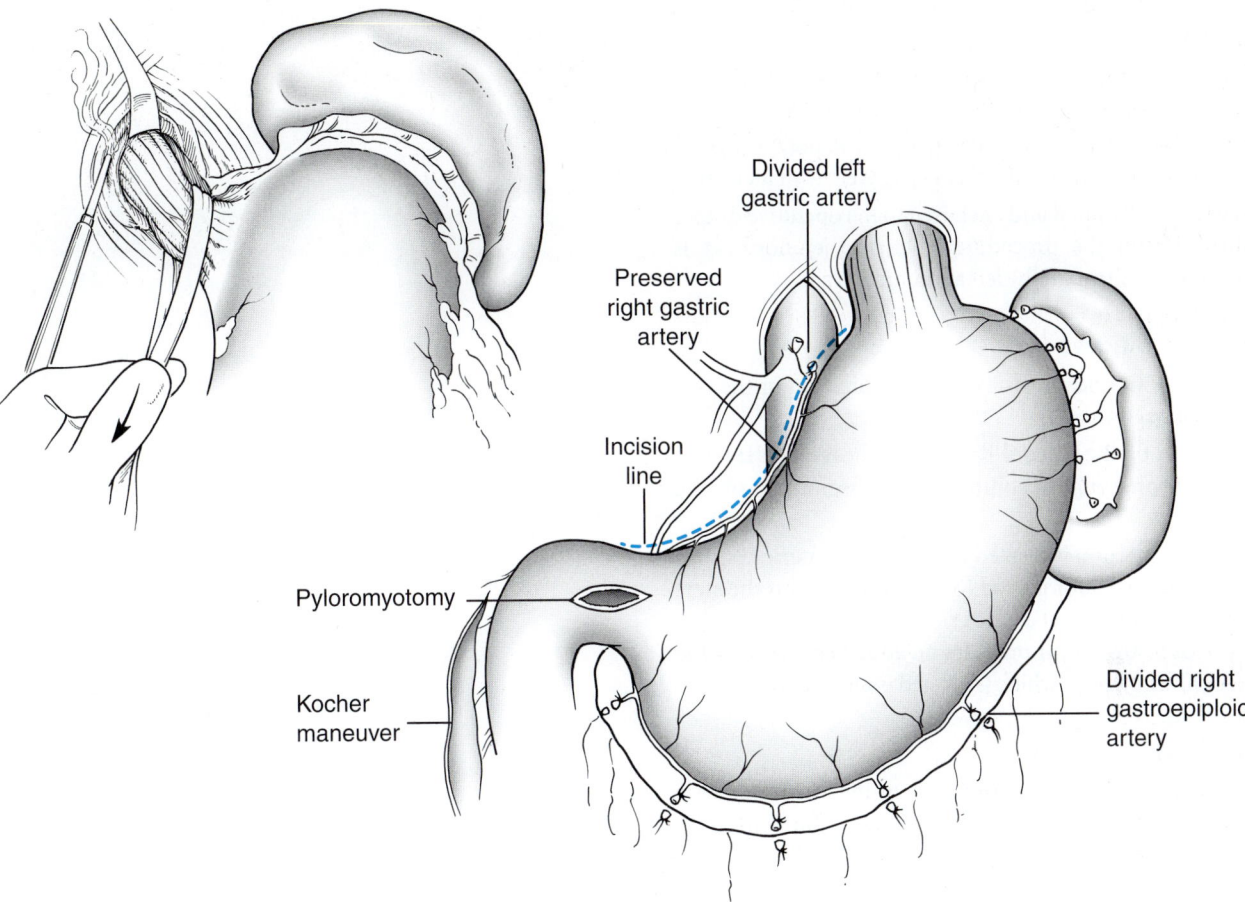

Figure 5-2

- The gastrohepatic omentum is then incised, taking care to preserve the right gastric artery.
- The left gastric artery and vein are divided between clamps and doubly ligated, avoiding injury to the celiac axis.
- The artery is ligated and divided at its origin from the celiac axis, sweeping any adjacent lymph nodes toward the stomach.
- Throughout this dissection, the surgeon should be mindful of aberrant vascular anatomy, particularly an aberrant left hepatic artery arising from the left gastric artery, which might need to be preserved.
- To maximize the reach of the stomach superiorly, a generous Kocher maneuver is performed, and the duodenum is mobilized sufficiently so that the pylorus can be grasped and moved to the level of the xiphoid process medially.
  - Two traction sutures are placed, one at the superior and one at the inferior pole of the pylorus.
  - A 2-cm long pyloromyotomy is created, beginning 1.5 cm on the gastric side and extending through the pylorus and onto the duodenum for 0.5–1 cm.
- This is performed using the cutting current of a needle-tipped electrocautery device and a fine-tipped vascular mosquito clamp to dissect the gastric and duodenal submucosa away from the overlying muscle.
- The pylorus is marked with two metallic silver clips on the traction sutures for future radiographic localization.
- Downward traction is placed on the Penrose drain encircling the esophagogastric junction.
- The diaphragmatic hiatus is progressively dilated manually until the surgeon's hand can be inserted into the posterior mediastinum through the hiatus.
- A narrow Deaver retractor is placed into the hiatus to allow visualization, division, and ligation of the lateral attachments of the distal half of the esophagus.
- Gentle blunt dissection is used in combination with electrocautery and a long right-angled clamp to expose the lateral esophageal attachments and mobilize the distal 5–10 cm of the lower esophagus.
- The low posterior mediastinum is gently packed with a gauze "lap pack" as attention is now turned to the neck.

- A feeding jejunostomy tube should be placed in all patients.
  - A 14 French rubber jejunostomy tube is inserted approximately 8–10 inches beyond the ligament of Treitz.
  - This is secured in place using two 4-0 polypropylene purse-string sutures and a 4-cm long Weitzel maneuver.
  - The tube is clamped and anchored to the operative drapes until later in the procedure when the jejunostomy is brought out through the left abdominal wall.

Cervical Phase

- **Figure 5–3:** Cervical incision and mobilization of the cervical esophagus.
  - Palpation of the cricoid cartilage indicates the level of the cricopharyngeal sphincter, the beginning of the esophagus.
  - A 5–7 cm incision is created along the left anterior border of the sternocleidomastoid (SCM) muscle from the sternal notch to the level of the cricoid cartilage. An incision superior to this point provides no added exposure of the cervical esophagus, which is located inferior to the cricoid cartilage.
  - The platysma muscle is incised.
  - The fascia along the anterior edge of the SCM muscle is incised in the direction of the wound, and the SCM muscle is retracted laterally to expose the omohyoid muscle.

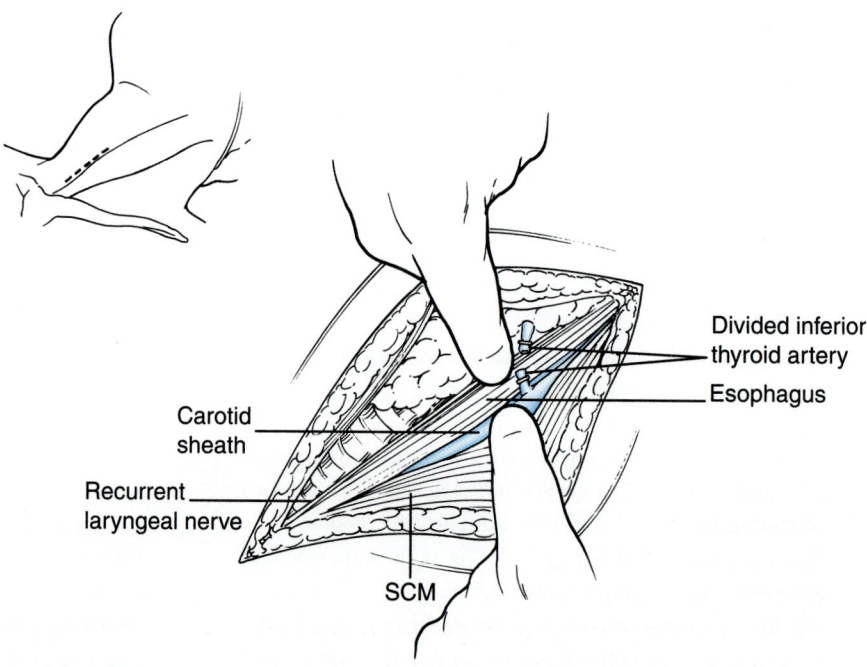

Figure 5–3

- The omohyoid muscle and its contiguous fascial sheath are divided, exposing the underlying carotid sheath.
- The SCM muscle and carotid sheath and its contents are gently retracted laterally, while the larynx, thyroid, and trachea are retracted medially using only a finger. Hand-held retractors should not be used for this purpose to prevent injury to the recurrent laryngeal nerve lying in the tracheoesophageal groove.
- The middle thyroid vein is divided.
- The inferior thyroid artery, which is always found at the level of the cricoid cartilage and upper esophageal sphincter, is identified, divided, and ligated. The dissection is carried directly posterior until the prevertebral fascia is identified.
- Blunt finger dissection into the superior mediastinum separates the cervical and upper thoracic esophagus from the prevertebral fascia.
- Upward retraction on the cervical esophagus by a finger placed gently along the tracheoesophageal groove elevates the upper thoracic esophagus from the superior mediastinum into the cervical wound, and sharp dissection posterolateral to the tracheoesophageal groove is used to free the anterior surface of the esophagus away from the trachea.
- The cervical esophagus is encircled with a 1-inch Penrose drain. With upward traction on the Penrose drain, the cervical esophagus is mobilized circumferentially to the level of the carina by the surgeon's index finger, which is kept directly against the esophagus.

Mediastinal Dissection

- **Figure 5–4A:** Posterior mobilization of the intrathoracic esophagus.
  - Back in the abdomen, working through the diaphragmatic hiatus, the surgeon palpates the esophagus to assess its mobility and establish that transhiatal resection is feasible.
  - The surgeon inserts one hand through the diaphragmatic hiatus posterior to the esophagus.
  - The hand is advanced superiorly, keeping as close to the spine as possible along the prevertebral fascia.
  - At the same time, the cervical esophagus is gently retracted anteriorly and medially using the rubber Penrose drain.
  - A "sponge-on-a-stick" is inserted through the cervical incision behind the esophagus. By advancing the sponge stick inferiorly, the esophagus is dissected free from the prevertebral fascia.
  - Working upward from the diaphragmatic hiatus and downward through the cervical incision, posterior mobilization of the esophagus is completed using a combination of finger dissection and dissection with the sponge stick.

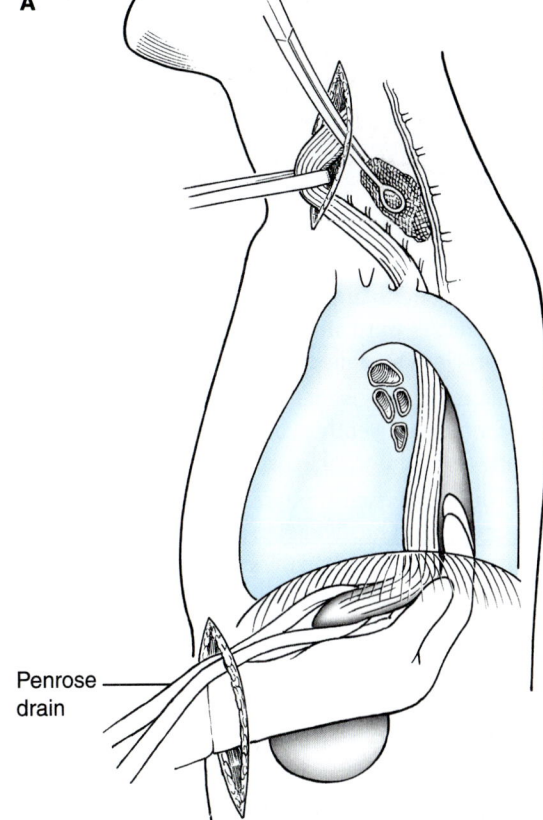

Figure 5–4A

- The sponge stick is advanced downward until it meets the surgeon's hand inserted through the diaphragmatic hiatus.
- At this point, a 28 French Argyle Saratoga sump catheter is placed through the cervical incision into the mediastinum along the dissected path to evacuate blood.

■ **Figure 5–4B:** Anterior mobilization of the intrathoracic esophagus.
- While the esophagogastric junction is retracted inferiorly with its encircling Penrose drain, the surgeon places his or her hand against the anterior esophagus, palm downward.
- The hand is advanced into the mediastinum, gently dissecting the esophagus from the posterior pericardium and the carina.
- The cervical esophagus is retraced superiorly and laterally, and the surgeon places his or her hand against the anterior wall of the esophagus.
- The hand is advanced inferiorly with two fingers dissecting along the wall of the anterior esophagus to free the esophagus from the posterior membranous trachea.
- Care must be taken to avoid injury to the trachea during this process.
- With the anterior and posterior esophageal attachments divided, the cervical esophagus is gently retracted superiorly into the cervical wound as the lateral attachments of the upper esophagus are progressively swept away by blunt dissection.
- Approximately 5–8 cm of the upper thoracic esophagus is circumferentially mobilized in this fashion.

■ Attention is then turned to the abdominal field.
- The previously placed lap pad is removed from the posterior mediastinum.
- The hand is inserted palm downward through the diaphragmatic hiatus and advanced along the anterior esophagus until the circumferentially mobilized upper thoracic esophagus can be identified by palpation.
- The remaining lateral esophageal attachments and vagal branches are gently avulsed by drawing the hand inferiorly along the esophagus in a "raking" motion.
- If difficulty is encountered in this dissection, the upper sternum can be divided to provide exposure of the upper thoracic esophagus in the superior mediastinum and division of its lateral attachments under direct visualization.
- Throughout the mediastinal dissection, intra-arterial blood pressure is monitored with a radial artery catheter to avoid prolonged hypotension due to displacement of the heart.

■ Once the entire thoracic esophagus has been mobilized, the nasogastric tube is withdrawn to a level above the upper esophageal sphincter.

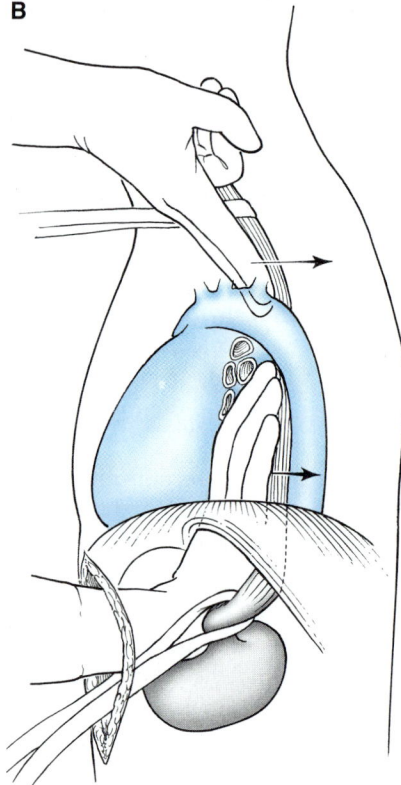

Figure 5–4B

- The cervical esophagus is elevated out of the wound and divided approximately 8–10 cm distal to the upper sphincter using a GIA surgical stapler.
  - Approximately 5 cm of excessive cervical length should be left to ensure a tension-free reconstruction.
- The thoracic esophagus and stomach are then delivered downward through the diaphragmatic hiatus, and the sump catheter is advanced down into the posterior mediastinum from the neck incision.
- A narrow Deaver retractor is inserted into the diaphragmatic hiatus to allow the surgeon to inspect the mediastinum for bleeding and the mediastinal pleura for injury that indicates the need for a chest tube.
- If the pleura has been violated, a 28 French chest tube is inserted in the appropriate anterior axillary line in approximately the sixth intercostal space, sutured in place, and connected to an underwater seal chest tube suction system.
- The posterior mediastinum is packed again with a large gauze abdominal lap pad to control minor bleeding, and the cervical wound is covered with a moist pack as the surgeon returns to the abdomen for preparation of the gastric conduit.

Creation of the Gastric Conduit and Abdominal Closure

- **Figure 5–5A:** Preparing the gastric conduit.
  - With the mobilized stomach and attached esophagus placed on the patient's anterior chest wall, the site along the greater curvature of the stomach that will reach most superior is identified by gently pulling the fundus toward the cervical incision.
  - Once this point is identified, it is continuously retracted superiorly, as the fat along the lesser curvature is cleared between clamps and ligated at the level of the second "crow's foot."
  - The upper stomach is progressively divided by sequential applications of the GIA stapler, starting at the lesser curvature and working toward the fundus.
  - Traction on the fundus during this maneuver must be maintained to straighten the stomach sufficiently to reach the neck.
  - The proximal stomach is divided approximately 5 cm distal to the esophagogastric junction, and the specimen is passed off of the field. The staple line along the lesser curve of the stomach is oversewn with a running 4-0 polypropylene Lembert stitch.
- **Figure 5–5B:** Completed gastric conduit.
  - The completed gastric conduit should reach 4–5 cm above the left clavicle.

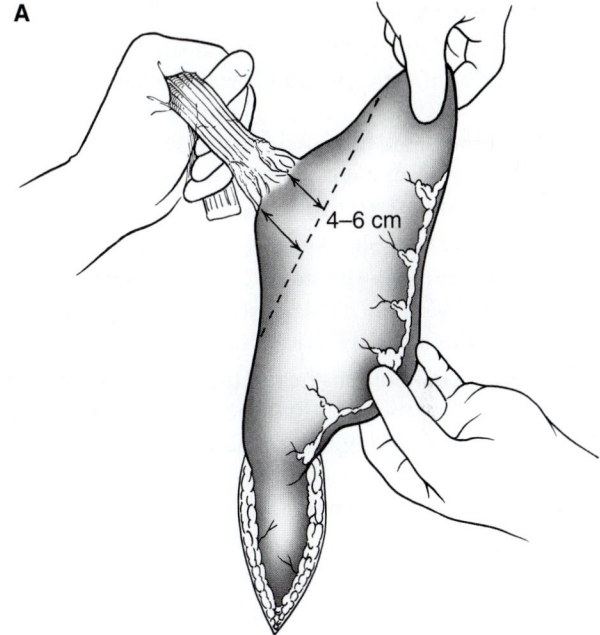

Figure 5–5A

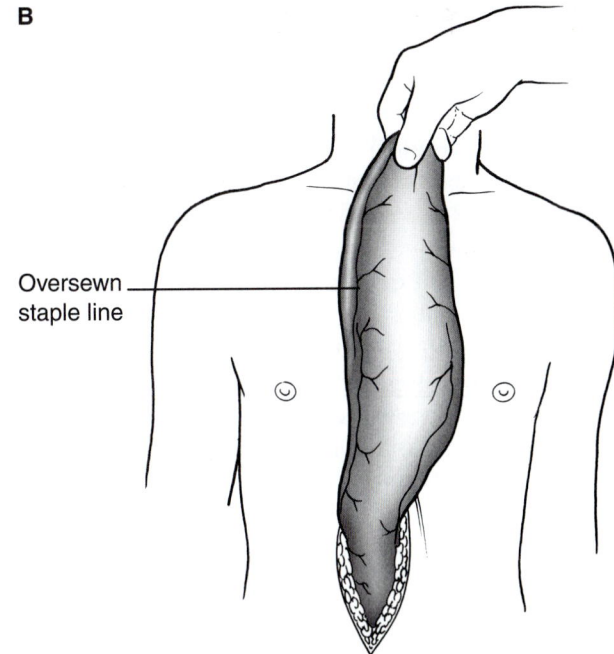

Figure 5–5B

- **Figure 5–6:** Delivery of the gastric tip into the cervical wound in preparation for the anastomosis.
  - Using a narrow Deaver retractor to expose the diaphragmatic hiatus, the superior tip of the gastric fundus is placed through the hiatus.
  - The surgeon's hand should remain on top of the stomach, gently guiding it upward through the posterior mediastinum, underneath the aortic arch and into the superior mediastinum.
  - When the gastric fundus can be palpated in the superior mediastinum with a finger inserted through the cervical incision, a Babcock clamp is inserted into the superior mediastinum and the gastric tip gently grasped. The jaws of the clamp are not completely closed to minimize trauma to the gastric tip.
  - The gastric tip should not be pulled into the cervical wound, but rather the stomach pushed upward and the tip guided with the hand inserted through the diaphragmatic hiatus into the cervical wound.
  - The surgeon should ensure that the stomach is not twisted by noting that the staple line along the lesser curvature of the stomach is facing toward the patient's right side and by palpating the stomach through the diaphragmatic hiatus and the cervical incision.
  - The gastric tip should remain pink and without evidence of ischemia throughout the remainder of the procedure.
  - The position of the stomach in the neck wound is maintained by packing a small moistened gauze pad into the thoracic inlet alongside the stomach to prevent it from retracting downward into the mediastinum.
- Attention is redirected to the abdomen, which is inspected for hemostasis.
- After delivery of the gastric conduit into the cervical incision, the pyloromyotomy will lie 3–4 cm below the level of the diaphragmatic hiatus.
  - The diaphragmatic hiatus is closed loosely using one or two interrupted No. 1 silk sutures until three fingers slide easily alongside the stomach in the hiatus.
  - Additionally, one or two interrupted 3-0 silk sutures are placed between the anterior gastric wall and the adjacent hiatus to discourage migration of a loop of small intestine through the hiatus into the chest.
- Finally, the left lobe of the liver is returned to its anatomic location, and the triangular ligament is sutured over the hiatus to prevent future herniation of abdominal contents.
- The jejunostomy tube is brought out of the left upper abdominal wall through a separate stab incision and tacked to the adjacent peritoneum using interrupted 3-0 silk sutures.
  - The jejunostomy tube is secured to the skin using a 2-0 polypropylene suture.

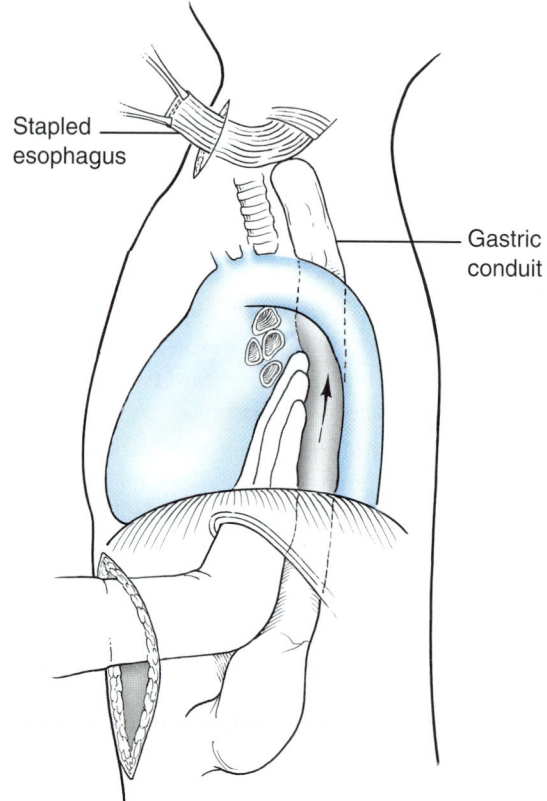

Figure 5–6

- The abdomen is then closed using No. 1 looped PDS suture on the muscle fascia, running 2-0 chromic catgut suture on the subcutaneous tissue, and running 3-0 nylon suture on the skin.
- The abdominal incision is isolated from the field with a sterile towel to prevent wound contamination by oral flora, which can occur once the cervical esophagus is opened for performance of the anastomosis.
- A sterile drape is placed over the abdominal field.

Cervical Esophagogastric Anastomosis

- **Figure 5–7A-F:** Creation of the cervical esophagogastric anastomosis.
  - After closure of the abdomen, attention is turned to the cervical wound.
  - The tip of the divided cervical esophagus is grasped with an Allis clamp and retracted superiorly and to the right.
  - The anterior wall of the stomach is grasped using a Babcock clamp, and the staple line is rotated more medially.
  - A seromuscular traction suture is placed in the anterior gastric wall to elevate the stomach into the wound, the cervical esophagus is aligned with the stomach, and the site of the anastomosis selected.
  - A 1.5-cm vertical gastrotomy is created in the anterior gastric wall to allow later insertion of a 3-cm Endo-GIA staple cartridge (Figure 5–7A).
  - The cervical esophageal staple line is amputated obliquely, allowing for enough redundancy to accommodate later retraction of the stomach into the thoracic inlet (Figure 5–7B).
  - The staple line is then sent for pathologic examination as the proximal esophageal margin.
  - Two stay sutures are placed, one at the anterior tip of the divided esophagus and the other between the posterior end of the divided esophagus and the superior end of the gastrotomy (Figure 5–7C).
  - These stay sutures align the back wall of the cervical esophagus and the front wall of the stomach for construction of the anastomosis.
- An Endo-GIA-30 stapler is placed in the stomach as the traction sutures are drawn inferiorly, gently pulling the stomach and esophagus downward as the stapler is advanced inward and closed (Figure 5–7D).
  - Two lateral suspension sutures of 4-0 Vicryl are placed between the cervical esophagus and the stomach on either side of the anastomosis to alleviate tension on the anastomosis.
  - The stapler is fired and removed, thereby creating a 3-cm-long side-to-side stapled esophagogastric anastomosis.
  - The previously placed 16 French nasogastric tube is guided across the anastomosis and into the intrathoracic stomach.

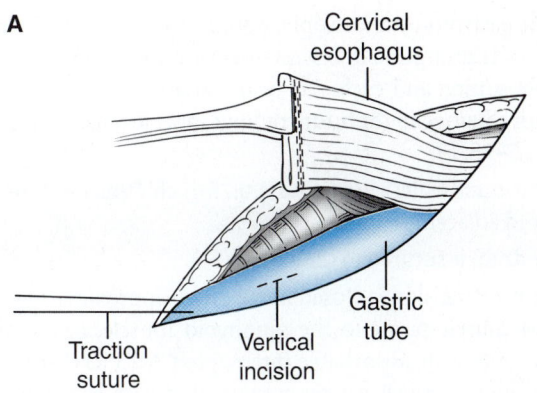
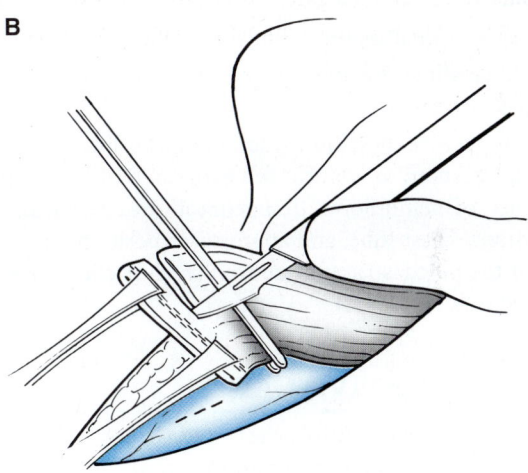
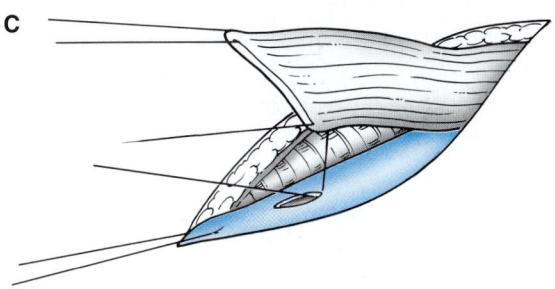
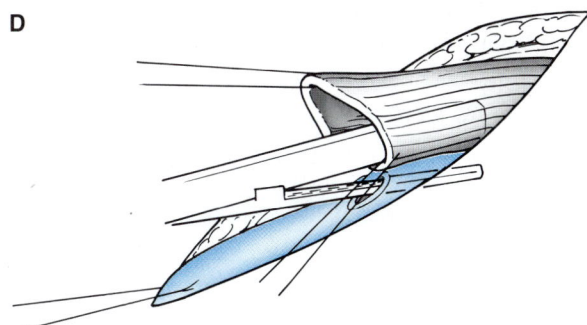

Figure 5–7A–D

- The gastrotomy and esophagotomy are closed in two layers of running and interrupted 4-0 monofilament absorbable suture, and each side of the anastomosis is marked with a hemoclip for future radiographic localization (Figure 5–7E, F).
- The wound is irrigated, and a 0.25-inch Penrose drain is placed adjacent to the anastomosis.
- The drain is sutured to the skin.
- The neck incision is closed loosely by reapproximating the SCM muscle fascia to the omohyoid muscle, fascia, and platysma using absorbable interrupted 3-0 Vicryl sutures, and the skin edges are reapproximated with running 4-0 nylon.
- **Figure 5–8:** Final anatomic position of the gastric conduit.
- Sterile dressings are applied, and the thoracostomy tubes are placed on suction.
- A postoperative chest radiograph should be obtained in the operating room to confirm full expansion of both lungs, absence of hemothorax or pneumothorax requiring an additional chest tube, and appropriate positioning of the tip of the nasogastric tube above the silver clips marking the pylorus.

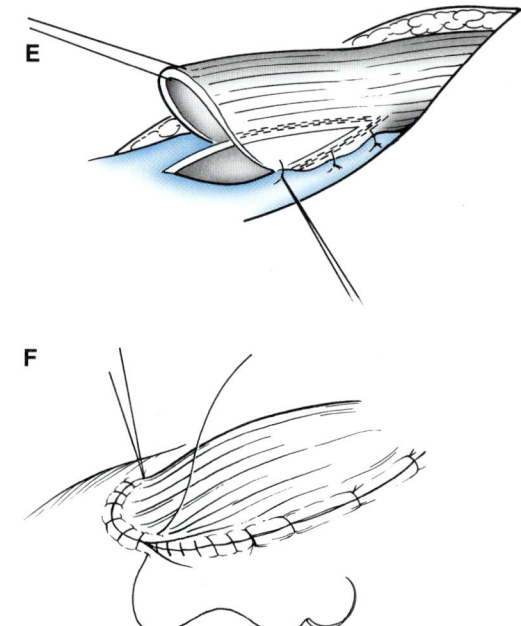

Figure 5–7E–F

POSTOPERATIVE CARE

- Immediate postoperative chest radiograph while the patient is in the operating room to exclude unrecognized pneumothorax or hemothorax.
- Extubation in the operating room and initiation of epidural anesthesia.
- Early use of an incentive spirometer within several hours of awakening from anesthesia.
- Early ambulation beginning on postoperative day (POD) 1.
- Ice chips by mouth (not to exceed 30 mL/h) for throat comfort until the nasogastric tube is removed on POD 3.
- Initiation of oral liquids on POD 4, with progressive daily advancement to full liquids, then mechanical soft (pureed) diet, and a soft diet by POD 7.
- Initiation of jejunostomy tube feedings on POD 3 and tapering as oral intake increases.
- Monitoring for resolution of ileus.
- Barium swallow examination on POD 7 to document integrity of the anastomosis, adequate gastric emptying through pylorus and hiatus, and absence of obstruction at the jejunostomy site.
- If oral intake is poor, nocturnal jejunostomy tube feeding supplementation can be used.
- If the patient is eating well and has no complications, the jejunostomy tube can be removed 4 weeks postoperatively during follow-up examination.

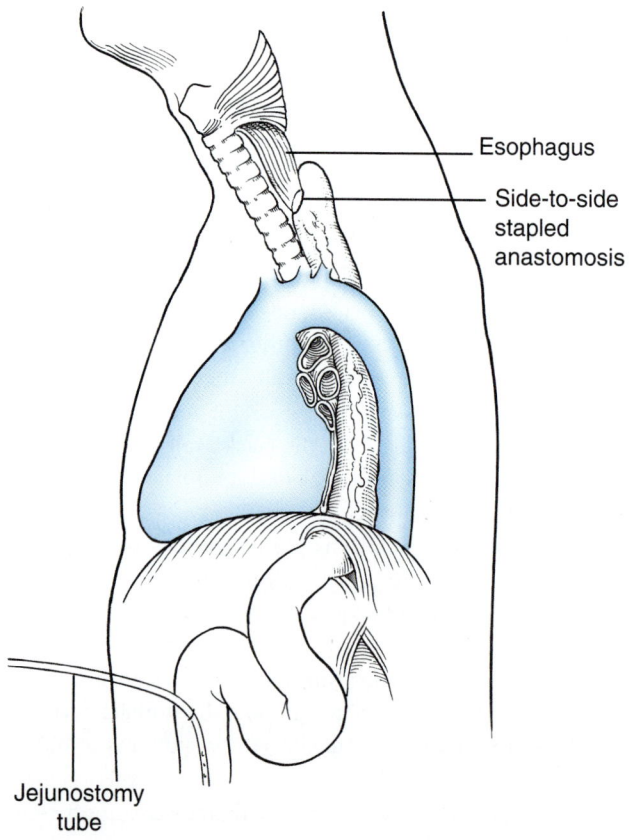

Figure 5–8

POTENTIAL COMPLICATIONS

Intraoperative
- Pneumothorax.
- Hemothorax.
- Uncontrollable mediastinal bleeding (< 1%).
- Need for thoracostomy tubes due to entry into pleural cavity (75%).
- Iatrogenic splenectomy (3%).
- Membranous tracheal laceration (< 1%).
- Injury to the gastric or duodenal mucosa during pyloromyotomy (< 2%).

Early Postoperative
- Recurrent laryngeal nerve injury (< 1–2%) causing hoarseness and difficulty swallowing.
- Chylothorax (1%).
- Cardiac arrhythmia (atrial fibrillation).
- Sympathetic pleural effusion.
- Pneumonia and atelectasis (2%).
- Cervical esophagogastric anastomotic leak (4%).
- Gastric tip necrosis (1%).
- Dysphagia.
- Regurgitation.
- Postvagotomy "dumping."
- Anastomotic stricture requiring dilation.
- Delayed gastric emptying due to incomplete pyloromyotomy, narrowing of the diaphragmatic hiatus, or jejunostomy tube site obstruction.

Late
- Cervical anastomotic stricture.
- Diaphragmatic hernia.
- Small bowel obstruction due to torsion at the jejunostomy tube site (< 1%).

PEARLS AND TIPS
- Marking the pyloromyotomy and cervical esophagogastric anastomosis with hemoclips allows for visualization on postoperative imaging to assess the position of the stomach in the chest and gastric emptying.
- Use only a fingertip to retract the cervical esophagus, thyroid, and trachea medially during mobilization of the cervical esophagus. To minimize the chance of injury to the recurrent laryngeal nerve, do not place metal retractors against the tracheoesophageal groove.
- Minimize gastric trauma during mobilization and particularly to the gastric tip so that a healthy stomach can be anastomosed to the esophagus, reducing the risk of postoperative anastomotic leak.
- When creating the gastric conduit, preserve as much of the stomach as possible to maximize collateral circulation. Repeatedly assess the color and viability of the stomach after mobilization of the stomach, when the gastric tube is delivered into the cervical wound, and after the closure of the diaphragmatic hiatus to be certain that there is no venous congestion or ischemia from mechanical causes.
- Avoid use of suspension sutures to tack the gastric tip to the prevertebral fascia because of the risk of vertebral osteomyelitis.
- Use a radial artery catheter to monitor for intraoperative hypotension, particularly during the mediastinal dissection. Hypotension can be caused by cardiac displacement or hemorrhage from injury to mediastinal structures.
- Aggressive preoperative conditioning with abstinence from cigarette smoking, regular use of an incentive spirometer, and walking are rewarded by a less complicated postoperative course.

REFERENCES
Orringer M. Transhiatal esophagectomy without thoracotomy. *Operative Techniques in Thoracic and Cardiovascular Surgery.* 2005;10:63–83.

Orringer MB, Marshall B, Chang AC, et al. Two thousand transhiatal esophagectomies: changing trends, lessons learned. *Ann Surg.* 2007;246:363–372.

Orringer MB, Marshall B, Iannettoni MD. Eliminating the cervical esophagogastric anastomotic leak with a side-to-side stapled anastomosis. *J Thorac Cardiovasc Surg.* 2000;119: 277–288.

CHAPTER 6

Operative Management of Gastric Lesions

Erika L. Newman, MD, and Michael W. Mulholland, MD, PhD

INDICATIONS
- Malignant tumors.
- Benign tumors.
- Intractable bleeding.
- Chronic ulceration and inflammation.

CONTRAINDICATIONS

Absolute
- Inability to completely resect primary cancer.
- Distant metastases.

Relative
- High operative risk because of age or comorbidities.

INFORMED CONSENT
- Operative mortality rates range from 3%–7%.
- Resection of the spleen, pancreas, or colon may be required if a gastric tumor has invaded adjacent organs.

Expected Benefits
- Surgical treatment of gastric malignancy with curative intent.
- Resolution of bleeding or obstruction from benign or malignant gastric tumors or disease processes.

Potential Risks
- Anastomotic leak.
- Wound infection.
- Pancreatic fistulae.
- Intra-abdominal abscesses.

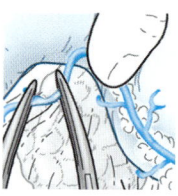
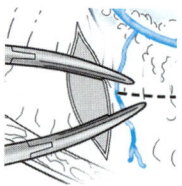
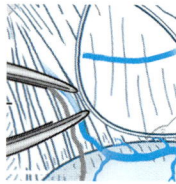
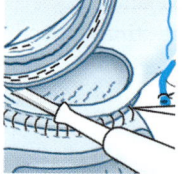
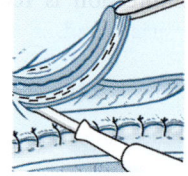
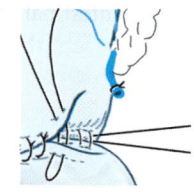
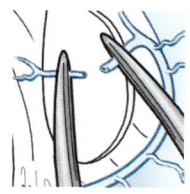
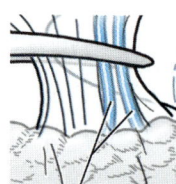
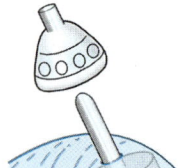

EQUIPMENT

- A self-retaining retractor is necessary for optimal exposure.
- Gastrointestinal anastomosis (GIA), thoracoabdominal (TA), and end-to-end anastomosis (EEA) staplers are often used for resection and reconstruction, and should be available.

PATIENT PREPARATION

- All patients should undergo fiberoptic endoscopy when neoplasm is suspected, and the diagnosis should be confirmed by multiple biopsies.
- Preoperative tests should be performed to determine whether distant metastases are present.
  - Abdominal and pelvic CT scans, endoscopic ultrasound, or laparoscopy may be required for adequate staging.
- A first- or second-generation cephalosporin is adequate as antibiotic prophylaxis for most gastric operations.
- Deep venous thrombosis prophylaxis should be administered.
- Bowel preparation is only useful in complicated cases when intestinal decompression is required and may serve to lessen the bacterial load if an intestinal resection is required.
- Electrolyte and coagulation deficits should be corrected before operation.

PATIENT POSITIONING

- The patient should be supine, with the operating surgeon on the right side of the patient.
- An upper midline incision is made from the xiphoid to the umbilicus to enter the abdomen.
  - Reverse Trendelenburg positioning facilitates exposure.
- Once the abdomen has been entered, a routine exploration should be performed and a nasogastric tube placed by the anesthetist.

PROCEDURE

Overview and Surgical Anatomy

- **Figure 6–1A-C:** Overview of surgical options for resection of gastric lesions.
  - For lesions involving the cardia of the stomach, esophagogastrectomy with esophagogastrostomy is performed (Figure 6–1A). A thoracotomy combined with laparotomy may be required. To ensure blood supply to the gastric remnant, the right gastroepiploic vessels are preserved.
  - For lesions in the body of the stomach, total gastrectomy with esophagojejunostomy is typically performed (Figure 6–1B).

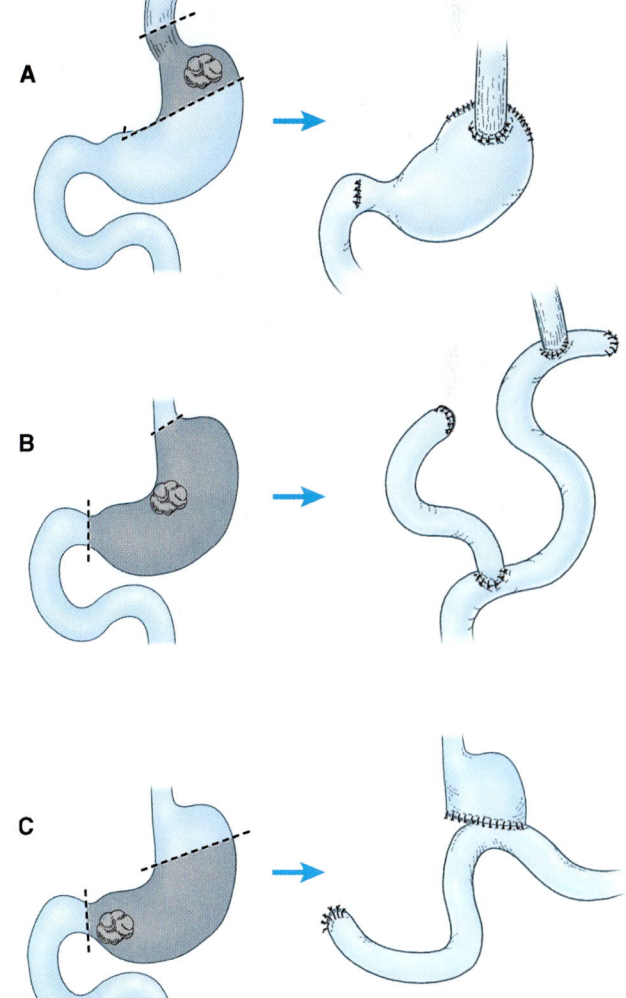

Figure 6–1A–C

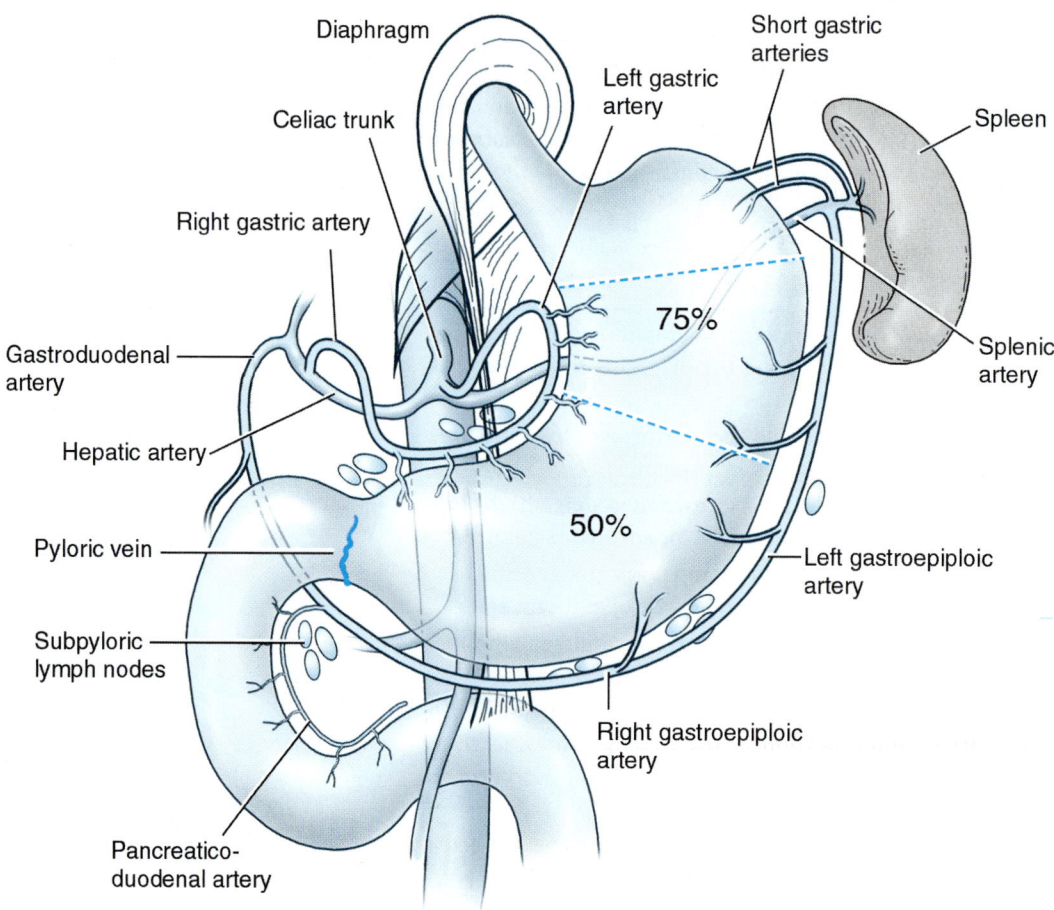

Figure 6–2

- For antral lesions, subtotal gastrectomy with gastrojejunal reconstruction is performed (Figure 6–1C).
- **Figure 6–2:** Surgical anatomy of the stomach.
  - The esophagus terminates in the stomach after penetrating the diaphragm at the esophageal hiatus.
  - The stomach is divided into the fundus, body, and antrum based on differences in mucosal histology.
  - The fundus lies to the left and superior to the esophagogastric junction.
  - The junction of the body and antrum is approximately 6–8 cm proximal to the pylorus along the lesser curvature, to a point one-third the distance from the pylorus to the esophagogastric junction along the greater curvature.
  - Subtotal gastrectomy resects up to 75% of the stomach, and resection is defined as distal if at least 50% remains after resection.

Distal and Subtotal Gastrectomy

- For distal lesions, distal or subtotal gastrectomy has an equivalent oncologic result and fewer complications when compared with total gastrectomy.
- A partial gastrectomy begins with a full Kocher maneuver that mobilizes the duodenum.
- The lesser sac must then be entered to allow early evaluation of the posterior stomach and to aid in division of the greater omentum. With cephalad retraction of the greater omentum, the avascular plane above the transverse colon is entered to the left of the midline, avoiding disruption of the middle colic vessels.
- **Figure 6–3:** The gastrocolic omentum is then dissected from the stomach. The dissection begins at the pylorus with ligation of the right gastroepiploic artery and continues along the greater curvature. In the circumstances of benign disease, the gastroepiploic vessels may be preserved.
- **Figure 6–4:** For 50% resection, the dissection ends halfway between the pylorus and the esophagogastric junction, sparing the left gastroepiploic artery and the short gastric vessels. For a subtotal or 75% resection, the left gastroepiploic artery and a portion of the short gastric vessels are divided.
- The tissue attachments of the posterior antrum are then separated from the anterior pancreas and the base of the transverse mesocolon.
- **Figure 6–5:** The gastrohepatic ligament is incised, and the lesser curvature is dissected.
- **Figure 6–6:** The right gastric vessels are ligated close to the stomach. If the pylorus is inflamed, care must be taken in this area to avoid injury to both the hepatic artery and the common bile duct.
- **Figure 6–7:** The proximal duodenum is divided carefully, avoiding injury to the common bile duct.
- **Figure 6–8:** The proximal stomach is divided with a TA-90 or a GIA stapler.
- **Figure 6–9:** The gastric staple line is oversewn at the superior portion with either a continuous or running suture. Traction sutures may be used at either end of the stapled closure to prevent retraction of the gastric remnant from the operative field.

Gastric Reconstruction for Distal and Subtotal Gastrectomy

- **Figure 6–10A-C:** Billroth I/Gastroduodenostomy.
  - For gastroduodenostomy reconstruction, the duodenum is apposed to the inferior gastric staple line (Figure 6–10A). Posterior seromuscular sutures are placed using interrupted silk sutures. The stapled end of the duodenum and the inferior gastric staple line are then excised using electrocautery.

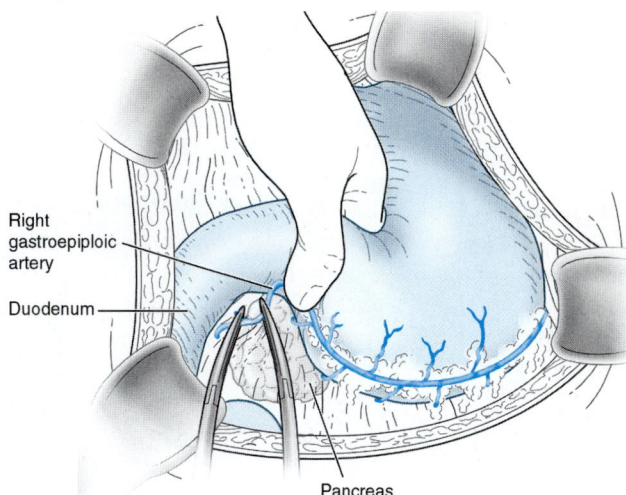

Figure 6–3

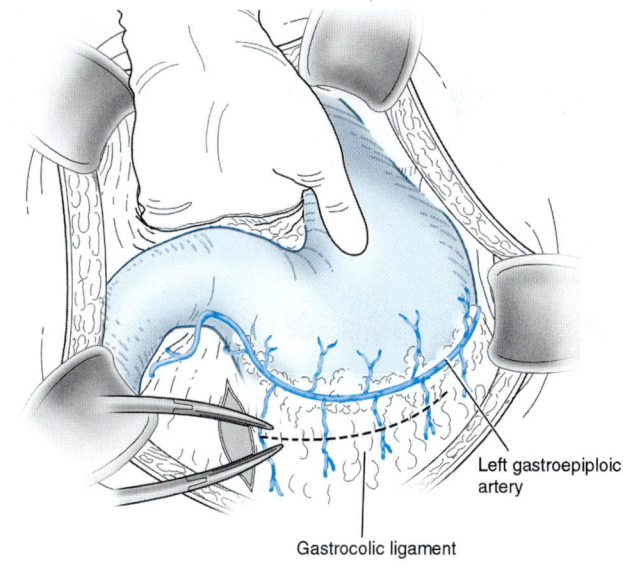

Figure 6–4

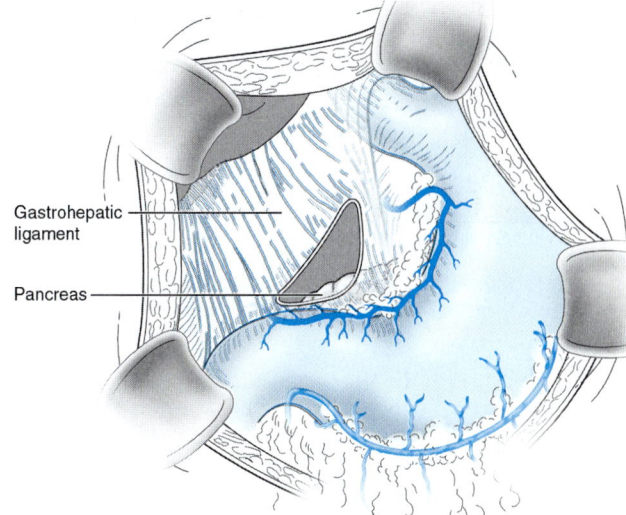

Figure 6–5

46 • Current Procedures: Surgery

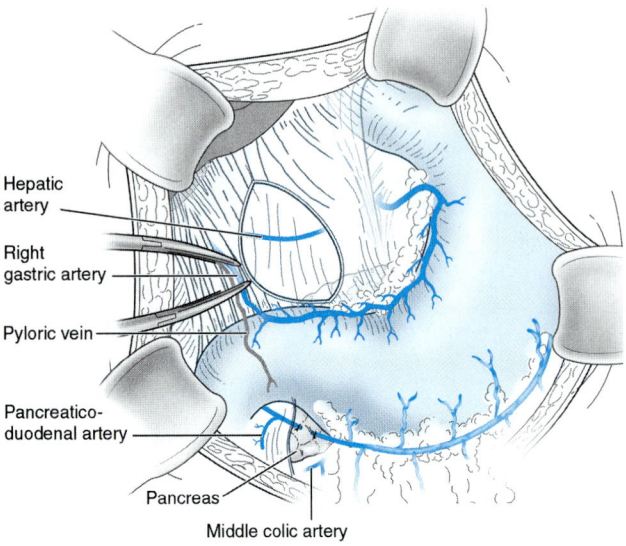

Figure 6–6

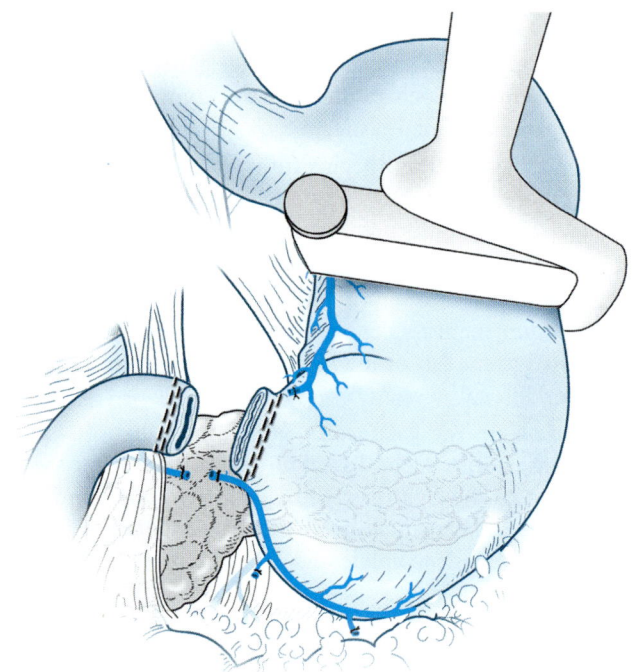

Figure 6–8

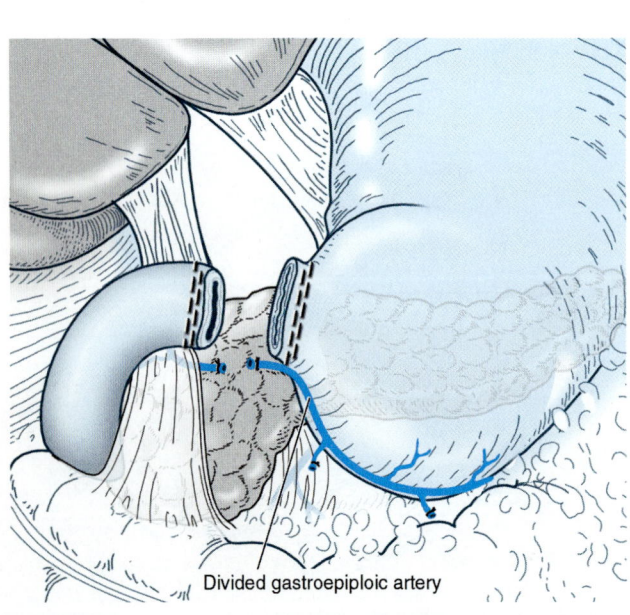

Figure 6–7

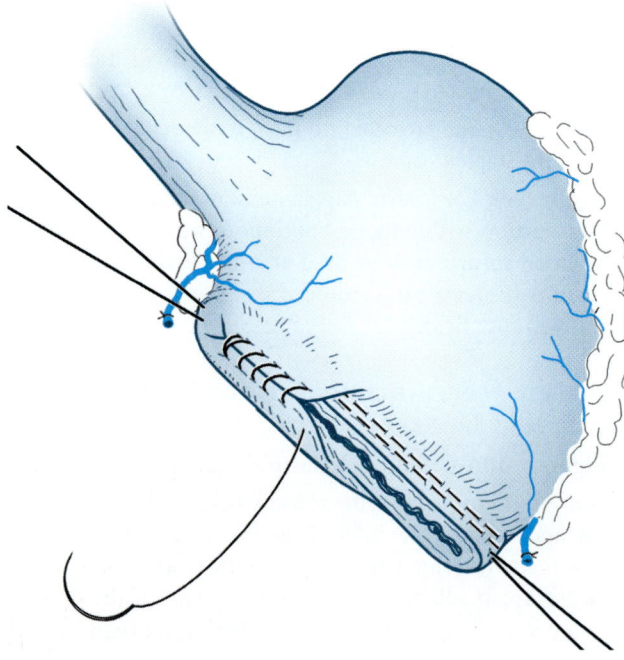

Figure 6–9

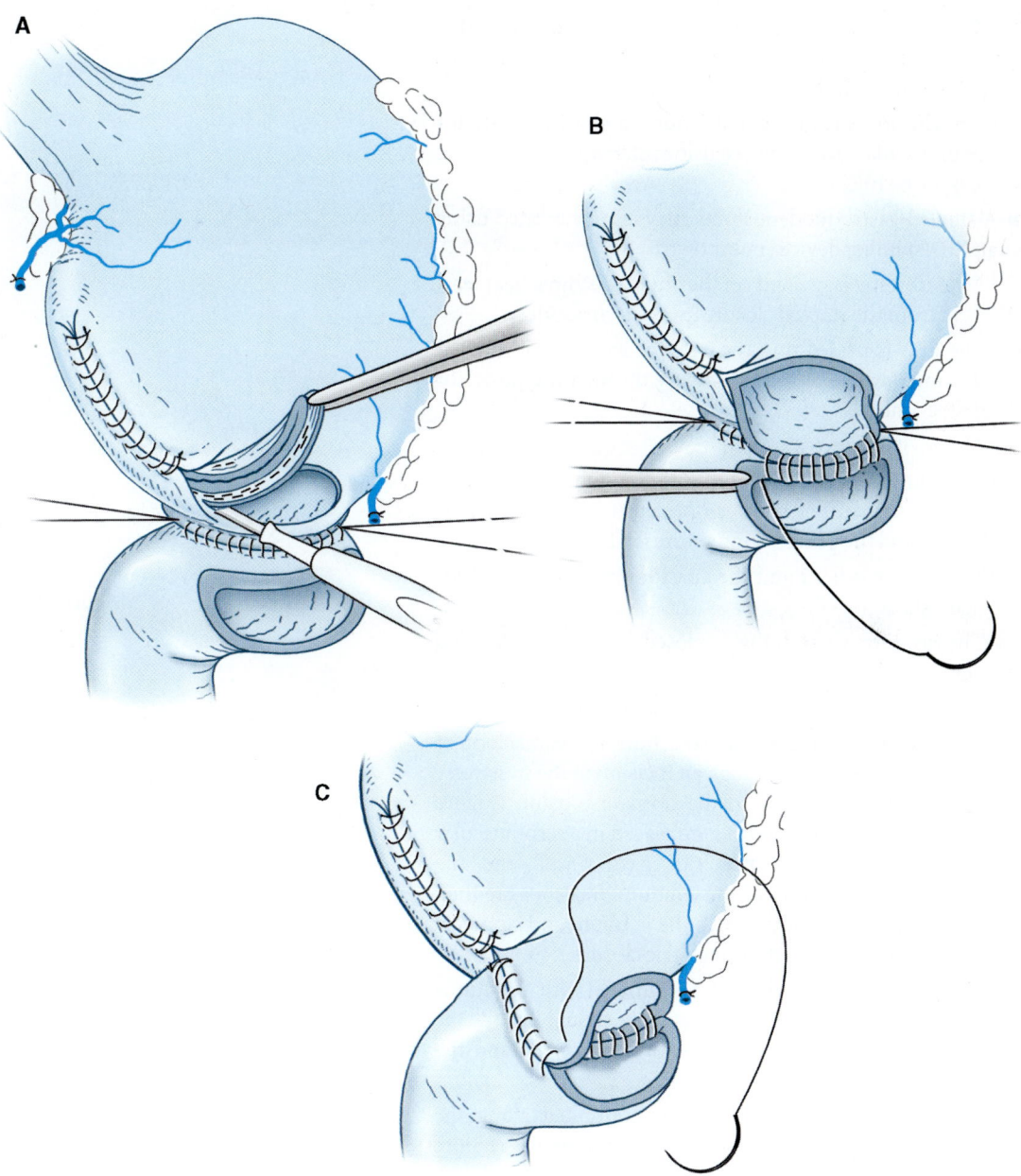

Figure 6-10A-C

- All layers of the duodenum and stomach are incorporated in the inner mucosal closure, using a continuous absorbable suture (Figure 6–10B).
- The closure is continued anteriorly and a final anterior seromuscular layer is placed using interrupted silk sutures (Figure 6–10C).

■ A stapled gastroduodenostomy may also be created using an EEA stapling device (not shown).
- A gastrotomy is created on the anterior stomach, at least 3 cm from the stapled closure using electrocautery.
- The EEA is passed into the anterior gastrotomy without the anvil, with the rod advancing through the posterior gastric wall.
- The anvil is then reattached.
- The EEA anvil is introduced into the duodenum after a purse-string suture has been placed using an automatic device, and the purse-string suture is tied.
- The stapler is fired and the anastomosis is inspected for hemostasis.
- The anterior gastrotomy is closed using a TA stapling device.

■ **Figure 6–11A-D:** Billroth II/Gastrojejunostomy.
- For gastrojejunostomy reconstruction, a proximal loop of jejunum is delivered through an incision in the transverse mesocolon or anterior to the transverse colon (Figure 6–11A). Interrupted sutures are placed in a seromuscular fashion between the posterior gastric wall and the antimesenteric border of the jejunum. Incisions are then created with electrocautery in the jejunum and stomach, partially excising the stapled gastric closure.
- The posterior mucosal closure is initiated with a continuous absorbable suture. Corner stitches should include the anterior gastric wall, the posterior gastric wall, and the jejunum (Figure 6–11B).
- The posterior mucosal suture is continued along the length of the anterior aspect of the anastomosis (Figure 6–11C).
- An anterior layer of interrupted nonabsorbable sutures completes the closure (Figure 6–11D).

■ A stapled gastrojejunostomy may also be created using a GIA stapling device (not shown).
- The anastomotic site on the posterior gastric wall is usually 2–3 cm proximal from the stapled closure.
- The GIA limbs are inserted in matching gastrotomy and antimesenteric enterotomy incisions are made with electrocautery.
- The staple line is inspected for hemostasis, and the GIA defect is closed using a TA stapler.

■ A gastrojejunostomy may also be created in a Roux-en-Y fashion (see Figures 6–17 to 6–19).

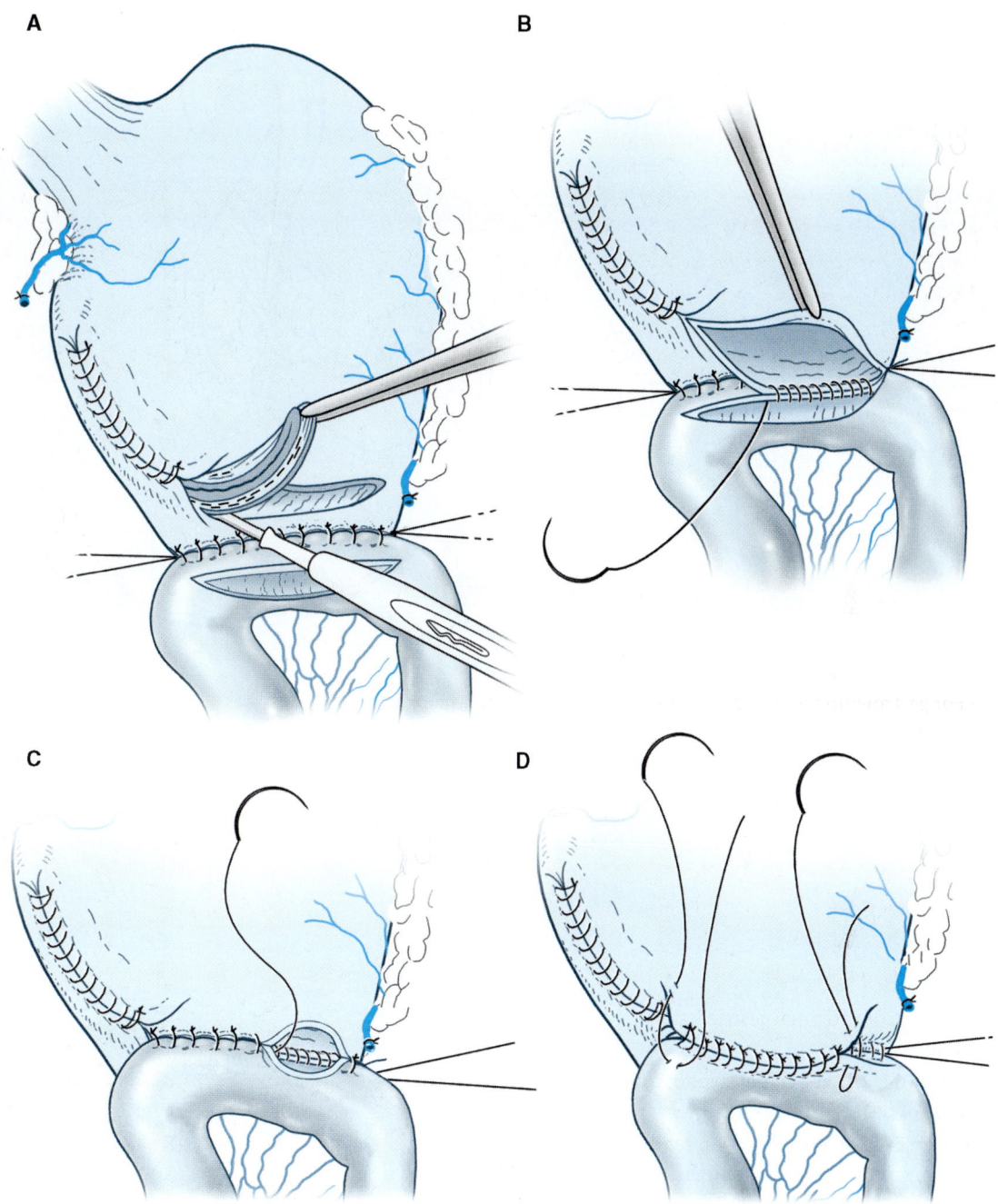

Figure 6-11A-D

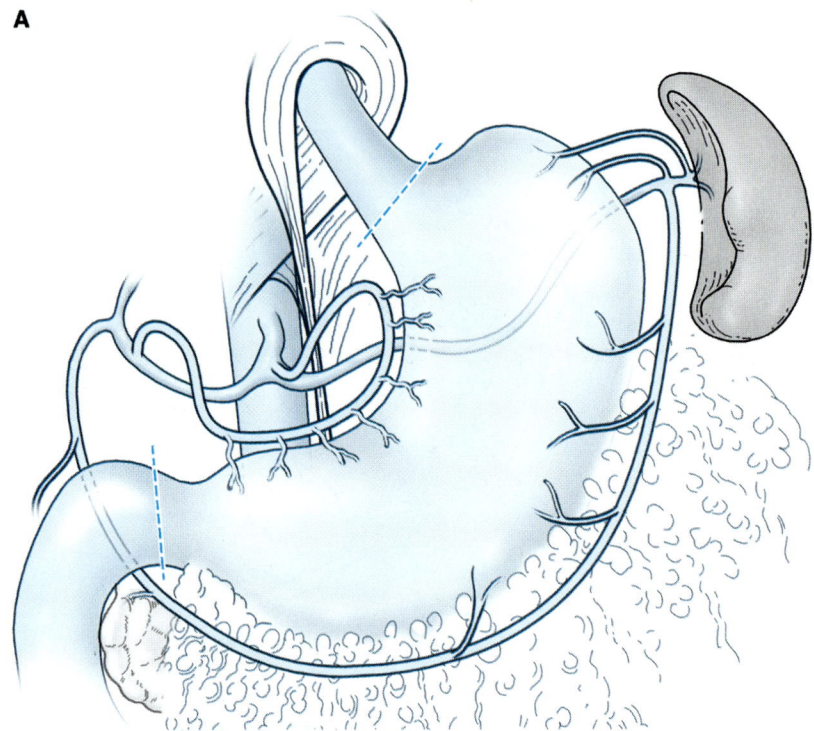

Figure 6–12A

Total Gastrectomy

- For large or proximal gastric lesions, a total gastrectomy is required.
- **Figure 6–12A:** The initial steps of total gastrectomy mirror those of distal gastrectomy.
- **Figure 6–12B:** The dissection requires a complete omentectomy and continues along the length of the greater curvature, to include the left gastroepiploic artery and the short gastric vessels (if the neoplasm does not involve the spleen).
- **Figure 6–13:** Division of the gastrohepatic ligament.
  - The right gastric artery is ligated, and if the inferior phrenic vein is encountered it can be controlled with clamps and ligated.
  - The dissection is continued proximally by dividing the peritoneum overlying the esophagus.
- **Figure 6–14:** The stomach is then retracted cephalad to expose the left gastric artery. The vascular pedicle is encircled and clamps are placed. It is important to avoid injury to the nearby pancreas.

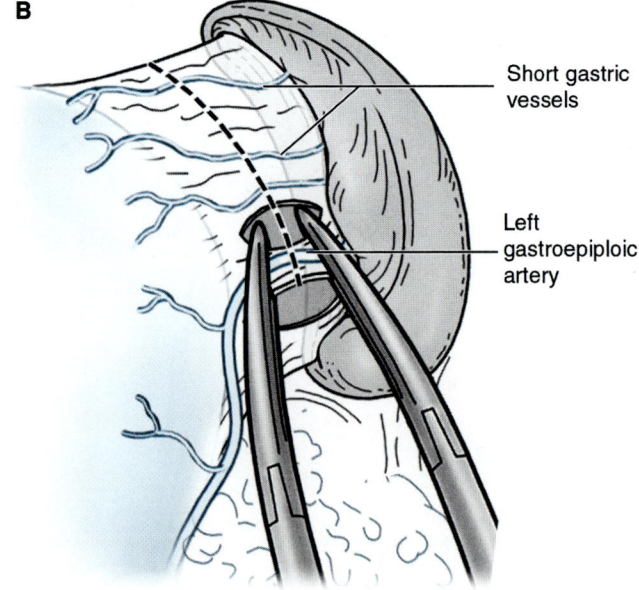

Figure 6–12B

Chapter 6 : Operative Management of Gastric Lesions • 51

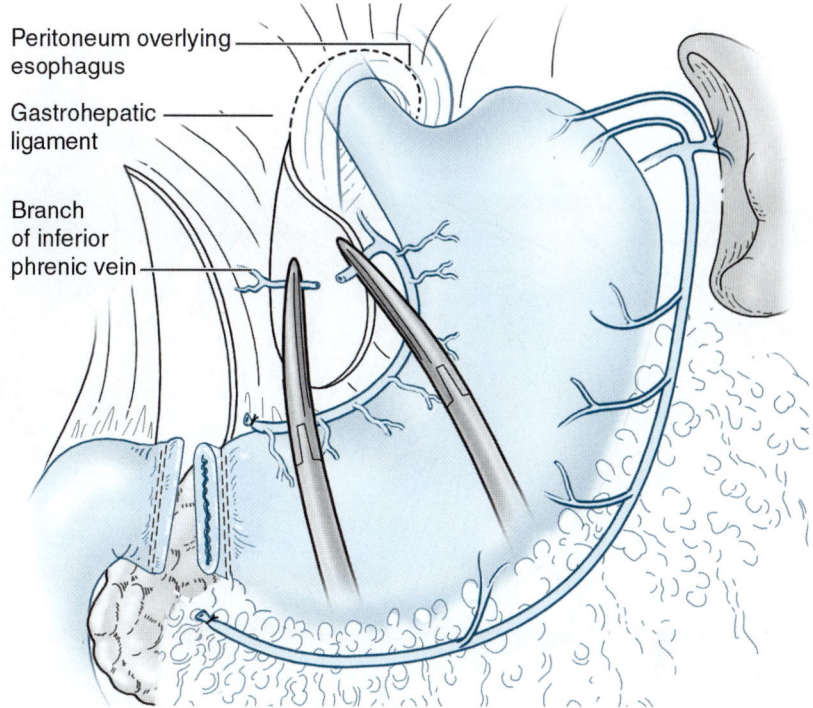

Figure 6-13

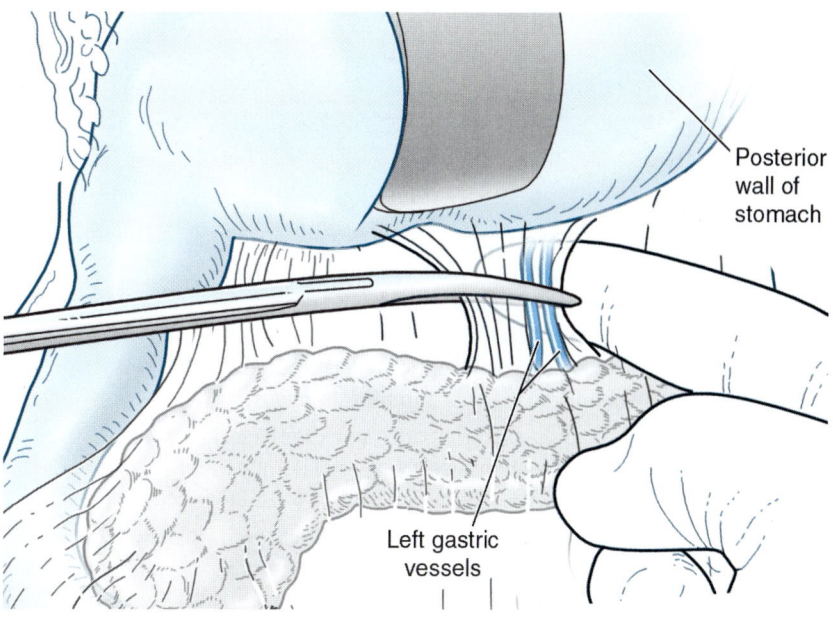

Figure 6-14

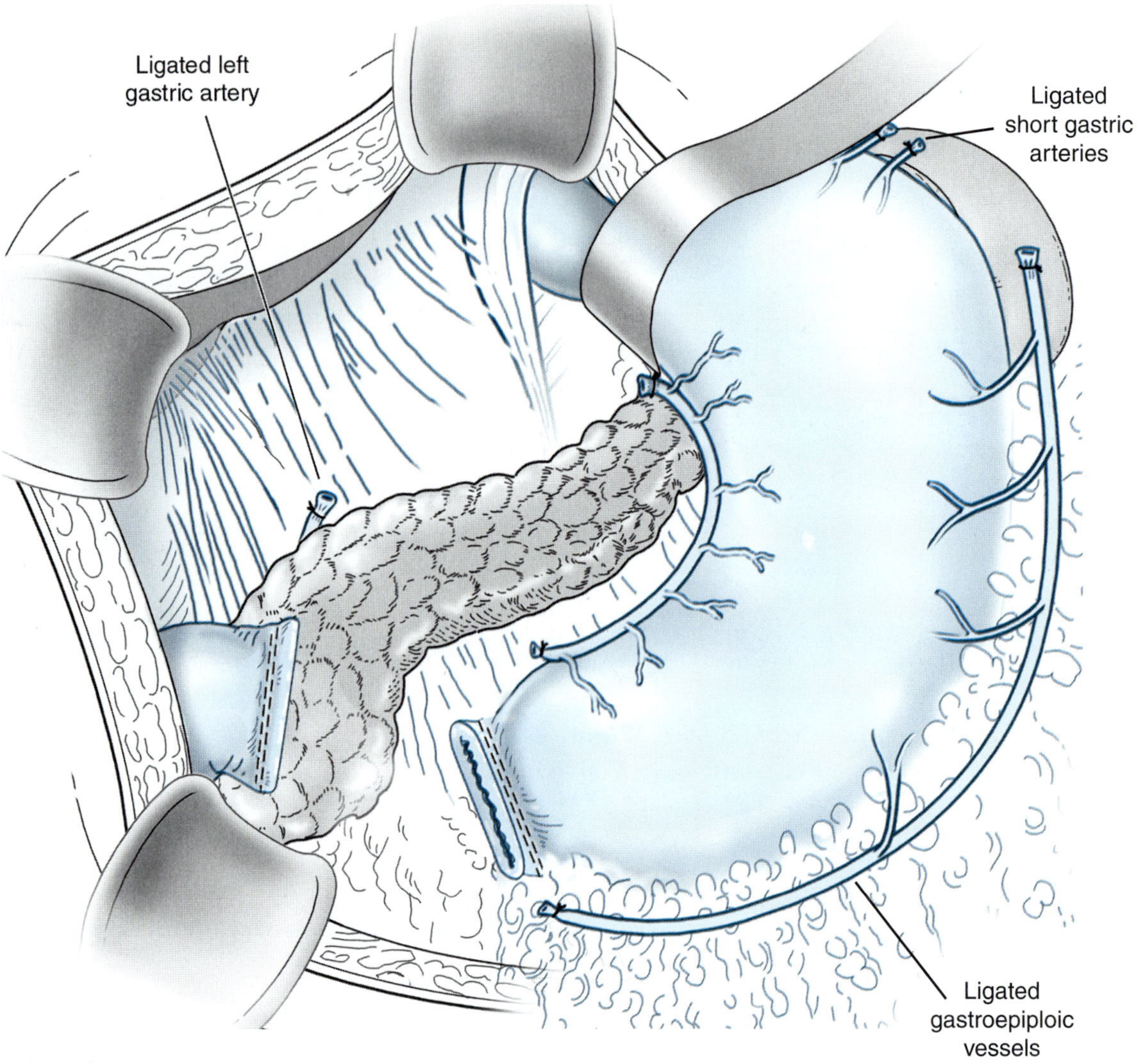

52 • Current Procedures: Surgery

Figure 6–15

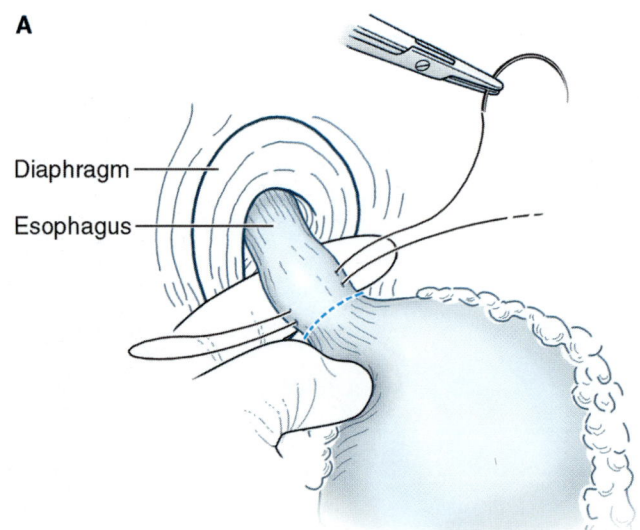

Figure 6–16A

- **Figure 6–15:** When the entire stomach has been mobilized, the surgeon can inspect the distal esophagus and determine whether additional esophageal length is required. Mobilization of the distal esophagus within the mediastinum may be required if the neoplasm extends into the esophagus.
- **Figure 6–16A, B:** Once satisfied that adequate esophageal length has been achieved, stay sutures are placed laterally in the distal esophagus to prevent retraction (Figure 6–16A).
  - The esophagus is transected, and the stomach is removed.
  - A purse-string suture is placed in the distal esophagus using monofilament suture in preparation for the esophagojejunal anastomosis (Figure 6–16B).

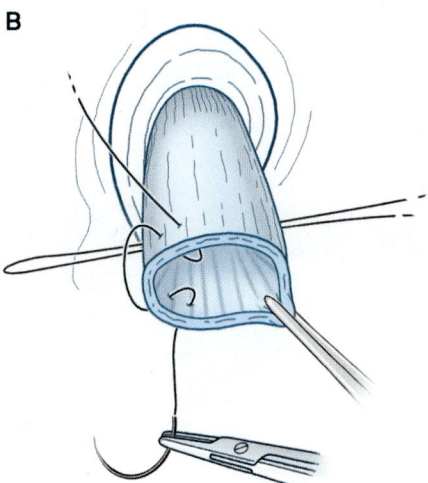

Figure 6–16B

Gastric Reconstruction for Total Gastrectomy

- **Figure 6–17A-C:** Roux-en-Y esophagojejunostomy.
  - The proximal jejunum is divided approximately 10–20 cm distal to the ligament of Treitz (Figure 6–17A).
  - An opening is made in the transverse mesocolon to the left of the middle colic vessels above the ligament of Treitz (Figure 6–17B).
  - The Roux limb/distal end of the transected jejunum is passed in a retrocolic fashion to the area of the distal esophagus (Figure 6–17C). The Roux limb must be placed carefully, without angulation or tension.

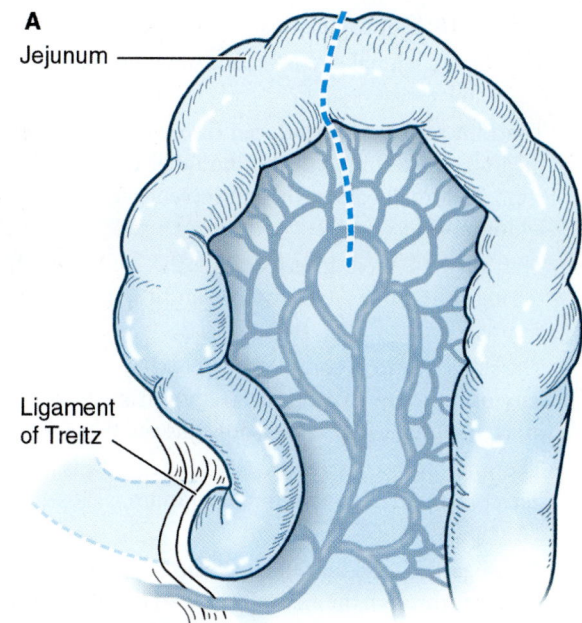

Figure 6–17A

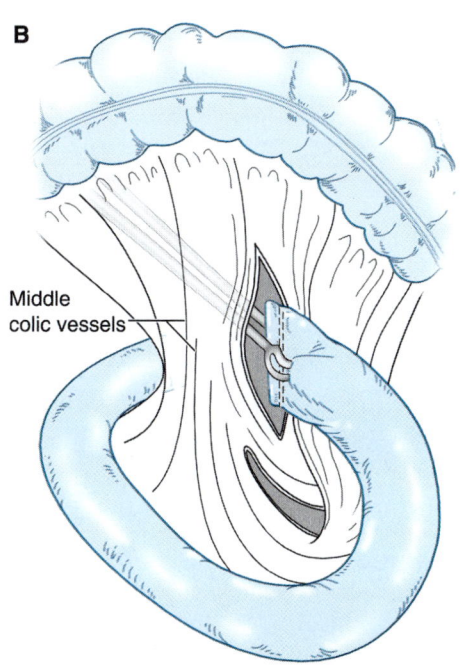

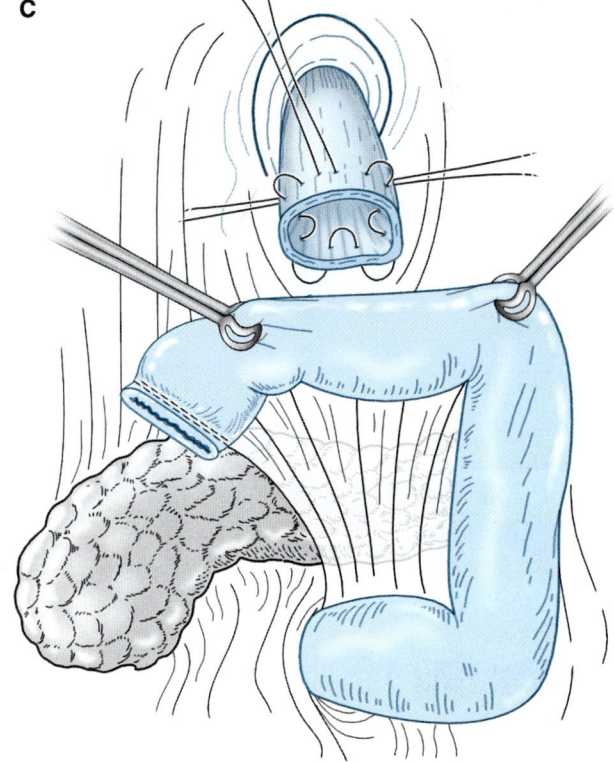

Figure 6–17B, C

- **Figure 6–18:** Esophagojejunal anastomosis.
  - The stapled jejunal end is excised to permit passage of an EEA stapler.
  - The EEA stapler is introduced through the open end of the Roux-en-Y limb. The rod should be positioned to exit 3 cm proximally along the antimesenteric border of the jejunum.
  - The anvil is then inserted into the distal esophagus through the purse-string suture and the purse-string is secured.
  - The stapler is fired, completing an end-to-side esophagojejunostomy. The EEA device is removed and inspected for intact tissue rings from the esophagus and the jejunum.
  - The anastomosis is inspected for hemostasis, and the defect of the EEA device in the jejunum is closed with a TA stapler.
  - A nasogastric tube may then be placed with the surgeon's guidance through the anastomosis and may be used to test for anastomotic integrity after the operative field has been filled with saline. The absence of bubbling after air insufflation of the anastomosis suggests an intact suture line.

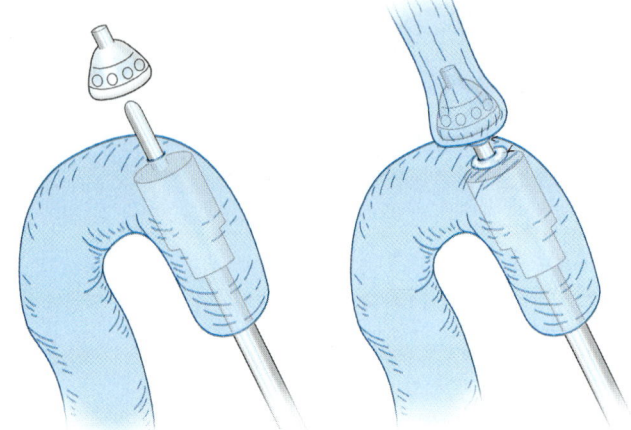

Figure 6–18

- **Figure 6–19A, B:** Completion of Roux-en-Y reconstruction.
  - The completed esophagojejunal anastomosis is shown (Figure 6–19A).
  - Intestinal continuity is restored by an end-to-side enteroenterostomy, approximately 50 cm distal to the esophagojejunal anastomosis (Figure 6–19B). The mesenteric defect is closed to prevent internal herniation.

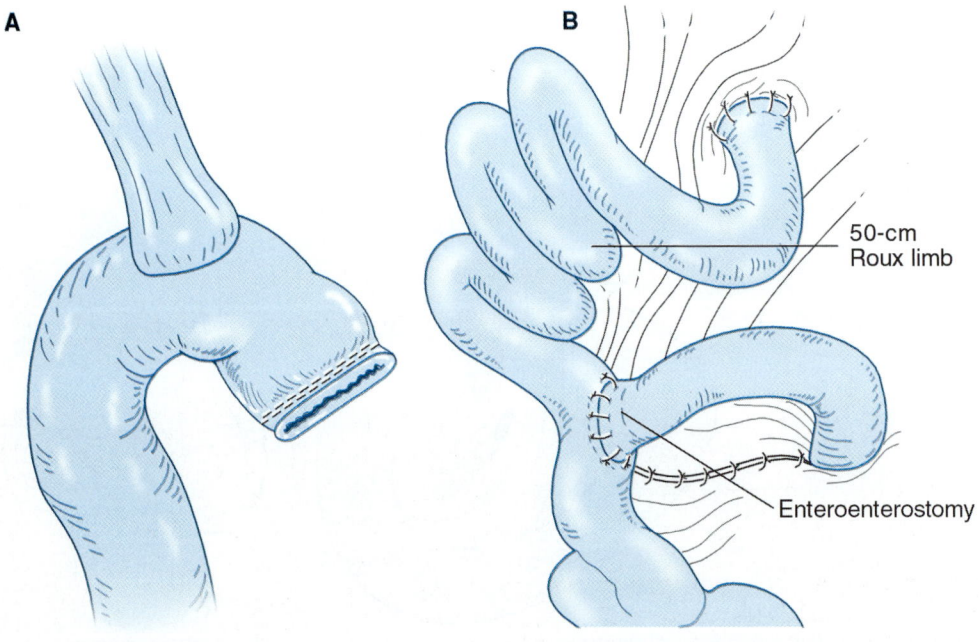

Figure 6–19A–B

Lymph Node Distribution for Gastric Cancer: Figure 6–20

- For a potentially curative resection of gastric cancer, en bloc resection of the lymph node groups draining the primary tumor should also be performed. This should include omental, pyloric, and lesser curvature lymph nodes.
- For lesions of the proximal stomach and along the greater curvature, splenectomy should also be considered to include the splenic hilar nodes.
- For adequate TNM staging, a minimum of 15 lymph nodes must be excised and examined histopathologically before assigning an exact N-classification.
- Anatomic gastric nodal groups have been described as:
  - N1 (lesser and greater curvature perigastric nodes).
  - N2 (splenic, left gastric, celiac axis nodes).
  - N3 (distant hepatoduodenal and root of mesentery nodes).
  - N4 (distant aortic and middle colic areas).
- Gastric resection has been classified as:
  - D0: Removal of involved stomach and less than all relevant N1 nodes.
  - D1: Removal of involved stomach or the entire stomach, complete omentectomy, and all N1 lymph nodes (safe standard).
  - D2: Excision of omental bursa along with the front leaf of the transverse mesocolon, and removal of all N1 and N2 lymph nodes; splenectomy is also required.
  - D3: Resection of above structures, as well as N3 and N4 nodes.
- More radical surgery (beyond D1) has not been shown to increase survival in western countries and may lead to higher complication rates.

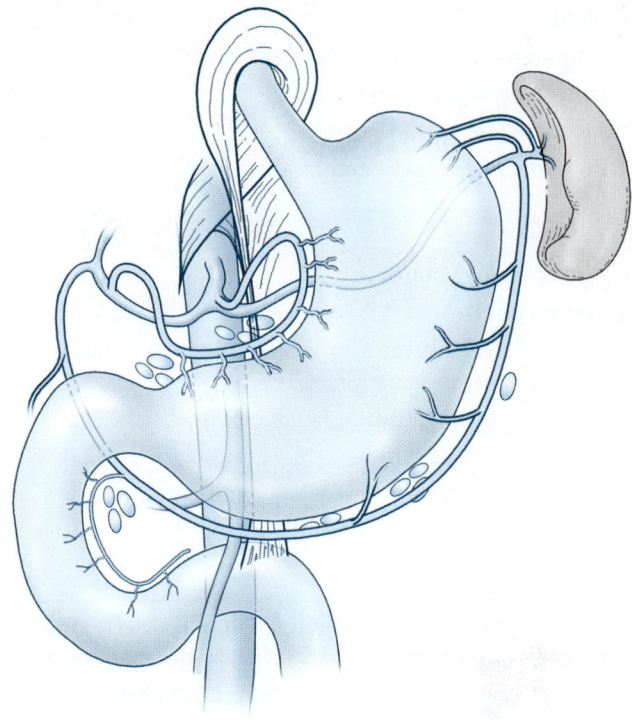

Figure 6–20

POSTOPERATIVE CARE

- Nothing by mouth.
- Monitoring for return of bowel function.
- Early nutritional support.
  - Parenteral or jejunal feedings are not routinely necessary but may be considered for delayed bowel function or delayed emptying.
  - Postgastrectomy diet (six or more small meals daily, high protein, low carbohydrate, decreased liquids with meals).

POTENTIAL COMPLICATIONS

Early

- Complications from general anesthesia.
- Wound infection.
- Anastomotic leak.

- Bleeding.
- Subphrenic or intra-abdominal abscess and peritonitis.
- Early dumping syndrome.
- Acute afferent loop syndrome.
- Rupture of duodenal stump.

Late
- Late dumping syndrome.
- Obstruction.
- Marginal ulcer disease (in jejunum no more than 2 cm from gastrojejunal anastomosis).
- Pernicious anemia (caused by vitamin B_{12} deficiency).
- Alkaline reflux gastritis.
- Chronic afferent and efferent loop syndromes.

PEARLS AND TIPS
- The extent of gastric resection required is determined by the ability to obtain microscopic disease-free margins.
- For distal gastrectomy, the dissection ends halfway between the pylorus and the esophagogastric junction, sparing the left gastroepiploic artery and short gastric vessels.
- For subtotal resection, the left gastroepiploic artery and a portion of the short gastric vessels are divided.
- For total gastrectomy, the dissection includes the right and left gastroepiploic arteries, and the right and left gastric vessels.
- In western countries, extensive lymph node resection for gastric cancer has not been shown to increase survival rates and may have more complications. A D1 resection is considered a safe standard in the United States.

REFERENCES
Ajani J, Bekalii-Saab T, D'Amico TA, et al. Gastric Cancer. In: NCCN Practice Guidelines in Oncology, v.1.2006. Available at: http://www.nccn.org/professionals/physician_gls/PDF/gastric.pdf.

Bell RH Jr, Rikkers LF, Mulholland MW, eds. *Digestive Tract Surgery*. Philadelphia, PA: Lippincott-Raven Publishers; 1996.

Braasch JW, Sedgewick CE, Veidenheimer MC, Ellis FH Jr, eds. *Atlas of Abdominal Surgery*. Philadelphia, PA: WB Saunders; 1991.

Sabiston DC Jr, ed. *Atlas of General Surgery*. Philadelphia, PA: WB Saunders; 1994.

Zinner MJ, Schwartz SI, Ellis H, eds. *Maingot's Abdominal Operations*. Stamford, CT: Appleton & Lange; 1997.

CHAPTER 7

Surgery of the Hiatus

C. J. Lee, MD, and Jonathan F. Finks, MD

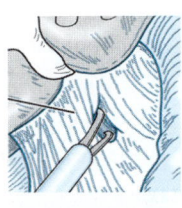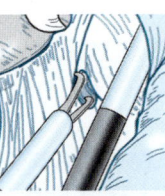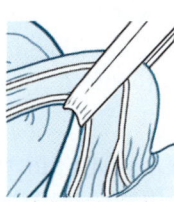
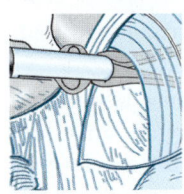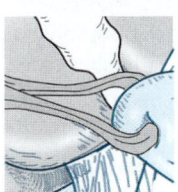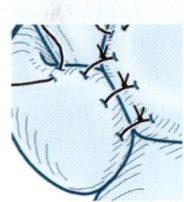
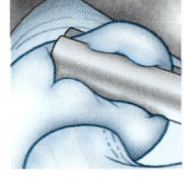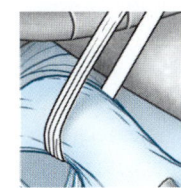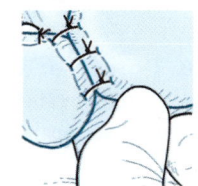

INDICATIONS

Laparoscopic and Open Nissen Fundoplication

- Evidence of gastroesophageal reflux disease (GERD) plus:
  - Sequelae of GERD refractory to medical therapy (eg, esophageal strictures, Barrett's esophagus, recurrent aspiration, or pneumonia).
  - Persistent reflux symptoms despite maximal medical therapy.
  - Paraesophageal hernia.

Laparoscopic and Open Paraesophageal Hernia Repair

- Objective evidence of paraesophageal herniation.
- Many patients are asymptomatic and a large number of cases are found incidentally.

CONTRAINDICATIONS

Absolute

- Inability to tolerate general anesthesia.
- Uncorrectable coagulopathy.

Relative

- Numerous previous abdominal operations (for laparoscopy).
- Previous esophageal or hiatal surgery (for laparoscopy).
- For morbidly obese patients with GERD, consider bariatric surgery rather than Nissen fundoplication.

INFORMED CONSENT

Laparoscopic and Open Nissen Fundoplication

A. Expected Benefits

- Approximately 80–90% long-term control of reflux symptoms.
- Cessation of medical antireflux therapy may be possible postoperatively.

- Treatment of extraesophageal reflux symptoms such as aspiration.

B. Potential Risks
- Esophageal perforation and splenic injury (< 1% of patients).
- Wrap migration into the chest (up to 10% of patients).
- Dysphagia (common early in the postoperative period but diminishes over time; 10–15% of patients experience occasional mild dysphagia in the first few weeks after the operation but only 1–2% require esophageal dilation).
- Excess gas and bloating (common), which usually resolve with time.
- Conversion from laparoscopic to open fundoplication (occurs < 5% of the time).

Laparoscopic and Open Paraesophageal Hernia Repair

A. Expected Benefits
- Prevention of strangulation, volvulus, incarceration, bleeding, and perforation of the herniated stomach.
- Many patients with paraesophageal hernias also have a defective lower esophageal sphincter; therefore, an antireflux procedure or fundoplication is also typically performed at the time of operation with the expected benefits listed earlier.

B. Potential Risks
- Mortality rate of up to 50% for patients presenting with acute surgical emergencies related to the hernia; this occurs in up to 17% of patients with paraesophageal hernias.
- Conversion from laparoscopic to open repair (approximately 3–5%).
- Surgical complications include:
  - Surgical site infection.
  - Bleeding.
  - Injury to the esophagus and stomach.
  - Early disruption of the repair, with recurrence rates as high as 20–40%.
  - Complication rates vary widely from 2–17%.

EQUIPMENT
- Laparoscopic instrument set including:
  - Straight (0 degree) and angled laparoscopes (30 or 45 degree).
  - Atraumatic liver retractor.
  - Atraumatic grasping instruments.
  - Bipolar or monopolar electrosurgical devices.
  - Ultrasonic dissector.
- General instrumentation set in case of conversion to open procedure.

PATIENT PREPARATION

Laparoscopic and Open Nissen Fundoplication
- A 24-hour pH test is the gold standard to confirm the presence of gastroesophageal reflux but is not mandatory in patients with esophagitis and typical symptoms (heartburn, regurgitation).
- Before surgery, all patients should undergo upper endoscopy to rule out Barrett esophagus and malignancy.
- Esophageal manometry is required in all patients preoperatively to rule out severe motility disorders (eg, achalasia or scleroderma).
- An upper gastrointestinal contrast study may be useful to define the anatomy in patients with hiatal hernia.

Laparoscopic and Open Paraesophageal Hernia Repair
- All patients should have a barium esophagram for diagnosis and anatomic delineation.
- Upper endoscopy is necessary to rule out malignancy.
  - This often demonstrates a second orifice adjacent to the gastroesophageal junction, with gastric rugae ascending into the hernia upon retroflexion in the stomach.
  - Anatomic distortion of the stomach may make it difficult to identify and cannulate the pylorus.
- Symptomatic patients may undergo 24-hour pH monitoring and esophageal manometry, although some degree of dysmotility is common in patients with long-standing paraesophageal herniation.
- A thorough cardiopulmonary workup should be completed for all patients.

PATIENT POSITIONING
- After induction of general anesthesia and endotracheal intubation, the patient is placed supine with legs abducted or in modified lithotomy position.
- Placing the table at about 30 degrees reverse Trendelenburg further optimizes patient positioning and exposure of the esophageal hiatus.
- **Figure 7–1:** The surgeon stands between the patient's abducted legs, and the assistant usually stands to the patient's left side.
- Video monitors are positioned at the head of the table.
- A nasogastric or orogastric tube is inserted for gastric decompression.

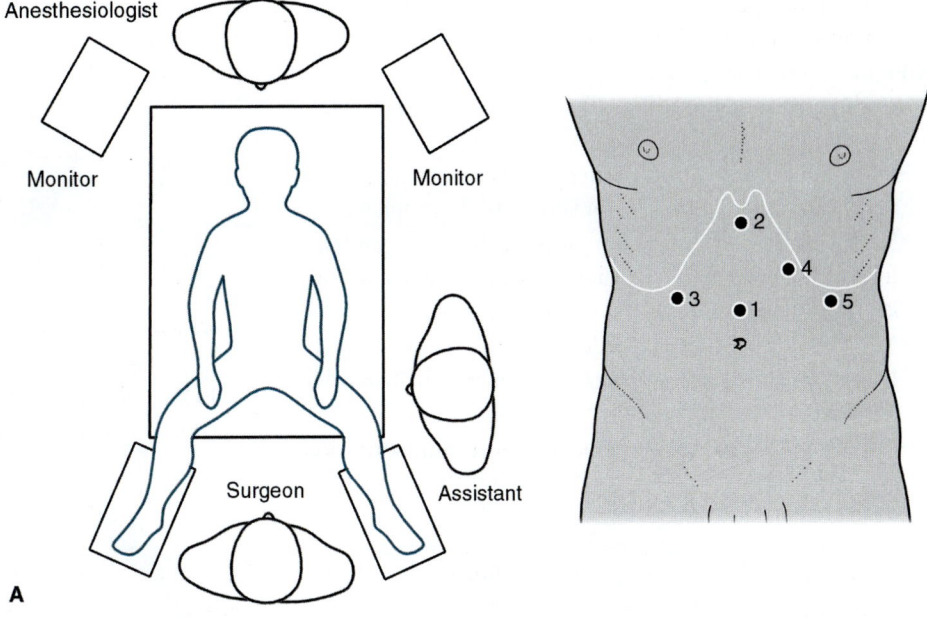

Figure 7–1A

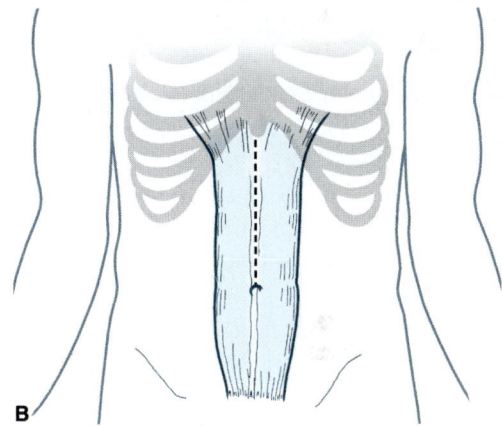

Figure 7–1B

PROCEDURE

Laparoscopic and Open Nissen Fundoplication

- An open or closed technique may be used to access the peritoneal cavity.
- Port placement for laparoscopic Nissen fundoplication (Figure 7–1A):
  - A 10-mm camera port is placed midline, typically above the umbilicus.
  - A 5- or 10-mm port is placed midline below the xiphoid for insertion of the liver retractor.
  - A 5-mm port and a 10-mm port are placed below the right subcostal margin and left upper epigastrium, respectively. These will function as the surgeon's working ports.
  - A 5-mm assistant's port is placed in the left anterior axillary line, just below the costal margin.
  - If laparoscopy is not feasible, a midline incision is made extending from the xiphoid to the umbilicus (Figure 7–1B).
- **Figure 7–2:** Appropriate retraction is obtained on the left lobe of the liver to expose the gastrohepatic ligament; the stomach is retracted caudally and to the left.
  - Hiatal exposure is begun by dividing the gastrohepatic ligament just superior to the hepatic branch of the vagus nerve.
  - An accessory left hepatic artery may accompany the hepatic branch of the vagus nerve in up to 12% of patients and should be preserved or, if necessary, divided between surgical clips.

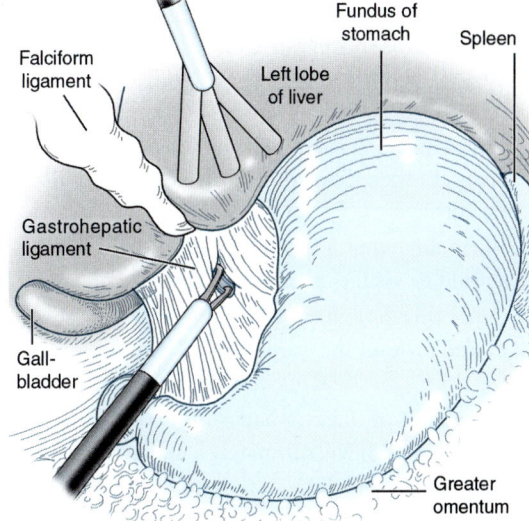

Figure 7–2

- The gastrohepatic ligament is divided up to the level of the right crus of the diaphragm.
■ **Figure 7–3:** The phrenoesophageal and phrenogastric attachments (hiatus sling fibers) are then carefully released.
  - During this dissection, the anterior vagus nerve is identified running along the anterior surface of the esophagus.
  - As the hiatus sling fibers are dissected free, the caudate lobe of the liver, the right crus of the diaphragm, and the esophageal hiatus should be exposed.
  - Mobilization of the right side of the esophagus is first begun by establishing a plane between the right crus and the esophagus with blunt dissection.
  - While right lateral retraction is maintained on the right crus, the esophagus and paraesophageal tissues are gently swept to the left.
  - As the distal esophagus is mobilized, the posterior vagus nerve is identified and is swept along with the esophagus to the left.
  - The dissection should allow for mobilization of the esophagus in a cephalad direction as far as possible, and caudally to the decussation of the crura.
■ **Figure 7–4:** Once the right side of the esophagus is adequately mobilized, attention is directed to mobilizing the left side of the esophagus.
  - The left diaphragmatic crus is freed from the phrenoesophageal attachments. This maneuver creates a retroesophageal window that allows for posterior dissection of the esophagus.
  - The gastrosplenic ligament or spleen, or both, should be seen from the right side as adequate posterior dissection is completed.
■ The remainder of the retroesophageal dissection (and the mediastinal dissection) is performed after mobilization of the stomach.
■ The entire fundus is mobilized using ultrasonic dissection to divide the short gastric vessels, beginning approximately 10 cm from the angle of His and extending up to the left crus.
■ The posterior attachments between the stomach and pancreas are then divided to complete the mobilization of the fundus.
■ With adequate posterior dissection, the caudate lobe should be visible from the left side.
■ Once this mobilization is complete, a Penrose drain is placed around the esophagus to help with retraction during the mediastinal dissection.
■ Dissection of the esophagus into the mediastinum is performed, which will ultimately lengthen the abdominal portion of the esophagus.

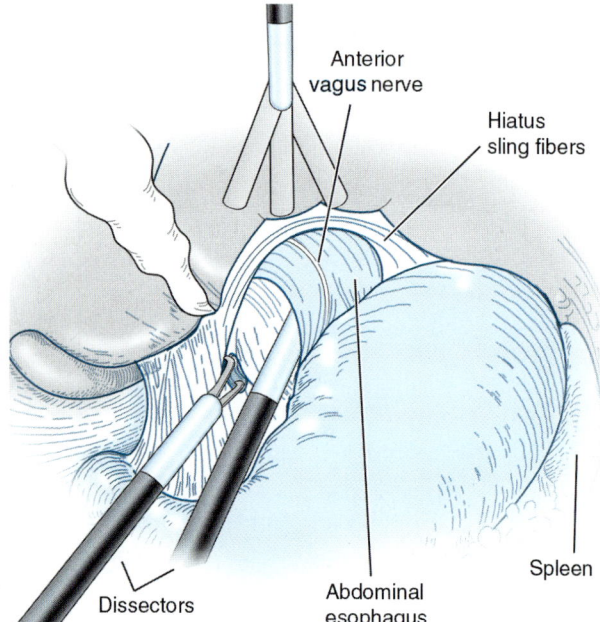

Figure 7–3

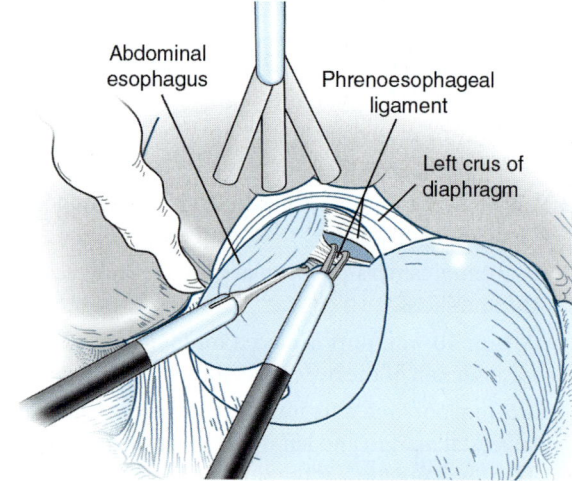

Figure 7–4

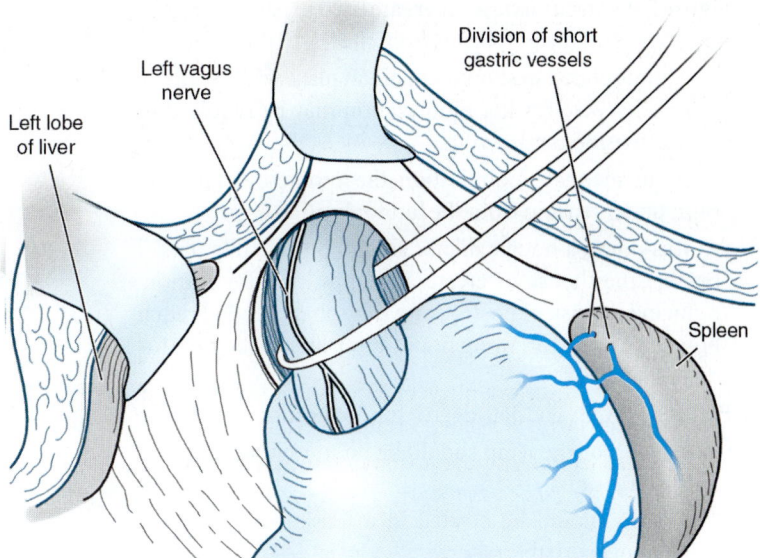

Figure 7–5

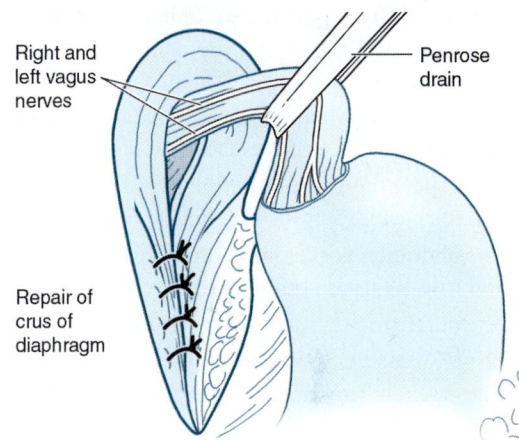

Figure 7–6

- The distal portion of the esophagus should be at least 3 cm long without tension. If the length of the esophagus below the diaphragm is < 3 cm, an esophageal lengthening procedure, such as a Collis gastroplasty, should be performed.
- Careful attention is made in identifying the vagus nerves, and more importantly the left pleura, which can be inadvertently injured during this dissection.
- **Figure 7–5:** This diagram shows the exposure of the hiatus as seen during an open Nissen fundoplication.
  - As the distal esophagus is mobilized, the short gastric vessels are divided with the ultrasonic dissector to free the gastric fundus.
  - Upon mobilization of the distal esophagus and gastric fundus, a Penrose drain is passed through the retroesophageal window and around the esophagus.
  - The Penrose drain is then used to apply caudal left lateral as well as anterior traction on the esophagus to expose the origin of the diaphragmatic crura at the hiatus.
- **Figure 7–6:** The hiatal defect is subsequently repaired by placing interrupted, nonabsorbable sutures to reapproximate the crura posterior to the esophagus.
  - In the case of a large hiatal hernia, mesh cruroplasty may reduce the risk of wrap herniation.
- **Figure 7–7:** The mobilized gastric fundus is then brought through the retroesophageal window.

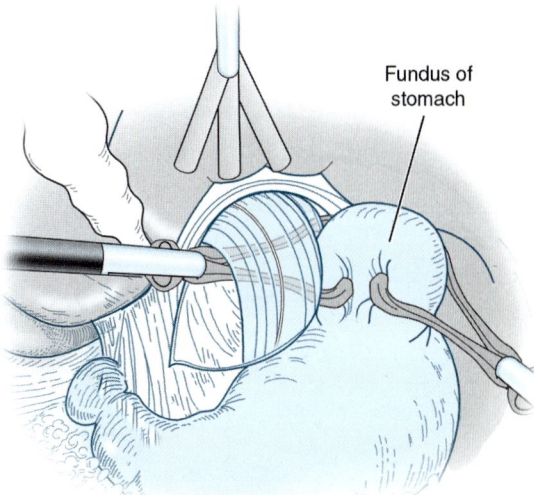

Figure 7–7

- **Figure 7–8:** Atraumatic graspers are used to pass the gastric fundus behind the esophagus from the left to the right.
  - The fundoplication should remain in place without being held; otherwise further mobilization may be required to release tension on the wrap.
  - Without adequate mobilization, the lower esophagus will twist under tension from the fundoplication.
  - At this point, a bougie dilator should be carefully placed by the anesthetist to create a "floppy" fundoplication, reducing the risk of postoperative dysphagia. A 56 French bougie is used for women and a 60 French bougie for men.
- **Figure 7–9A, B:** The 360-degree fundoplication is created.
  - The length of the wrap should be no more than 2 cm on the lower esophagus.
  - The wrap should be created in a tension-free manner using nonabsorbable sutures.
  - Deep seromuscular bites of the fundus should be taken, approximating the leading edge of the wrapped fundus to the gastric fold right of the esophagus. Sutures should also incorporate the anterior esophageal wall to anchor the wrap and prevent slippage (Figure 7–9A).
  - Some surgeons may choose to place an additional anchoring suture to the crura as shown in Figure 7–9B.
- With the wrap completed, the liver retractor is removed, and the liver is examined for injury.
- The abdomen is examined carefully to ensure hemostasis and rule out occult bowel injury.
- The ports are then removed under direct vision, and pneumoperitoneum is released.
- The fascia of any port sites larger than 5 mm should be closed with sutures. Midline incisions are closed in standard fashion.

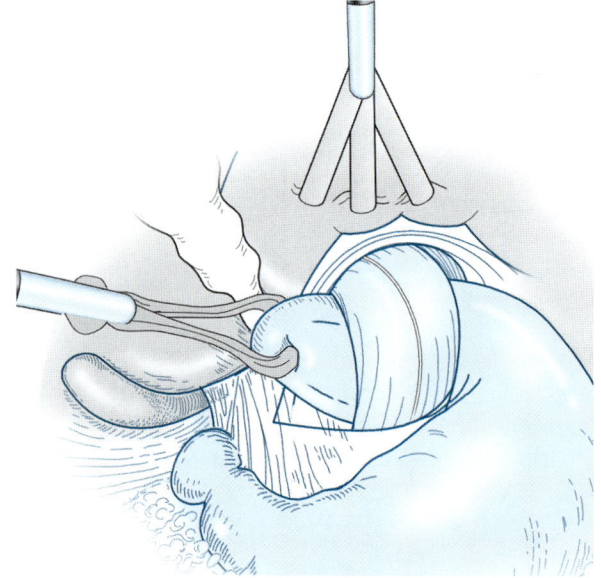

Figure 7–8

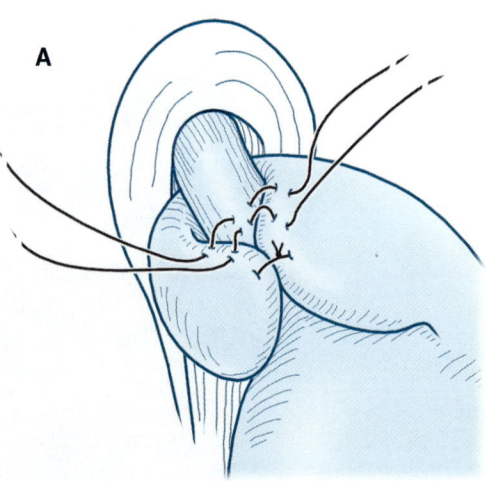
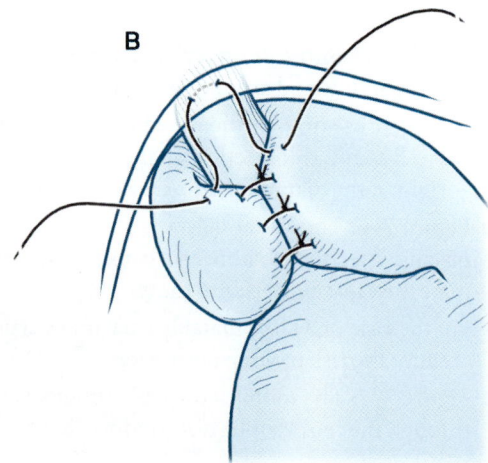

Figure 7–9

Laparoscopic and Open Paraesophageal Hernia Repair

- Paraesophageal hernia constitutes approximately 5% of all hiatal hernias.
  - Type III: the most common type of paraesophageal hernia (approximately 85%), involving herniation of both the fundus and the gastroesophageal junction into the mediastinum.
  - Type II: only the fundus herniates through the diaphragm while the gastroesophageal junction remains in the abdomen.
- Paraesophageal hernia repair can be divided into four major components:
  - Exposure of the hiatus and hernia reduction.
  - Dissection of the diaphragmatic crura and excision of the hernial sac.
  - Repair of diaphragmatic crura.
  - Fundoplication.
- Port placement for the procedure is similar to that for laparoscopic Nissen fundoplication (see Figure 7–1).
- Figure 7–10: A liver retractor is placed to retract the left lobe of the liver.
  - The herniated viscera should be visible and is reduced into the abdomen using atraumatic graspers.
  - If extensive adhesions are encountered, meticulous sharp dissection should be used to mobilize structures.
  - To further facilitate exposure of the hiatus, the gastrohepatic ligament should be divided, being wary of the possible presence of an aberrant hepatic artery.
  - Once the stomach has been reduced, the hernial sac should be visible anterior to the esophagus.

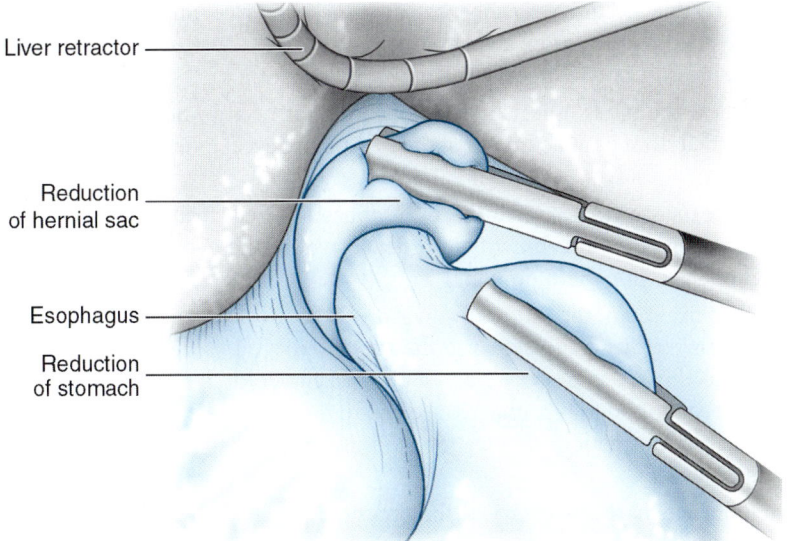

Figure 7–10

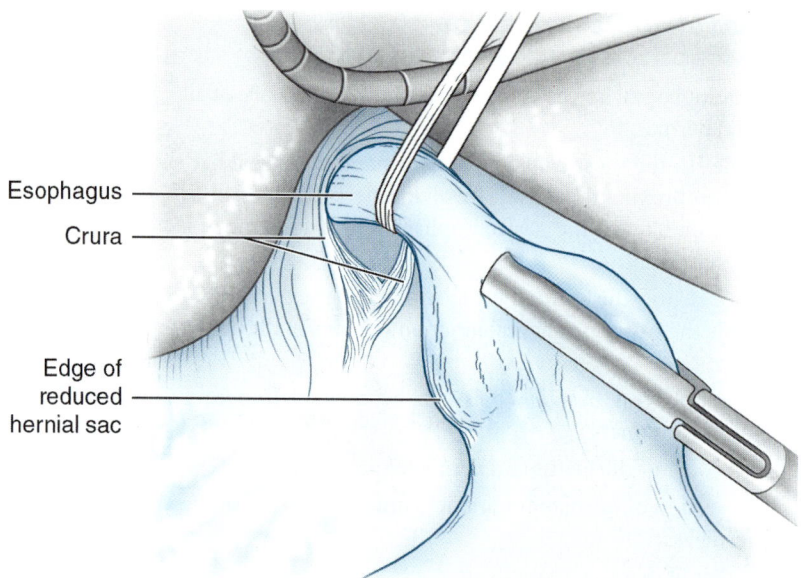

Figure 7-11

- To avoid injury to the lesser curvature vessels, which may lie close to the right crus, dissection of the hernial sac begins at the left crus.
- The sac is divided sharply away from the crus and opened anteriorly, taking care to avoid injury to the anterior vagus and esophagus.
- **Figure 7–11:** Once an avascular plane has been identified, the peritoneal sac is bluntly dissected away from the mediastinal fascia and completely reduced into the abdomen, ending with its attachments to the right crus.
- Care must be taken to avoid injury to the pleura. If pleural injury does occur, a red rubber catheter can be inserted into the pleural cavity from the abdomen in order to equalize the pressure and reduce the risk of tension capnothorax.
- Unless the sac is especially bulky, it does not need to be divided from its attachments at the gastroesophageal junction.
- Once the sac has been reduced, the esophagus is freed from its mediastinal attachments in order to reduce the distal esophagus into the abdomen.
- Mobilization of the fundus by division of the short gastric vessels may facilitate access to the retroesophageal space. Once this space has been developed, a Penrose drain is looped around the esophagus (see Figure 7–6) to give gentle anterior traction allowing for exposure posterior to the esophagus.
- Blunt and sharp dissection with the ultrasonic dissector is then used to divide the posterior attachments to the esophagus.
  - Care must be taken to avoid injury to the esophagus and posterior vagus nerve.

- The hiatus should be well exposed and both leaflets of the crura should be clearly visible upon completion of the posterior esophageal dissection.
■ If at least 3 cm of distal esophagus cannot be reduced without tension into the abdomen, an esophageal lengthening procedure, such as a stapled-wedge gastroplasty, should be performed.
■ **Figure 7–12:** The crural defect is generally repaired posteriorly with several interrupted nonabsorbable sutures. The size of the defect determines the number of sutures needed.
  - The surgeon should be aware of the close medial location of the aorta during the repair.
  - If the crural leaflets are thin, pledgeted sutures are indicated to reduce the risk of tearing.
  - Bites of the crura that are at least 1 cm or larger should be taken.
  - Reinforcement of the closure by anchoring mesh to the posterior crura may reduce the risk of hernia recurrence; however, care must be taken to avoid mesh erosion into the esophagus.
  - A 55–60 French bougie dilator can be passed with extreme care to ensure that the repair is not too tight.
■ **Figure 7–13:** If the short gastric vessels have not already been divided, this should be done to mobilize the fundus and ensure a tension-free fundoplication. A 2-cm tension-free wrap is performed with interrupted nonabsorbable suture to approximate the fundal folds. Full-thickness bites of the stomach are incorporated with an anchoring bite of the anterior esophagus.
■ **Figure 7–14:** A gastropexy may be performed, especially if a fundoplication was not performed.
  - The superior fundus is anchored with interrupted nonabsorbable suture to the crura and the diaphragm.
  - The body of the stomach is then anchored to the anterior abdominal wall, often with placement of a gastrostomy tube.
  - After careful inspection of the crural repair and the fundoplication, the ports are removed under direct visualization.
  - The fascia of port sites 10 mm or larger are closed with interrupted absorbable sutures.
  - Pneumoperitoneum is evacuated.
  - Midline incisions are closed in standard fashion if an open procedure was performed.

POSTOPERATIVE CARE

Laparoscopic and Open Nissen Fundoplication

■ Antiemetics should be administered to prevent early postoperative vomiting as this can lead to disruption of the crural closure and migration of the wrap into the chest.

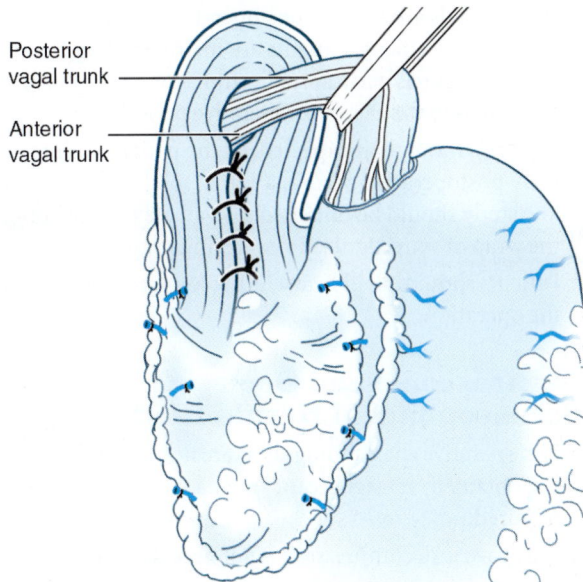

Figure 7-12

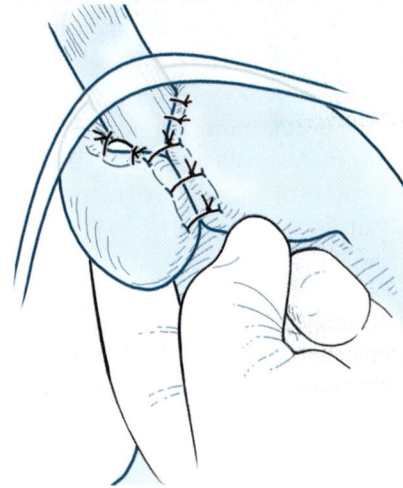

Figure 7-13

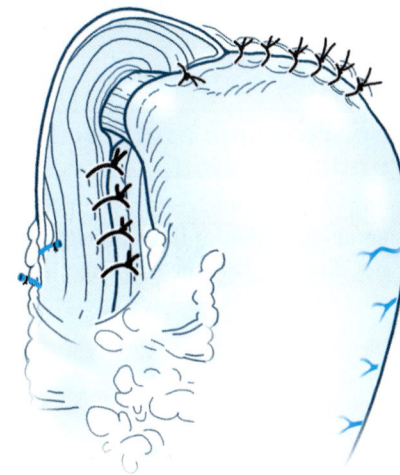

Figure 7-14

- Clear liquids are allowed postoperatively and a soft diet on postoperative day 1. Patients are maintained on a soft diet for 2–4 weeks as perifundoplication edema can narrow the esophagus in the early postoperative period.
- If pain is more than expected, or the patient vomits in the early postoperative period, a water-soluble contrast swallow study should be obtained to evaluate for disruption of the wrap or unrecognized visceral injury.
- Patients should avoid heavy lifting for 4–6 weeks following the operation.

Laparoscopic and Open Paraesophageal Hernia Repair

- Postoperative chest radiographs are not routine but should be obtained if significant mediastinal dissection was required.
- Nasogastric decompression is not necessary.
- Clear liquids are allowed postoperatively and a soft diet on postoperative day 1, if tolerating liquids well. Patients are maintained on a soft diet for the first 2–4 weeks as edema-related dysphagia is common in the early postoperative period.
- If pain is more than expected, or the patient vomits in the early postoperative period, a water-soluble contrast swallow study should be obtained to evaluate for disruption of the wrap or unrecognized esophageal and gastric injury.
- Patients should avoid heavy lifting for 4–6 weeks following the operation.

POTENTIAL COMPLICATIONS

- Pleural injury and pneumothorax.
- Esophageal and gastric perforation.
- Splenic injury.
- Wrap disruption or intrathoracic migration (Nissen fundoplication).
- Early disruption of repair (paraesophageal hernia repair).

PEARLS AND TIPS

Laparoscopic and Open Nissen Fundoplication

- To prevent esophageal injury, perform careful circumferential dissection of the esophagus under direct vision. Do not directly grasp the esophagus and avoid use of thermal energy when close to the esophagus.
- Take care to identify and avoid injury to the anterior and posterior vagus nerves.
- A minimum of 3 cm of esophagus must rest within the abdomen without tension.

Laparoscopic and Open Paraesophageal Hernia Repair

- Be prepared to perform an esophageal lengthening procedure in the event of a shortened esophagus.
- The hernial sac must be completely reduced from the mediastinum to help avoid recurrence.
- Consider mesh reinforcement of the crural closure to reduce risk of recurrence.
- Use caution during dissection to avoid injury to the pleura, esophagus, and vagus nerves.
- Carefully monitor airway pressures and end-tidal CO_2 and have a low index of suspicion for unrecognized pleural injury.

REFERENCES

DeMeester TR, Bonavina L, Albetucci M. Nissen fundoplication for gastroesophageal reflux disease: evaluation of primary repair in 100 consecutive patients. *Ann Surg.* 1986;204:9–20.

Edye MB, Canin-Endres J, Gattorno F, Salky BA. Durability of laparoscopic repair of paraesophageal hernia. *Ann Surg.* 1998;228:528–535.

Frantzides CT, Carlson MA. Laparoscopic versus conventional fundoplication. *J Laparoendosc Surg.* 1995;5:137–143.

Peters JH, DeMeester TR, Crookes P, et al. The treatment of gastroesophageal reflux disease with laparoscopic Nissen fundoplication: prospective evaluation of 100 patients with "typical" symptoms. *Ann Surg.* 1998;228:40–50.

Perdikis G, Hinder RA, Filipi CJ, et al. Laparoscopic paraesophageal hernia repair. *Arch Surg.* 1997;132:586–589.

CHAPTER 8

Emergency Operations for Peptic Ulcer Disease

Susan Tsai, MD, and Michael W. Mulholland, MD, PhD

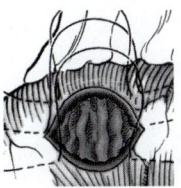 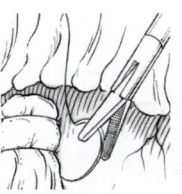 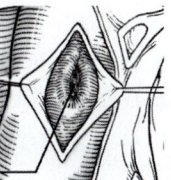

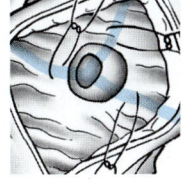 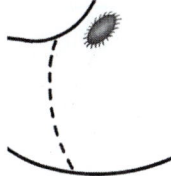

INDICATIONS

General
- Duodenal or gastric ulcer.
- Bleeding.
- Perforation.

Vagotomy for Bleeding Duodenal Ulcer
- With current antacid therapies, indications have become more selective.
  - Chronic ulcers that are *Helicobacter pylori*–negative and have failed medical therapies.
  - NSAID dependence or noncompliance.
  - Previous *H pylori* treatment failure.
  - Previous ulcer complication.

CONTRAINDICATIONS

Absolute
- Inability to tolerate general anesthesia.
- Uncorrectable coagulopathy.

Relative
- Factors that may influence the aggressiveness of the surgical procedure:
  - Age.
  - Preexisting comorbidities.
  - Shock.
  - Delay in diagnosis.
  - Large ulcer size.
  - Noncompliance with medical therapy or risk factor modification.
  - Previous *H pylori* treatment failure.
  - Failed vagotomy and drainage procedure.

INFORMED CONSENT

Expected Benefits
- Control of bleeding and repair of perforation may be accomplished by various surgical options; however, with current antacid medication and triple-therapy treatment of *H pylori*, the surgical options are routinely less radical.
- Historically ulcer recurrence is < 2% for vagotomy and antrectomy, and 10% for vagotomy and pyloroplasty.
- Triple therapy eradicates *H pylori* in 90% of patients completing therapy.

Potential Risks
- Recurrent ulceration.
- Pancreatitis.
- Leak.
- Wound infection, intra-abdominal abscess.
- Delayed gastric emptying.
- Dumping syndrome.

EQUIPMENT
- General instrumentation set.
- Laparoscopic instrument set including 10-mm 30-degree laparoscope; 5-mm, 10-mm, and 15-mm ports; 5-mm needle holder; 5-mm atraumatic grasper; and clip applier.
- Gastrointestinal anastomosis (GIA) stapler.

PATIENT PREPARATION
- Fluid and electrolyte resuscitation.
- Nasogastric suction or Ewald gastric lavage tube as necessary.
- Systemic antibiotics.
- For bleeding ulcers, surgery is generally preceded by previous attempts at endoscopic therapies.
  - Performance of initial endoscopy within 24 hours of bleeding has been associated with improved outcome.
  - Risk of rebleeding after endoscopic therapy is 10–30%.
  - Endoscopic retreatment has a success rate of 50–70%.
  - Failure of endoscopic therapy has been associated with advanced age, large ulcer, active hemorrhage, and hypotension.
- For perforated ulcers, diagnosis is made by history, physical examination, and radiographic imaging demonstrating free air or fluid. Risk factors associated with operative mortality include medical comorbidities, preoperative shock, and long-standing perforation (> 48 hours).

PATIENT POSITIONING
- After induction of general anesthesia and endotracheal intubation, the patient is placed supine.

PROCEDURE

Perforated Duodenal Ulcer

A. Open Graham Patch

- **Figure 8–1:** The right upper quadrant may be accessed through an upper midline incision.
  - The lesser curvature of the stomach is followed to the pylorus. The perforation is usually along the anterior wall of the duodenum. If this is not the site, the remaining anterior stomach, intra-abdominal esophagus, and lesser sac are explored.
  - Three or four nonabsorbable sutures are placed through the edge of the defect, approximately 0.5–1.0 cm from the edge of the perforation. The suture line should start and stop 0.5 cm from the apices of the perforation.
  - The stitch is brought through the wall on one side and the needle tip should pass through the perforated defect and through the contralateral wall. These stitches should be left untied. All sutures should be placed before being tied.
- **Figure 8–2:** Adjacent omentum is placed over the perforation site.
  - The sutures are tied to secure the omental patch in place. It is important that the stitches secure the patch in place, without causing ischemia.
  - It is not necessary for the ulcer to be sewn shut.
  - The abdomen is copiously irrigated with a large volume of warm saline.

B. Laparoscopic Graham Patch

- The patient is placed supine with arms abducted.
- A 10-mm infraumbilical port is inserted and a 10-mm laparoscope is introduced. The patient is placed in reverse Trendelenburg position.
- Once the perforation is identified, a 5-mm port may be inserted on the patient's right and a 15-mm port on the left abdomen, approximately 20 cm from the site of perforation. These ports serve as the working ports.
- Three 2-0 Vicryl sutures cut to 30 cm are used for intracorporeal suturing. The sutures are placed in the same manner as previously described for open repair, starting with the most inferior stitch.
- Each stitch should be taken in two bites to ensure that an adequate amount of tissue is taken on each side of the perforation.
- The suture ends are held by a single metal clip to form a loop. The needles are cut and removed. In a similar manner, the most superior stitch is placed.
- The middle suture is inserted last to avoid crossing of the sutures under the perforation. The ends are not clipped.
- The patient is placed in Trendelenburg position and a tongue of omentum is positioned over the perforation without tension.

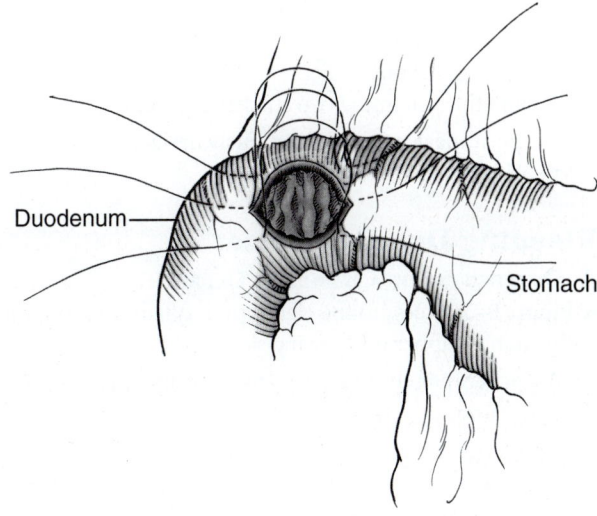

Figure 8–1

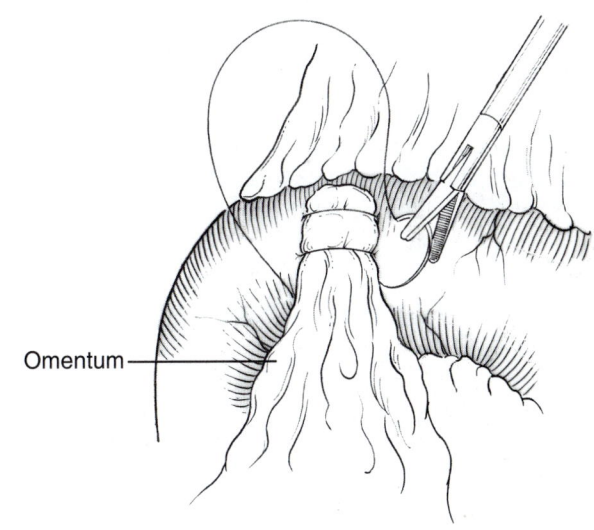

Figure 8–2

- The uppermost stitch is tied first using intracorporeal knot tying.
- The patient is repositioned in reverse Trendelenburg position and the remaining two stitches are secured.
- The peritoneal cavity is copiously irrigated with warm saline.

Bleeding Duodenal Ulcer

A. Oversewing of a Bleeding Ulcer

- **Figure 8–3:** Access to the right upper quadrant is obtained through an upper midline incision.
  - A Kocher maneuver is performed for mobilization of the duodenum.
  - The pyloric vein may be used as a landmark of the pylorus.
  - Two 2-0 silk stay sutures are placed at the 3 o'clock and 9 o'clock positions adjacent to the planned duodenotomy to aid exposure of the posterior wall.
  - A longitudinal incision is made on the anterior surface of the duodenum.
  - When an actively bleeding ulcer is identified, digital pressure may be used to control of bleeding.
  - The most likely source of bleeding is posterior duodenal erosion into the gastroduodenal complex, involving the gastroduodenal artery and the transverse pancreatic branch.
- **Figure 8–4:** Three U-stitches of 2-0 silk suture are placed to control the gastroduodenal artery proximally and distally and to include the transverse pancreatic branch medially. It is important to identify the common bile duct prior to placing these stitches.

B. Truncal Vagotomy and Pyloroplasty

- Pyloroplasty.
  - Two 2-0 silk stay sutures are placed superior and inferior to the pylorus.
  - A 2-cm longitudinal incision is made on each side of the pylorus through all layers of the anterior wall using electrocautery.
  - The duodenum and stomach can be explored through this incision. Oversewing of the bleeding ulcer is performed as described earlier.
  - The longitudinal incision is then closed transversely in a Heineke-Mikulicz fashion in one layer with full-thickness interrupted 3-0 silk sutures.
- Truncal vagotomy.
  - After the pyloroplasty has been completed, the left lobe of the liver is retracted away from the esophageal hiatus.
  - Downward traction on the greater curvature of the stomach may aid exposure.

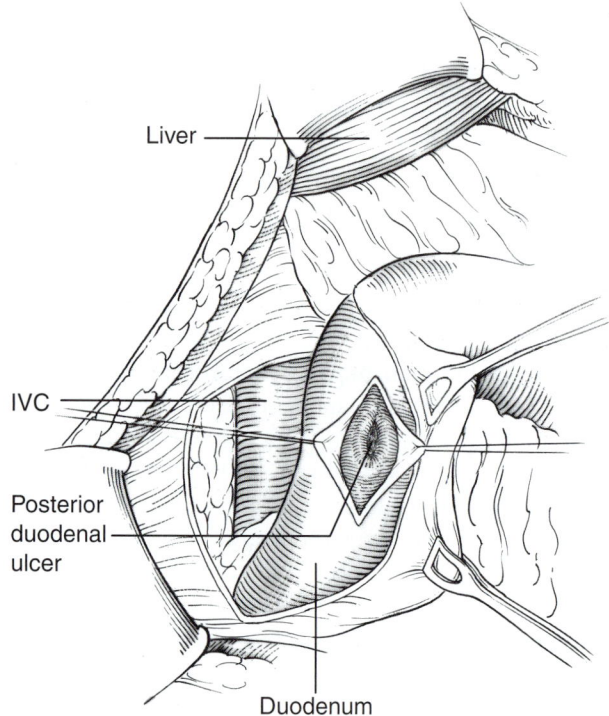

Figure 8–3

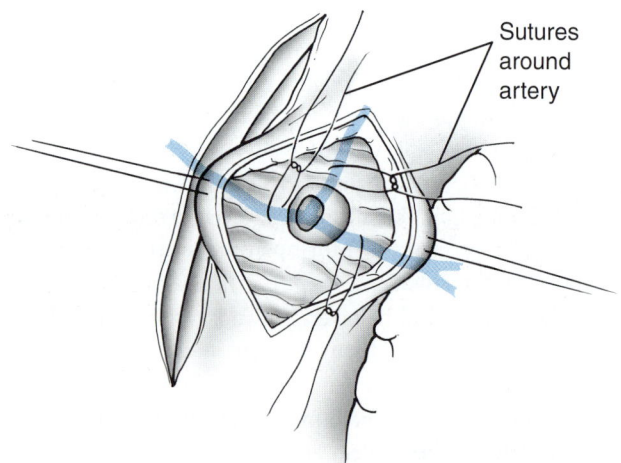

Figure 8–4

- The diaphragmatic peritoneal covering is incised transversely and, using blunt dissection, the esophagus is dissected circumferentially. The esophagus should be dissected 5 cm above the gastroesophageal junction to fully identify all vagal branches.
- The anterior vagal trunk is located anterior to the esophagus between the 12 o'clock and 2 o'clock positions and is usually closely adherent to the esophagus.
- The posterior vagal trunk is located between the 6 o'clock and 8 o'clock positions. It is usually some distance from the esophagus and thus is more difficult to identify.
- Once both nerves are identified, they should be dissected free. Medium clips are placed approximately 2 cm apart and the nerves are divided. The nerves should be sent for histologic confirmation.
- The lower 5 cm of the esophagus should then be cleared of all nerve fibers. If the hiatus admits two or more fingers, a cruroplasty should be performed with 0 silk suture to narrow the hiatus to the size of 1 fingerbreadth.

Gastric Ulcers

- **Figure 8–5A-D:** Classification of gastric ulcers.
  - Type I: most common; occurs along lesser curvature, usually at the incisura angularis.
  - Type II: usually two ulcers, in the body of the stomach and in the duodenum.
  - Type III: prepyloric.
  - Type IV: least common; occurs high on the lesser curvature near the gastroesophageal junction.
  - Types I, IV: not related to acid production.
  - Types II, III: related to acid hypersecretion.
- Unstable patient.
  - In an unstable patient with a bleeding gastric ulcer, an anterior gastrotomy with oversewing of the ulcer is acceptable. Biopsy specimens of the ulcer should be obtained for pathologic examination and histologic *H pylori* confirmation.
  - Perforated gastric ulcers in unstable patients may be managed with a Graham patch.
  - Aggressive postoperative anti-acid therapies should be administered.
- Stable patient.
  - Bleeding or perforated type II or III gastric ulcer may be managed using antrectomy with truncal vagotomy and Billroth I or II reconstruction. Antrectomy with Billroth I or II reconstruction and medical therapy with proton pump inhibitors postoperatively is also acceptable.
  - Bleeding or perforated type I gastric ulcers may be managed using distal gastrectomy with Billroth I or II reconstruction. There is no need for vagotomy.

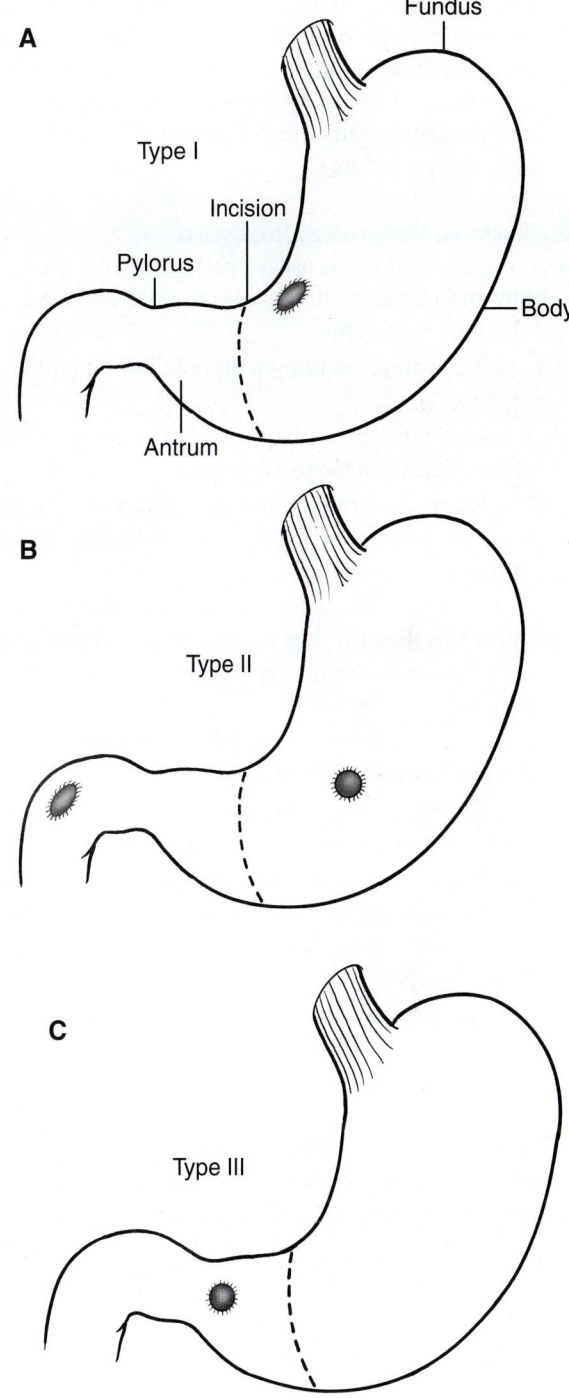

Figure 8–5A–C

- Bleeding type IV gastric ulcers may be managed using gastrotomy with oversewing of the ulcer. Recurrent or perforated type IV ulcers may require resection of the gastric antrum and body up to the gastroesophageal junction and reconstruction with a Roux-en-Y limb of jejunum (Csendes procedure).

A. Truncal Vagotomy and Antrectomy

- A truncal vagotomy is usually performed after the gastrectomy and reconstruction has been completed. The procedure is reviewed earlier.
- To perform an antrectomy, a supraumbilical midline incision is used.
  - A Kocher maneuver is performed to assess the suitability of the duodenum for anastomosis.
  - The lesser sac is entered through division of the gastrocolic ligament at the middle of the greater curvature of the stomach.
  - The posterior wall of the stomach is inspected. The gastrocolic ligament is then divided close to the gastric wall for a short distance in preparation for subsequent resection and anastomosis.
  - The dissection is carried along the greater curvature of the stomach toward the duodenum.
  - The right gastroepiploic vessels are identified and divided close to their origin from the gastroduodenal artery.
  - The dissection is then carried along the lesser curvature of the stomach. The right gastric artery can be identified at the superior border of the proximal duodenum. It should be divided close to the duodenal wall.
  - The duodenum is divided using a GIA stapler.
  - The stomach is divided using the GIA stapler at approximately a 45-degree angle from the lesser curvature. We prefer to oversew the staple line with 3-0 silk Lembert sutures. A short segment of the staple line toward the greater curvature is preserved for the anastomosis.
- **Figure 8–6A:** Billroth I anastomosis.
  - A Billroth I reconstruction can be attempted if the duodenal stump is not inflamed and is mobile enough to permit a tension-free anastomosis.
  - Two 3-0 silk stay sutures are placed through the lesser curvature of the stomach to the antimesenteric duodenal wall, and similarly through the greater curvature of the stomach to the medial duodenal wall.
  - A row of 3-0 silk stay sutures is then placed in the posterior wall of the anastomosis.
  - The gastric and duodenal anastomotic staple lines are removed using electrocautery.
  - A 3-0 double-armed Vicryl suture is used for a continuous running inner layer.

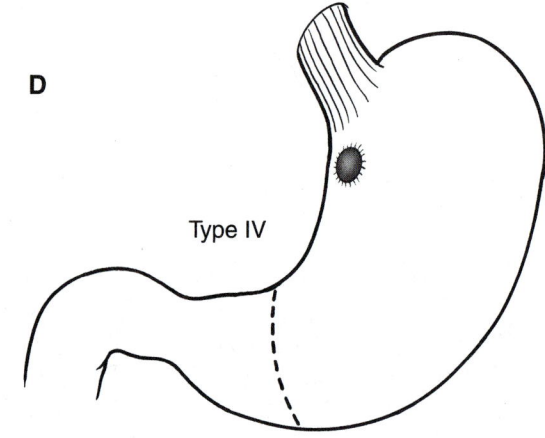

Figure 8–5D

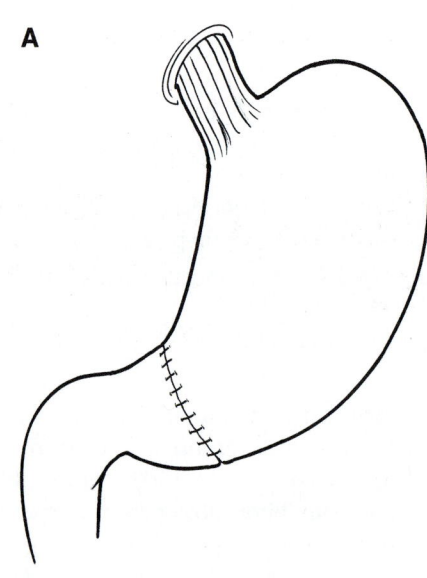

Figure 8–6A

- To complete the double-layer anastomosis, the anterior wall is then reinforced using interrupted 3-0 silk sutures. The stay sutures are also tied.

■ **Figure 8–6B:** Billroth II anastomosis.
- If there is concern about excessive inflammation or scarring of the duodenum, or if it appears that a Billroth I reconstruction would be under tension, a Billroth II reconstruction can be performed.
- We prefer to oversew the duodenal staple line with interrupted 3-0 Lembert silk suture, provided it does not cause additional ischemia.
- The first or second portion of the jejunum is mobilized and placed in a retrocolic fashion opposite the greater curvature of the stomach. The jejunum may be placed in an isoperistaltic or antiperistaltic fashion. Two 3-0 silk stay sutures placed at the ends help to align the stomach and jejunum.
- Interrupted 3-0 silk sutures are placed along the posterior gastric wall to the antimesenteric border of the jejunum.
- The equal length anastomotic staple lines are removed using electrocautery.
- A 3-0 double-armed Vicryl suture is used for a continuous running inner layer. The anterior wall is then reinforced using interrupted 3-0 silk sutures. The stay sutures are tied.
- The anastomosis is then delivered beneath the transverse mesentery and is secured in this position with sutures from the mesentery to the gastric wall.

B. CSENDES PROCEDURE

■ Type IV gastric ulcers are typically within 2 cm of the gastroesophageal junction and are not associated with a high-acid environment. Resection of this lesion therefore involves resection of the lesser curvature of the stomach with preservation of much of the greater curvature of the stomach.

■ Reconstruction after resection of the lesser curvature poses a problem in that the standard gastrojejunostomy would narrow the distal esophagus.

■ **Figure 8–7A, B:** The initial part of this procedure is as described earlier for an antrectomy. However the line of resection extends along the lesser curvature up to the esophagus.
- A Roux-en-Y jejunal loop is created and brought up in an antecolic fashion.
- The jejunum is anastomosed to the entire opening in the stomach, including the opening in the distal esophagus. This enlarges the circumference of the distal esophagus.

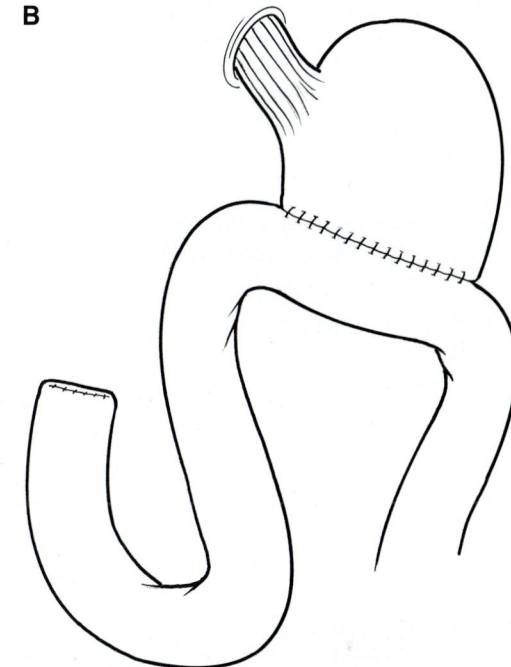

Figure 8–6B

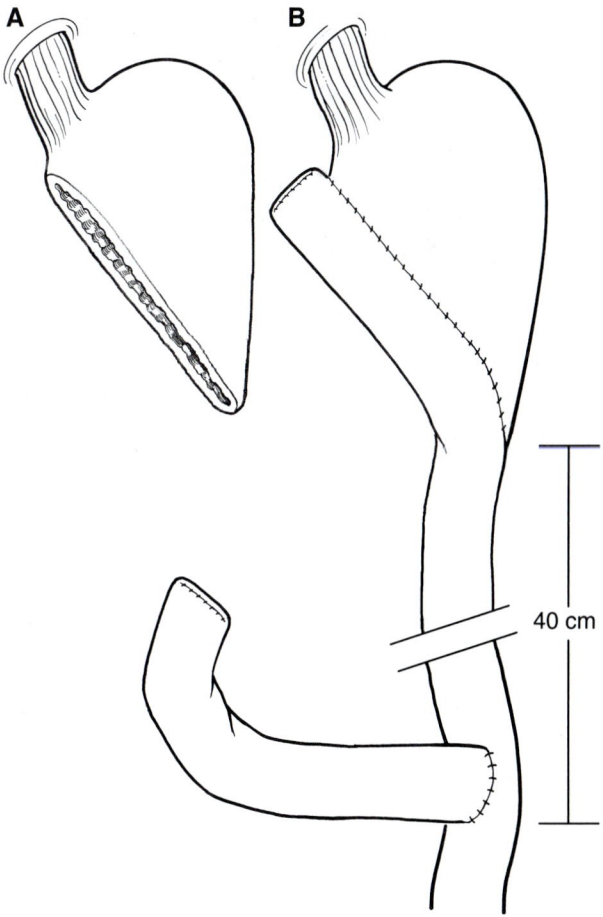

Figure 8–7A–B

POSTOPERATIVE CARE

- All patients with complicated duodenal or gastric ulcers should undergo workup for *H pylori* by serum, fecal testing, urease testing, or biopsy. Those who are positive for *H pylori* should undergo 14 days of triple therapy. Endoscopy may be performed 4–6 weeks post-procedure to document ulcer response to therapy.
- All patients with duodenal, type II, or type III gastric ulcers should receive aggressive anti-acid pharmacologic therapies with proton pump inhibitors or H_2 blockers.
- NSAIDs should be avoided when possible. The synthetic prostaglandin analogue misoprostol decreases the incidence of recurrent bleeding when NSAIDs cannot be discontinued.
- Generally, the nasogastric tube may be left in place until the output is < 1 L/day. Subsequently the diet may be advanced accordingly. Postvagotomy patients are not routinely placed on antidumping diets.
- If the patient continues to have severe pain, fevers, or persistent gastric ileus, CT scan with oral contrast should be considered to evaluate for leak or undrained abscess. Alternatively, a water-soluble upper gastrointestinal contrast study may be performed to evaluate for an anastomotic leak.

POTENTIAL COMPLICATIONS

- Anastomotic leak.
- Duodenal leak.
- Injury to the common bile duct.
- Bleeding (splenic injury or suture line bleeding).
- Postsurgical gastroparesis.
- Gastric outlet obstruction.
- Small bowel obstruction after Billroth II reconstruction (migration of the jejunal limbs above the transverse mesentery).
- Dumping syndrome.
- Afferent loop syndrome, intussusception.
- Cancer in the gastric remnant.

PEARLS AND TIPS

Graham Patch

- Do not attempt to approximate the edges of the perforation with sutures. If the tissue is friable, this may cause more damage. In addition, the omental patch is more secure when applied to the open defect.
- When performing this procedure laparoscopically, place the inferior stitch first as this will help serve as a point of retraction.

Oversewing of a Duodenal Ulcer

- It is important to identify the course of the common bile duct as it passes under the first and second portions of the duodenum. If necessary the ampulla may be probed with a silver tip probe to identify the structure as the hemostatic stitches are placed.

Truncal Vagotomy and Pyloroplasty

- Avoid repetitive entrances and exits of hands, drains, and instruments around the gastroesophageal junction to prevent inadvertent injuries.
- Downward traction on the stomach with the surgeon's hand may be more effective that the use of a Penrose drain.
- Initial identification of the posterior vagus nerve may be made more effectively by palpation than by visualization.

Truncal Vagotomy and Antrectomy

- Careful attention to identification the portal triad is important when performing an antrectomy as these structures may be injured inadvertently during the resection.
- If closure of the duodenal stump is difficult or precarious, a catheter duodenostomy may be employed. A T tube may be placed through a separate opening in the duodenal wall and secured with two purse-string sutures. An additional drain may be placed in the area. Both tubes are then brought out through the abdominal wall.

REFERENCES

Fischer J, Bland K, Callery M, et al, eds. *Mastery of Surgery,* 5th ed. Philadelphia, PA: Lippincott, Williams, & Wilkins; 2006.

Lam P, Lam M, Hui E, et al. Laparoscopic repair of perforated duodenal ulcers. *Surg Endosc.* 2005;19:1627–1630.

Millat B, Fingerhut A, Borie F. Surgical treatment of complicated duodenal ulcers: controlled trials. *World J Surg.* 2000;24:299–306.

Millat B, Hay JM, Valleur P, et al. Emergency surgical treatment for bleeding duodenal ulcer: oversewing plus vagotomy versus gastric resection, a controlled randomized trial. *World J Surg.* 1993;17:568–574.

Rokkas T, Karameris A, Mavrogeorgis A, et al. Eradication of Helicobacter pylori reduces the possibility of rebleeding in peptic ulcer disease. *Gastrointest Endosc.* 1995;41:1–4.

CHAPTER 9

Surgical Therapies for Morbid Obesity

John B. Ammori, MD, and Jonathan F. Finks, MD

INDICATIONS
- Body mass index (BMI) > 40.
- BMI between 35 and 40 and presence of such comorbid conditions as severe obstructive sleep apnea, pickwickian syndrome, obesity-related cardiomyopathy, degenerative joint disease, diabetes mellitus, hypertension, and hyperlipidemia.
- Failed dietary attempts at weight loss.

CONTRAINDICATIONS
Absolute
- Active substance abuse.
- Severe psychiatric disorders.
- Pregnancy.
- Untreated esophagitis.

Relative
- BMI < 35.
- Age younger than 18 years.
- Age older than 60 years.
- Desire to become pregnant within 2 years.

INFORMED CONSENT
Expected Benefits
- Loss of 50–80% of excess weight.
- Improvement of comorbid factors.

Potential Risks
- Overall mortality < 1%.
- Anastomotic leak (1%).
- Anastomotic stricture (5–10%).
- Wound complications (infection, hernia) more common with open surgery (15–20%) than with laparoscopic procedure (2–5%).

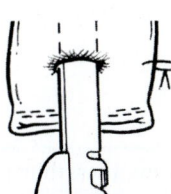 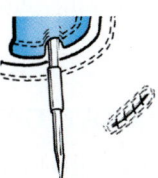 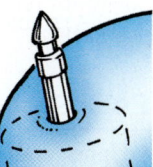
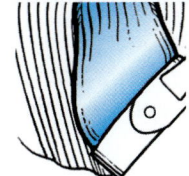

- Systemic complications of major surgery (pneumonia, venous thromboembolism, and cardiovascular events).

EQUIPMENT
- Operating table capable to accommodate the morbidly obese patient.
- Extra-large sequential compression device (SCD) stockings.
- For laparoscopic surgery, video telescopic equipment with two monitors and extra-long instruments (laparoscope, graspers, staplers, ultrasonic dissector, suction/irrigator).
- For gastric bypass procedure, end-to-end anastomosis (EEA) stapler.

PATIENT PREPARATION
- Upper endoscopy if indicated by symptoms (heartburn, regurgitation, dysphagia, epigastric pain, anemia).
- Right upper quadrant ultrasound to rule out cholelithiasis if indicated by symptoms.
- Cardiovascular evaluation.
- Psychiatric evaluation.
- Nutritionist evaluation.

PATIENT POSITIONING
Open Operation
- The patient should be supine with arms abducted and extended.

Laparoscopic Operation
- The patient should be supine with arms abducted and extended.
- Split-leg position is preferable.
- Contact and pressure points should be padded.
- The patient must be well secured to the operating table.

PROCEDURE
Roux-en-Y Gastric Bypass: Open and Laparoscopic
- **Figure 9–1:** The typical port placement for a laparoscopic approach.
- Following port placement, the abdomen is explored.
- The jejunum is divided approximately 30–40 cm from the ligament of Treitz and the alimentary (Roux) limb is tagged with Penrose drain.
- **Figure 9–2:** Creation of a side-to-side stapled enteroenterostomy 100–150 cm from the stapled end of the alimentary limb.

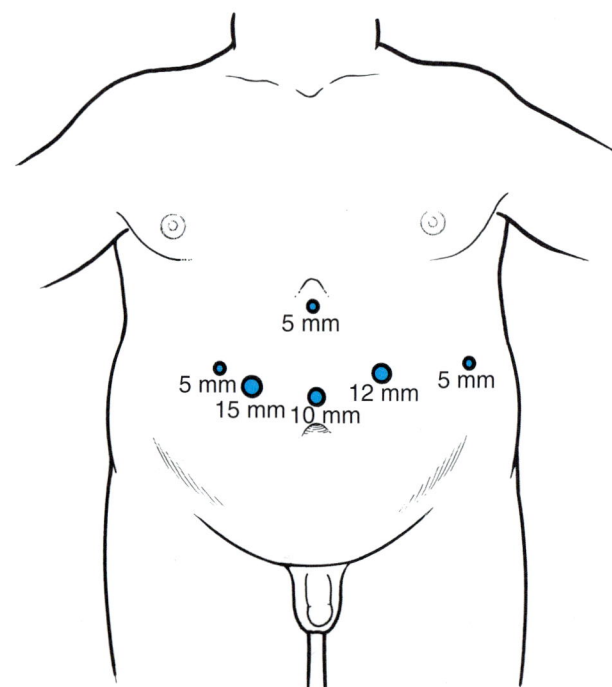

Figure 9–1

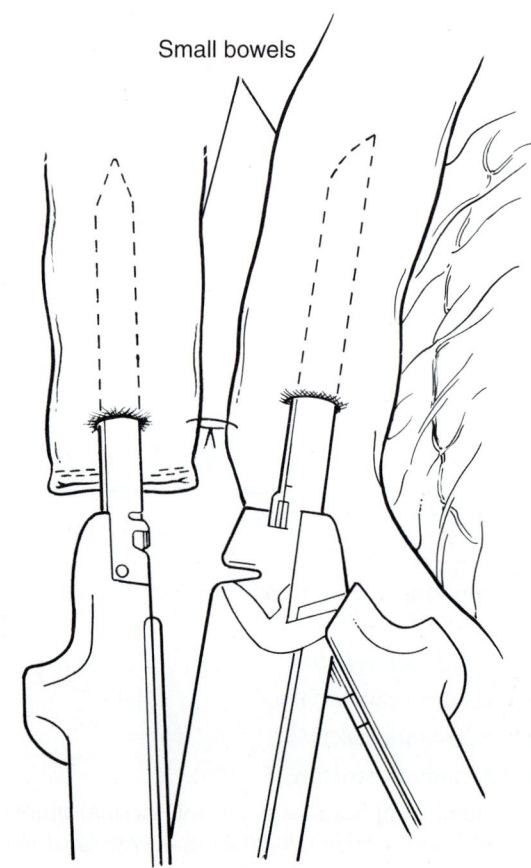

Figure 9–2

- The mesenteric defect is closed with permanent sutures.
- The omentum is divided with an ultrasonic dissector.
- A Nathanson liver retractor is used to elevate the left lateral segment, exposing the proximal stomach.
- The patient is placed into steep reverse Trendelenburg position.
- Peritoneal attachments between the diaphragm and the cardia at the angle of His are bluntly divided.
- The lesser omentum is incised at the pars flaccida portion and divided up to the proximal lesser curvature with an endoscopic stapler.
- A gastrotomy is made in the body of the stomach with an ultrasonic dissector. This will be closed with an endoscopic stapler after anvil introduction.
- The anvil from a 25-mm EEA stapler is introduced through the 15-mm port site and inserted into the gastrotomy. The anvil tip is brought out through the proximal stomach, near the lesser curvature, between the first and second lesser curvature vessels.
- **Figure 9–3:** Creation of a lesser curvature–based proximal gastric pouch with serial firings of the endoscopic stapler.
  - The anvil is placed into the stomach via the gastrotomy and pierced through the proximal gastric wall.
  - The gastrotomy is then stapled, and a 30-mL gastric pouch is created below the anvil.
- The alimentary limb is brought into an antecolic, antegastric position.
- The stapled end of the alimentary limb is opened with the ultrasonic dissector.
- **Figure 9–4:** The 25-mm EEA stapler is introduced through the 15-mm port site.
  - The stapler is inserted into the cut end of the alimentary Roux limb and advanced 5–6 cm.
  - The stapler is opened with the spike exiting the antimesenteric portion of the bowel and readied to connect with the anvil in the gastric pouch.

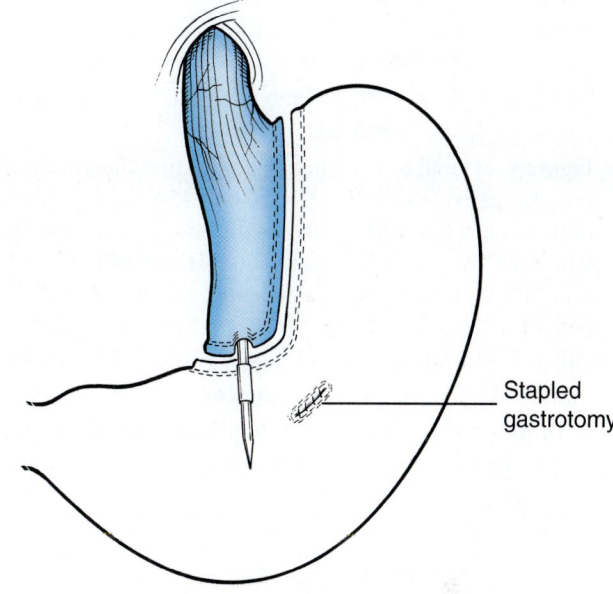

Figure 9–3

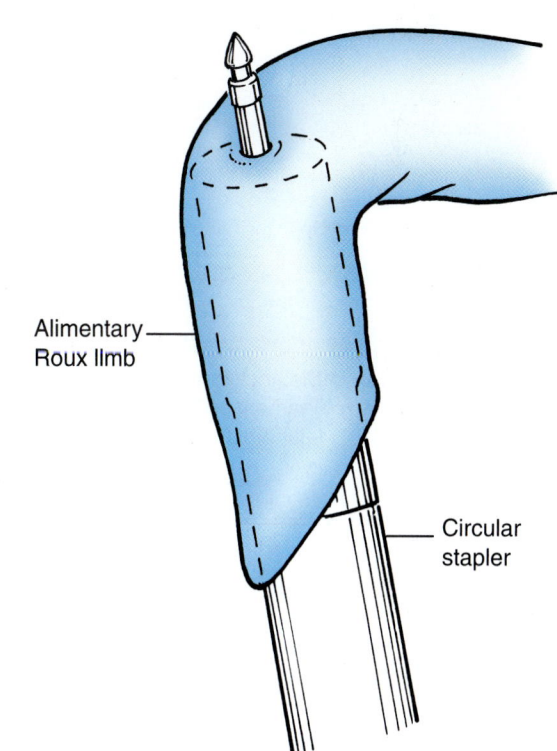

Figure 9–4

- **Figure 9–5:** The anvil and stapler are mated, taking care that no extraneous tissue comes between the stomach and bowel. The stapler is then fired and removed from the abdomen, and the donuts are assessed for integrity.
- The end of the alimentary limb is divided with an endoscopic stapler and removed.
- **Figure 9–6:** Final reconstruction results in a 100-cm Roux limb for patients with a BMI < 50 or a 150-cm Roux limb for patients with a BMI > 50. The distance between the ligament of Treitz and the jejunojejunostomy will similarly range from 30 cm to 100 cm depending on the BMI of the patient.
- Upper endoscopy is then performed to rule out an anastomotic leak and to assess for hemostasis.
- A 10-mm Jackson-Pratt drain is placed posterior to the gastrojejunostomy and brought out through the right lateral port site.
- The fascia of the 15-mm port site is closed with interrupted absorbable sutures.

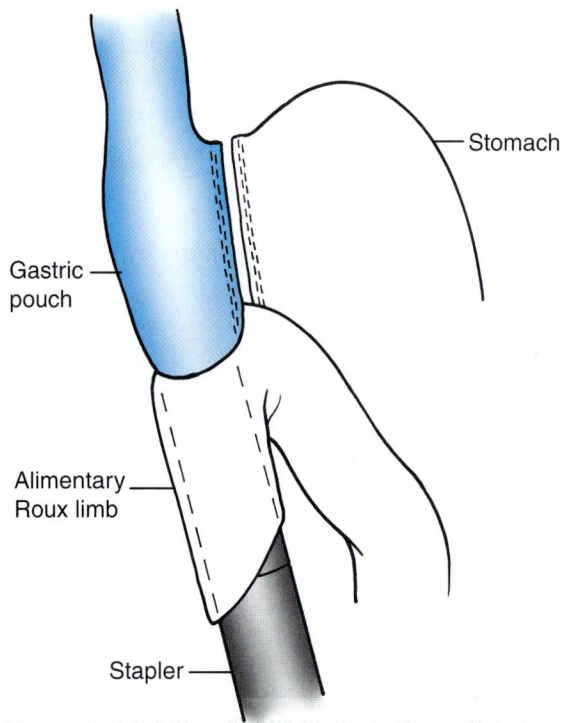

Figure 9–5

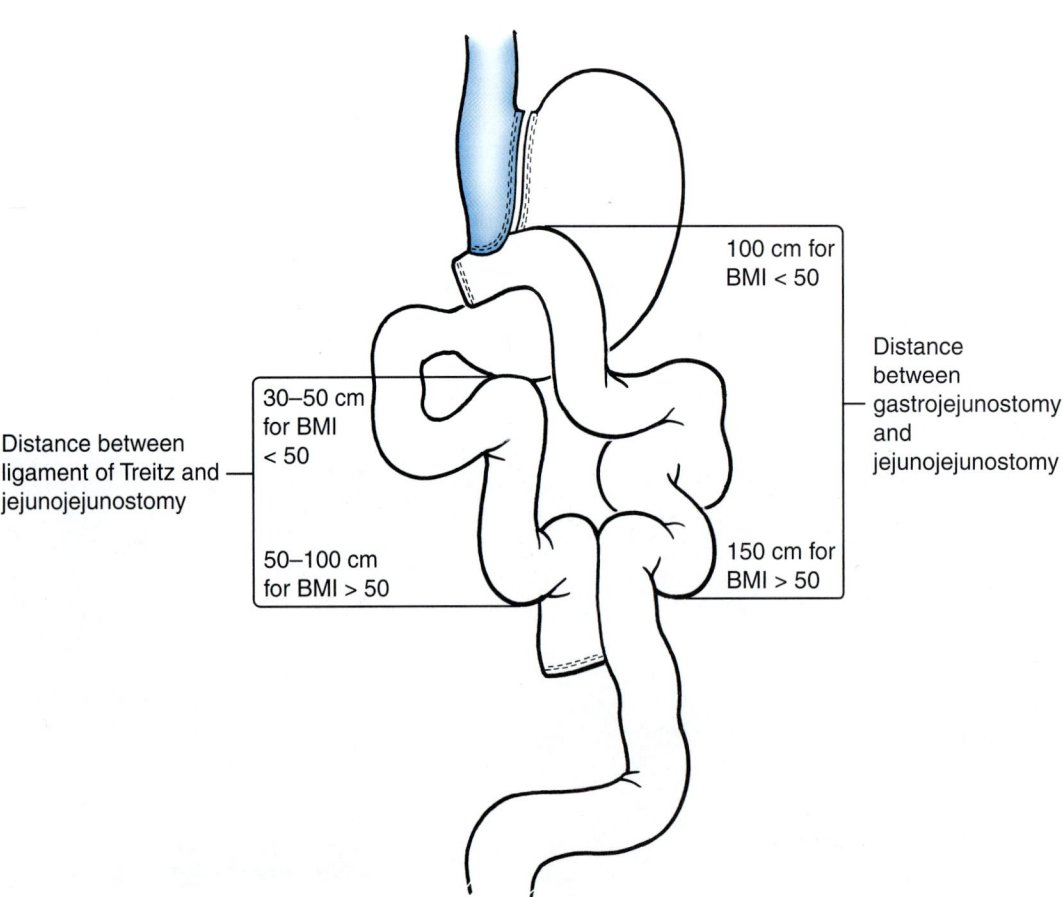

Figure 9–6

Laparoscopic Adjustable Gastric Band

- **Figure 9–7:** Laparoscopic port placement for gastric band procedure.
- A Nathanson liver retractor is used to elevate the left lateral segment of the liver, exposing the proximal stomach.
- Attachments between the diaphragm and the cardia at the angle of His are bluntly divided.
- The gastroesophageal fat pad is excised with an ultrasonic dissector.
- The lesser omentum is divided with an ultrasonic dissector beginning at the pars flaccida portion and extending toward the diaphragm to expose the right crus.
- The peritoneum overlying the right crus is incised at approximately the level of the crural decussation.
- A bowel grasper from the right lateral port is passed posterior to the esophagogastric junction, emerging at the angle of His.
- The band is inserted into the abdomen through the 15-mm port. The band tubing is pulled around the stomach using the retrogastric grasper.
- **Figure 9–8:** The band tubing is fed through the buckle until the flanges are through and the band is locked. The band should rotate easily around the stomach.
- An anterior fundoplication is performed with nonabsorbable suture. Interrupted gastrogastric sutures are placed to cover the band, beginning at the leftmost portion of the fundus and advancing toward the right. Care must be taken to avoid tension and prevent any part of the fundoplication from covering the buckle of the band.
- The band tubing is brought out through the 15-mm port and secured. The liver retractor and remaining ports are then removed and the abdomen is deflated.
- The end of the tubing is removed and the tubing is mated to the access port. The port is anchored to the anterior rectus fascia lateral to the 15-mm port site with four interrupted permanent sutures. The incision is then closed in layers.

POSTOPERATIVE CARE

- An upper gastrointestinal study with water-soluble contrast is obtained on postoperative day 1 for the following reasons:
  - To rule out obstruction or leak from the gastrojejunostomy following Roux-en-Y gastric bypass (open and laparoscopic).
  - To rule out perforation or obstruction.
  - To document pouch size and band position following adjustable gastric band placement.
- Early ambulation is encouraged.

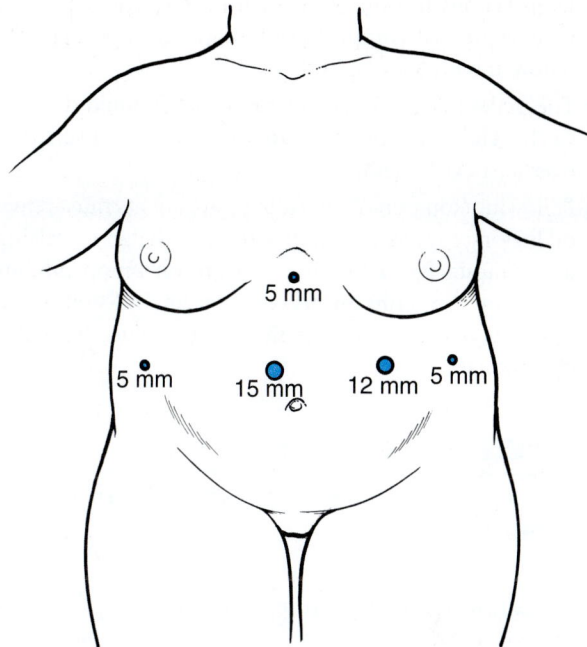

Figure 9–7

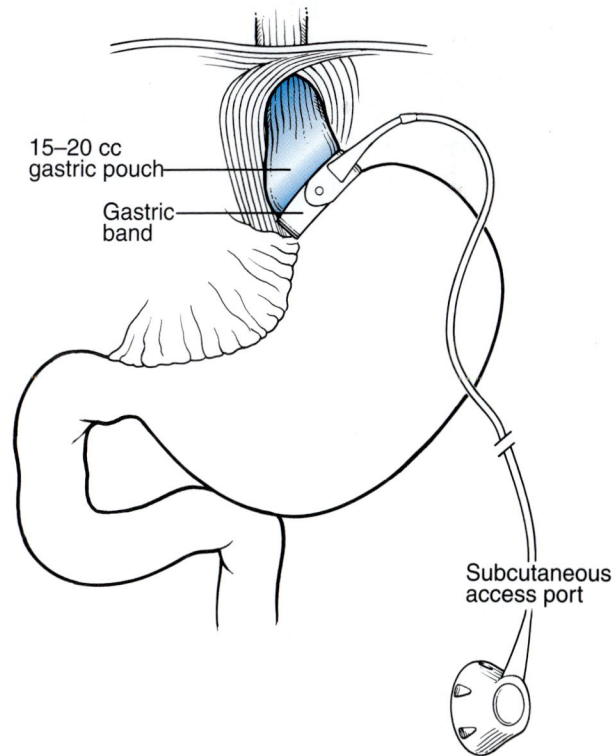

Figure 9–8

- Deep venous thromboembolism prophylaxis is provided with sequential compression devices and unfractionated or low-molecular-weight heparin.
- The patient is discharged home on a full liquid diet for 2 weeks. The diet is advanced to pureed and then solid food over the next 4 weeks.
- Following Roux-en-Y gastric bypass, patients must remain on lifelong supplementation with a multivitamin, calcium, and vitamin B_{12}. They receive a proton pump inhibitor (PPI) for 3 months to prevent marginal ulceration and ursodeoxycholic acid for 6 months to reduce the risk of cholelithiasis.

POTENTIAL COMPLICATIONS

Roux-en-Y Gastric Bypass: Open and Laparoscopic

- Anastomotic leak.
  - Occurs within 10 days postoperatively.
  - May be treated either conservatively or surgically.
- Stomal stenosis.
  - Occurs as a late complication, usually within 4–6 weeks of surgery.
  - Most patients respond to endoscopic dilation.
  - Refractory cases require operative revision.
- Marginal ulceration.
  - Occurs in 5–10% of patients.
  - Patients have epigastric pain or upper gastrointestinal bleeding, or both.
  - Perforation is less common but has been reported.
  - Usually responds to PPI but may require endoscopic or surgical intervention.
- Internal hernia.
  - May occur as an early or late complication in 3–5% of patients.
  - Patients typically present with acute or chronically intermittent obstructive symptoms.
  - Treatment is surgical.
- Incisional hernia (may occur in up to 15% of open operations).

Laparoscopic Adjustable Gastric Band

- Acute esophageal obstruction.
- Gastric prolapse ("slipped band") and pouch dilation.
- Band erosion.
- Esophageal dilation or dysmotility.
- Port and tubing complications (eg, breakage, migration, infection).

PEARLS AND TIPS

Roux-en-Y Gastric Bypass: Open and Laparoscopic

- A checklist of important operative steps (eg, closure of the gastrotomy, removal of the spike) should be maintained by the circulating nurse to avoid missed steps.
- Care must be taken to correctly identify alimentary and biliary limbs and to prevent twisting of the mesentery. This should be checked and rechecked.
- The mesenteric defect should be completely closed with permanent suture.
- The angle of His must be clearly identified during creation of the proximal pouch to prevent injury to spleen or esophagus.

Laparoscopic Adjustable Gastric Band

- Passage of the bowel grasper behind the esophagogastric junction should occur without any resistance. If resistance is encountered, withdraw the grasper and reinsert it 5–10 mm caudad.
- Complete excision of the gastroesophageal fat pad is important to reduce the risk of esophageal obstruction and facilitate placement of the fundoplication sutures.
- Avoid placement of the fundoplication over the buckle of the band to minimize the risk of band erosion.
- Carefully anchor the port to the anterior fascia lateral to the 15-mm port to prevent port migration or rotation.
- Late port site infections indicate band erosion until proven otherwise.

REFERENCES

McGrath V, Needleman BJ, Melvin WS. Evolution of the laparoscopic gastric bypass. *J Laparoendosc Adv Surg Tech.* 2003;13:221–227.

NIH conference. Gastrointestinal surgery for severe obesity. Consensus Development Conference Panel. *Ann Intern Med.* 1991;115:956–961.

Ren CJ, Fielding GA. Laparoscopic adjustable gastric banding: surgical technique. *J Laparoendosc Adv Surg Tech.* 2003;13: 257–263.

CHAPTER 10

Enteral Access

Kerianne H. Quanstrum, MD, and Richard E. Burney, MD

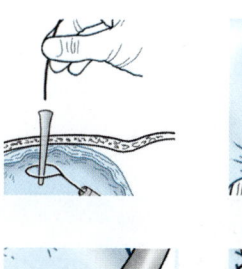
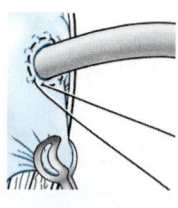
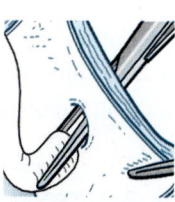
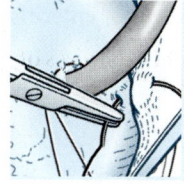
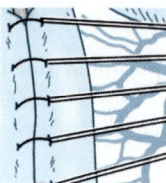
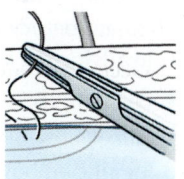

INDICATIONS

Gastrostomy

- Long-term (> 4–6 weeks) gastric feeding required under the following circumstances:
  - Patient is unable to swallow.
  - Oral feeding is precluded.
  - Oral intake alone is inadequate.
- Long-term gastric decompression.
- Intolerance to nasogastric or Dobbhoff tube, or both.
  - In cases requiring access to the gastric lumen for < 4–6 weeks, a nasogastric or Dobbhoff tube generally suffices.
- Percutaneous endoscopic gastrostomy (PEG) is the procedure of choice, when feasible, for gastrostomy placement alone. If the stomach is not accessible percutaneously or if gastrostomy is performed at the time of another upper abdominal operation, an open technique is used.

Witzel Jejunostomy

- Secondary procedure during extensive upper digestive tract surgery (eg, esophagectomy, total gastrectomy) to enable early enteral feeding, particularly when recovery is expected to be long and potentially complicated.
- Sole procedure in patients in whom oral feeding is precluded and postpyloric feeding is desired (eg, patients with duodenal trauma, gastroparesis, or pancreatitis).

CONTRAINDICATIONS

Gastrostomy

A. Absolute

- Absence of stomach (subtotal gastrectomy, transhiatal esophagectomy with gastric pullup).
- For PEG, esophageal obstruction. (Stamm gastrostomy remains feasible.)
- For PEG, lack of access to esophagus (eg, trismus, teeth wired shut). (Stamm gastrostomy remains feasible.)

B. Relative
- Severe gastroesophageal reflux or incompetent lower esophageal sphincter.
- Anatomy that prevents direct apposition of the stomach with the abdominal wall (eg, interposition of an enlarged liver; severe kyphoscoliosis).
- For PEG, morbid obesity. (Stamm gastrostomy remains feasible.)
- Ascites.
- Irreversible coagulopathy.

Witzel Jejunostomy
A. Absolute
- Distal intestinal obstruction.
- Small bowel dysmotility.

B. Relative
- Hostile abdomen (adhesions, malignancy).
- Inflammatory bowel disease or postradiation enteritis involving the jejunum.
- Ascites.
- Irreversible coagulopathy.
- Significant bowel wall edema.
- Severe immunodeficiency.

INFORMED CONSENT
Gastrostomy
A. Expected Benefits
- Permits gastric feeding or decompression more conveniently and comfortably than by nasogastric tube.

B. Potential Risks
- Gastric leak.
- Injury to adjacent organs, including colon, small intestine, and liver.
- Gastrocutaneous fistula.
- Bleeding.
- Infection.
- Risks inherent to sedation or general anesthesia.
- Metastatic oropharyngeal cancer rarely occurs at the PEG site (< 1% occurrence), and usually occurs in rapidly progressive disease with other sites of metastasis.

Witzel Jejunostomy
A. Expected Benefits
- Provides a means for enteral feeding that bypasses the stomach and upper digestive system.

B. Potential Risks
- Damage to surrounding structures, including bowel wall injury.
- Enteroenteric or enterocutaneous fistula.
- Bleeding.
- Infection.
- Risks inherent to general anesthesia.

EQUIPMENT
Percutaneous Endoscopic Gastrostomy
- Upper gastrointestinal endoscope.
- PEG kit (commercially available).

Stamm Gastrostomy
- 18–22 French Malecot, Pezzer, or equivalent catheter, such as a 20 French Ponsky replacement PEG tube.

Witzel Jejunostomy
- 12–16 French red rubber catheter.

PATIENT PREPARATION
Percutaneous Endoscopic Gastrostomy
- Thorough history and physical examination are generally sufficient to rule out the presence of conditions that would preclude or contraindicate the procedure.
- There must be sufficient space between incisors to pass an endoscope without compromising the airway.
- In the case of previous abdominal surgery or an otherwise questionable abdominal examination, a limited abdominal CT scan can be obtained to determine whether direct apposition of the stomach and anterior abdominal wall is possible.
- Nothing by mouth for 4 hours before the procedure.
- Antibiotic prophylaxis is optional.

Stamm Gastrostomy and Witzel Jejunostomy
- Same as for any major abdominal operation.
- Both procedures are most easily performed under general anesthesia.
- Alternate methods of anesthesia such as deep sedation and local anesthesia can be performed in special circumstances.

PATIENT POSITIONING
Percutaneous Endoscopic Gastrostomy
- The patient should be supine.
- The head of the bed may be elevated to 45 degrees as the scope is passed, but the best percutaneous access to the stomach is achieved when the patient is fully supine.

Stamm Gastrostomy and Witzel Jejunostomy

- The patient should be supine.

PROCEDURE

Percutaneous Endoscopic Gastrostomy

- The patient is given intravenous conscious sedation before beginning the procedure.
- A nurse assistant should monitor the blood pressure, pulse, and oxygenation.
- The posterior pharynx is anesthetized with a topical agent. A bite block is placed between the incisors.
- The upper gastrointestinal endoscope is passed through the pharynx and esophagus and into the stomach.
- The stomach is insufflated with air.
- The anterior wall of the stomach is localized through the left upper quadrant abdominal wall by gentle digital palpation, transillumination, or both.
- Gentle pressure of a finger on the abdominal wall should visibly depress the stomach on endoscopic view.
- The best gastrostomy site is usually left subcostal, near the midclavicular line. It is helpful to mark the skin at the desired puncture site.
- **Figure 10–1A:** Following sterile preparation and draping, local anesthetic is injected first intradermally and then into the muscle and peritoneum through which the tube will pass at an angle perpendicular to the skin.
- A few moments is allowed for the anesthetic to take effect. A scalpel is then used to make an 8–10-mm incision in the skin.
- **Figure 10–1B:** A needle/cannula is passed through this abdominal wall incision and into the stomach. Entry into the gastric lumen is observed through the endoscope.
  - A snare passed through the endoscope is looped around the cannula. The needle may be removed or retracted from the cannula.
  - A guidewire is passed through the cannula into the gastric lumen, where it is grasped by the snare.
  - The snare holding the guidewire and the endoscope are pulled out together through the patient's mouth.
  - At the end of this maneuver, the guidewire provides a continuous pathway through the mouth, esophagus, gastric lumen, and abdominal wall (see Figure 10–1C).
  - An alternative method, if a suitable snare is not available, is to pass the guidewire through the accessory channel of the endoscope and directly out through the cannula.
- **Figure 10–1C:** The tapered end of the special percutaneous gastrostomy tube is threaded completely over the wire that exits from the patient's mouth.

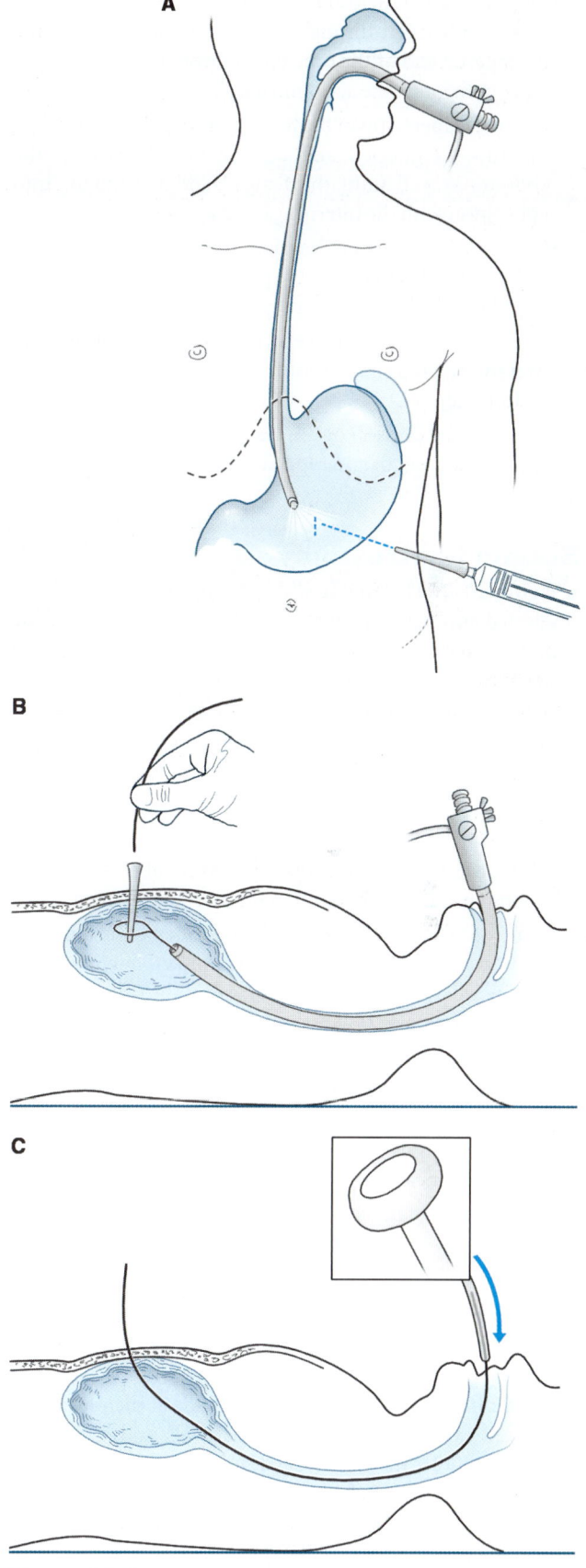

Figure 10–1

- The guidewire is held at the flanged end of the tube as the wire is pulled out through the abdominal wall, bringing the tapered end of the tube down through the esophagus and out through the abdominal wall.
- Once the tapered tip of the tube emerges through the skin, the tube is grasped and quickly pulled through the abdominal wall until the flanged end is brought into apposition with the internal gastric wall.
- Counterpressure is held against the anterior abdominal wall during this maneuver to prevent the abdominal wall from being pulled up and away from the stomach.
- The tube is secured in place by sliding an external crossbar over the tapered end of the tube until it is snug against the abdominal wall.
- The external portion of the gastrostomy tube is cut to an appropriate length and capped with an adapter.

Stamm Gastrostomy

- **Figure 10–2:** The site at which to bring out the tube is selected and marked approximately 3 cm to the left of the midline and 2–3 cm below the costal margin. Following sterile preparation and draping, a 5–6-cm midline incision is then made at the level of the chosen gastrostomy site.
- Once the peritoneal cavity is entered, the stomach is identified.
  - The tube should be placed as proximally as possible in the stomach.
  - The greater curvature of the stomach is pulled downward gently with Babcock clamps until resistance is met.
- A gastrotomy site is chosen on the anterior gastric wall near the greater curvature. Placement is checked to ensure that this site will reach the abdominal wall at the exit site previously chosen.
- **Figure 10–3:** An absorbable or nonabsorbable purse-string suture is placed at the site chosen for the gastrostomy and left untied.
  - A gastrotomy is made in the center of the purse-string using electrocautery.
  - Penetration to mucosa is confirmed and the edges of the gastrotomy are held with Allis clamps while the tube is inserted into the stomach through the gastrotomy.
  - The purse-string suture is tied down.
  - A second purse-string suture is placed around the first for further security (not shown).
- **Figure 10–4:** A stab wound is then made at the previously marked exit site on the abdominal wall, and a clamp is pushed bluntly through the abdominal wall, entering peritoneum at least 2 cm from the midline fascial incision. The external end of the tube is pulled partway through this opening.

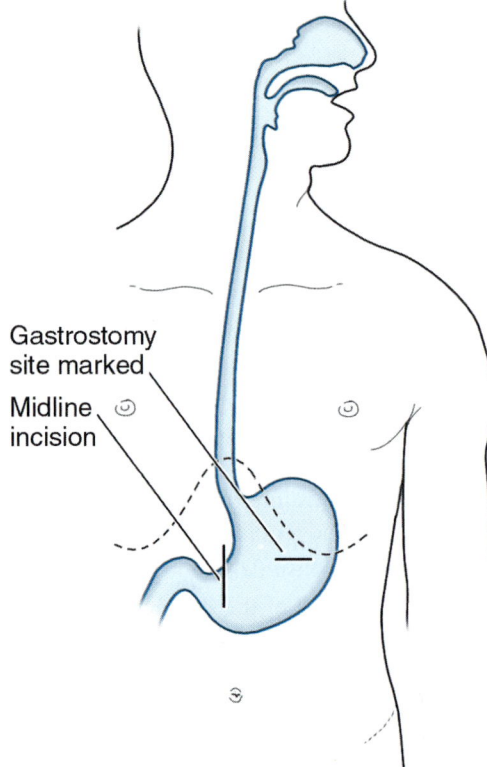

Figure 10–2

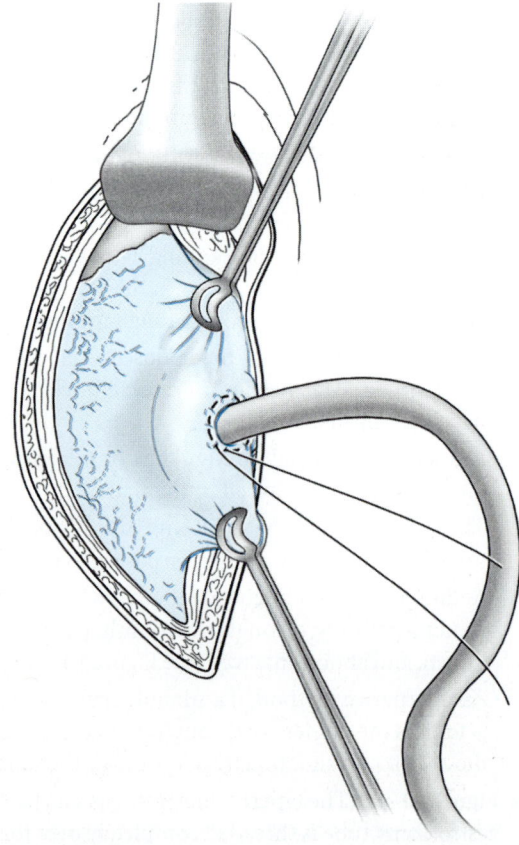

Figure 10–3

- **Figure 10–5:** The free intra-abdominal portion of the tube is used to manipulate the stomach while four sutures are placed to secure the stomach to the abdominal wall.
- **Figure 10–6:** After the sutures are placed, the tube is pulled completely through the abdominal wall apposing the stomach to the abdominal wall's underside, and the sutures are tied down. The external portion of the tube is anchored to the skin with an external crossbar, suture, or both.
- Finally, the original midline incision is closed.

Witzel Jejunostomy

- If jejunostomy is the sole procedure being performed, a short midline incision is made in the abdomen.
- Once the peritoneum has been entered, the small bowel is identified and traced to the ligament of Treitz.
- A loop of jejunum approximately 20 cm from the ligament of Treitz is brought up into the wound.
- **Figure 10–7:** A 3-0 absorbable or nonabsorbable purse-string suture is placed in the antimesenteric wall of the jejunum at the planned enterotomy site and left loose. A second purse-string suture may be placed concentrically around the first; this is also left loose.
- **Figure 10–8:** The catheter is brought onto the field and placed through an enterotomy made in the center of the purse-string sutures into the bowel lumen.
  - The tube is advanced a distance of 8–10 cm or more and the purse-string sutures are tied down.
  - A Witzel serosal tunnel is created by bringing the bowel wall over the tube for a distance of 4–6 cm proximal to its insertion site using a series of interrupted Lembert seromuscular 3-0 silk sutures.
  - The tube, including its insertion site into the small bowel, is completely invaginated in this way with great care taken not to overly narrow the lumen of the jejunum at the site of tube entry and Witzel tunnel.
  - The external end of the catheter is brought out through a stab wound in the abdominal wall.
- **Figure 10–9:** The jejunum is anchored to the peritoneum using interrupted 3-0 silk sutures for a length of 2–3 cm proximal to the serosal tunnel in order to prevent volvulus around the tube.
- The external portion of the catheter is secured to the skin with nylon suture or other external fixation device.
- Finally, the original midline incision is closed.

Alternative Techniques

- A jejunostomy tube can also be placed using the needle catheter technique.
  - A 9 French catheter is passed via a needle/cannula through the abdominal wall, through a submucosal tunnel in the jejunal wall, and then into the jejunal lumen.

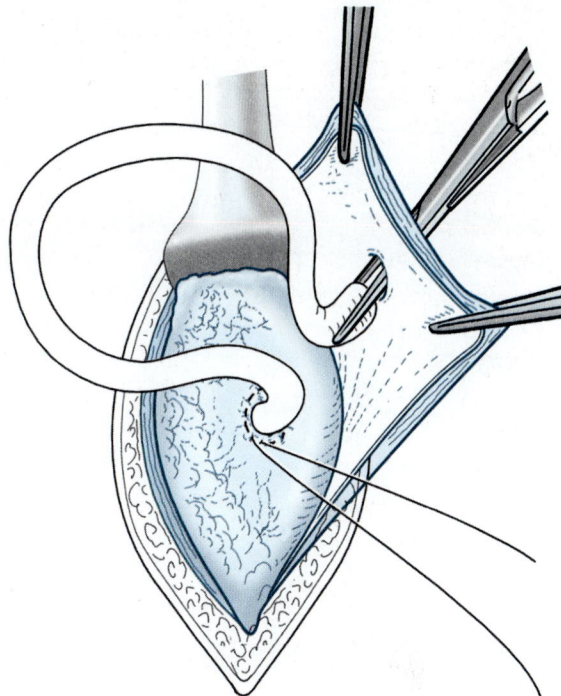

Figure 10–4

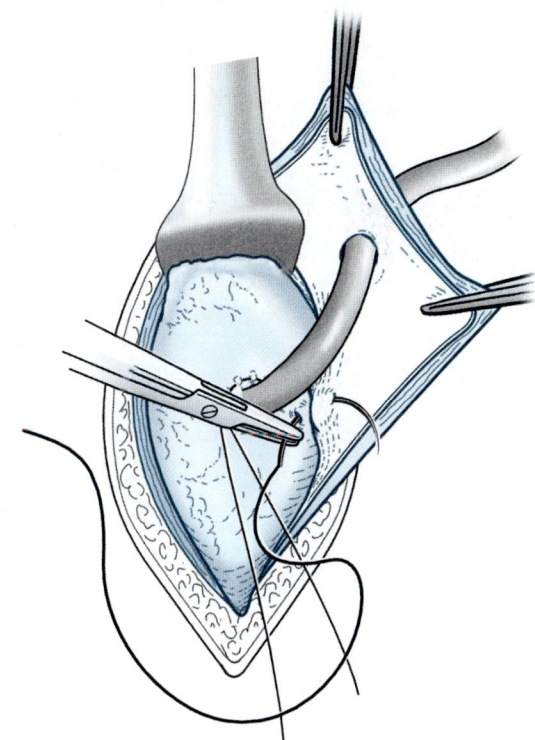

Figure 10–5

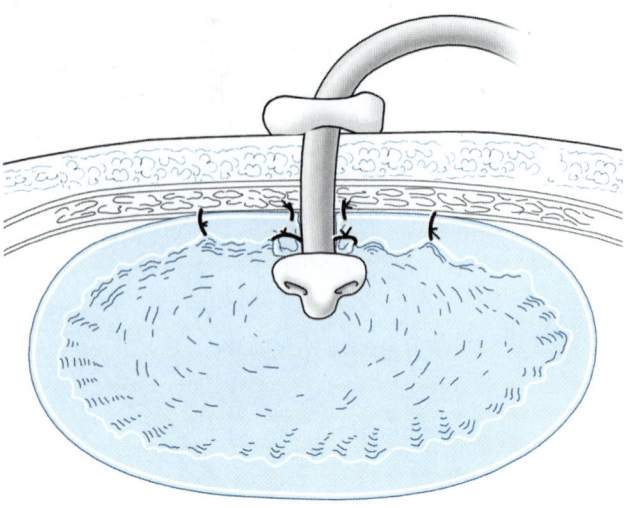

Figure 10–6

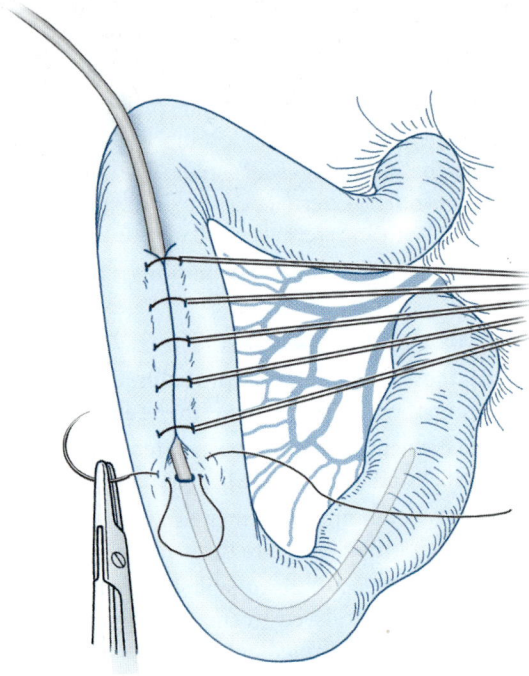

Figure 10–8

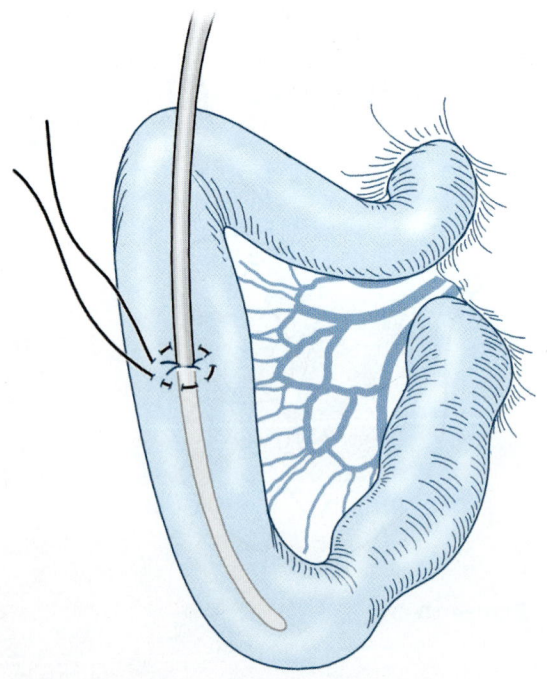

Figure 10–7

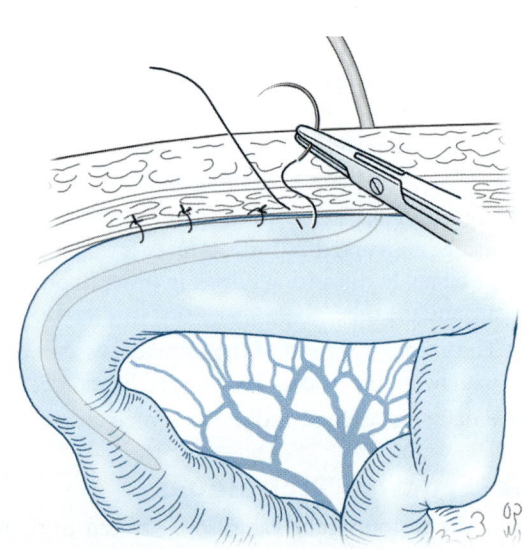

Figure 10–9

- The jejunum is sutured to the anterior abdominal wall to prevent volvulus around the catheter insertion site.
- Although this technique is simple and can be performed quickly, it has a higher complication rate than standard jejunostomy. The small catheter is more prone to clogging and kinking and is difficult to replace, making it unsuitable for long-term use. There have also been reports of serious infections occurring after needle catheter jejunostomy.

- If a patient has a gastrostomy and postpyloric feedings are desired, a gastrojejunostomy (G-J) extension tube can be used.
  - The original gastrostomy tube is removed and a G-J tube is inserted.
  - Under endoscopic control, the jejunal extension is threaded through the gastrostomy portion of the G-J tube and placed in the fourth portion of the duodenum.

POSTOPERATIVE CARE

Percutaneous Endoscopic Gastrostomy
- A percutaneous gastrostomy may be used for medication administration immediately and for feeding within 6–12 hours. The patient should be instructed that the retention bar, which is initially snug, may be loosened slightly after 24–48 hours.

Stamm Gastrostomy
- Unlike a PEG, an open gastrostomy tube is connected to gravity drainage for 12–24 hours before being used for feeding. This allows for verification that gastric emptying is taking place.

Witzel Jejunostomy
- The jejunostomy tube can be used immediately following the procedure.
- Tube feedings should be started slowly, at one-fourth or one-half strength, to avoid osmotically induced ischemic injury.

POTENTIAL COMPLICATIONS

Gastrostomy
- Intraperitoneal leakage of gastric contents.
- External leakage of gastric contents around the tube, especially if the tube is too loose or if the tube has been placed in the antrum rather than the body of the stomach.
- Gastric outlet obstruction if the tube has been placed distally in the stomach and occludes the pylorus.
- Puncture of the colon, small intestine, or liver (greater risk with PEG).
- Cellulitis or subcutaneous abscess at the tube exit site.
- Accidental dislodgment of the tube.

Witzel Jejunostomy
- Failure to place the tube in the proximal jejunum.
- Rotation or volvulus of the small bowel around the jejunostomy site.
- Bowel obstruction due to narrowing and edema at the site of tube entry and Witzel tunnel.
- Kinking of the tube at the tube insertion site.
- Intraperitoneal leakage at the jejunostomy site.
- Intra-abdominal or subcutaneous abscess formation.
- Enterocutaneous fistula.

PEARLS AND TIPS

Percutaneous Endoscopic Gastrostomy
- The procedure may be done in an endoscopy suite or at the bedside in an ICU. However, if the patient is poorly cooperative (eg, developmentally disabled) or cannot protect his or her airway, the procedure is best done in an operating room with full anesthesia support.
- It is helpful to have a Dobbhoff tube already in place to follow when passing the endoscope in patients who cannot swallow effectively or in those whose oropharyngeal anatomy is distorted by tumor or prior operation.
- If the external crossbar is too tight, the risk of infection is increased. If the site is painful or if infection develops around the tube, the crossbar should be loosened to relieve pressure on the skin and to permit drainage.
- Free air may be seen on a chest film after a PEG is placed. This does not necessarily imply leakage. A contrast study through the tube is the best way to rule out a gastric leak.
- When there is uncertainty about the patient's anatomy, obtain a contrast study to locate the stomach anatomically and determine suitability for the procedure. A blind puncture should not be done.

Stamm Gastrostomy
- It is technically much easier to place the second purse-string suture in the stomach after the tube has been inserted and the first purse-string suture tied down. Lifting the stomach wall by gently pulling up on the tube facilitates placement of the second purse-string suture.
- It is technically easier to place the sutures securing the stomach to the abdominal wall before the stomach is pulled up tight against it. Initially pulling the gastrostomy tube only halfway through the exit site facilitates circumferential suture placement.

- If using a Malecot or similar tube, an external crossbar can be fashioned by cutting a segment of a large red Robinson catheter and trimming a small hole on each side through which to pull the gastrostomy tube. A silastic crossbar is included with the Ponsky tube.
- A Foley catheter can be used if nothing else is available, but it is not durable and gastric contents tend to leak around the tube.
- If the stomach cannot be brought to the abdominal wall, a Witzel technique can be used to place the gastrostomy tube, obviating the need for gastropexy (see later discussion).
- It is always best to bring the tube out through a separate stab wound rather than through the midline incision.

Witzel Jejunostomy

- Jejunostomy tubes are easily pulled out because they do not have an inner flange. If this occurs shortly after tube placement, it can be difficult to reinsert the tube because the Witzel tunnel closes down rapidly. Fluoroscopy may be helpful for attempting reinsertion.
- If using a red rubber catheter for the jejunostomy tube, cut the tip off of the tube so that exchange over a guidewire is possible if the tube clogs in the early postoperative period.
- Supplemental free water must be given in addition to tube feedings, particularly if tube feedings are hyperosmolar. Do not start with full-strength tube feedings.

REFERENCES

Cruz I, Mamel JJ, Brady PG, Cass-Garcia M. Incidence of abdominal wall metastasis complicating PEG tube placement in untreated head and neck cancer. *Gastrointest Endosc.* 2005;62:708–711.

Johnston WD, Lopez MJ, Kraybill WG, Bricer EM. Experience with a modified Witzel gastrostomy without gastropexy. *Ann Surg.* 1982;195:692–699.

Rolandelli RH, Bankhead R, Boullata JL, Compher CW, eds. *Clinical Nutrition—Enteral and Tube Feeding,* 4th ed. Philadelphia, PA: Elsevier Saunders, 2005.

Rombeau JL, Caldwell MD, Forlaw L, Guenter PA, eds. *Atlas of Nutritional Support Techniques.* Boston: Little, Brown, 1989.

Shellito PC, Malt RA. Tube gastrostomy. Techniques and complications. *Ann Surg.* 1985;201:180–185.

Tapia J, Murguia R, Garcia G, et al. Jejunostomy: techniques, indications, and complications. *World J Surg.* 1999;23:596–602.

CHAPTER 11

Laparoscopic Cholecystectomy

Kevin Tri Nguyen, MD, PhD, and John D. Birkmeyer, MD

INDICATIONS

- Biliary colic.
- Chronic cholecystitis.
- Acute cholecystitis.
- Acalculous cholecystitis.
- Gallstone pancreatitis.
- Choledocholithiasis.

CONTRAINDICATIONS

Absolute

- Inability to tolerate an operation under general anesthesia (eg, patients with end-stage cardiopulmonary disease or hemodynamic instability).
- Suspicion of gallbladder cancer based on preoperative imaging.

Relative

- Pregnancy (first or third trimester).
- Previous abdominal operations precluding laparoscopic access.
- Cirrhosis, portal hypertension, or bleeding disorders.

INFORMED CONSENT

Expected Benefits

- Patients with gallstone pancreatitis or biliary obstruction from choledocholithiasis risk recurrent complications if the gallbladder is not removed.
  - Biliary colic will most likely recur unless the gallbladder is removed.
  - Acute cholecystitis may progress to gallbladder necrosis and possibly sepsis unless cholecystectomy is performed.

Potential Risks

- Possible complications include:
  - Bleeding (from the cystic artery stump, gallbladder fossa, abdominal wall, omental or mesenteric adhesions).

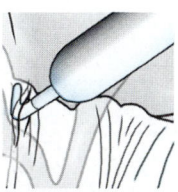 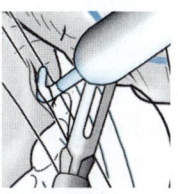 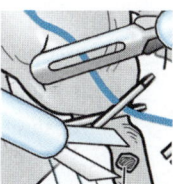
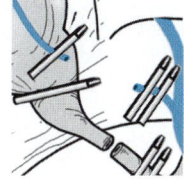 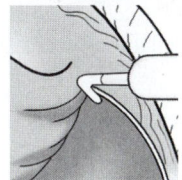 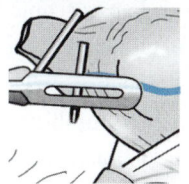
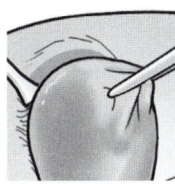 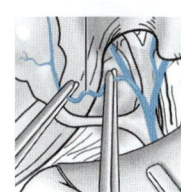 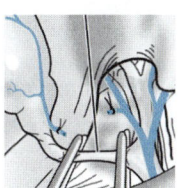

- Surgical site infection (either superficial or deep).
- Bile leak (most likely from the cystic duct stump), biliary tract injury, or both.
- Bowel injury.
- Systemic complications of abdominal surgery (pneumonia, venous thromboembolism, and cardiovascular events).
- Postoperative choledocholithiasis.

EQUIPMENT

- Standard laparoscopic equipment:
  - 5-mm and 10-mm trocars, 5-mm or 10-mm 30-degree laparoscope.
  - Atraumatic graspers.
  - Electrocautery instrument (hook or spatula).
  - Maryland dissector.
  - Clip applier.
  - Laparoscopic scissors.
- Other equipment available as necessary:
  - Suction-irrigator.
  - Disposable specimen retrieval bag.
  - Cholangiography equipment.

PATIENT PREPARATION

- Abdominal ultrasound and liver function tests.
- Preoperative endoscopic retrograde cholangiopancreatography (ERCP) for patients with clinical, laboratory, or radiographic evidence of choledocholithiasis. (Some surgeons with advanced laparoscopy experience may prefer laparoscopic common duct exploration.)
- Cardiopulmonary evaluation as needed.
- Anesthesiology consultation as needed.
- Nothing by mouth for 6 hours before surgery.
- Prophylactic antibiotics for patients with acute cholecystitis. (Although preoperative antibiotics are recommended by many surgeons, their benefit in patients with uncomplicated biliary colic or chronic cholecystitis has not been established.)

PATIENT POSITIONING

- The patient should be supine with the arms perpendicular to the body or tucked to the side.
- After general anesthesia, the abdomen is prepped from nipple to pubis and sterilely draped.
- The primary surgeon stands on the patient's left side, while the assistant stands on the patient's right.

PROCEDURE

- General anesthesia is used.
- A small periumbilical incision is made, with the location and orientation depending on the patient's body habitus and cosmetic considerations. Although most surgeons employ a closed technique to establish pneumoperitoneum and initial access (usually with a Veress needle), an open technique is also appropriate.
- **Figure 11–1:** Port positions:
  - 5-mm (preferred) or 10-mm port in the periumbilical position for a 5-mm or 10-mm laparoscopic scope.
  - 10-mm port in the subxiphoid position with the intra-abdominal portion located to the right of the falciform ligament.
  - 5-mm port 2 fingerbreadths below the costal margin and close to the midclavicular line, to position the port over the gallbladder intra-abdominally.
  - 5-mm port laterally along the anterior axillary line for gallbladder fundus retraction.
- The laparoscope is used to explore the abdomen for adhesions and potential injuries that may have occurred during port placement (the subxiphoid and subcostal ports are placed under direct visualization to minimize risk of injury).
- **Figure 11–2:** A ratcheted grasper is inserted through the lateral 5-mm port to retract the gallbladder fundus in cephalad fashion.
  - If the gallbladder is too distended to be grasped, it may be first decompressed with a needle or using the suction device.
  - An atraumatic grasper is inserted through the middle 5-mm port to retract the gallbladder infundibulum laterally, exposing the anteromedial aspect of the triangle of Calot.
  - The primary surgeon uses a two-handed technique and begins the dissection.
  - Adhesions to the body of the gallbladder are released using blunt or sharp dissection, as appropriate.
  - A hook cautery is used to carefully incise the peritoneum overlying the triangle of Calot, continuing along the medial aspect of the proximal gallbladder.
- **Figure 11–3:** As the infundibulum is retracted superomedially, peritoneum overlying the posterolateral aspect of the triangle of Calot is similarly incised using hook cautery.
- **Figure 11–4:** All remaining connective tissue is dissected out of the triangle of Calot using blunt dissection and hook cautery as needed to fully mobilize the gallbladder infundibulum.
- **Figure 11–5:** The cystic duct is dissected free.
- **Figure 11–6:** The cystic artery is dissected free.

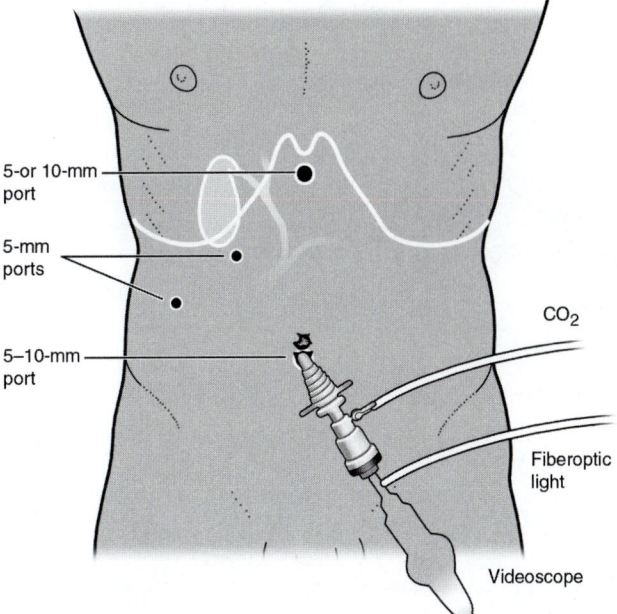

Figure 11–1

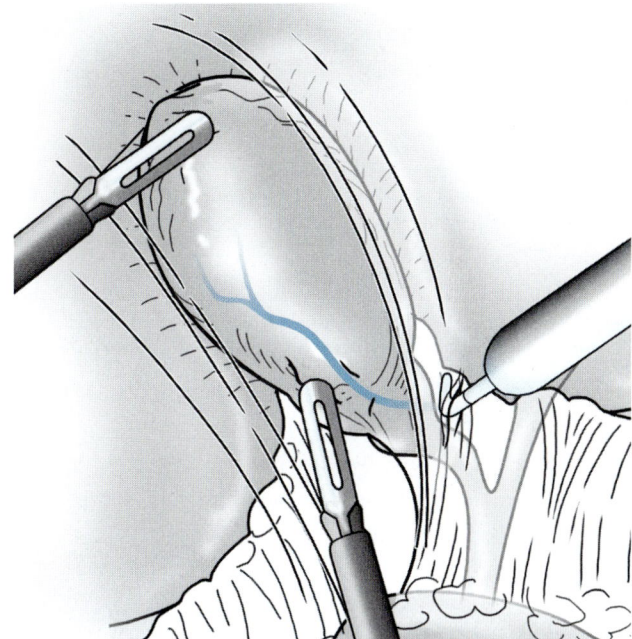

Figure 11–2

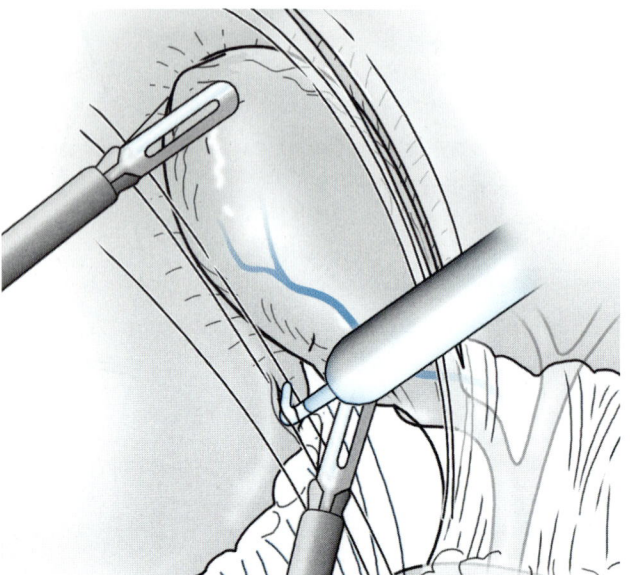

Figure 11-3

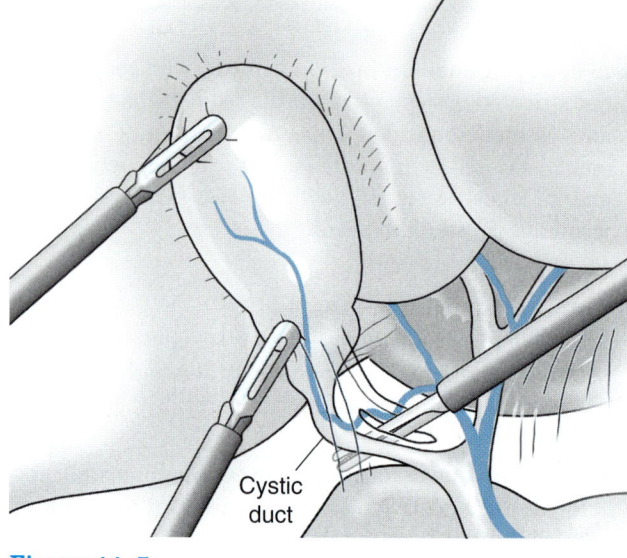

Figure 11-5

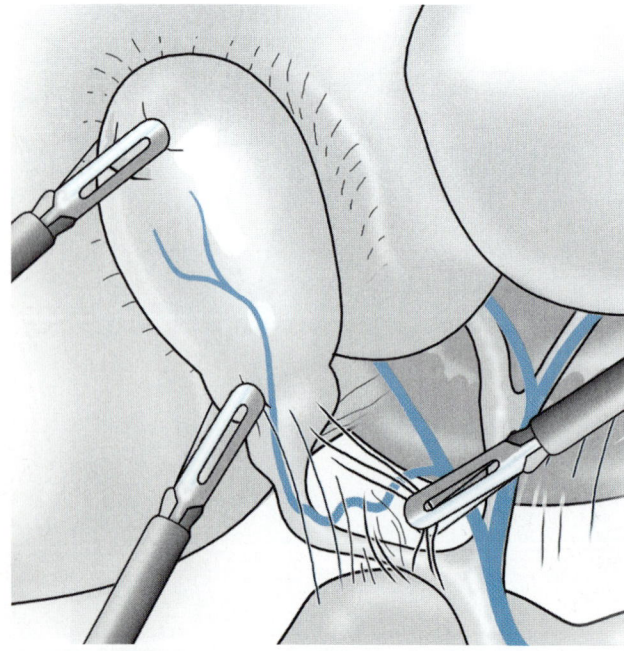

Figure 11-4

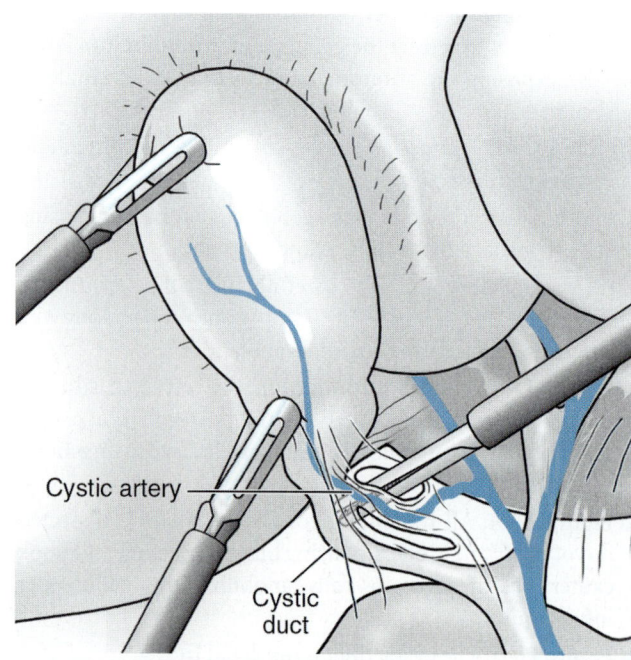

Figure 11-6

- At this point, only two tubular structures (the cystic duct and artery) remain connected to the proximal gallbladder; this represents the "critical view of safety."
- **Figure 11–7:** If a cholangiogram is to be performed, a clip is applied on the cystic duct at the junction to the infundibulum. An anterolateral cystic ductotomy is made just distal to the clip.
- **Figure 11–8:** A cholangiogram catheter is inserted through the ductotomy and secured using either clips or a cholangiogram clamp.
  - The whole system should be flushed with 2–3 mL of saline before placement of the cholangiocatheter as well as initially upon placement in the cystic duct to remove any air bubbles, which might produce an artifact on the cholangiogram.
  - Approximately 15–20 mL of contrast dye diluted 1:1 with saline is injected under fluoroscopy with the table tilted slightly to the left. The contrast is injected slowly at first to visualize the distal common bile duct and then at higher pressures and volumes to visualize the entire biliary tree.
  - An adequate cholangiogram requires visualization of the biliary tree proximal to the biliary bifurcation (revealing both right and left hepatic ducts and branches) and evidence of dye passage into the duodenum.
  - If common bile duct stones are identified, they can be managed via laparoscopic bile duct exploration or postoperative ERCP, depending on surgeon preference and experience.
- **Figure 11–9:** After the cholangiogram, the cystic duct is double clipped proximal to the ductotomy and divided. The cystic artery is likewise divided between the previously placed clips.
- **Figure 11–10:** The gallbladder is then dissected out of the gallbladder fossa using hook cautery.
- **Figure 11–11:** The gallbladder is retrieved via the umbilical or subxiphoid port, depending on surgeon preference. A disposable specimen bag may be used for this purpose, particularly in cases of acute cholecystitis or gallbladder perforation during dissection (to prevent stone spillage).
- The ports are removed under direct vision to evaluate for potential bleeding.
- If a 10-mm trocar is used at the umbilicus, the residual fascial defect is closed with interrupted 0 Vicryl sutures. The fascia at the epigastric trocar site is closed in similar fashion.
- **Figure 11–12A:** Open cholecystectomy is performed through a 10–15-cm right subcostal incision.
- A Bookwalter retractor is used to retract the liver and bowel, exposing the gallbladder.
- **Figure 11–12B:** An antegrade approach is used to dissect the gallbladder out of the gallbladder fossa from the fundus down toward the porta hepatis.

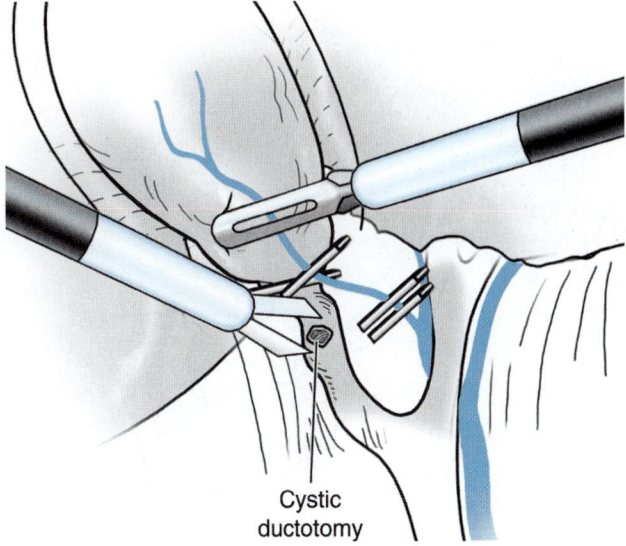

Figure 11–7

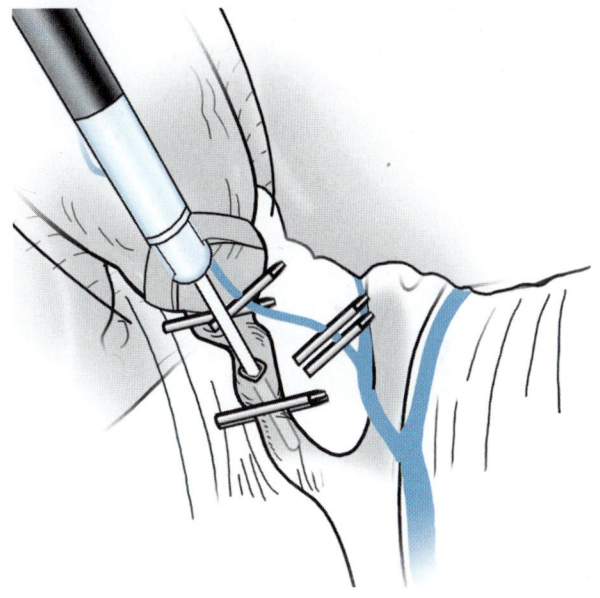

Figure 11–8

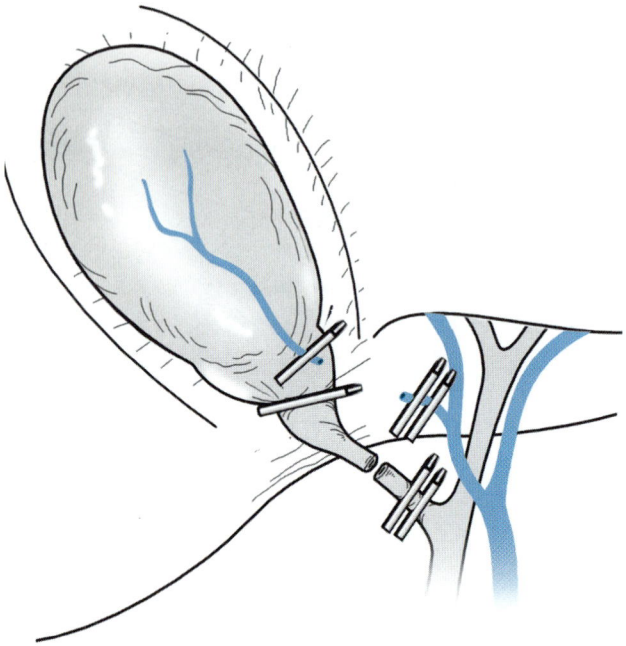

Figure 11–9

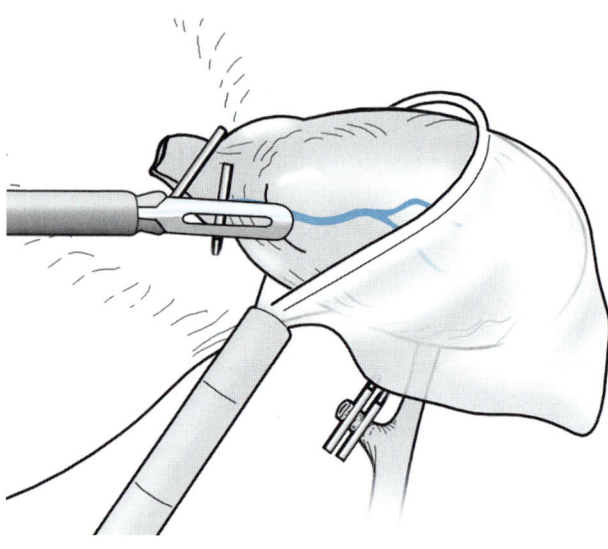

Figure 11–11

- The triangle of Calot is exposed just as in the laparoscopic approach.
- **Figure 11–12C:** The cystic artery is identified and ligated
- **Figure 11–12D:** The cystic duct is isolated and ligated.

POSTOPERATIVE CARE

- Orogastric tubes and Foley catheters, if placed preoperatively, are removed at the end of the procedure.
- Diet is advanced as tolerated.
- Oral pain medications are prescribed.
- Patients undergoing laparoscopic cholecystectomy are typically discharged on the day of surgery; open cholecystectomy usually requires a short hospital stay (eg, 1–3 days).
- Ambulation should be initiated as soon as possible.

POTENTIAL COMPLICATIONS

- Veress needle or trocar injury to great vessels or bowel.
  - Must be recognized early and repaired, either laparoscopically or after conversion to open surgery, depending on the injury and the surgeon's experience.
- Bile leak.
  - May occur from the cystic duct stump or a bile duct injury to the common bile duct.
  - Patients usually present several days after cholecystectomy with symptoms that include abdominal pain, fever, nausea, anorexia, and jaundice.
  - Evaluation should include ultrasound to evaluate for free abdominal fluid and, if the diagnosis remains uncertain, HIDA scan to demonstrate biliary extravasation.

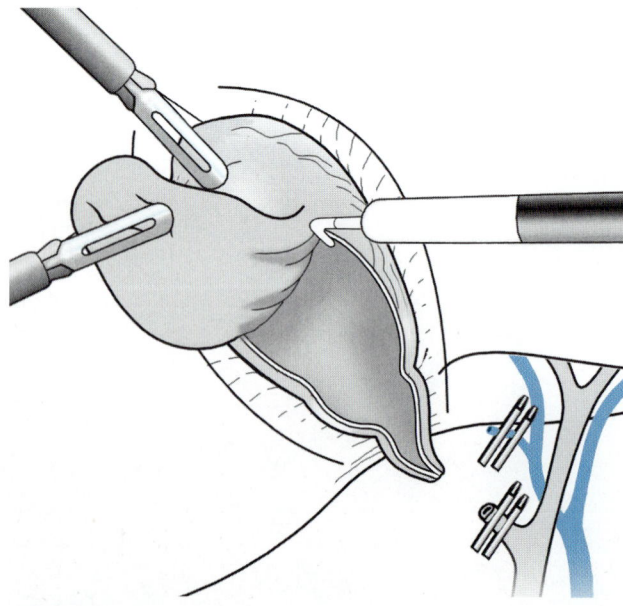

Figure 11–10

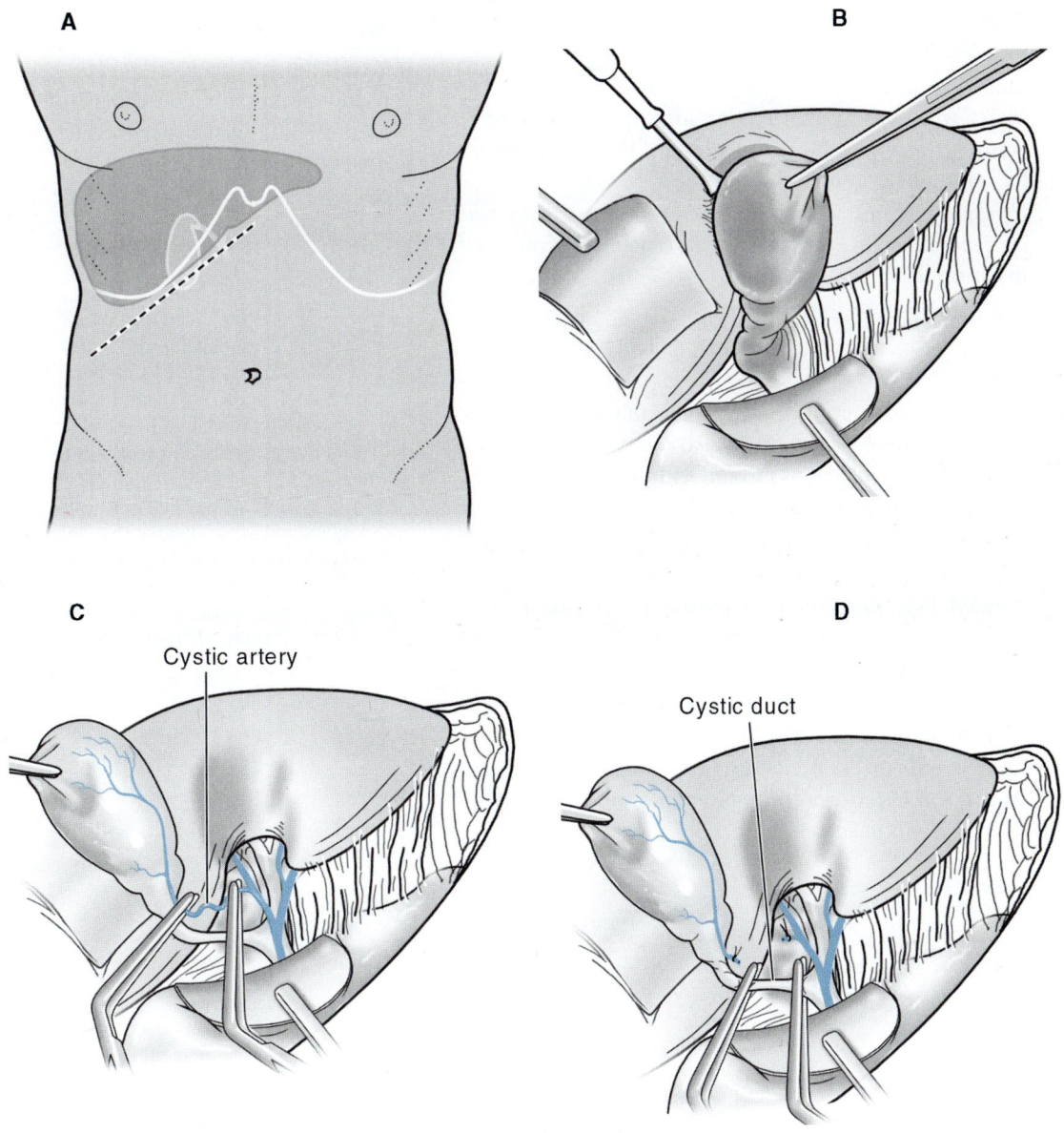

Figure 11-12A-D

- Treatment includes percutaneous abdominal drain placement for biloma and ERCP with stenting, sphincterotomy, or both.
- Failure to control the bile leak with ERCP implies the need for reoperation (laparoscopic or open), with repair depending on the etiology of the leak.
- Bile duct injury.
  - Most frequently occurs because of misidentification of anatomic structures (common bile duct or aberrant right hepatic duct mistaken for the cystic duct).
  - Can also result from overzealous use of electrocautery or clips to control bleeding in the region of the porta hepatica,

or due to excessive traction on the cystic duct and common bile duct during dissection.
- Management depends on the nature and severity of the injury, when it is recognized (intraoperatively vs postoperatively), and the relative experience of the surgeon with biliary reconstruction techniques.
- In some circumstances, patients are best managed by prompt referral to a tertiary medical center with expertise in hepatobiliary surgery.

■ Retained spilled stones.
- Spillage of stones occurs in more than 10% of laparoscopic cholecystectomies.
- Although rarely resulting in serious complications (eg, intra-abdominal abscess), spilled stones should be retrieved as completely as possible using a specimen bag.

■ Retained common bile duct stones.
- Patients may present with abdominal pain, jaundice, light-colored stools, dark urine, pancreatitis, cholangitis, elevated liver function tests (bilirubin, alkaline phosphatase, transaminases), or dilated common bile duct or intrahepatic ducts on ultrasound.
- Primary management consists of ERCP for stone clearance and sphincterotomy.
- Laparoscopic or open bile duct exploration, depending on surgeon experience, is required in unusual instances where ERCP is unsuccessful.

PEARLS AND TIPS

■ To minimize risks of bile duct injury, use the "critical view" technique to clear the triangle of Calot and completely identify and isolate the cystic duct and artery before dividing these structures.

■ Obtain a cholangiogram if the anatomy cannot be precisely identified.

REFERENCES

Colletti LM. Complications of Biliary Surgery. In: Mulholland MW, Doherty GM, eds. *Complications in Surgery*. Philadelphia, PA: Lippincott Williams & Wilkins; 2006:423–462.

Massarweh NN, Flum DR. Role of intraoperative cholangiography in avoiding bile duct injury. *J Am Coll Surg*. 2007;204:656–664.

Nakeeb A, Ahrendt SA, Pitt HA. Calculous Biliary Disease. In: Mulholland MW, Lillemoe KD, Doherty GM, et al, eds. *Greenfield's Surgery: Scientific Principles & Practice*, 4th ed. Philadelphia, PA: Lippincott Williams & Wilkins; 2006:978–999.

Strasberg SM. Avoidance of biliary injury during laparoscopic cholecystectomy. *J Hepatobiliary Pancreat Surg*. 2002;9: 543–547.

CHAPTER 12

Management of Complex Biliary Stone Disease

Richard V. Ha, MD, and Charles E. Binkley, MD

INDICATIONS

Open Common Bile Duct Exploration

- Clearance of biliary obstruction due to calculus disease if endoscopic techniques (eg, endoscopic retrograde cholangiopancreatography) are unavailable, have failed, or are not feasible due to patient anatomy or status.

Transduodenal Sphincteroplasty

- Impacted stone at the ampulla of Vater.
- Previous attempt at common bile duct exploration.
- Most often performed at the time of cholecystectomy when common bile duct exploration has failed to clear a stone impacted in the distal common bile duct.

Choledochoduodenostomy

- Unresectable malignant distal common bile duct obstruction, as a palliative procedure.
- Benign strictures of the distal common bile duct.
- Salvage drainage procedure in the presence of large primary stones or numerous stones in the distal common bile duct.

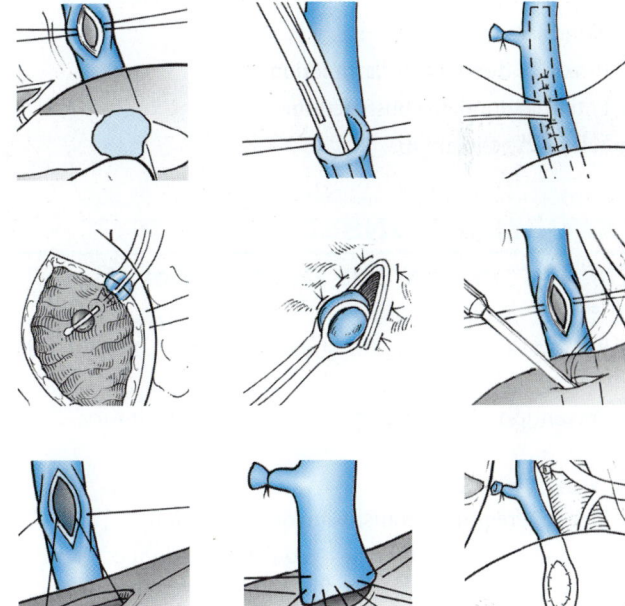

CONTRAINDICATIONS

Open Common Bile Duct Exploration

A. ABSOLUTE
- None.

B. RELATIVE
- Previous biliary bypass.

Transduodenal Sphincteroplasty

A. ABSOLUTE
- None.

B. Relative
- Fibrotic ampulla.
- Inability to pass a 3-mm probe through the ampulla.
- Abnormal-appearing ampulloduodenal junction on cholangiography.
- Common bile duct diameter > 2 cm.
- Long common bile duct stricture.

Choledochoduodenostomy
A. Absolute
- Duodenal obstruction.

B. Relative
- Primary resection of the obstructing lesion or clearance of the obstructing calculi.
- Nondilated bile duct.
- Proximal duodenal inflammation.
- Potential duodenal obstruction.
- Sclerosing cholangitis.

INFORMED CONSENT

Open Common Bile Duct Exploration
A. Expected Benefits
- Removal of the stone (or stones) from the common bile duct.
- Prevention of cholangitis and cholestatic liver injury.

B. Potential Risks
- Bleeding requiring transfusion or reoperation.
- Retained bile duct stones requiring prolonged T-tube drainage, additional procedures by interventional radiology, or possible additional surgical intervention.
- Bile leak requiring prolonged T-tube drainage.
- Iatrogenic injury to the biliary tree or duodenum.
- Surgical site infection requiring drainage or antibiotics.

Transduodenal Sphincteroplasty
A. Expected Benefits
- Removal of the stone (or stones) from the distal common bile duct.
- Prevention of cholangitis and cholestatic liver injury.

B. Potential Risks
- Bleeding requiring transfusion or reoperation.
- Bile leak requiring prolonged drainage, drain placement, or reoperation.
- Duodenal leak.
- Iatrogenic injury to the bile duct or duodenum.
- Pancreatitis.
- Biliary stricture.
- Surgical site infection requiring incision and drainage or antibiotics.

Choledochoduodenostomy
A. Expected Benefits
- Restoration of enteric biliary drainage.
- Prevention of cholangitis and cholestatic liver disease.

B. Potential Risks
- Bleeding requiring transfusion or reoperation.
- Bile leak requiring prolonged drainage, drain placement, or reoperation.
- Surgical site infection requiring drainage or antibiotics.
- Conversion to choledochojejunostomy if choledochoduodenostomy cannot be performed.

EQUIPMENT

Open Common Bile Duct Exploration
- Cholangiography catheter with occluding balloon.
- Contrast material, diluted to half strength if necessary.
- Imaging capability for intraoperative cholangiography, either fluoroscopy or plain film.
- Flexible choledochoscope with a working port and Dormia basket for stone extraction.
- Glassman stone extractors.
- Fogarty biliary catheter.
- No. 14 or 16 French T-tube.
- Bakes biliary dilators.

Transduodenal Sphincteroplasty
- Surgical magnification loupes may be beneficial.
- No. 14 French T-tube.

Choledochoduodenostomy
- No special equipment required.

PATIENT PREPARATION
- Nothing by mouth the evening before surgery.
- Magnetic resonance cholangiopancreatography may be useful to define biliary anatomy.
- Serum transaminases, total bilirubin, alkaline phosphatase, coagulation studies (PT, PTT). Coagulopathies should be treated with vitamin K, fresh frozen plasma, or both, accordingly.
- Anesthesiology consultation as needed.
- Preoperative broad-spectrum antibiotics.

PATIENT POSITIONING

- For all procedures, the patient should be supine.

PROCEDURE

Open Common Bile Duct Exploration

- General anesthesia with endotracheal intubation is required.
- Open common bile duct exploration is most often performed at the time of cholecystectomy.
- Incision and exposure:
  - A right upper quadrant incision is made parallel to the right costal margin. This is approximately 3 fingerbreadths below the costal margin and should extend from the right of midline to the right anterior axillary line.
- If not previously completed, a cholecystectomy is performed.
- Using an abdominal retractor, the liver is elevated superiorly and the small bowel is packed inferiorly.
- A Kocher maneuver is performed to mobilize the first and second portions of the duodenum.
- Intraoperative cholangiography through the cystic duct stump should be performed before beginning common bile duct exploration in order to define the location and extent of calculi.
- **Figure 12–1:** The common bile duct is identified and its anterior aspect is dissected in preparation for longitudinal choledochotomy.
  - If the location of the common bile duct is in question, cholangiography or aspiration of bile will confirm its identity.
  - Stay sutures of 4-0 silk are placed on either side of the planned incision on the anterior wall of the common bile duct.
  - A 1.0–1.5-cm incision is made longitudinally immediately distal to the cystic duct along the anterior aspect of the common bile duct between the previously placed 4-0 silk sutures.
  - If not previously done, cholangiography should be performed.
  - The common bile duct should be palpated from the choledochotomy distally through the head of the pancreas. Any palpable calculi may be "milked" proximally for extraction through the choledochotomy.
- **Figure 12–2:** Several maneuvers can be used to clear calculi from the bile duct.
  - Bakes biliary dilators can be used to gently dilate the bile duct and aid in stone retrieval.
  - A Fogarty balloon catheter can be passed through the choledochotomy distally and through the ampulla. The catheter can then be withdrawn back into the distal

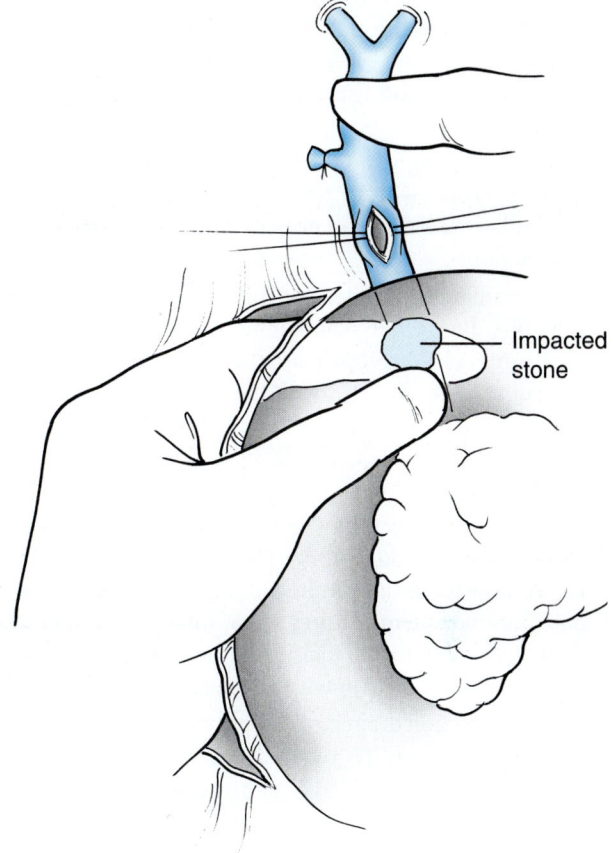

Figure 12–1

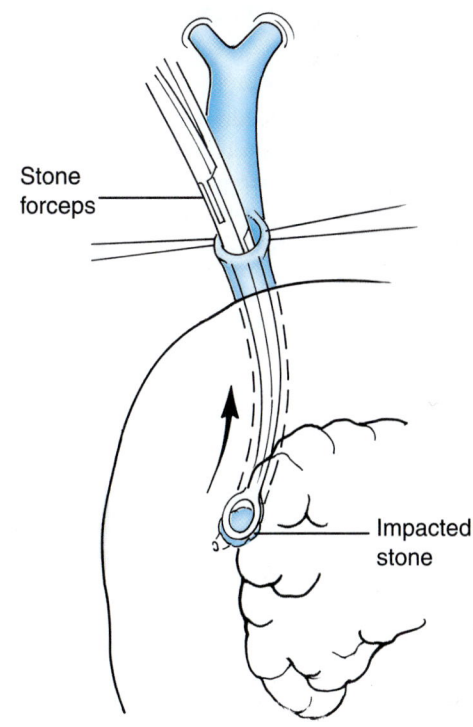

Figure 12–2

common bile duct and the balloon inflated to drag stones proximally and through the choledochotomy. Care must be taken to avoid either duodenal or biliary injury by excessive force on the catheter or overinflation of the balloon.
- Choledochoscopy can be performed using a flexible choledochoscope with a working port through which a Dormia wire basket can be placed for stone retrieval and extraction.
- A Glassman stone extractor may be passed distally into the bile duct, while maintaining tactile feedback of the instrument by direct palpation. The surgeon may be able to palpate the stone through the anterior duodenal wall and place it into the stone extractor to be removed.

■ **Figure 12–3:** After the stone is extracted and a completion cholangiogram is performed confirming complete clearance of the bile duct, a 14 or 16 French T-tube is inserted through the choledochotomy. The choledochotomy is then closed over the T-tube limbs with interrupted 4-0 absorbable monofilament sutures. The tube is brought out through a separate stab incision in the anterior abdominal wall and connected to gravity drainage.
- A closed suction drain is placed posterior to the bile duct.

Transduodenal Sphincteroplasty

■ General anesthesia with endotracheal intubation is required.
■ Sphincteroplasty is most often performed at the time of cholecystectomy when common bile duct exploration has failed to clear a stone impacted in the distal common bile duct.
■ Incision and exposure:
- A right upper quadrant incision is made parallel to the right costal margin. This is approximately 3 fingerbreadths below the costal margin and should extend from the right of midline to the right anterior axillary line.
■ If not previously completed, a cholecystectomy is performed.
■ Using an abdominal retractor, the liver is elevated superiorly and the small bowel is packed inferiorly.
■ A Kocher maneuver is performed to mobilize the first and second portions of the duodenum.
■ Intraoperative cholangiography through the cystic duct stump should be performed in order to define the location and extent of calculi.
■ **Figure 12–4:** Stay sutures of 4-0 silk are placed and a 1.0–1.5-cm anterior choledochotomy is performed in preparation for common bile duct exploration.

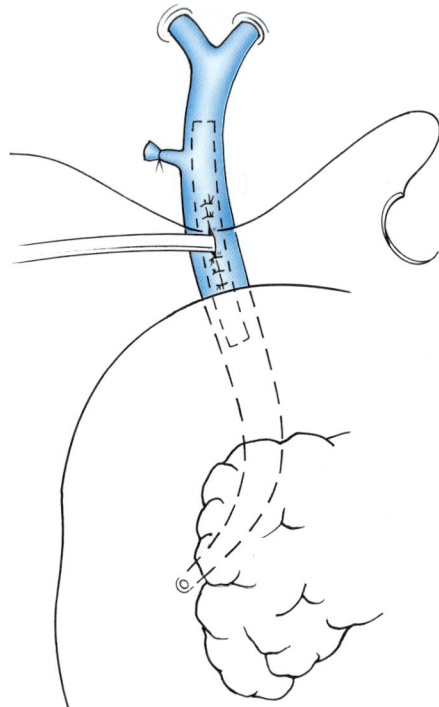

Figure 12–3

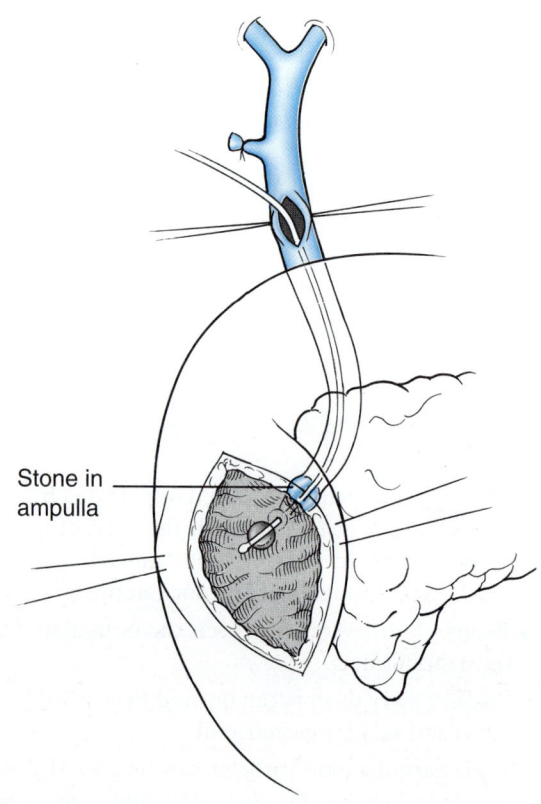

Figure 12–4

- If not previously done, cholangiography and common bile duct exploration should be performed.
- A Fogarty balloon catheter or a fine probe is placed through the choledochotomy and distally through the ampulla in order to identify the ampulla for duodenotomy.
- Stay sutures of 2-0 silk are placed on either side of the planned longitudinal duodenal incision.
- Using needle tip electrocautery, a 5-cm longitudinal duodenotomy is performed, centered directly over the ampulla.

■ **Figure 12–5A:** Adequate exposure of the ampulla is required. If anterograde placement of either a fine probe or Fogarty biliary catheter was not possible, retrograde placement should be attempted to reliably identify the course of the common bile duct for sphincterotomy.

- Surgical magnification loupes may prove beneficial, particularly in identification of the pancreatic duct.
- Using needle tip electrocautery, the ampulla is opened for a distance of 4–5 mm in the 11 o'clock position.
- The cut edge of the ampulla is approximated to the duodenum using 4-0 or 5-0 interrupted absorbable monofilament sutures.
- The pancreatic duct should be identified and any injury to it avoided.

■ **Figure 12–5B:** The ampulla can be incised with cautery another 4–5 mm with placement of sutures to approximate the ampulla to the duodenum as previously performed.

- The stone is either extracted through the opened sphincter or pushed proximally to be removed through the choledochotomy.

■ **Figure 12–5C:** The sphincteroplasty is completed and the pancreatic duct identified.

- The duodenotomy is closed longitudinally in two layers. A running 3-0 braided absorbable suture is used for the inner layer followed by interrupted 3-0 silk sutures placed in a Lembert fashion. Care is taken not to narrow the duodenum.
- As with a common bile duct exploration, a T-tube should be placed and the choledochotomy closed as previously described.
- A closed suction drain should be placed lateral to the duodenotomy.
- The abdominal wall is closed in a routine manner.

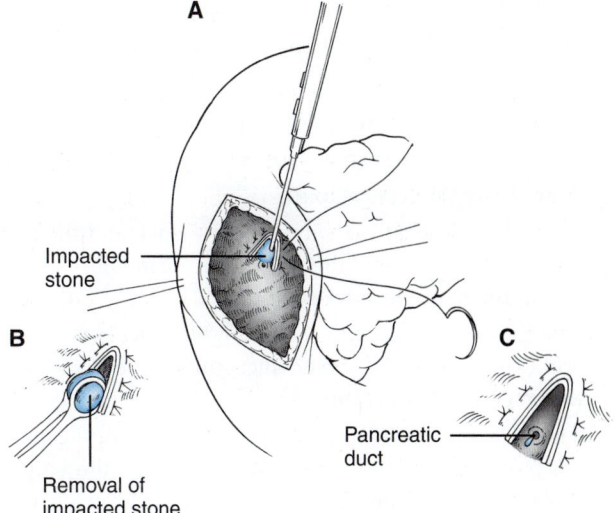

Figure 12–5A–C

Choledochoduodenostomy

- General anesthesia is required.
- Incision and exposure:
  - A right subcostal or an upper midline incision is made.
  - General abdominal exploration is performed.
- **Figure 12–6:** Cholecystectomy.
  - A generous Kocher maneuver is performed and the first and second portions of the duodenum are mobilized from the foramen of Winslow distally.
  - The anterior aspect of the common bile duct is dissected and exposed from the cystic duct stump to the proximal extent of the obstruction.
  - The surgeon should ensure that the duodenum can be easily elevated to the common bile duct, allowing a tension-free anastomosis.
  - Stay sutures of 4-0 silk are placed on either side of the planned anterior longitudinal choledochotomy.
  - A 2–2.5-cm longitudinal incision is made, centered on the anterior common bile duct below the cystic duct entrance.
  - If the procedure is performed for biliary calculi, the common bile duct is palpated for stones and "milked" proximally for removal. A common bile duct exploration can also be performed through the choledochotomy.
  - A 1.5–2.0-cm longitudinal incision is made on the adjacent anterior aspect of the proximal duodenum.
- **Figure 12–7:** The anastomosis is begun using 4-0 absorbable monofilament sutures by placing corner anchoring sutures between the midportion of the choledochotomy and the edges of the duodenotomy in order to "tent" the anastomosis open. These should be tied on the outside.
  - The anastomosis should employ full-thickness bites of both the bile duct and the duodenum in order to effect a duct-to-mucosa approximation.
  - The posterior anastomosis is continued by approximating the distal portion of the choledochotomy to the superior edge of the duodenotomy, using interrupted 4-0 absorbable monofilament sutures.
  - Waiting until the entire back row of sutures is placed before they are tied may aid in forming the anastomosis.
- **Figure 12–8:** Complete the anastomosis between the bile duct and duodenum by placing the anterior row of sutures. These are then tied and cut.

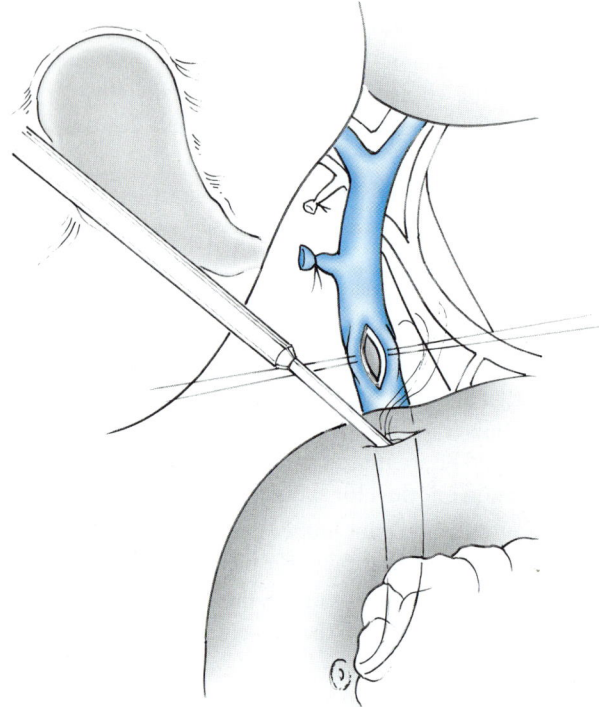

Figure 12–6

Chapter 12 : Management of Complex Biliary Stone Disease • 103

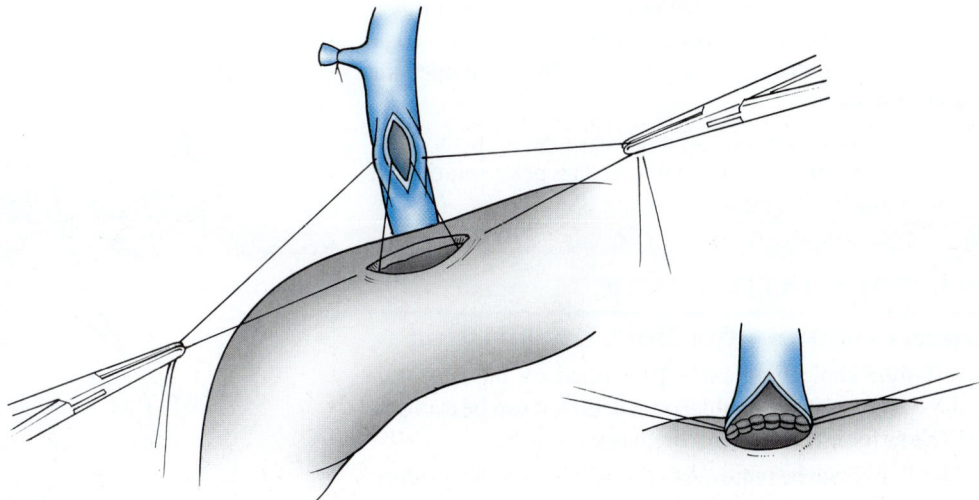

Figure 12-7

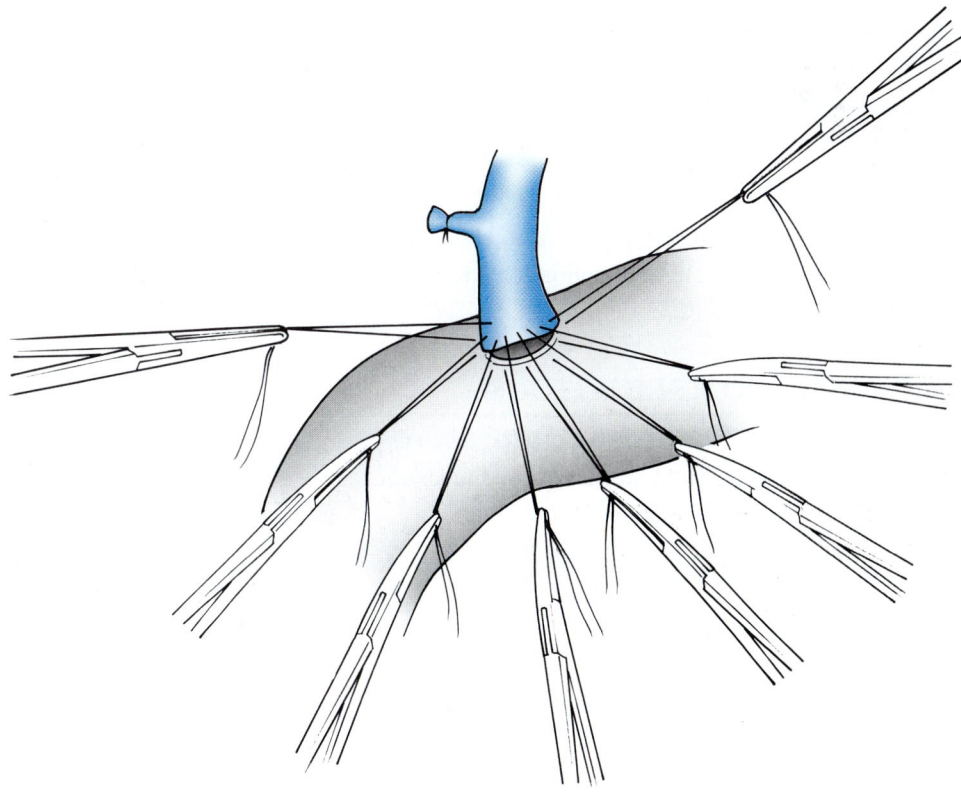

Figure 12-8

- **Figure 12–9:** The completed anastomosis is shown utilizing the longitudinal choledochotomy made at a right angle to the longitudinal duodenotomy in order to tent open the anastomosis.
  - A closed suction drain may be placed adjacent to the anastomosis. It can be removed several days postoperatively if there is no bile in the drain.

POSTOPERATIVE CARE

Open Common Bile Duct Exploration
- A T-tube cholangiogram is performed on postoperative day 3. If there is no residual obstruction, it can be clamped to allow for internal biliary drainage.
- The T-tube can be removed in the office 3–4 weeks postoperatively.
- If there are retained calculi, the T-tube tract can be used for stone extraction by interventional radiology.

Transduodenal Sphincteroplasty
- Nasogastric decompression via low continuous wall suction should be continued for 3–5 days to allow for resolution of transient duodenal obstruction from duodenal edema.
- After the nasogastric tube is removed, with the return of bowel function, clear liquids can be started and the diet advanced as tolerated.
- If no bilious output occurs after resumption of diet, the drain can be removed.

Choledochoduodenostomy
- If no bilious output is noted, the drain can be removed a few days after the procedure.
- A nasogastric tube attached to low continuous wall suction should be continued for 3–4 days postoperatively. With the resolution of ileus, it can be discontinued and the diet advanced as tolerated.

POTENTIAL COMPLICATIONS

Open Common Bile Duct Exploration
- Iatrogenic injury to the common bile duct or duodenum.
- Retained stone despite exploration.
- Bile leak from the T-tube.
- Cholangitis.
- Excessive bile loss requiring fluid replacement.

Transduodenal Sphincteroplasty
- Iatrogenic injury to the pancreatic duct, bile duct, or duodenum.
- Bile leak, duodenal leak, or pancreatic leak.
- Wound infection or intra-abdominal abscess.

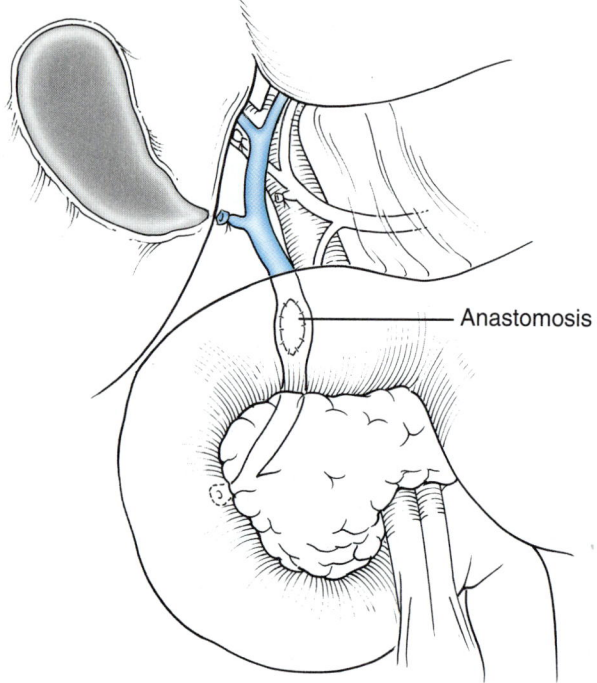

Figure 12–9

Choledochoduodenostomy
- Bile leak.
- Stenosis of the anastomosis.
- "Sump" syndrome, which affects 1% of patients, occurs when debris collects in the distal segment of the bile duct below the anastomosis. This can cause obstruction of the anastomosis or even pancreatitis.

PEARLS AND TIPS
Open Common Bile Duct Exploration
- If there is evidence of bile leak (bile in the closed suction drain) or obstruction (elevated transaminases, bilirubin, jaundice) after the T-tube is clamped, immediately reinstitute gravity drainage and obtain a cholangiogram.
- If there is any sign of cholangitis, reconnect the T-tube to gravity drainage and start broad-spectrum antibiotics.

Transduodenal Sphincteroplasty
- A combination of manipulation through the sphincteroplasty and choledochotomy may be required for severely impacted stones.
- To avoid injury, identify the pancreatic duct early.

Choledochoduodenostomy
- A double-layer anastomosis is unnecessary and may narrow the anastomotic orifice.
- If the duodenum does not mobilize despite extensive Kocherization, a choledochojejunostomy may be a better choice.

REFERENCES

Carboni M, Negro P, D'Amore L, Proposito D. Transduodenal sphincteroplasty in a laparoscopic era. *World J Surg.* 2001;25:1357–1359.

Ellison CE, Carey LC. Cholecystostomy, Cholecystectomy, and Intraoperative Evaluation of the Biliary Tree. In: Baker RJ, Fischer JE, eds. *Mastery of Surgery,* 5th ed. Philadelphia, PA: Lippincott Williams & Wilkins; 2006.

Ellison CE, Melvin WS, Moon SG. Current Application of Lateral Choledochoduodenostomy and Transduodenal Sphincteroplasty. In: Baker RJ, Fischer JE, eds. *Mastery of Surgery,* 5th ed. Philadelphia, PA: Lippincott Williams & Wilkins; 2006.

Girard RM, Legros G. Retained and recurrent bile duct stones. Surgical or nonsurgical removal? *Ann Surg.* 1981;193:150–154.

Hutter MM, Rattner DW. Open Common Bile Duct Exploration: When Is It Indicated? In: Cameron JL, ed. *Current Surgical Therapy,* 8th ed. St Louis, MO: Mosby; 2004.

Madura JA, Madura JA II, Sherman S, Lehman GA. Surgical sphincteroplasty in 446 patients. *Arch Surg.* 2005;140:504–512.

CHAPTER 13

Management of Bile Duct Injuries and Biliary Strictures

Amit K. Mathur, MD, and James A. Knol, MD

INDICATIONS

- Iatrogenic biliary injuries associated with laparoscopic cholecystectomy (most common), or other foregut operations.
- Operative approach depends on the time the injury is diagnosed (eg, immediately, early [≤ 4 weeks after injury], or late [> 4 weeks after injury]).
  - If the patient is hemodynamically stable, immediate biliary reconstruction is indicated when an injury is identified intraoperatively during a laparoscopic cholecystectomy or other operation and a hepatobiliary surgeon is available to perform the repair.
  - For patients with early or late injuries, operative management typically requires delayed biliary reconstruction with a biliary-enteric anastomosis.
- The aim of operative intervention is definitive treatment of patients with iatrogenic common bile duct or more proximal biliary injuries after the residual inflammation from the acute injury has resolved.
- If the injury has been thoroughly evaluated and the biliary system has been sufficiently decompressed and drained for 6 weeks or more, reconstruction is required if a biliary stricture persists or if biliary-enteric discontinuity remains.

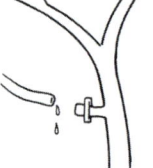 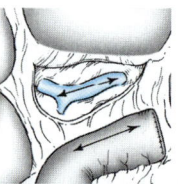 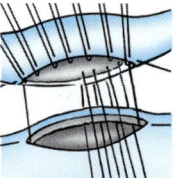
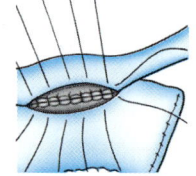 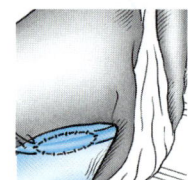

CONTRAINDICATIONS

Biliary Decompression

- Few contraindications exist for biliary decompression. This may be achieved using a percutaneous transhepatic approach or endoscopic retrograde-guided stent placement. Rarely, operative decompression may be required.

PERCUTANEOUS TRANSHEPATIC APPROACH
A. Absolute
- Active coagulopathy.

B. Relative
- Hepatic malignancy.
- Hydatid disease.

- Ascites.
- Contrast-related anaphylaxis.

ENDOSCOPIC RETROGRADE APPROACH
A. Absolute
- Patients who cannot cooperate with the study.

B. Relative
- Active or recent acute pancreatitis.
- Recent myocardial infarction.
- Severe cardiopulmonary disease.

Biliary Stricture Dilation
- Contraindications depend on approach (transhepatic or endoscopic retrograde), as outlined earlier.

Biliary Reconstruction
A. ABSOLUTE
- Incomplete preoperative evaluation.
- Inability to tolerate general anesthesia.
- Surgeon's lack of expertise in performing complex biliary reconstruction.

B. RELATIVE
- Acute cholangitis.
- Early biliary injury without adequate biliary drainage (< 6 weeks).

INFORMED CONSENT
Biliary Stenting, Drainage, and Dilation
A. EXPECTED BENEFITS
- Treatment of life-threatening cholangitis.
- Treatment of biliary stricture.
  - In patients with short strictures (< 2 cm), biliary stenting with successive dilation may successfully resolve the stricture without operative reconstruction.
- Prevention of cholestatic liver injury in situations where cholestasis cannot be definitively relieved within 2–4 weeks.
- In patients with bilirubin > 20 mg/dL, biliary decompression allows recovery of liver function prior to operative therapy.
- Assists in identification of hilar bile ducts at the time of operative biliary reconstruction.

B. POTENTIAL RISKS
- Bleeding.
- Biliary sepsis.
- Pancreatitis.
- Damage to liver or adjacent structures.
- Failure of drainage.
- Need for periodic stent changes until reconstruction.
- Need for additional interventions or procedures.

Biliary Reconstruction
A. EXPECTED BENEFITS
- Internal drainage of obstructed bile flow by providing enteric drainage of the biliary tree.
  - Correction of biliary strictures results in decreased risk of biliary cirrhosis, cholangitis, intrahepatic gallstones, hepatic abscesses, portal hypertension, and resulting progressive liver failure.
  - Alleviation of strictures also lessens the risk of future development of cholangiocarcinoma.

B. POTENTIAL RISKS
- Late failure of reconstruction resulting in biliary cirrhosis, cholangitis, intrahepatic gallstones, hepatic abscesses, portal hypertension, and resulting progressive liver failure.
- Need for additional invasive or operative procedures.
- Usual postoperative complications (eg, infection, injury to adjacent structures, cardiopulmonary complications).

EQUIPMENT
Biliary Injury Evaluation
- Access to CT, percutaneous transhepatic cholangiogram (PTC), diagnostic and therapeutic endoscopic retrograde cholangiopancreatogram (ERCP), magnetic resonance cholangiopancreatogram (MRCP), and intraoperative cholangiogram are imperative.

Biliary Reconstruction
- General instrumentation set.
- Vascular instrumentation should be available.
- Intraoperative ultrasound.
- Gastrointestinal anastomosis (GIA) stapler.
- Self-retaining retractor.
- Intraoperative cholangiogram capability (C-arm, contrast, cholangiogram catheters).
- Device to divide liver parenchyma.
- Choledochoscope should be available.

PATIENT PREPARATION
Preoperative Evaluation
- **Figure 13–1:** Management algorithm for patients with suspected biliary injury, based on timing of diagnosis.
  - Management of iatrogenic injuries depends on the time at which they are diagnosed. A combination of imaging

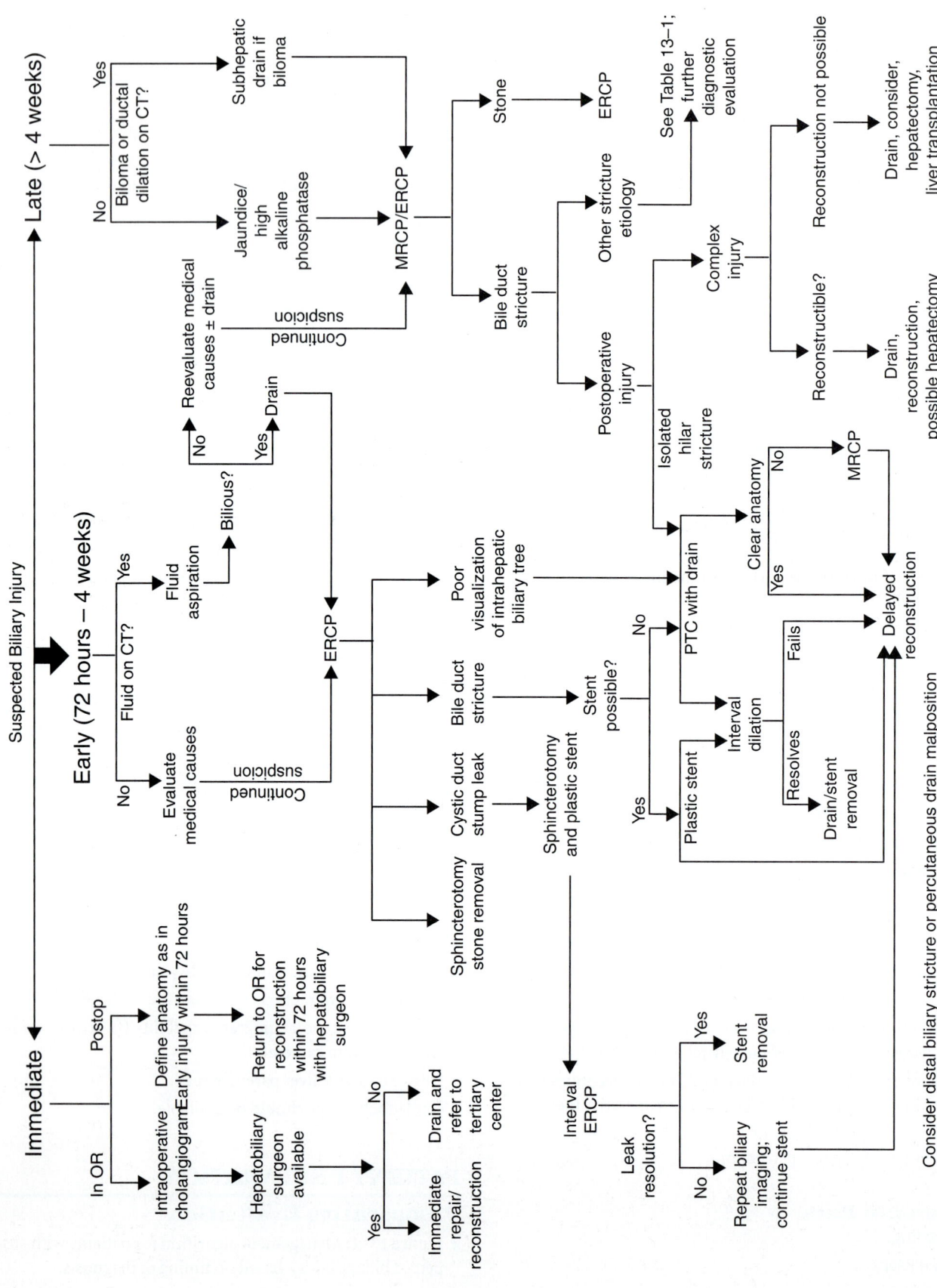

Figure 13–1. Management algorithm for patients with suspected biliary injury, based on timing of diagnosis.

studies may be required to properly understand the anatomy of the injury.
- Complete diagnostic evaluation is necessary for successful reconstruction.
- The goal of preoperative therapeutic interventions is to relieve biliary obstruction, drain bilomas, and assist in identification of hilar bile ducts for a future reconstructive operation.

■ External or internal biliary drainage, as warranted by type of injury.
- Treatment of sepsis and recurrent cholangitis is the goal of therapy.
- Common duct strictures may be stented via an endoscopic retrograde approach.
- Patients with more proximal strictures may benefit from both external and internal biliary drainage with interval dilation over time and delayed reconstruction.
- A transected common duct requires external biliary drainage.
- All bilomas and bile leaks should be drained.

■ Concomitant injuries to the hepatic vasculature may also be present, and may require preoperative angiographic evaluation.

■ Review of operative reports from the index operation and direct discussion with the initial surgeon may improve understanding of the injury.

■ Patients presenting with a stricture late after biliary surgery should be evaluated for other potential stricturing processes (**Table 13–1**), which should be ruled out before proceeding with operative intervention.

At the Time of Elective Biliary Reconstruction

■ Preoperative nutritional supplementation, if necessary.
■ Intraoperative placement of a Foley catheter.
■ Intraoperative placement of nasogastric suction.
■ External or internal biliary drains in the right ductal system often exit very far laterally and do not necessarily need to be included in preparation of the operative field.
■ Left-sided external or internal biliary drains should be included in preparation of the operative field.
■ Care should be taken not to manipulate these tubes while positioning the patient. The skin sutures anchoring the left-sided catheter should be loosened to maintain catheter position during the operation, as elevation of the anterior abdominal wall can dislodge left-sided catheters during the dissection.
■ Prophylactic antibiotics.
■ Pharmacologic deep vein thrombosis prophylaxis.

PATIENT POSITIONING

■ The patient should be supine with biliary drainage catheters positioned as outlined earlier.

Table 13–1. Causes of extrahepatic biliary stricture.

Ampullary adenoma	Infectious: viral, *Clonorchis sinensis*
Ampullary carcinoma	
Biliary adenoma	Mirizzi syndrome
Blunt or penetrating trauma	Pancreatic adenocarcinoma
Cholangiocarcinoma	Postoperative stricture
Cholangiohepatitis	Primary sclerosing cholangitis
Choledocholithiasis	Radiation therapy-related
Chronic pancreatitis	Retroperitoneal fibrosis
Crohn disease	Stenosis at sphincter of Oddi
Duodenal adenocarcinoma	Toxic drugs
Duodenal ulcers	

Source: Based on information in Lillemoe KD. Biliary Injuries and Strictures and Sclerosing Cholangitis. In: Mulholland MW, Lillemoe KD, Doherty GM, et al, eds. *Greenfield's Surgery: Scientific Principles & Practice,* 4th ed. Philadelphia, PA: Lippincott Williams & Wilkins; 2006:999–1014.

PROCEDURE

Classification of Biliary Injuries

- Postoperative strictures are related to multiple direct causes, including cautery-related burn injury to the biliary tree, transection or sharp injury to the common bile duct or the right or left hepatic ducts, stapling of the bile duct, ischemia-related injury due to vessel ligation, or a combination of these injury types.
  - Complex injuries may or may not be surgically reconstructible.
- **Figure 13–2A–H:** Strasberg classification of biliary injuries.
- Type A injuries (Figure 13–2A) are reserved for cystic duct stump leaks, which are usually managed with very good results via a combination of sphincterotomy and endoscopically placed plastic stents.
  - Interval ERCP is conducted after 4–6 weeks.
  - Stents may be removed if the leak has resolved, as outlined in Figure 13–1.
- Type B (Figure 13–2B) and C (Figure 13–2C) injuries involve the division of an aberrant right hepatic duct. Type B injuries involve ligation of the aberrant proximal duct, but type C injuries involve persistent biliary leak through the aberrant duct from the right hepatic lobe.
  - Most laparoscopic cholecystectomy-related biliary injuries involve division of the bile duct going to the right anterior liver, which aberrantly inserts onto the common duct instead of inserting as the first radical of the right hepatic duct.
  - Operative strategies for these types of injury are dictated by the amount of liver dependent on biliary drainage through that duct.
  - If the biliary flow through the transected duct is low, this duct may be electively ligated. The patient should subsequently be followed for the development of cholangitis.
  - Large hepatic segments with significant flow through this duct may need biliary reconstruction or hepatic resection.
  - Reconstruction can be considered if the bile duct is at least 1 cm in length and > 3 mm in diameter.
  - If reconstruction is not feasible, the liver segments at risk should not be salvaged.
- Type D (Figure 13–2D) injuries represent a lateral injury to the common hepatic duct. These may resolve with stenting and dilation, depending on the anatomy of the injury and the size of the defect in the duct.
  - Large defects usually require reconstruction.
- Type E injuries are subclassified into five injury types, according to the Bismuth classification.
  - E1 and E2 (Figure 13–2E) injuries involve common hepatic duct transection.
  - E3 (Figure 13–2F) and E4 (Figure 13–2G) injuries are complex hilar injuries, and may also be associated with hepatic artery injuries.

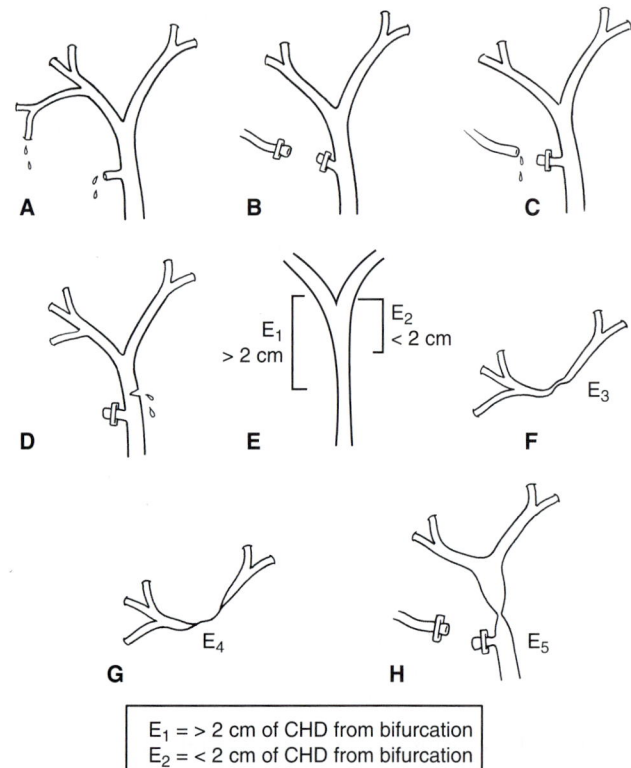

E_1 = > 2 cm of CHD from bifurcation
E_2 = < 2 cm of CHD from bifurcation

Figure 13–2 A–H

- E5 (Figure 13–2H) injuries involve strictures of the common hepatic duct with an associated stricture or injury to an aberrant right sectorial duct.
- Biliary reconstruction, depending on the exact anatomy of the injury and viability of the remaining bile ducts, may involve a single biliary-enteric anastomosis or multiple anastomoses.

Injuries Identified at the Index Operation

- If an injury is suspected during a laparoscopic cholecystectomy, an intraoperative cholangiogram should be performed to identify the exact nature and extent of the injury.
- Consideration of immediate reconstruction should only be entertained by surgeons with sufficient training and experience in managing complex operative and nonoperative hepatobiliary problems.
- The area should be widely drained with Jackson-Pratt or Blake drains. Proximal bile ducts should be marked, if possible, with careful attention to avoid worsening the injury.
- Retrograde external biliary drainage catheters should be avoided.
- A hepatobiliary surgeon or a tertiary referral center should be contacted and the patient transferred as quickly as possible. Reconstructions performed for even complex injuries within 72 hours have been successful in our experience.
- The relevant workup (as outlined in Figure 13–1) should be performed expeditiously to enable the patient to proceed to a well-planned reconstruction within 72 hours.
- For biliary reconstruction, a retrocolic Roux-en-Y biliary-enteric anastomosis is our preferred method, and is described later.

Delayed Reconstruction

- The right upper quadrant and the liver hilum can be accessed through a variety of incisions. We attempt to use a previous incision, otherwise a Kocher incision or upper midline offers adequate exposure.
- Right upper quadrant and upper abdominal adhesions may be present and should be taken down sharply.
- Careful dissection of the hepatoduodenal ligament is necessary.
- Palpation of the porta hepatis for the biliary catheters assists in identification of the injured bile ducts in a scarred field. Intraoperative ultrasound may be helpful in identifying the hepatic artery and portal vein.
- The bile duct should be dissected sharply in a distal to proximal direction.
- Large lymphatics should be ligated.
- Careful attention must be paid to avoid injuring or ligating hepatic artery branches, which often run anterior to the right and left bile ducts.
  - In particular, the left hepatic artery travels anterior to the left hepatic duct.
  - Right hepatic arteries may also run anterior to the right duct but may have been ligated at the index operation due to misidentification.
- The Roux limb is constructed by dividing the jejunum and its mesentery approximately 15–20 cm from the ligament of Treitz. A GIA stapler is used to divide the bowel, and the crossing mesenteric vessels are ligated with silk sutures.
- The hepatic flexure of the colon is mobilized in the usual fashion.
- A window is opened behind the hepatic flexure of the colon, anterior to the duodenum, between the middle colic and right colic arteries.
- The Roux limb is delivered to the liver hilum through this window, with careful attention to avoid twisting the mesentery.
- **Figure 13–3:** Dissection of the biliary tree at the liver hilum. The injured bile ducts are visible and have been dissected with the assistance of preoperatively placed biliary catheters.
- The distal common bile duct is suture-ligated or oversewn.
- The Roux limb is also pictured, and is placed without tension near the hilum of the liver against the transected bile duct.
- Depending on the type of injury, exploration of the distal common bile duct prior to ligation may be warranted.
  - The goal is to identify and treat choledocholithiasis in the distal duct.
  - This may be achieved by incising the duct and inserting a choledochoscope, visually inspecting the duct, and removing the stones. The duct may then be closed.

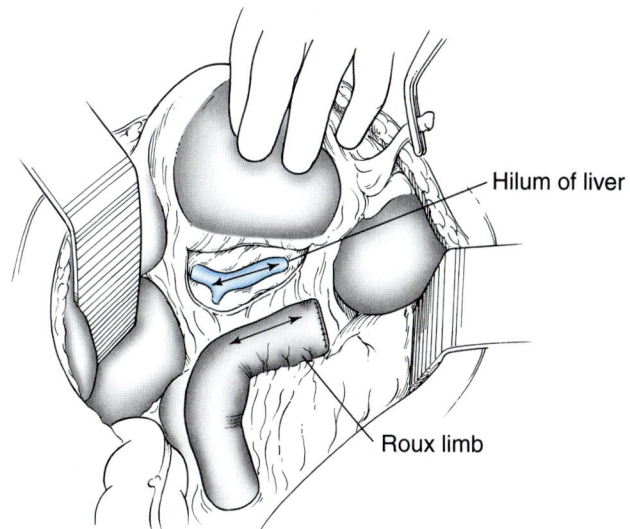

Figure 13–3

- Splitting the liver may be necessary if adequate length or exposure of the bile duct is not achieved. This division is very helpful in accessing the right anterior bile duct.
  - Dissection proceeds proximally along the interlobar plane anterior to the hilum.
  - A short distance of liver dissection may yield sufficient bile duct length and exposure for reconstruction.
- Preoperatively placed external or internal biliary drains can be helpful if maintained postoperatively in several situations.
  - Postoperative edema may cause poor bile drainage, and external drainage may be warranted.
  - Anastomotic leaks or strictures may develop, requiring external biliary drainage and stenting.
  - Technically difficult biliary-enteric anastomosis may lead to these situations.
  - Interrogation of the anastomosis may be clinically warranted postoperatively, and catheter access to the biliary tree is extremely helpful.
  - The preoperative external or internal biliary drain is transected approximately 1–2 cm proximal to the intended anastomosis or may be retained through the anastomosis.
- Bile cultures should be obtained upon entering the proximal biliary tree.
- **Figure 13–4A:** The biliary-enteric anastomosis. Creation of the anastomosis involves a few key points:
  - Bile duct spatulation.
  - Biliary-enteric alignment.
  - Tension-free approximation.
  - Every attempt should be made to maximize the circumference of the biliary-enteric anastomosis by spatulating the bile duct. This may be accomplished by incising the bile duct longitudinally on the anterior aspect of the bile duct. Careful attention should be paid to avoid shortening the length of the duct.
  - The bowel is aligned with the spatulated duct and sharply incised in the diameter of the duct on its antimesenteric surface.
  - We do not recommend spatulating the right and left ducts and syndactylizing them for long distances (> 1 cm) proximal to the anastomosis. Syndactylizing the right and left hepatic ducts only at the point where they are closest will allow a single large anastomosis, rather than two small ones.
  - The anastomosis is performed in an interrupted fashion using 4-0 PDS sutures. The anterior sutures should be placed on the bile duct first, with the needles left on. These sutures may act as a handle to expose the posterior wall.
  - The posterior wall is then completed, and the knots are tied in the lumen after all the back row stitches are placed.
- **Figure 13–4B:** Front wall of the biliary-enteric anastomosis.
  - Once the back wall is complete, the front wall is closed in a similar fashion. The knots are tied on the outside.

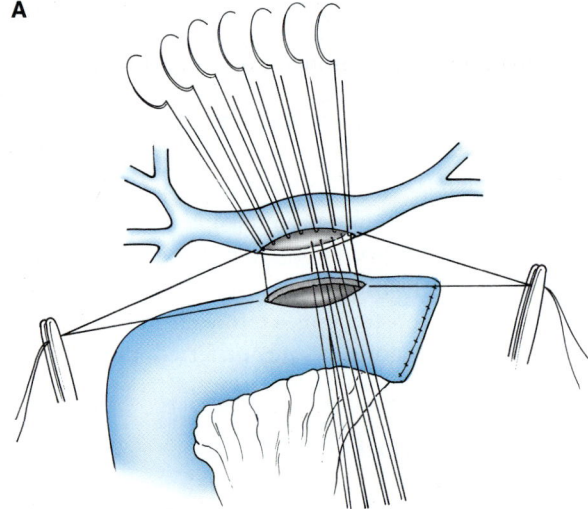

Figure 13–4A

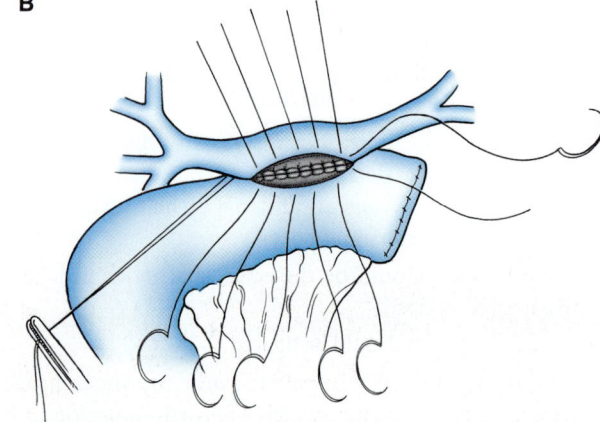

Figure 13–4B

- **Figure 13–5:** Roux-en-Y hepaticojejunostomy. The use of tacking sutures from the Roux limb to the liver capsule anteriorly reduces tension on the bowel.
  - The mesocolon should also be tacked to the serosa of the Roux limb to prevent internal hernias.
  - The enteroenterostomy is constructed 40 cm from the anastomosis, which may be performed using a hand-sewn or stapled technique.
  - A 10-mm Jackson-Pratt drain is typically used, and is placed in Morrison's pouch. The drain is not placed against the anastomosis.
  - If internal or external biliary drains have been removed in the operating room, and the exit tracts from the liver are exposed, drains are placed near these holes. These tracts drain bile until they heal, and drains placed in the operating room control these leaks well.

POSTOPERATIVE CARE

Antibiotics
- Systemic antibiotics are administered and tailored according to the bile culture from the operating room sample.

Deep Vein Thrombosis Prophylaxis
- Pharmacologic deep vein thrombosis prophylaxis is routine with subcutaneous unfractionated or low-molecular-weight heparin.
- Early ambulation should be encouraged.

Drain Management
- Drains are monitored for bilious output and are removed if bilious drainage is not present following advancement to a regular diet.
- Persistent bilious drain output (drain fluid bilirubin level > 3.0 mg/dL) should warrant cholangiography on or after postoperative day 4.
  - If an anastomotic leak is detected, the external or internal biliary drains can be exchanged if needed, and advanced past the anastomosis. Percutaneous drains control the ongoing peritoneal contamination.
  - After 6 weeks, cholangiography should be repeated. If the leak has resolved, the drains can be removed.

Biliary Duct Catheters
- External or internal biliary drain catheters should be removed 6 weeks after surgery if there is no evidence of an anastomotic leak.
- If a leak is suspected, cholangiography should be performed through the biliary drain catheter. If a leak is present, the drain catheter should be exchanged for an appropriately sized catheter, and it should be advanced through the anastomosis.
- After 6 more weeks, a repeat cholangiogram should be performed. If the leak has resolved, the catheters can be removed.

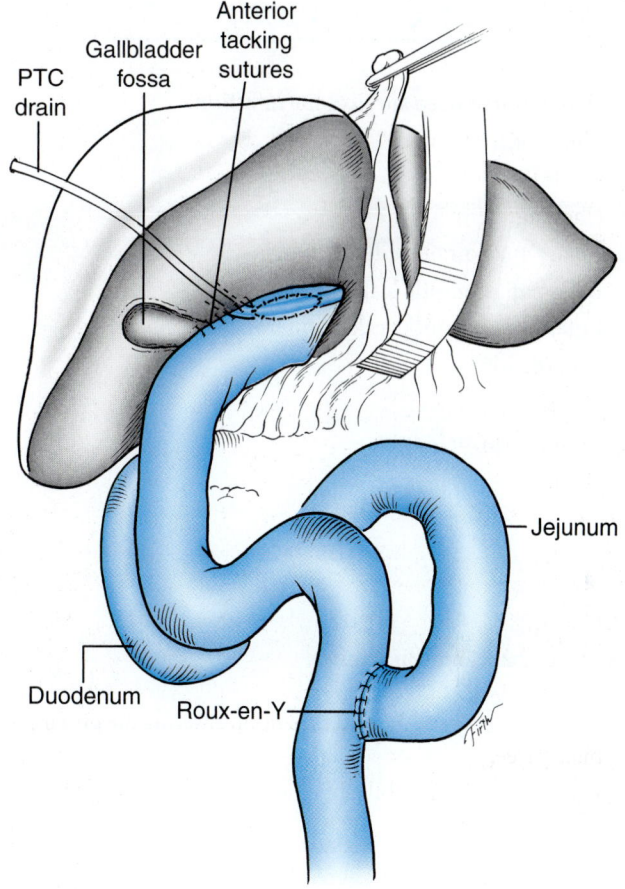

Figure 13–5

POTENTIAL COMPLICATIONS

Early
- Superficial or deep surgical site infection.
- Bleeding.
- Bile leak.
- Cholangitis.
- Biliary anastomotic edema.
- Biliary anastomotic leak.
- Enteric anastomotic leak or enterocutaneous fistula.
- Pancreatitis.
- Sepsis.
- Multiple organ failure.
- Death.

Late
- Stricture.
- Cholangitis.
- Intrahepatic bile duct stones.
- Liver abscess.
- Varices.
- Biliary cirrhosis.
- Portal hypertension.
- Further biliary injury related to ischemia or technical issues from repeated attempts at reconstruction, resulting in non-reconstructible anatomy. These patients should be referred for liver transplant evaluation.

PEARLS AND TIPS

- Reconstruction of iatrogenic biliary injuries that are diagnosed during the index operation should only be undertaken by hepatobiliary surgeons, or those who have training or expertise in the operative and nonoperative management of complex hepatobiliary problems.
  - Wide drainage and expedient contact of a referral center or appropriately trained or experienced surgeon is warranted and optimally done while in the operating room with the patient on the table.
  - Clear communication with receiving surgeons is imperative.
- Nonoperative management of the iatrogenic biliary injuries aims to identify the extent of the injury anatomically, followed by biliary decompression with drainage to prevent ongoing cholestatic liver injury and provide relief of cholangitis.
- Some short segment strictures may be managed nonoperatively with PTC tube or ERCP-placed stents and interval dilation, with reasonable rates of resolution.
- Metal wall stents should not be used in the biliary tree for benign strictures.
- Identification of the injured bile duct is difficult in an inflamed or scarred liver hilum; preoperative PTC or endobiliary drain placement facilitates this maneuver.
- Appropriate biliary drainage and delayed operation lead to the best results from biliary reconstruction.
- Retrocolic Roux-en-Y biliary-enteric anastomosis is the preferred approach for reconstruction. Anastomotic tension can be relieved by securing the Roux limb to the liver capsule.
- Spatulation of the bile duct decreases the risk of postoperative anastomotic strictures.
- Maintenance of the external or internal biliary drain is useful for potential evaluation of bile leaks.

REFERENCES

Cameron JL, Sandone C. *Atlas of Gastrointestinal Surgery*, 2nd ed, vol 1. Hamilton, ON: BC Decker; 2007.

Colletti LM. Complications of Biliary Injury. In: Mulholland MW, Doherty GM, eds. *Complications in Surgery*. Philadelphia, PA: Lippincott Williams & Wilkins; 2006:999–1014.

Lillemoe KD. Biliary Injuries and Strictures and Sclerosing Cholangitis. In: Mulholland MW, Lillemoe KD, Doherty GM, et al, eds. *Greenfield's Surgery: Scientific Principles & Practice*, 4th ed. Philadelphia, PA: Lippincott Williams & Wilkins; 2006:1310–1334.

Strasberg SM. Avoidance of biliary injury during laparoscopic cholecystectomy. *J Hepatobiliary Pancreat Surg*. 2002;9:543–547.

CHAPTER 14

Hepatectomy

Theodore H. Welling, III, MD

INDICATIONS

- Metastasis (colon, breast, neuroendocrine).
- Hepatocellular carcinoma.
- Cholangiocarcinoma.
- Hepatoblastoma.
- Gallbladder carcinoma.
- Hepatic sarcoma.
- Adenoma.
- Biliary cystadenoma.
- Symptomatic hemangioma or focal nodular hyperplasia.
- Hepatic tumor of unknown etiology.

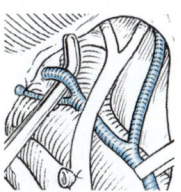 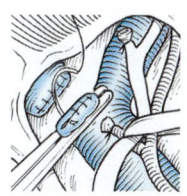 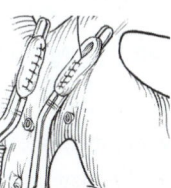
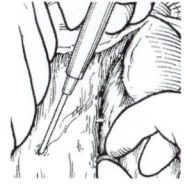 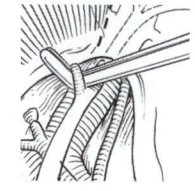 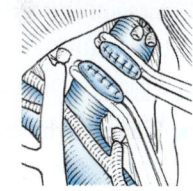
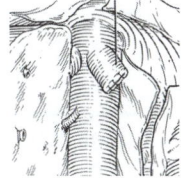 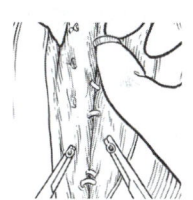 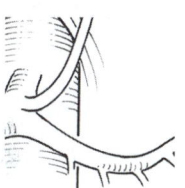

CONTRAINDICATIONS

- Distant metastatic disease for primary liver tumors.
- Presence of extrahepatic metastases for metastatic lesions (relative).
- Severe medical comorbidity.
- Inability to achieve negative margins.
- Insufficient estimated liver remnant following resection.
- Significant cirrhosis or portal hypertension.

INFORMED CONSENT

Expected Benefits

- Surgical treatment of primary and metastatic hepatic malignancies.
- Treatment of symptomatic benign hepatic mass.

Potential Risks

- Bleeding requiring reoperation or transfusion.
- Infection or abscess.
- Embolic events.
- Bile leak or stricture.
- Tumor recurrence.
- Possibility of unexpected findings intraoperatively.

- Need for additional tests or procedures.
- Hepatic dysfunction or failure.
- Death.

EQUIPMENT

- Intraoperative ultrasound equipment.
- Self-retaining retractor (eg, Omni or Thompson).
- Electrocautery, Cavitron Ultrasonic Surgical Aspirator (CUSA), Hydrojet, automatic clip applier, and possibly Tissue Link, LigaSure, or SonoSurg devices, depending on surgeon preference.

PATIENT PREPARATION

- Nothing by mouth the evening before surgery.
- Preoperative antibiotics.
- Adequate intravenous access (at least two > 16G intravenous lines and central venous pressure [CVP] line at the surgeon's discretion).
- Foley catheter.
- Orogastric tube decompression.
- Anesthesiology consultation and coordination.

PATIENT POSITIONING

- The patient should be supine with arms extended.

PROCEDURE

- **Figure 14–1:** Familiarity with hepatic segmental anatomy is important (Couinaud) to allow for resection planning along with intraoperative ultrasound.
- **Figure 14–2A, B:** Important vascular landmarks for planning of anatomic resections showing hepatic veins and main portal venous branches. Planes of transection for major hepatectomies are as follows:
  - Right lobectomy, right trisegmentectomy (extended right lobectomy) (Figure 14–2A).
  - Left lobectomy, left trisegmentectomy (extended left lobectomy), and left lateral segmentectomy (Figure 14–2B).
- **Figure 14–3:** Right hepatic lobectomy or extended right hepatic lobectomy. Identification and isolation of the right hepatic artery and right hepatic duct.
- **Figure 14–4:** Right hepatic lobectomy or extended right hepatic lobectomy. Identification of right portal vein.
  - Biliary and vascular structures can be divided before hepatic transection or after, depending on surgeon preference.
  - The portal vein should be oversewn with Prolene suture or secured with a vascular stapler.

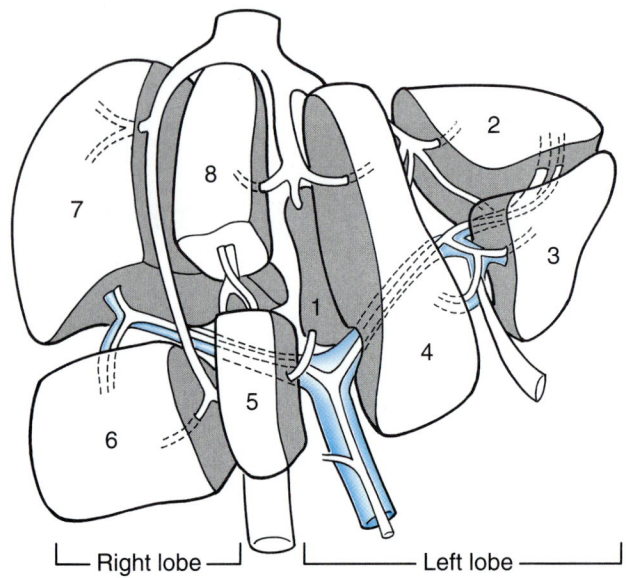

Figure 14–1

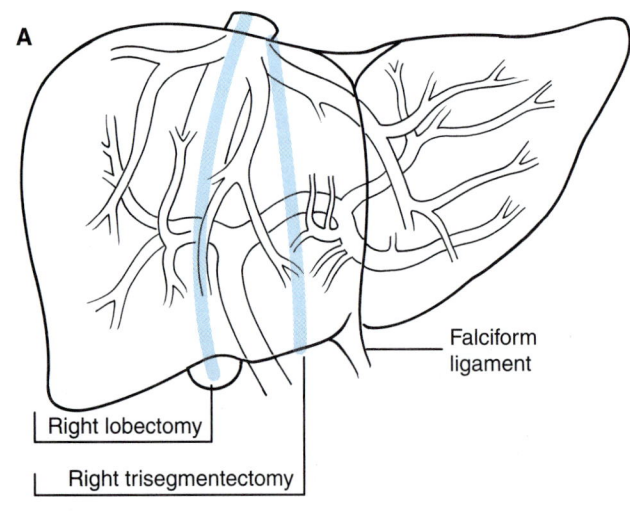

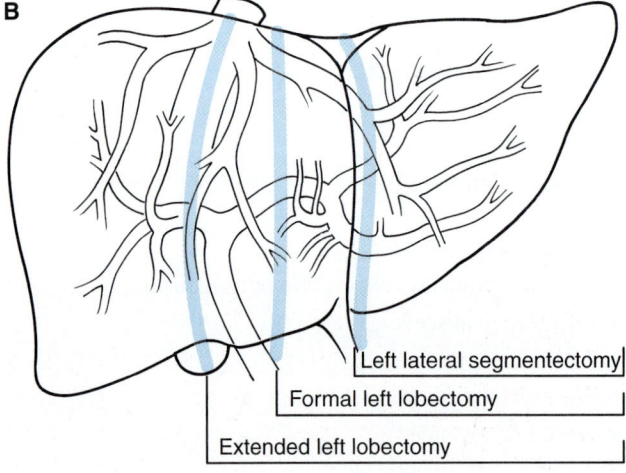

Figure 14–2A–B

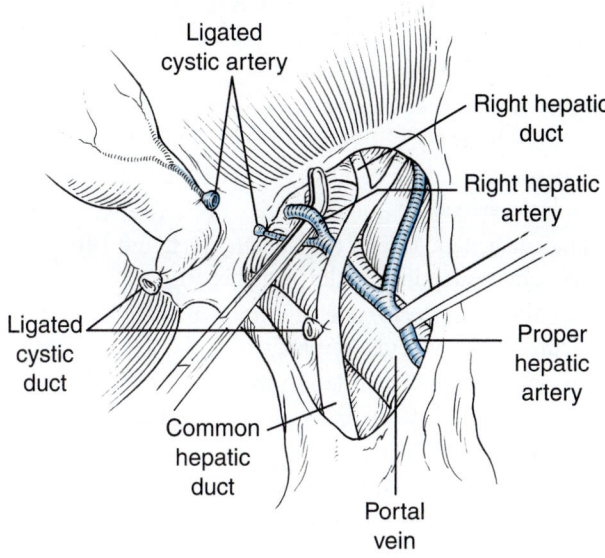

Figure 14–3

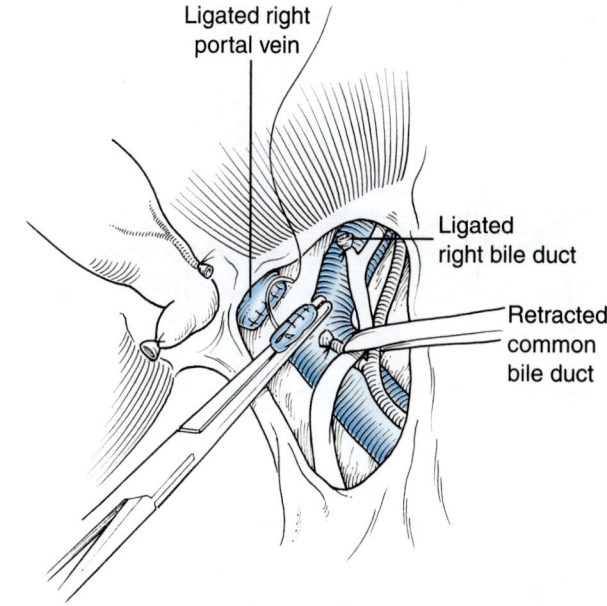

Figure 14–4

- **Figure 14–5:** Right hepatic lobectomy or extended right hepatic lobectomy.
  - Additional mobilization of the right hepatic lobe is performed by reflecting it lateral to medial.
  - Caudate hepatic vein branches as well as accessory right hepatic venous branches are ligated.
  - The right hepatic vein can be divided before or during parenchymal dissection and oversewn with Prolene or secured with a vascular stapler.
- **Figure 14–6:** Right hepatic lobectomy.
  - Parenchymal transection is performed by using vascular demarcation (if inflow is divided) or along the transection plane as detailed in Figure 14–2 (marked by ultrasound).
  - Transection is performed under intermittent inflow occlusion and maintaining a low CVP (3–7 mm Hg). Manual compression can also minimize blood loss from small hepatic veins.
  - Transection is initiated with electrocautery followed by CUSA or Hydrojet dissection to identify vascular or biliary radicals. These can be divided with autoclips, ligature, cautery, or Tissue Link device, depending on size.
- **Figure 14–7:** Right extended hepatic lobectomy.
  - Maneuvers are carried out as in Figures 14–3 through 14–5 with the addition of identification of portal branches to segment 4, which can be taken during parenchymal dissection or extrahepatically if desired.

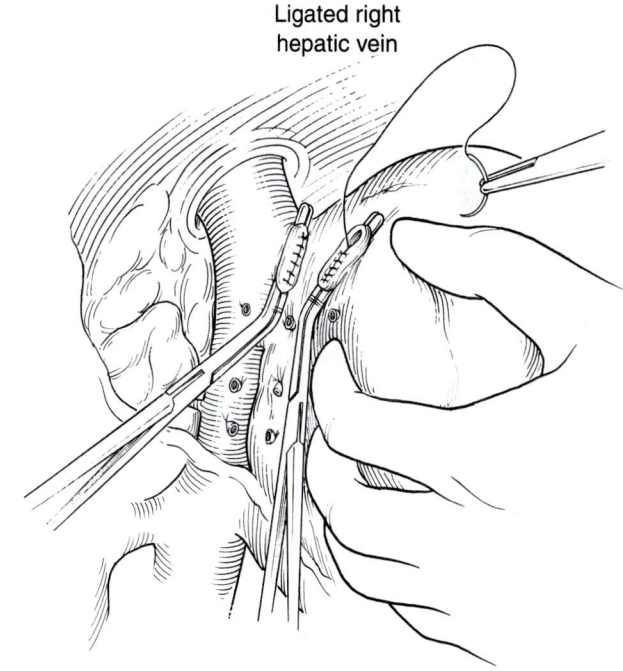

Figure 14–5

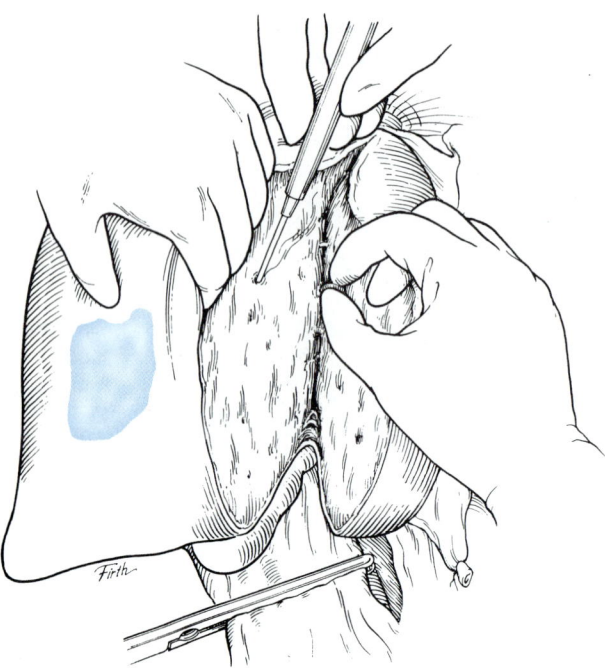

Figure 14–6

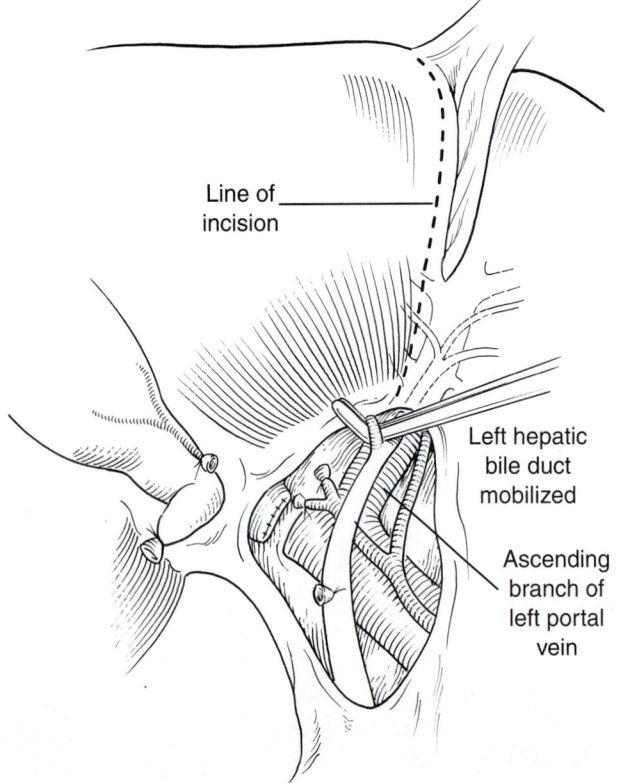

Figure 14–7

- The line of parenchymal dissection should proceed to the right of the falciform ligament, preserving the ascending branch of the left portal vein.
- **Figure 14–8:** Left hepatic lobectomy or extended left hepatic lobectomy.
  - The pars flaccida is divided, along with any accessory or replaced arterial anatomy.
  - The left hepatic artery, left hepatic duct, and left portal vein can be identified in the porta hepatis.
  - The left portal vein can be oversewn with Prolene or secured with a vascular stapler.
- **Figure 14–9:** Left hepatic lobectomy.
  - The parenchyma is divided as in Figure 14–6, with division of the left hepatic vein performed usually during parenchymal dissection and secured by oversewing with Prolene suture or securing with a vascular stapler.
- **Figure 14–10:** Left lateral segmentectomy.
  - No vascular dissection is required.
  - The parenchymal dissection plane should be along the medial side of the falciform ligament, preserving the ascending branch of the left portal vein.
- **Figure 14–11:** Hepatic artery perfusion catheter placement.
  - If regional chemotherapy is considered, the common and proper hepatic arteries are dissected free.
  - The left and right gastric arteries are ligated along with supraduodenal branches.
  - The distal gastroduodenal artery is ligated and cannulated proximally and secured in place such that the catheter tip is located at the orifice of the gastroduodenal artery.

POSTOPERATIVE CARE

- Adequacy of resuscitation should be monitored closely, and any concern for bleeding should be promptly evaluated.
- Assessment of liver function should be followed closely in the postoperative period (neurologic status, coagulation factors, liver function tests).
- Benzodiazepines and hepatotoxic medications should be avoided in the early postoperative period.
- Deep vein thrombosis prophylaxis should be provided.
- Oral diet can be advanced as tolerated; if not tolerated, other forms of enteral nutrition should be initiated.
- Close monitoring for possible complications is required (see later).

POTENTIAL COMPLICATIONS

- Bleeding.
- Bile leak.

Chapter 14 : Hepatectomy • 119

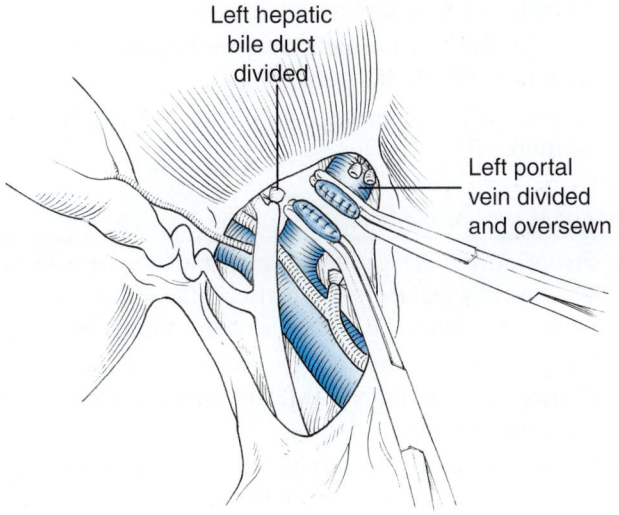

Figure 14–8

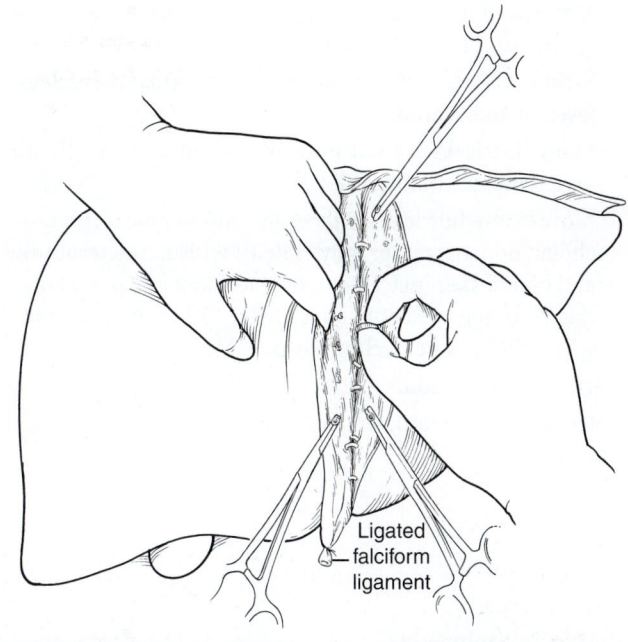

Figure 14–10

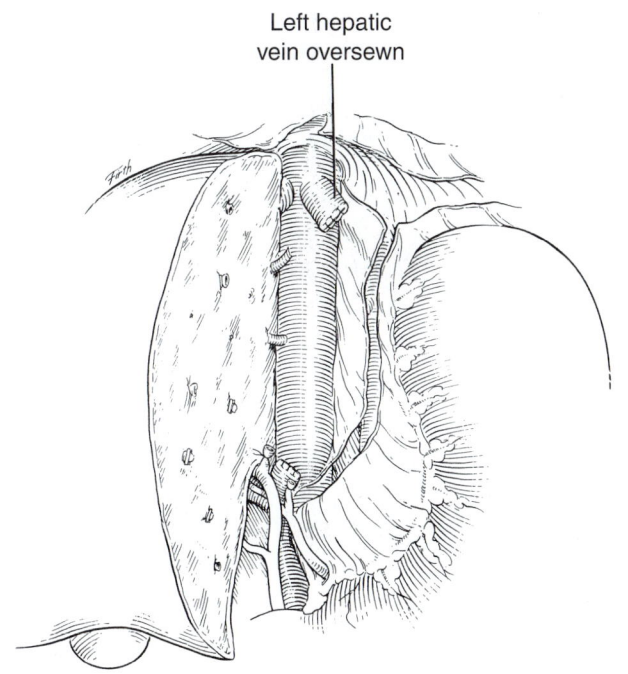

Figure 14–9

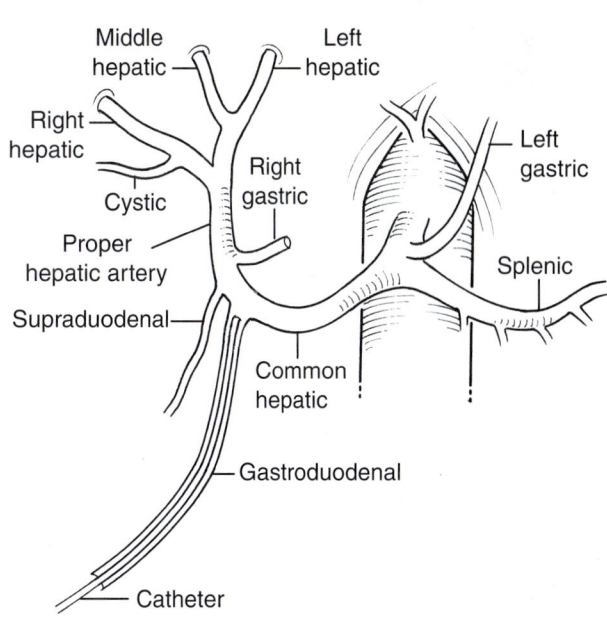

Branches of Hepatic Artery

Figure 14–11

- Manifested by bile staining in drains or evidence of cholestasis on liver function tests.
- Symptoms may involve increased abdominal pain, ileus, fever, or tachycardia.
- Many bile leaks are self limited and can be treated with percutaneous drainage alone.
- More severe bile leaks will require endoscopic retrograde cholangiopancreatography (ERCP) with sphincterotomy and biliary stent placement, or placement of a percutaneous transhepatic cholangiocatheter (PTC) in situations where ERCP is not technically possible.

■ Abscess or infection.

■ Hepatic dysfunction, which can be manifested by the following:
- Acidosis.
- Impaired mental status.
- Hypoglycemia.
- Coagulopathy.
- Hyperbilirubinemia.
- Transaminitis.
- Renal failure.
- Predisposition to infection.
- Care is primarily supportive, but evaluation should be performed to exclude major biliary or vascular complications.

■ Tumor recurrence.

■ Embolism (usually intraoperative).
- Can be diagnosed using intraoperative transesophageal echocardiography if necessary.
- Prevented by optimizing CVP during parenchymal dissection.

PEARLS AND TIPS

■ Preoperative imaging using CT angiography or triple phase CT is usually required. Alternatively MRI with contrast is useful, especially in cases of hepatocellular carcinoma.

■ Preoperative PTC cholangiogram or magnetic resonance cholangiopancreatogram (MRCP) may be required in cases of cholangiocarcinoma.

■ Perform portal lymph node dissection in cases of cholangiocarcinoma or gallbladder carcinoma.

■ Use of intraoperative ultrasound should be routine as it often alters the planned operative management.

REFERENCES

Blumgart LH, Fong Y, eds. *Surgery of the Liver and Biliary Tract*, 3rd ed. Philadelphia, PA: Saunders; 2006.

Knol JA. Complications of Hepatic Surgery. In: Mulholland MW, Doherty GM, eds. *Complications in Surgery*. Philadelphia, PA: Lippincott Williams & Wilkins; 2006.

Warren KW, Jenkins RL, Steele G, eds. *Atlas of Surgery of the Liver, Pancreas, and Biliary Tract*. Norwalk, CT: Appleton & Lange; 1991.

CHAPTER 15

Pancreaticoduodenectomy

Nicholas H. Osborne, MD, and Lisa M. Colletti, MD

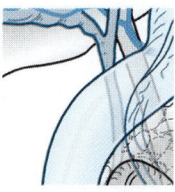 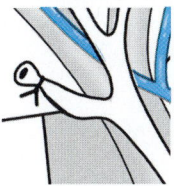 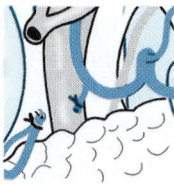
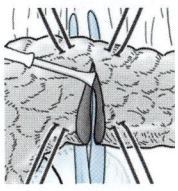 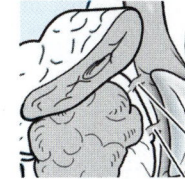 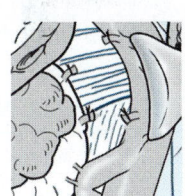
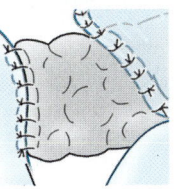

INDICATIONS

- Malignant lesions involving the head of pancreas, ampulla of Vater, distal end of the common bile duct, or duodenum.
  - Absence of metastasis.
  - Absence of arterial involvement.
- Refractory severe pain from chronic pancreatitis.
  - Refractory to medical therapy.
  - Repeat hospital admissions.
  - Majority of disease limited to the head of the pancreas.

CONTRAINDICATIONS

Absolute

- Evidence of metastatic disease.
- Evidence of para-aortic nodes outside the field of dissection.
- Involvement of the aorta or vena cava.
- Involvement of the superior mesenteric artery, hepatic artery, or celiac axis.

Relative

- Cardiopulmonary comorbidities.

INFORMED CONSENT

- Survival following resection of periampullary and pancreatic lesions depends on the site of the primary tumor and stage.
  - The overall 5-year survival rate is 20–30% but may be significantly better in patients with limited disease burden.
  - Using prognostic modeling, a patient with a well-differentiated small tumor (1 cm) and no nodal involvement would have a 50% 5-year survival.
  - A patient with a poorly differentiated lesion > 4 cm and 10 positive lymph nodes would have an estimated 10% 3-year survival rate.

Expected Benefits
- To remove malignancies involving the head of the pancreas, ampulla, distal common bile duct, or duodenum while restoring continuity of the biliary-pancreatic system.

Potential Risks
- Surgical site infections (superficial or deep, abscess).
- Bleeding.
- Pneumonia.
- Cardiovascular events.
- Venous thromboembolism.
- Delayed gastric emptying (15–40% of patients).
- Anastomotic leak (most commonly from the pancreaticojejunal anastomosis).
- Abscess.
- Biloma.
- Pseudocyst.
- Pancreatic fistulas.
- Incomplete resection and positive margins.

EQUIPMENT
- General surgery instrument tray.
- Self-retaining abdominal retractor to aid exposure.
- A surgical energy device (eg, harmonic scalpel or LigaSure) is useful for dividing the jejunal mesentery.
- Gastrointestinal anastomosis (GIA) stapler.
- Thoracoabdominal (TA) stapler.

PATIENT PREPARATION
- Assessment of tumor resectability.
  - Fine-cut (3-mm) pancreatic protocol CT.
  - MRI and magnetic resonance cholangiopancreatography (MRCP) can be useful to clarify the relationship of the tumor to the blood vessels and biliary system.
  - Endoscopic retrograde cholangiopancreatography (ERCP) should be reserved for patients with obstructive jaundice and no mass noted on CT.
  - ERCP with stent placement may be used for deeply jaundiced patients.
  - Endoscopic ultrasound (EUS) is helpful in assessing lymph node involvement and relationship to the major vasculature.
- Assessment of cardiovascular risk.

PATIENT POSITIONING
- The patient should be supine.
- The entire abdomen is shaved and prepped.

- The abdomen is entered through a midline incision or bilateral subcostal "Chevron" incision, depending on surgeon preference.

PROCEDURE

- The procedure can be divided into three stages: assessment of resectability, resection, and reestablishment of continuity.
- **Figure 15–1:** The round ligament and falciform ligaments are divided to provide adequate exposure.
  - A Kocher maneuver is performed initially to expose the proximal duodenum and pancreas and ensure that no direct extension of the tumor involves the aorta or inferior vena cava.
  - The duodenum is retracted medially under tension, and the peritoneum is incised along the lateral edge of the duodenum.
  - The retroperitoneum is entered carefully to avoid injury to the vena cava.
  - The gastrocolic omentum is divided and the lesser sac is entered to expose the anterior surface of the pancreas.

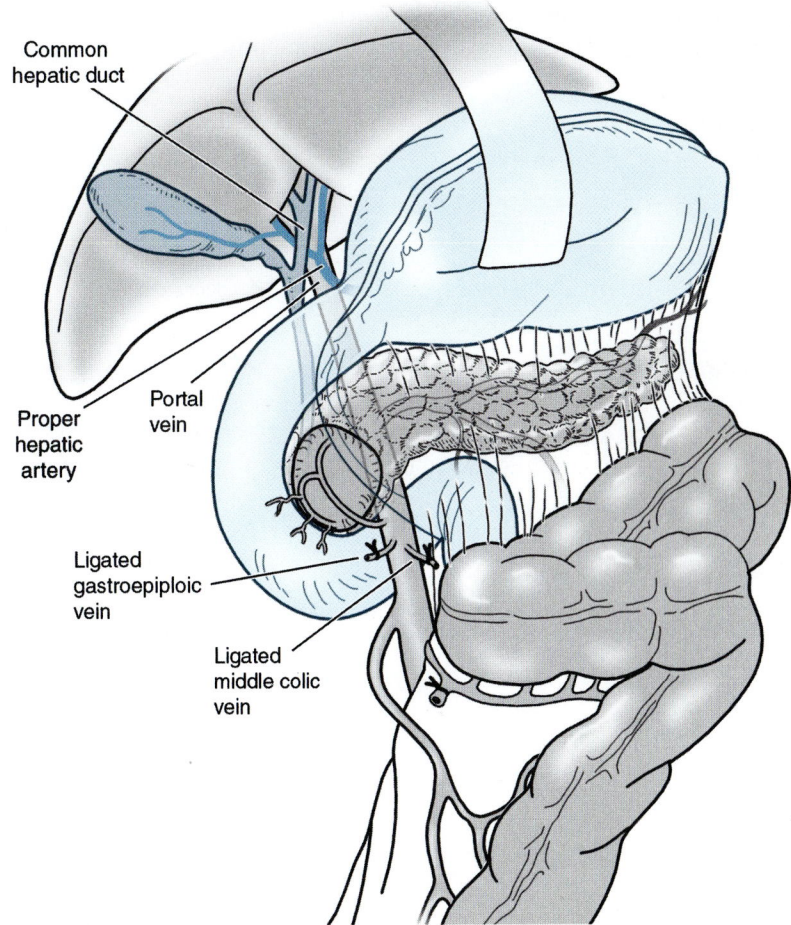

Figure 15–1

- The right and transverse colon is reflected completely down to expose the entire inferior portion of the pancreas. During this step the gastroepiploic vein is ligated and divided, and the middle colic vein can also be divided if necessary to facilitate exposure of the inferior border of the pancreas.
- A cholecystectomy is performed in the standard fashion.
- After appropriate exposure, the resectability of the lesion is assessed.

■ **Figure 15–2:** The hepatoduodenal ligament is dissected to expose the common bile duct and hepatic artery.
- The anterior surface of the portal vein is usually identified by careful dissection between the common bile duct and hepatic artery.
- The gastroduodenal artery should also be identified along the anterior surface of the pancreas, beneath the first portion of the duodenum, and its takeoff from the common hepatic artery should be carefully identified.
- The portal vein is freed from the posterior surface of the neck of the pancreas using careful blunt dissection.
- The middle colic vein should be identified and followed down to the inferior border of the pancreas to help identify the superior mesenteric vein, as shown in Figure 15–1.
- Additional careful dissection should be performed to create a "tunnel" under the neck of the pancreas, demonstrating

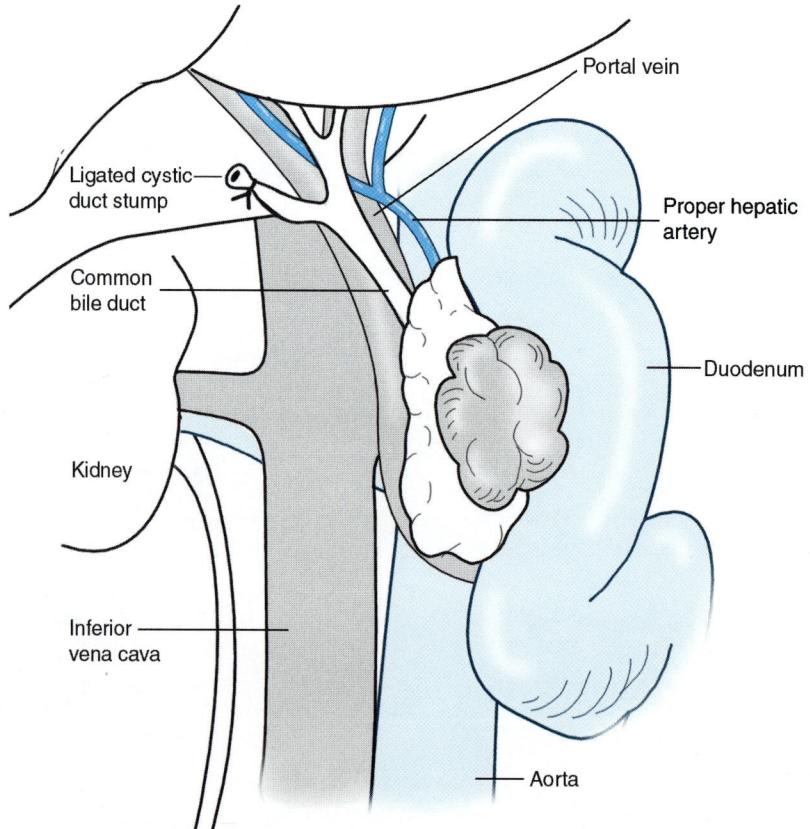

Figure 15–2

that the plane between the neck of the pancreas and the portal vein and superior mesenteric vein is free and that there is no evidence of tumor involvement.
- Alternatively, the right and transverse colon can be extensively mobilized, allowing identification of the superior mesenteric vein as it crosses over the third portion of the duodenum and goes under the neck of the pancreas.
- No further dissection, and more specifically, no structures should be divided prior to confirming that the vein is free of tumor involvement, unless the surgeon is prepared to proceed with en bloc vein resection.

■ **Figure 15–3:** The antrum of the stomach is stapled and divided using the landmarks of a Billroth I hemigastrectomy.
- The hepatic artery within the hepatoduodenal ligament is palpated and dissected free to identify the gastroduodenal and right gastric vessels, which can be doubly ligated and divided.
- Prior to division of the gastroduodenal artery, it is important to briefly occlude this artery ("pinch test") while palpating the hepatic artery to confirm that there is no decrease in the hepatic arterial flow.
- On occasion, in individuals with a celiac stenosis or other congenital arterial anomalies, the majority of the hepatic arterial blood flow may come via collateral vessels through the gastroduodenal artery. Although rare, hepatic necrosis can occur in these patients following division of the gastroduodenal artery. In such cases, a Whipple procedure is contraindicated unless hepatic arterial flow can be reestablished via other mechanisms, including possible arterial bypass or endovascular intervention.

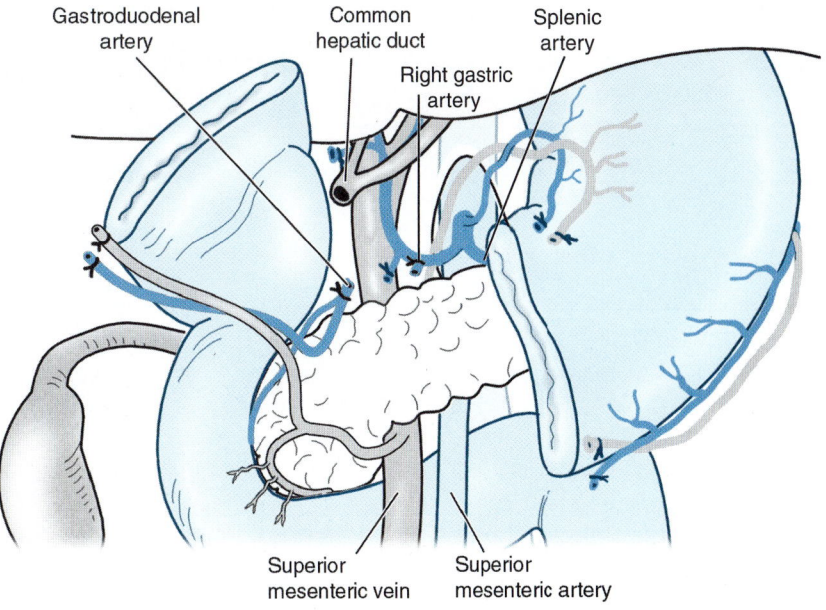

Figure 15–3

- The proximal stomach is packed away in the left upper quadrant, and the distal stomach is retracted inferiorly and to the right to aid exposure of the common bile duct.
- The common bile duct is divided and the distal end is ligated using a silk suture.
- The proximal common bile duct can be occluded temporarily with a Bulldog clamp.

■ **Figure 15–4:** The duodenum is dissected free from the ligament of Treitz.
- Multiple small feeding arteries and veins in the duodenal mesentery must be clamped and tied to minimize bleeding or sealed using a surgical energy device (eg, harmonic scalpel, LigaSure).
- The proximal jejunum is divided about 10 cm distal to the ligament of Treitz using a GIA stapler, and the jejunal mesentery is divided between clamps and ligated with silk sutures down to the level of the ligament of Treitz.

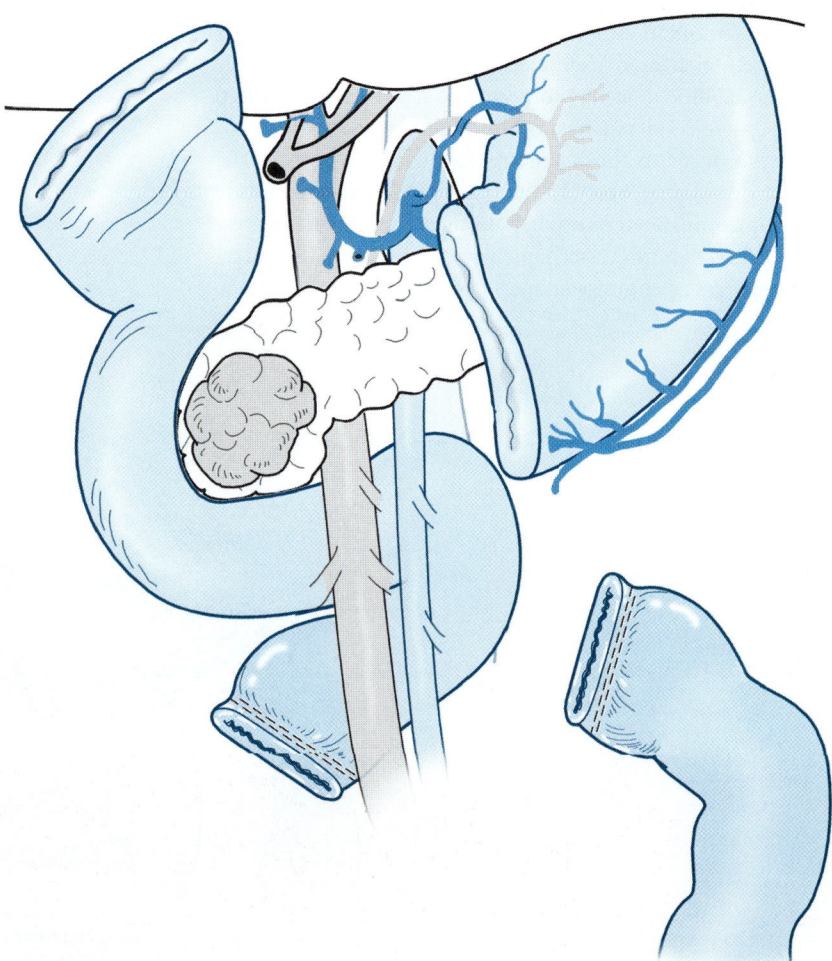

Figure 15–4

- The divided end of the jejunum can then be delivered beneath the mesentery of the small bowel.
- **Figure 15–5:** Hemostatic transfixion sutures are placed both inferiorly and superiorly in the pancreas body on either side of the line of planned transection.
  - The pancreas can be divided using electrocautery or sharply with a scalpel.
  - The pancreatic duct is identified, and any bleeding vessels are suture ligated with 4-0 or 5-0 Prolene.
- **Figure 15–6:** The uncinate process is dissected free from the superior mesenteric vein.
  - The superior and inferior pancreaticoduodenal veins are ligated and divided along with all other small branches that enter the lateral superior mesenteric and portal vein.

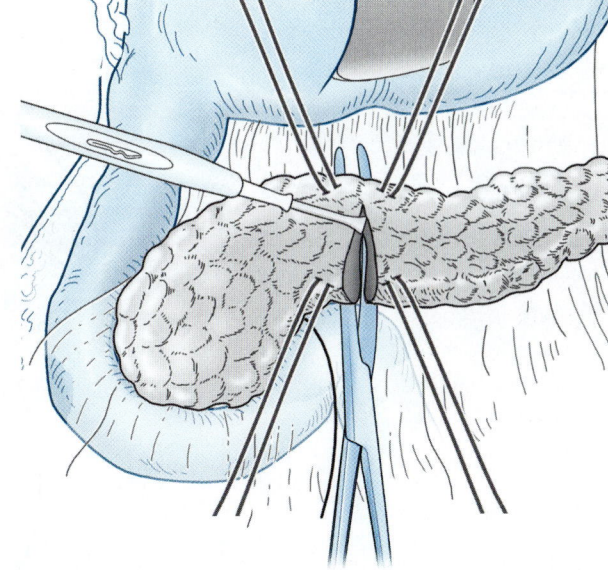

Figure 15–5

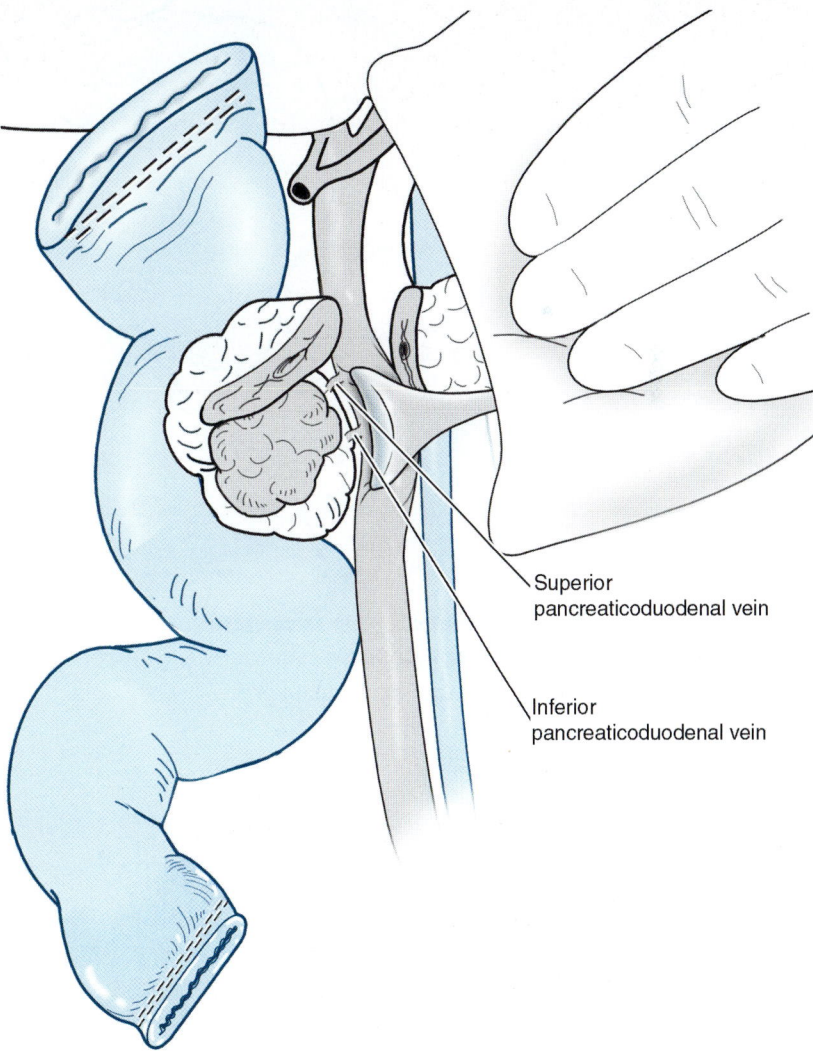

Figure 15–6

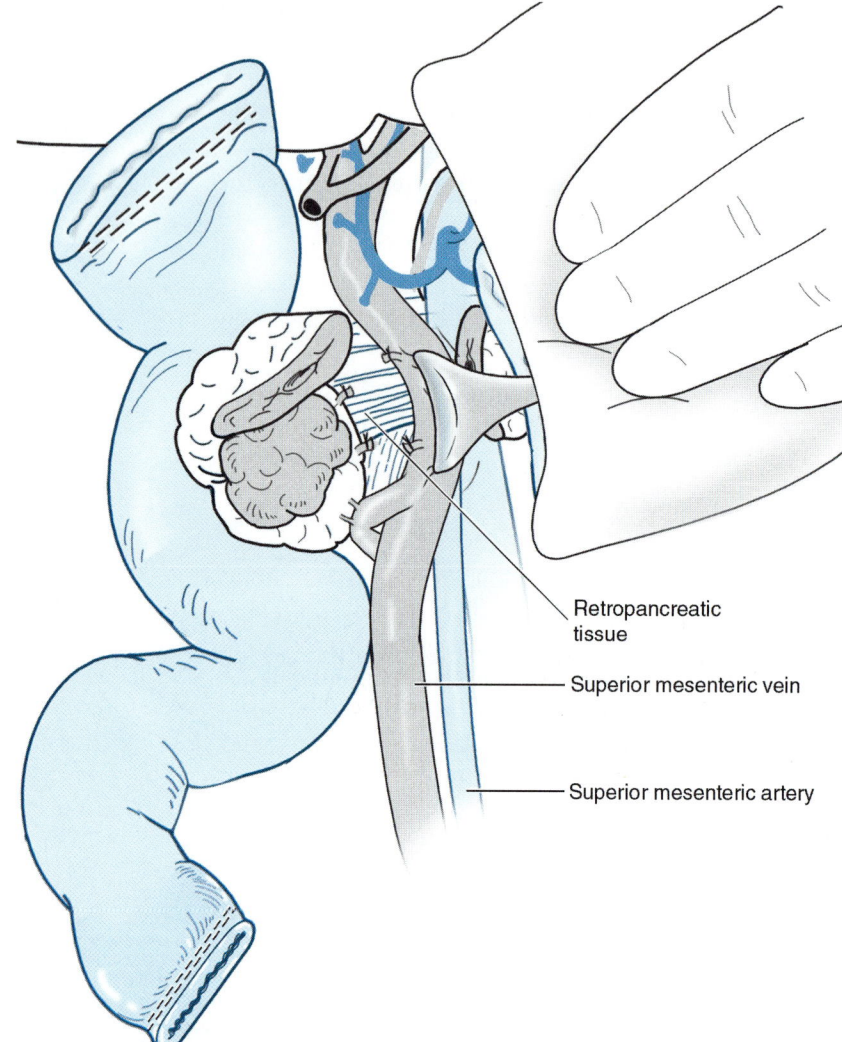

Figure 15–7

- **Figure 15–7:** The superior mesenteric vein is retracted medially, exposing the retropancreatic tissue.
  - The retropancreatic attachments to the uncinate process are then divided.
  - Either a TA stapler or traditional clamping and tying can be used. Clamping and tying is preferred for resection of malignancies. The TA stapler is preferred for benign disease.
  - The specimen, which should now be entirely free, should be sent for pathologic and frozen section examination of the biliary and pancreatic margins.
  - The retroperitoneal margin should be inked by the surgeon prior to sending the specimen for pathologic examination.

- **Figure 15–8:** The jejunal limb is delivered up to the right upper quadrant in a retrocolic fashion through an avascular window in the transverse mesocolon.
  - The pancreaticojejunostomy is performed using an end-to-side anastomosis.
  - The outer layer of the pancreaticojejunostomy is performed using interrupted 3-0 or 4-0 silk sutures between the capsule of the pancreas and the seromuscular layer of the jejunum.
  - The inner layer of the anastomosis is performed using interrupted absorbable suture (4-0 or 5-0 PDS or Vicryl) between the pancreatic duct and a full-thickness layer of jejunum.
  - Occasionally, a sterile 5 or 8 French pediatric feeding tube with extra side holes cut into it can be used to stent the pancreatic-jejunal anastomosis.
  - The choledochojejunostomy is subsequently performed in an end-to-side fashion using a singled layer of interrupted absorbable suture, such as 4-0 or 5-0 PDS or Vicryl.
  - The defect in the mesocolon is closed surrounding the delivered limb of jejunum to avoid internal herniation.
  - The gastrojejunostomy is then completed with an antecolic loop of jejunum and creation of a two-layered hand-sewn anastomosis.
  - The outer layer of the anastomosis is performed using interrupted seromuscular 3-0 silk sutures and the inner layer is a full-thickness running layer of 3-0 Vicryl or other absorbable suture.
  - The abdomen is copiously irrigated and two drains are placed within the abdominal cavity in apposition to the biliary and pancreatic anastomoses.
  - The midline incision is then closed using standard techniques.

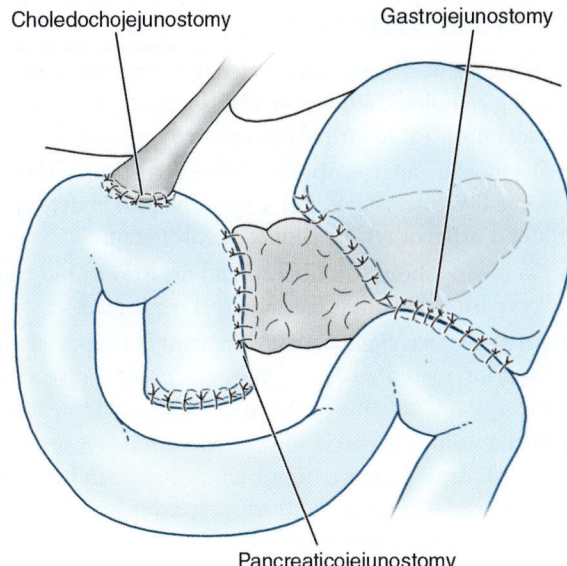

Figure 15–8

POSTOPERATIVE CARE

- Nothing by mouth with nasogastric tube decompression.
- Oral diet is advanced following removal of the nasogastric tube and once ileus has resolved, usually within 48–72 hours postoperatively.
- Monitoring of abdominal drain fluids for evidence of a biliary or pancreatic leak.

POTENTIAL COMPLICATIONS

- Delayed gastric emptying.
- Pancreatic leak.
- Surgical site infections.
- Gastroduodenal artery pseudoaneurysm.

PEARLS AND TIPS

- If metastatic disease is suspected but cannot be confirmed using radiologic studies or EUS, consider diagnostic laparoscopy prior to formal laparotomy.
- Diagnostic laparoscopy can detect carcinomatosis and some liver metastases, but it is not helpful in determining blood vessel or retroperitoneal involvement.
- No organs should be divided and no irreversible maneuvers performed until resectability is confirmed.
- If a patient has significant involvement of the portal vein or superior mesenteric vein, consider preoperative chemotherapy and radiation prior to an attempt at resection.
- Portal vein or superior mesenteric vein involvement does not render a patient's tumor unresectable, and an aggressive surgical approach with vein resection and reconstruction should be considered in appropriate patients.
- Perform a "pinch test" (eg, occlusion of the gastroduodenal artery) prior to division of the gastroduodenal artery to confirm that there is no significant arterial flow to the hepatic artery via collaterals through the gastroduodenal artery.

REFERENCES

Brennan MF, Kattan MW, Klimstra D, Conlon K. Prognostic nomogram for patients undergoing resection for adenocarcinoma of the pancreas. *Ann Surg.* 2004;240:293–298.

Nakeeb A, Lillemoe KD, Yeo CJ, Cameron JC. Neoplasms of the Exocrine Pancreas. In: Mulholland MW, Lillemoe KD, Doherty GM, et al, eds. *Greenfield's Surgery: Scientific Principles & Practice,* 4th ed. Philadelphia, PA: Lippincott Williams & Wilkins; 2006:861–879.

Simeone DM. Complications of Pancreatic Surgery. In: Mulholland MW, Doherty GM, eds. *Complications in Surgery.* Philadelphia, PA: Lippincott Williams & Wilkins; 2006:469–472.

CHAPTER 16

Distal Pancreatectomy

K. Barrett Deatrick, MD, and Gerard M. Doherty, MD

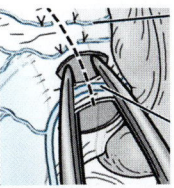 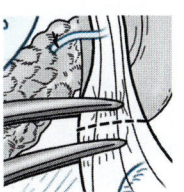 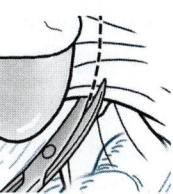
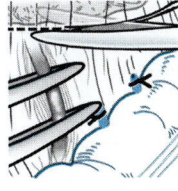 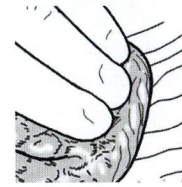 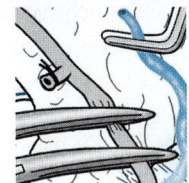
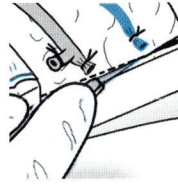 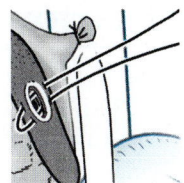

INDICATIONS

- Distal pancreatic solid mass.
  - Neuroendocrine tumor.
  - Pancreatic adenocarcinoma.
  - Solid neoplasm of indeterminate diagnosis.
- Distal pancreatic mucinous cystic neoplasms.
  - Asymptomatic, ≥ 3 cm in size.
  - Symptomatic, any size.
  - Presence of a solid component.
  - Dilated main pancreatic duct.
- Distal pancreatic symptomatic serous cystadenoma.
- Chronic calcific pancreatitis or small symptomatic pseudocyst limited to pancreatic tail (less common).

CONTRAINDICATIONS

Absolute

- Proximal mass requiring pancreatoduodenectomy.
- Known metastatic disease.
- Local invasion of structures that cannot be resected en bloc with the pancreas.
- Mass encasing mesenteric vessels, with loss of usual fat planes noted on preoperative imaging (CT, MRI, or endoscopic ultrasound [EUS]).
- Portal hypertension.

Relative

- Cardiopulmonary comorbidities.
- Splenic vein thrombosis.

INFORMED CONSENT

Expected Benefits

- Surgical cure of a neoplasm in the distal pancreas.
- Prevention of malignant transformation of mucinous cystic neoplasms.
- Treatment of symptomatic benign disease.

Potential Risks

- Surgical site infection, bleeding, and damage to adjacent structures.
- Removal of the spleen.
  - Should this be necessary, patients are at risk for the rare complication of post-splenectomy sepsis.
- Complications unique to operations on the pancreas include:
  - Postoperative pancreatitis.
  - Pancreatic leaks.
  - Pancreatic fistula formation.

EQUIPMENT

- No special equipment is needed.
- A self-retaining retractor helps facilitate exposure of the operative field.
- A surgical energy device (eg, harmonic scalpel, LigaSure) is extremely useful.
- Depending on surgeon preference, a surgical stapler may be used to transect the pancreatic tail. In that case, a thoracoabdominal (TA) or gastrointestinal anastomosis (GIA) stapler is used.

PATIENT PREPARATION

- Thorough preoperative evaluation is essential before undertaking this procedure.
- For symptomatic patients, delineation of the presenting symptoms and correlation of these symptoms with the mass in the pancreatic tail or body is critical.
- Potentially useful tests include:
  - Abdominal CT, ultrasonography.
  - Endoscopic retrograde cholangiopancreatography (ERCP) or EUS.
  - Magnetic resonance cholangiopancreatography (MRCP).
- For cystic neoplasms, cyst fluid is often obtained during EUS and analysis is performed to differentiate mucinous from serous cystic lesions and to determine cyst fluid CEA levels.
- Side branch versus main duct intraductal papillary mucinous neoplasms should be differentiated preoperatively using ERCP, MRCP, or EUS, if at all possible.
- Patients with persistent hypoglycemia and suspected insulinoma should receive glucose supplementation.
- Patients with refractory ulcers, elevated gastrin levels, and the suspicion of a gastrinoma should receive preoperative treatment for acid secretion and appropriate fluid and electrolyte supplementation.

- If splenectomy is planned, patients should undergo immunization for encapsulated organisms at least 2 weeks before surgery.

PATIENT POSITIONING

- The patient should be supine.
- The skin is prepared from the level of the nipples to the pubis, extending along the flank.
- The abdomen is entered through a midline incision.
- Alternatively, a bilateral subcostal incision may be used.

PROCEDURE

- **Figure 16–1:** Ligation of the short gastric vessels.
  - For resection of the distal pancreas, the standard approach is through an upper midline incision.
  - The pancreas is approached as in other pancreatic procedures through the lesser sac of the omentum.
  - The peritoneal covering along the inferior border of the pancreas is divided from the superior mesenteric vessels laterally toward the tail.
  - Vessels encountered in this space should be ligated and divided or sealed with the surgical energy device.
  - If concern exists for malignancy, then splenectomy is always performed; however, if pancreatectomy is being performed for benign disease, then spleen-preserving distal pancreatectomy is possible and the decision regarding splenectomy will be up to the surgeon.
  - If splenectomy is to be performed, the spleen is mobilized anteriorly and to the right, and off of the left kidney in the retroperitoneum (Gerota's fascia).
  - To mobilize the tail of the pancreas, the short gastric vessels that connect the splenic hilum with the greater curvature of the stomach must be isolated and divided.
  - This can be done either via standard division and ligation with fine silk sutures, or with the use of the surgical energy device.
- **Figure 16–2:** Division of the splenocolic ligament.
  - Once the spleen, still attached to the distal pancreas, has been liberated from the greater curvature of the stomach, its peritoneal attachment to the splenic flexure of the colon, the splenocolic ligament, must be divided.
  - The spleen is rotated gently to the right and clamps are placed across the splenocolic ligament, as shown.
  - The ligament itself is then divided sharply and the ends ligated.
- **Figure 16–3:** Mobilization of the spleen.
  - Once the splenocolic ligament has been divided, the spleen (attached to the tail of the pancreas) is rotated to the right.

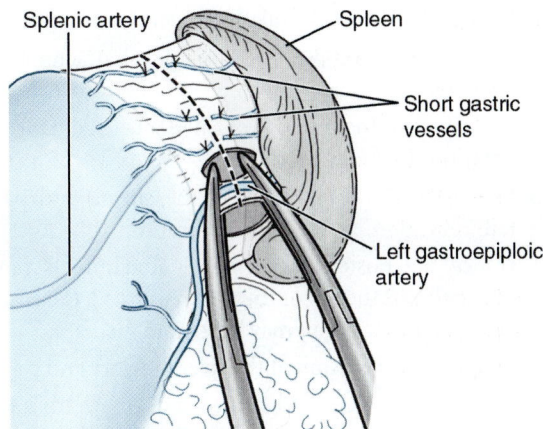

figure 16–1

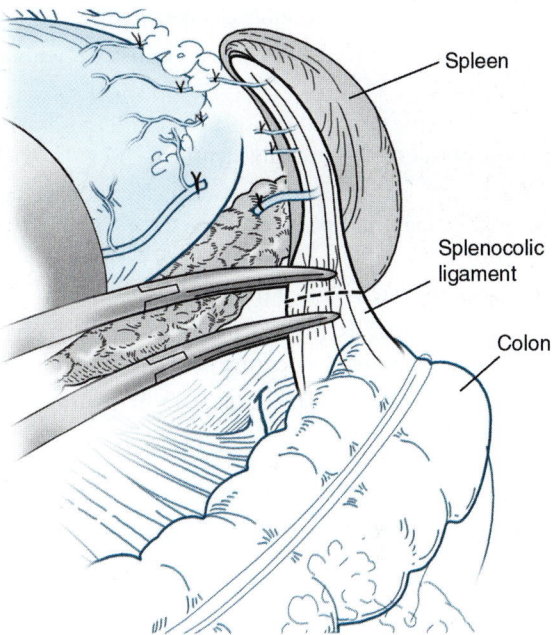

Figure 16–2

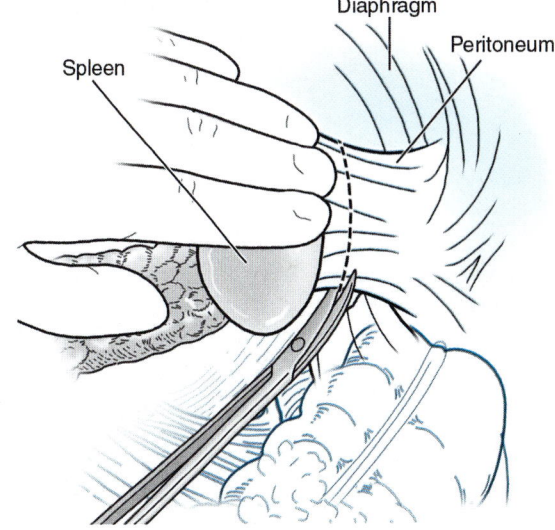

Figure 16–3

- **Figure 16–4:** Dissection along the inferior pancreatic margin.
  - The inferior and posterior peritoneal attachments of the pancreas are sharply divided.
  - The inferior mesenteric vein, if identified during this step, may be ligated and divided.
- **Figure 16–5:** Mobilization of the spleen and pancreatic tail.
  - Once the posterior peritoneal attachments have been divided and the tail of the pancreas freed, the entire distal portion of the organ may be rotated medially.
- **Figure 16–6:** Division of the splenic artery and vein.
  - The splenic artery is identified at its origin from the celiac trunk and traced distally along the posterior aspect of the gland.
  - It is encircled, then doubly clamped and ligated.
  - The proximal (celiac) portion is transfixed with a suture ligature.
  - The splenic vein is then isolated, and its confluence with the portal vein is carefully identified.
  - The vein is then divided between clamps, and the proximal (remaining) portion is oversewn with a 5-0 Prolene suture.
- **Figure 16–7:** Division of the pancreas.
  - The pancreas is rotated medially via traction on the splenic tail into the operative field.
  - A TA (shown) or GIA stapler can be used to divide the pancreas.

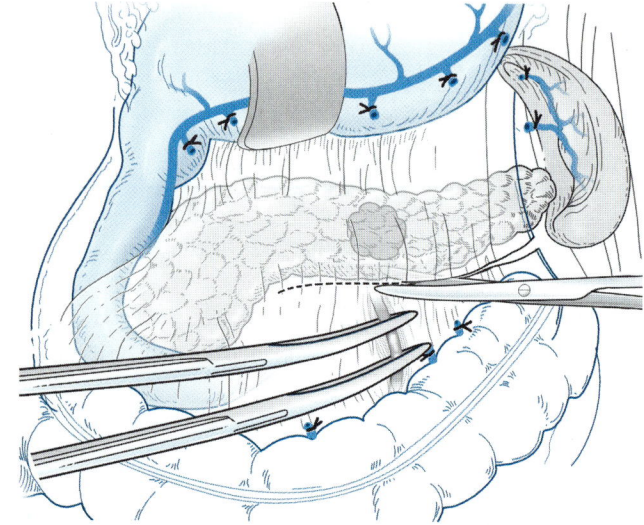

Figure 16–4

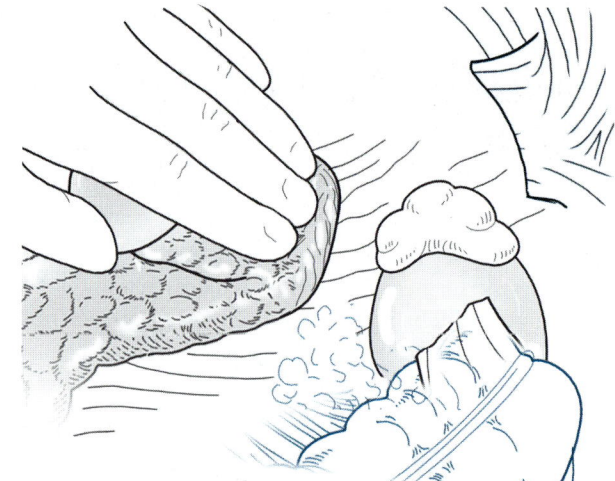

Figure 16–5

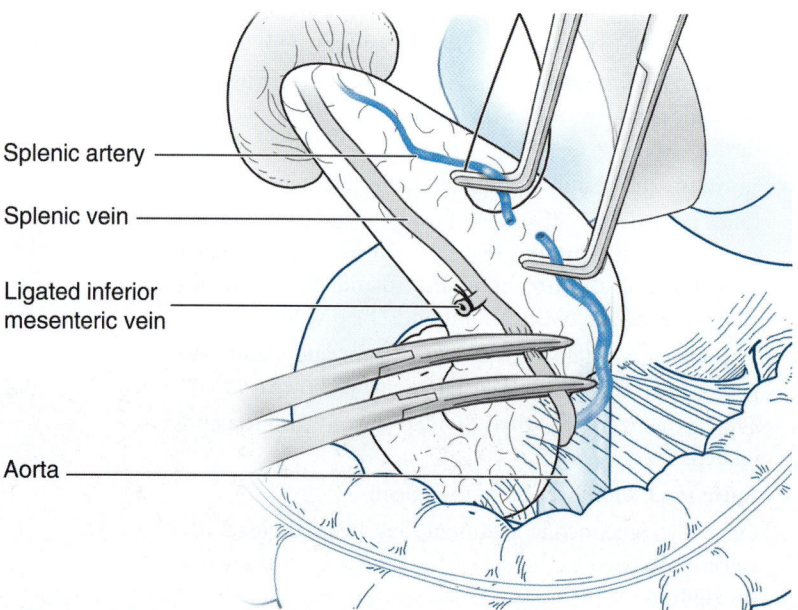

Figure 16–6

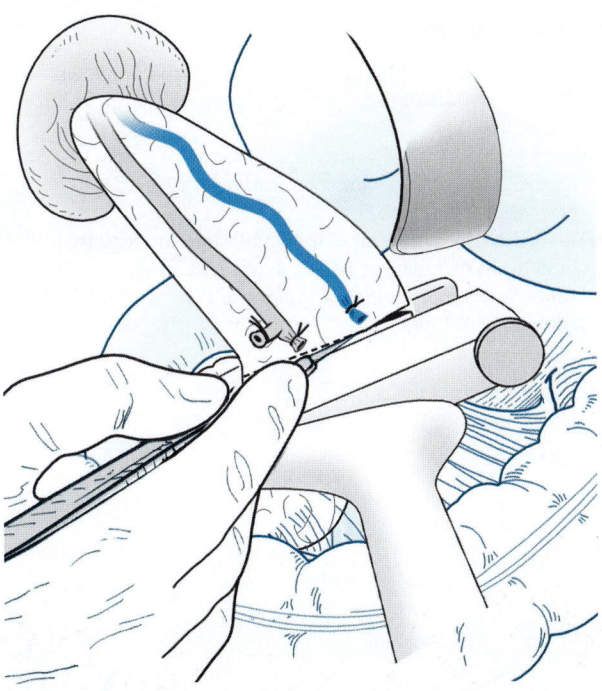

Figure 16–7

- If a TA stapler is used, the pancreas is then divided sharply using a scalpel.
- The duct should be oversewn and transfixed with a suture if visible.
- **Figure 16–8A, B:** Suturing the remainder of the pancreas.
  - If the pancreas is thick and a stapler cannot be used, it can be divided sharply with a scalpel or with a surgical energy device.
  - The duct is then transfixed with a suture (Figure 16–8A).
  - A row of interrupted mattress sutures is placed through the body of the residual pancreas and tied (Figure 16–8B).
  - Additional bites should be taken at sites of bleeding.
- Depending on surgeon preference, a drain can be left in the left upper quadrant near the transected pancreas, whether stapled or oversewn.

POSTOPERATIVE CARE

- Nothing by mouth with nasogastric tube decompression.
- Oral diet is resumed following removal of the nasogastric tube and resolution of postoperative ileus.

POTENTIAL COMPLICATIONS

- Pancreatic leak.
- Pancreatic fistula.
- Pancreatitis.
- Surgical site infection.
- Bleeding.

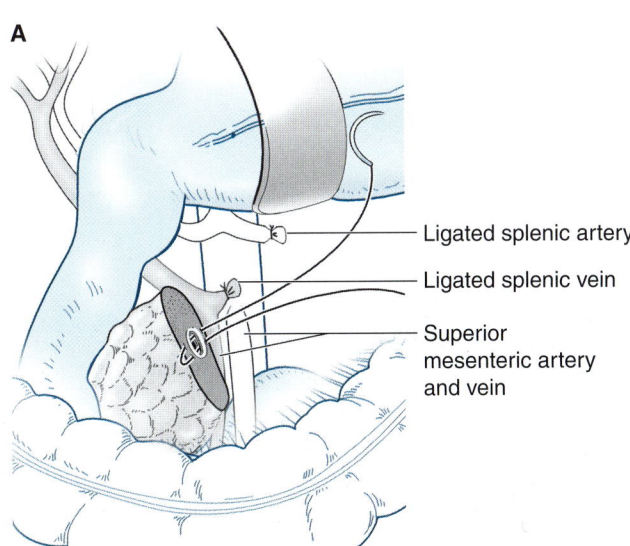
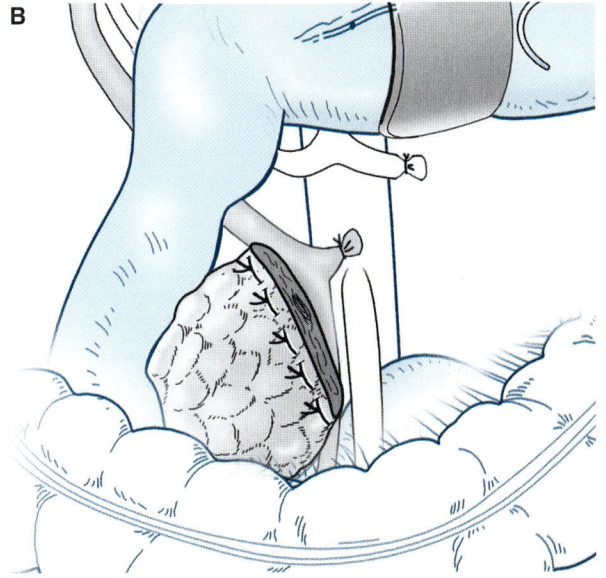

Figure 16–8A–B

PEARLS AND TIPS

- Intraoperative ultrasound can be useful if there is difficulty identifying the mass (cystic or solid) in the pancreas at the time of operation.
- To avoid inadvertent injury to the common hepatic artery, trace the splenic artery back to its origin from the celiac axis and visualize all branches prior to ligation of the splenic artery.
- For benign lesions, spleen-preserving distal pancreatectomy is possible and a medial-to-lateral approach is preferred.

REFERENCES

Bell RH Jr, Rikkers LF, Mulholland MW. *Digestive Tract Surgery: A Text and Atlas.* Philadelphia, PA: Lippincott-Raven Publishers; 1996.

Doherty GM, Way LW. Pancreas. In: Doherty GM, Way LW, eds. *Current Surgical Diagnosis and Treatment,* 12th ed. New York, NY: McGraw-Hill; 2005.

Riall TS, Yeo CJ. Neoplasms of the Endocrine Pancreas. In: Mulholland MW, Lillemoe KD, Doherty GM, et al, eds. *Greenfield's Surgery: Scientific Principles and Practice,* 4th ed. Philadelphia, PA: Lippincott Williams & Wilkins; 2006.

CHAPTER 17

Operative Management of Chronic Pancreatitis

Jules Lin, MD, and Diane M. Simeone, MD

INDICATIONS

Longitudinal Pancreaticojejunostomy
- Severe persistent pain from chronic pancreatitis.
  - Refractory to medical therapy.
  - Repeated hospital admissions.
- Dilated pancreatic duct > 8 mm in diameter.

Pancreatic Pseudocyst-Gastrostomy and Pseudocyst-Jejunostomy
- Persistent pancreatic pseudocyst present for > 6 weeks (ie, at which time the wall should be mature enough to hold sutures).

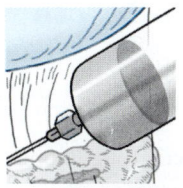 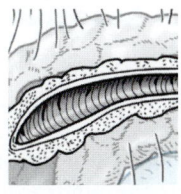 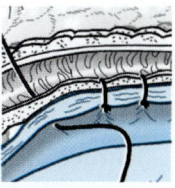
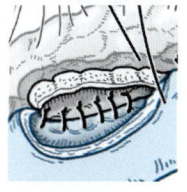 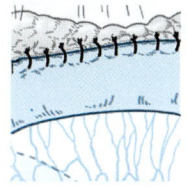 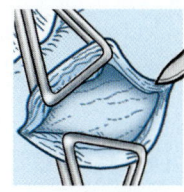
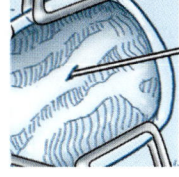 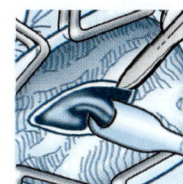 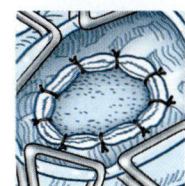

CONTRAINDICATIONS

Longitudinal Pancreaticojejunostomy

A. Absolute
- Absence of pain.
- Pancreatic cancer.
- Cirrhosis.

B. Relative
- Cardiopulmonary comorbidities.

Pancreatic Pseudocyst-Gastrostomy and Pseudocyst-Jejunostomy

A. Absolute
- Cystadenocarcinoma is a contraindication to enteric drainage and should be resected.
- Pseudocyst that has been present for < 6 weeks.

B. Relative
- Cardiopulmonary comorbidities.

INFORMED CONSENT

Expected Benefits: Longitudinal Pancreaticojejunostomy
- To provide pain relief while preserving pancreatic function.
- Pain is improved in 60–70% of cases.

Expected Benefits: Pancreatic Pseudocyst-Gastrostomy and Pseudocyst-Jejunostomy
- Pseudocysts generally do not resolve spontaneously if present for > 6 weeks; therefore, operative drainage is often entertained following that interval.

Potential Risks Associated with Both Procedures
- Surgical site infection (either deep or superficial).
- Bleeding.
- Systemic complications of major surgery (pneumonia, venous thromboembolism, and cardiovascular events).
- Pancreatic leaks and fistula, while possible, are relatively less common than with operations on less fibrotic pancreatic parenchyma.

EQUIPMENT
- No special equipment is required.
- A self-retaining retractor is useful to facilitate exposure of the operative field, and a gastrointestinal anastomosis (GIA) stapler for dividing the small bowel.

PATIENT PREPARATION
- A thorough preoperative workup is essential before recommending a pancreaticojejunostomy.
  - The goal is to confirm the diagnosis and rule out other causes of pain.
  - Sources other than the patient should confirm that he or she has abstained from alcohol use for a significant period of time.
  - The diameter of the pancreatic duct and location of the inflammation should be determined.
  - Any biliary or duodenal obstruction or pancreatic pseudocysts should be identified so that these conditions can be addressed concurrently.
- Potentially useful studies include:
  - Abdominal CT scanning.
  - Ultrasonography.
  - Endoscopic retrograde cholangiopancreatography (ERCP).
  - Magnetic resonance cholangiopancreatography.

- CT scans can show pancreatic ductal dilation as well as calcifications, pseudocysts, masses, and biliary dilation.
- If a pseudocyst is present, abdominal CT scan or ultrasonography can usually determine the size, chronicity, and location of the pseudocyst in relation to the stomach or duodenum.
- The patient's physiologic fitness should also be assessed.

PATIENT POSITIONING
- The patient should be supine.
- The abdomen is entered through a midline incision.

PROCEDURE
Longitudinal Pancreaticojejunostomy

- **Figure 17–1:** Abdominal CT in a patient with chronic pancreatitis shows a dilated pancreatic duct (arrow).
- **Figure 17–2:** Location of the pancreatic duct.
  - After entering the lesser sac, the stomach is reflected upward.
  - The posterior wall of the stomach may be adherent to the anterior surface of the pancreas due to peripancreatic inflammation.
  - After the adhesions are carefully divided, the pancreas is palpated to identify the pancreatic duct.
  - The dilated duct is aspirated with a 22-gauge needle.
  - If the duct cannot be identified, a Greenlee maneuver can be performed with an oblique incision made anteriorly near the junction of the body and tail until the duct is identified.

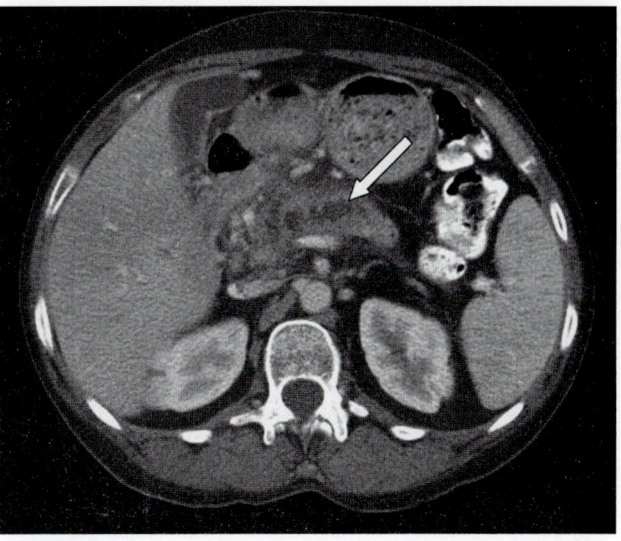

Figure 17–1

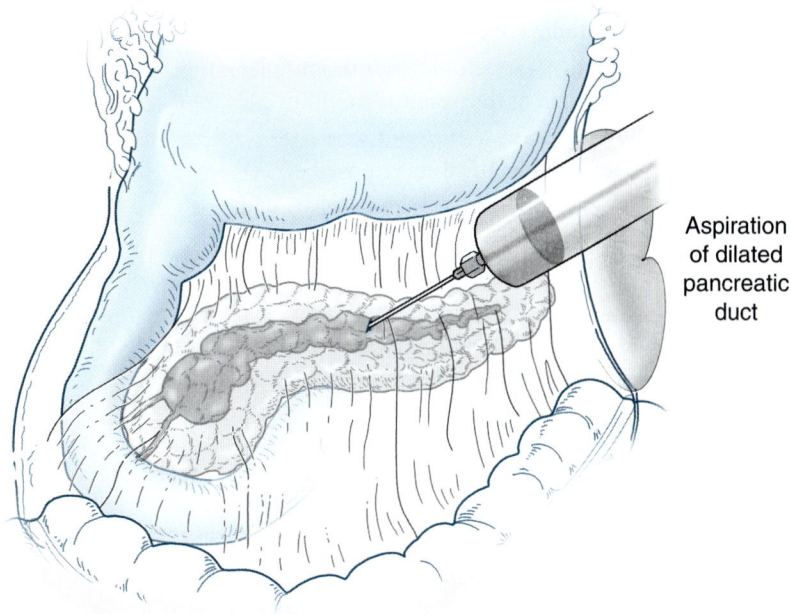

Figure 17–2

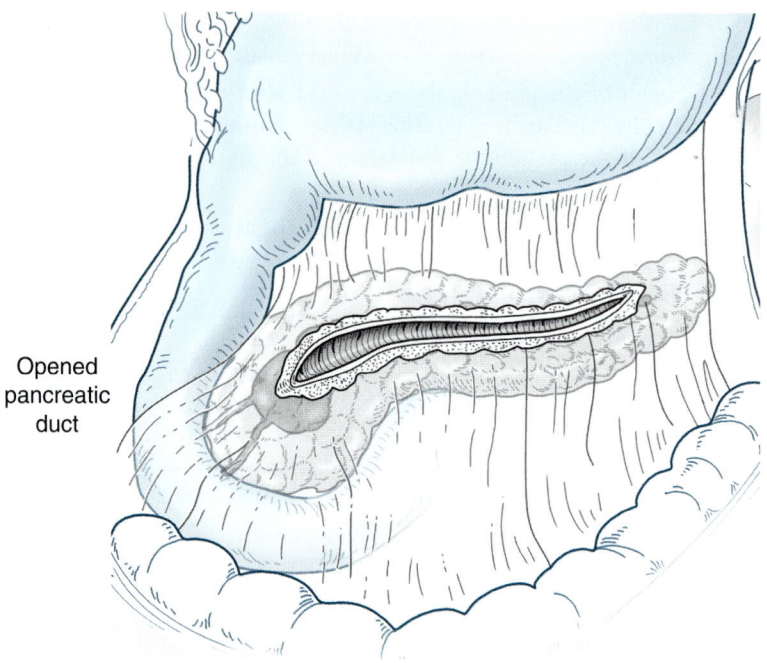

Figure 17–3

- Intraoperative ultrasound can also be used to identify the duct.
- Narrowing of the distal common bile duct occurs in 10–15% of cases of chronic pancreatitis and should be treated at the same time.
- Cholangiography typically shows a dilated common bile duct with a smooth elongated narrowing of the intrapancreatic bile duct.

■ **Figure 17–3:** After the dilated pancreatic duct has been identified, a longitudinal incision is made.
- The incision is then extended along the entire length of the duct from the tail of the pancreas to within 2–3 cm of the duodenum.
- Any debris or calculi identified are removed.
- The fibrotic pancreatic tissue is not well vascularized, although larger vessels are present near the duodenum.
- Hemostasis is obtained with electrocautery and suture ligatures.
- The Roux-en-Y limb is then prepared by dividing the jejunum approximately 20 cm from the ligament of Treitz using a linear GIA stapler.
- After the staple line is oversewn, the distal limb is brought through the transverse mesocolon and incised along the antimesenteric border.

■ **Figure 17–4:** The posterior wall of the anastomosis is formed with interrupted nonabsorbable sutures.
- The duct wall and overlying parenchyma are thickened and fibrotic and hold sutures well.

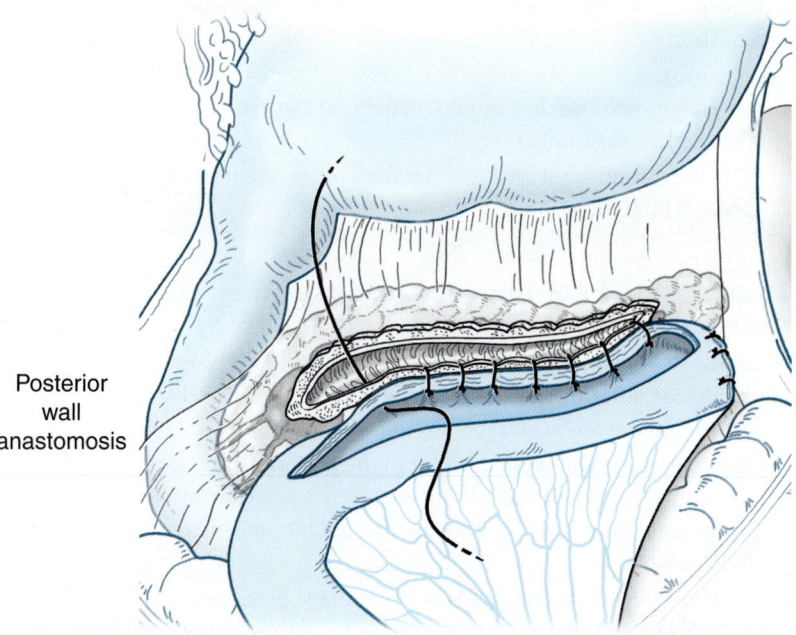

Figure 17-4

- Full-thickness bites are taken of the jejunum and the pancreatic duct with the overlying fibrotic pancreatic tissue.
- Some surgeons complete the anastomosis in two layers, with an additional layer incorporating the pancreatic capsule and seromuscular layer of the jejunum.

■ **Figure 17–5:** After the posterior layer has been finished, the anterior wall is completed in a similar fashion, taking full-thickness bites of the jejunum and the pancreatic duct with the overlying pancreatic tissue.

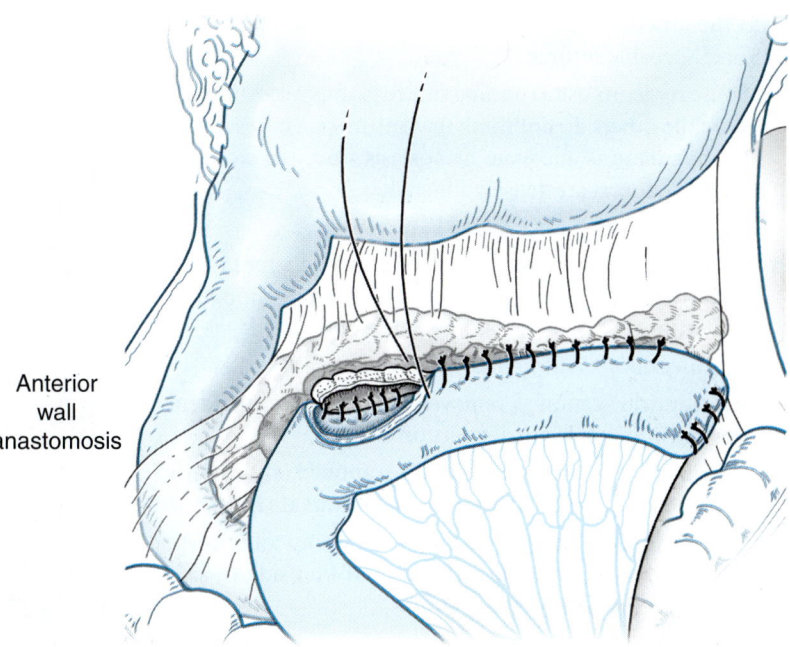

Figure 17-5

- **Figure 17–6:** The completed longitudinal pancreaticojejunostomy.
  - The proximal enteroenterostomy has been performed in an end-to-side fashion approximately 50 cm from the pancreatic anastomosis.
  - The Roux limb is sutured to the transverse mesocolon to prevent internal hernias.

Pancreatic Pseudocyst-Gastrostomy and Pseudocyst-Jejunostomy

- **Figure 17–7:** The abdominal CT scan shows a pancreatic pseudocyst anterior to the pancreatic body. This is closely adherent to the posterior aspect of the stomach (arrow).
  - A pancreatic pseudocyst adherent to the posterior wall of the stomach can be drained by a pseudocyst-gastrostomy when the cyst wall has matured sufficiently to be able to hold sutures.
- **Figure 17–8:** A 5-cm long gastrotomy is made in the anterior wall of the stomach. Care is taken to avoid the antrum.
- **Figure 17–9:** An 18-gauge needle is inserted through the posterior wall of the stomach to confirm the location and presence of the pseudocyst. A sample of the fluid is sent for cytologic testing.
- **Figure 17–10:** The common wall between the posterior stomach and anterior pseudocyst is incised and an elliptical section is removed and sent for frozen section analysis to rule out the presence of a cystic neoplasm (ie, cystadenoma or cystadenocarcinoma). The debris and fluid within the pseudocyst should be removed gently to prevent significant hemorrhage.
- **Figure 17–11:** The posterior wall of the stomach is sutured to the anterior wall of the pseudocyst using interrupted nonabsorbable sutures.
  - Some surgeons use a running suture to improve hemostasis while others do not think that sutures are necessary as long as there is adequate hemostasis since the stomach and pseudocyst are densely adherent.
  - The gastrotomy is then closed in two layers.
- **Figure 17–12:** When the pseudocyst is not adherent to the stomach or duodenum but the wall is mature enough to hold sutures, a cyst-jejunostomy can be performed.
  - The pseudocyst is aspirated with an 18-gauge needle.
  - An elliptical section is removed at the most dependent portion and sent for frozen section analysis.
  - The interior of the pseudocyst is examined, and biopsy specimens are obtained from any suspicious areas.
  - A Roux limb of jejunum is then brought up anterior to the transverse colon and anastomosed in a side-to-side fashion to the pseudocyst.

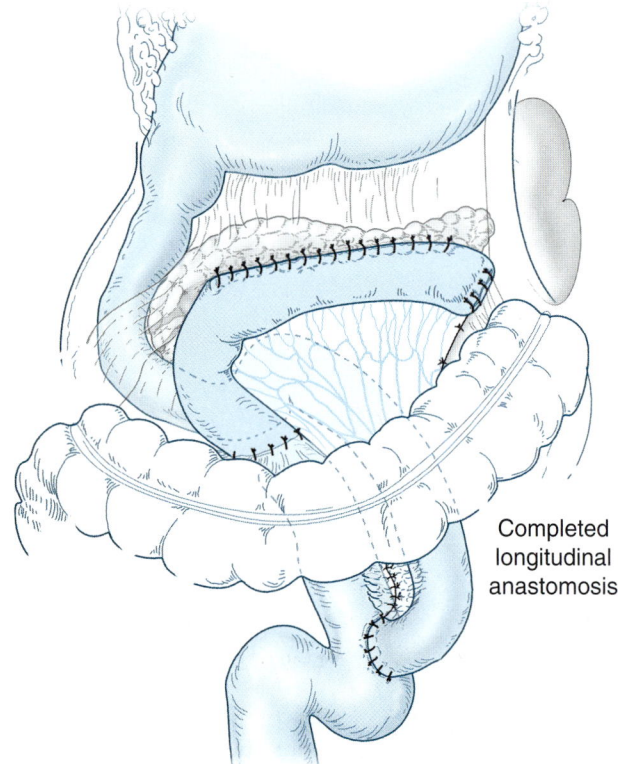

Figure 17–6

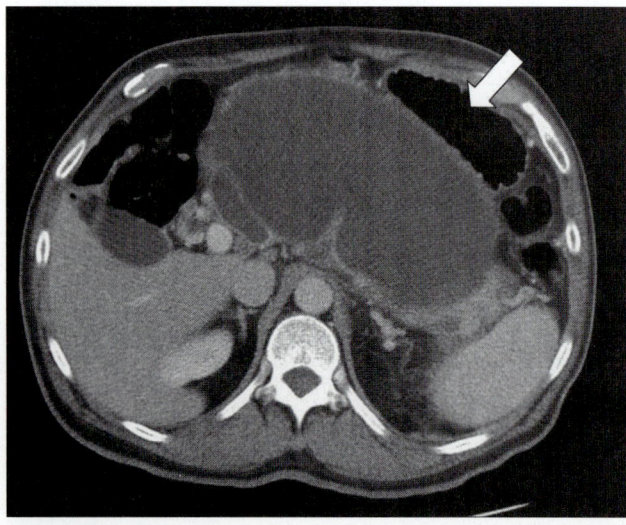

Figure 17–7

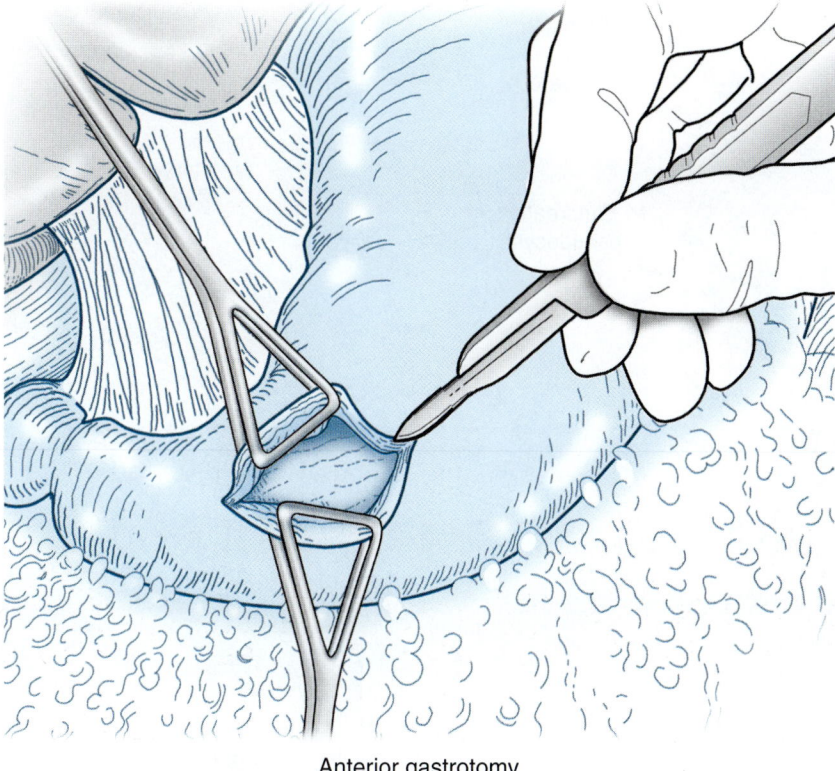

Figure 17-8

Anterior gastrotomy

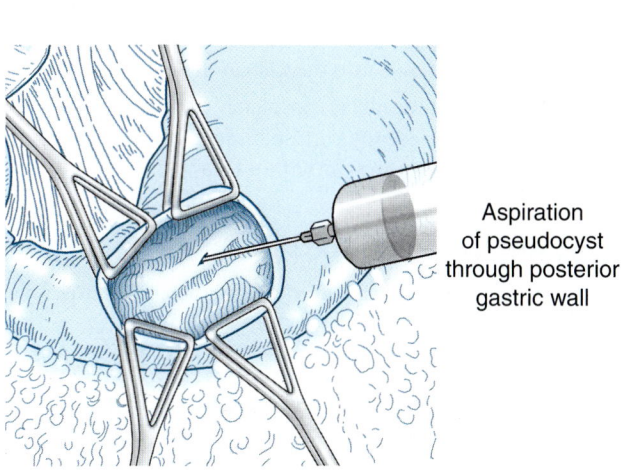

Figure 17-9

Aspiration of pseudocyst through posterior gastric wall

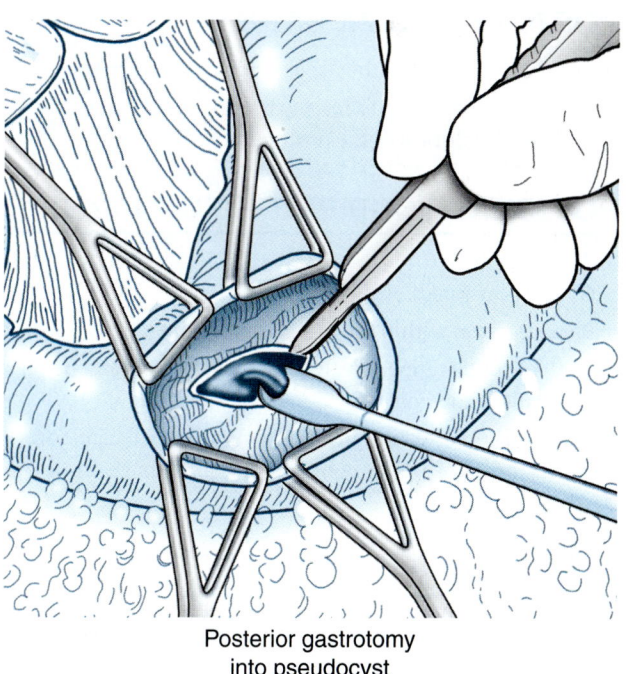

Figure 17-10

Posterior gastrotomy into pseudocyst

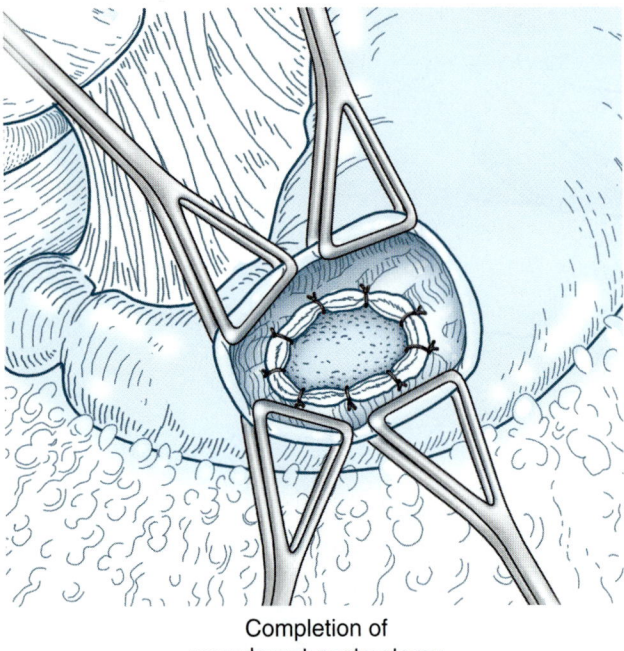

Completion of pseudocyst-gastrostomy

Figure 17–11

- Full-thickness bites are taken using interrupted nonabsorbable sutures.
- The mesenteric defect is then closed to prevent internal hernias.
- Large pseudocysts adherent to the stomach but extending well below the greater curvature of the stomach are better drained with cystojejunostomy than cystogastrostomy.

POSTOPERATIVE CARE

- Nothing by mouth with nasogastric tube decompression.
- Oral diet is advanced following removal of the nasogastric tube and resolution of the postoperative ileus.

POTENTIAL COMPLICATIONS

- Pancreatic leak.
- Surgical site infections.
- Bleeding from within the pseudocyst cavity.
  - Can occur intraoperatively or postoperatively and be very difficult to control.
  - Angiographic techniques (eg, embolization) can sometimes be effective in controlling hemorrhage from the pseudocyst cavity.

PEARLS AND TIPS

Longitudinal Pancreaticojejunostomy

- Operative pancreatography or intraoperative ultrasound can be used if there is difficulty identifying the pancreatic duct.

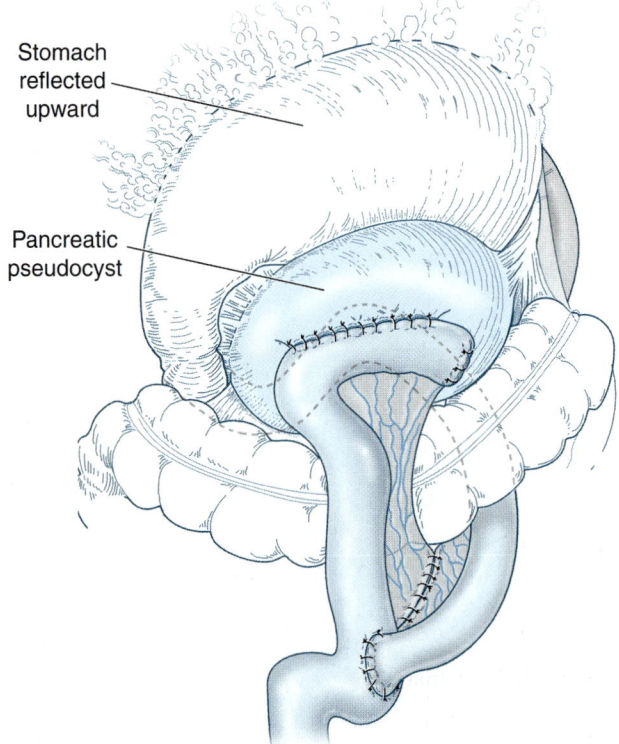

Completed Roux-en-Y pseudocyst-jejunostomy

Figure 17–12

- During division of the duct, a biliary probe or tip of a finger can be used to follow the path of the pancreatic duct.

Pancreatic Pseudocyst-Gastrostomy and Pseudocyst-Jejunostomy

- Be gentle with the internal surface of the cyst to avoid causing hemorrhage.
- Ensure that the cystogastrostomy opening is large enough to pass necrotic tissue into the gastrointestinal tract.
- The cyst resolves rapidly if completely drained, and esophagogastroduodenoscopy can document complete healing of the cystogastrostomy site within several days.

REFERENCES

Duval MK Jr. Caudal pancreaticojejunostomy for chronic relapsing pancreatitis. *Ann Surg.* 1954;140:775–785.

Frey CF. Pancreatic pseudocyst—operative strategy. *Ann Surg.* 1978;188:652–662.

Kohler H, Schafmayer A, Ludtke FE, et al. Surgical treatment of pancreatic pseudocysts. *Br J Surg.* 1987;74:813–815.

Puestow CB, Gillesby WJ. Pancreaticojejunostomy for chronic relapsing pancreatitis: an evaluation. *Surgery.* 1967;50:859.

CHAPTER 18

Splenectomy

Brett A. Almond, MD, PhD, and Kathleen M. Diehl, MD

INDICATIONS
- Splenic trauma with hemorrhage.
- Splenic cysts or splenic mass.
- Splenic abscess.
- Hematologic disorders.
  - Idiopathic thrombocytopenic purpura.
  - Hemolytic anemia.
  - Hereditary spherocytosis.
  - Other hereditary or autoimmune anemias.
- Severe hypersplenism.
- Perisplenic malignancy.
- Splenic artery aneurysm.
- Splenic vein thrombosis with left-sided portal hypertension.

CONTRAINDICATIONS
- Portal hypertension due to liver disease.
- Thrombocytopenia is not a contraindication of splenectomy.
  - Although preoperative transfusion is not recommended, intraoperative transfusion may be required should coagulopathic bleeding occur.

INFORMED CONSENT

Expected Benefits
- Cessation or prevention of life-threatening hemorrhage.
- Treatment of hematologic disorders, malignancy, or symptomatic mass or hypersplenism.

Potential Risks
- Post-splenectomy sepsis.
- Bleeding.
- Infection (wound or intra-abdominal abscess).
- Pancreatitis or pancreatic leak.
- Damage to surrounding structures (stomach, diaphragm, colon, etc).
- Recurrence of primary disease (thrombocytopenia, etc).

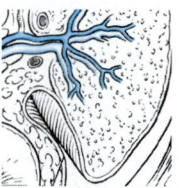 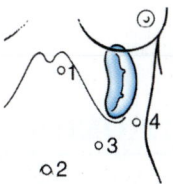 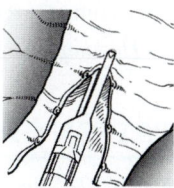
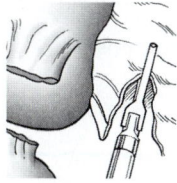 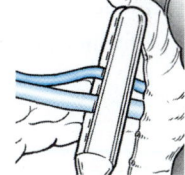 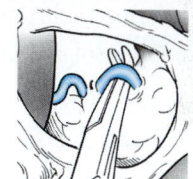
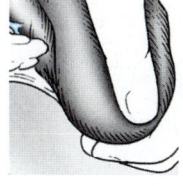 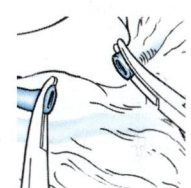 

EQUIPMENT

- Self-retaining retractor (eg, Bookwalter, Thompson, Upper Hand, etc).
- Bipolar cautery, LigaSure, harmonic scalpel, or similar instrument is needed for the laparoscopic procedure and may be used for the open procedure as well.

PATIENT PREPARATION

- Patients should be vaccinated against encapsulated organisms preoperatively.
  - Pneumococcus.
  - Meningococcus.
  - *Haemophilus influenzae*.

PATIENT POSITIONING

- Laparoscopic splenectomy is preferentially performed in the right lateral decubitus position but may also be performed with the patient supine.
- Open splenectomy is performed in the supine position.

PROCEDURE

Laparoscopic Splenectomy

- **Figure 18–1:** The gastrosplenic ligament contains the short gastric vessels and must be divided to obtain access to the splenic vessels, whereas the splenophrenic and splenorenal ligaments are relatively avascular.
- **Figure 18–2A, B:** Laparoscopic splenectomy can be performed either in the supine (Figure 18–2A) or right lateral decubitus (Figure 18–2B) positions using similar port placement. The lateral decubitus position is preferred.

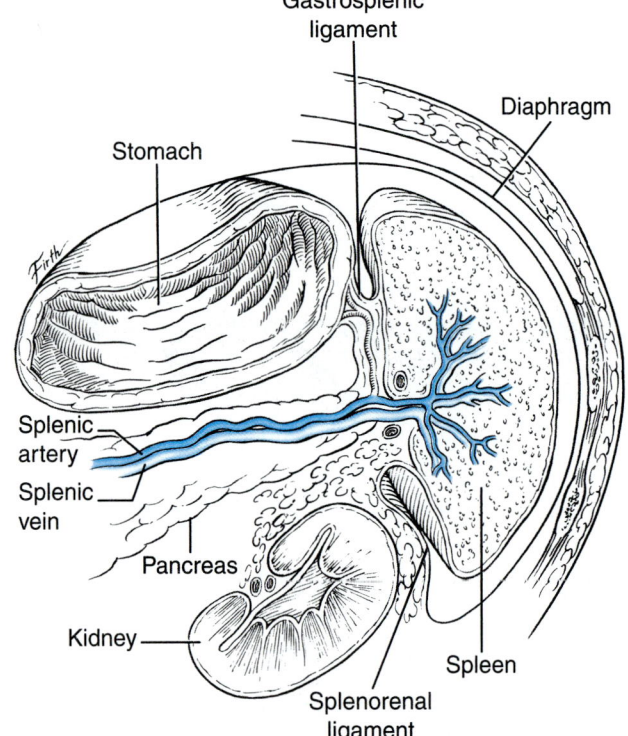

Figure 18–1

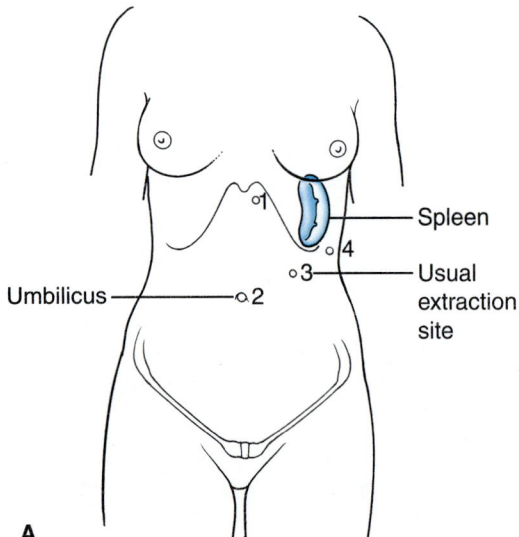

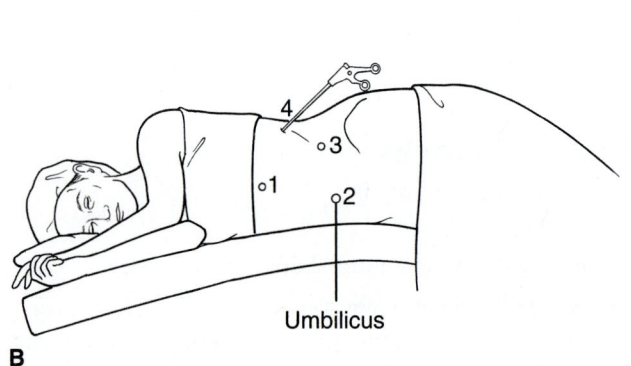

Figure 18–2A–B

- **Figure 18–3:** The gastrosplenic ligament is transected using bipolar cautery or harmonic scalpel to ensure hemostasis of the short gastric vessels, thereby obtaining access to the splenic vessels.
- **Figure 18–4:** Next, the relatively avascular splenocolic and splenorenal ligaments are divided along with the other attachments, freeing the spleen.
- **Figure 18–5:** A vascular stapler is used to divide the splenic artery and vein. The artery is always divided before the vein.
- The specimen is placed into an endoscopic retrieval bag. Depending on its size, the spleen may require maceration with a ring forceps or finger before it can be removed from the body.

Open Splenectomy

- **Figure 18–6:** Open splenectomy may be performed through a midline or left subcostal incision.

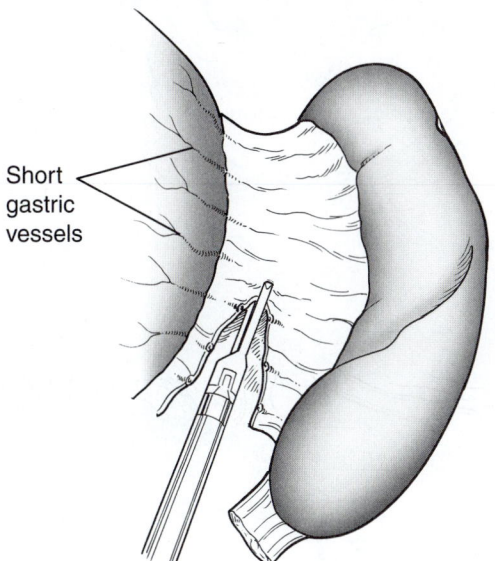

Figure 18–3

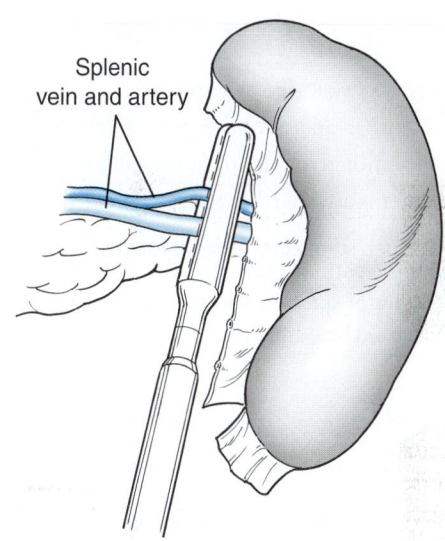

Figure 18–5

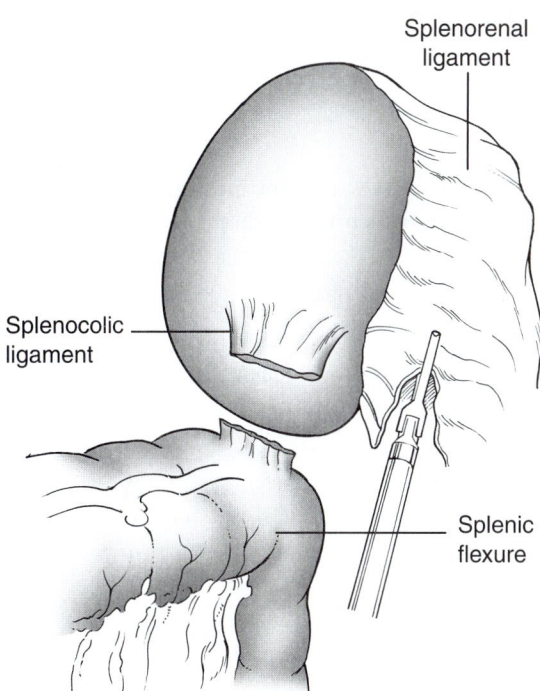

Figure 18–4

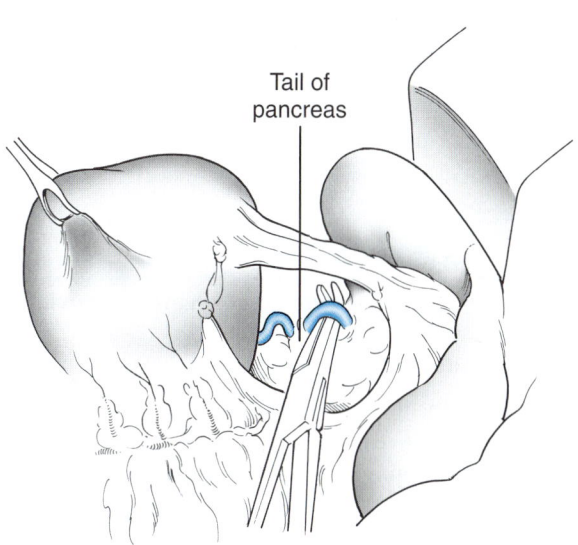

Figure 18–6

- To reduce intraoperative blood loss, some surgeons choose to begin by opening the lesser sac and ligating the splenic artery.
- **Figure 18–7:** The surgeon's left hand is passed laterally to the spleen, bluntly dissecting the splenophrenic and splenorenal ligaments, and mobilizing the spleen anteromedially into the wound.
- **Figure 18–8:** With the spleen fully mobilized, the splenic vessels are either taken between clamps and ligated or taken with a vascular stapler. Again, the artery is always ligated before the vein.
- Any remaining short gastric vessels or other attachments are divided, freeing the spleen from the abdomen.

POSTOPERATIVE CARE

- Nasogastric decompression.
  - For 12–36 hours after open splenectomy.
  - Optional for laparoscopic splenectomy.
- Diet is advanced as tolerated after removal of the nasogastric tube.
- If the patient has not been vaccinated preoperatively (eg, in cases of splenectomy for trauma or iatrogenic injury), this should be done promptly.

POTENTIAL COMPLICATIONS

- Postoperative bleeding or hemorrhage.
  - Classically associated with the short gastric vessels.
- Gastric injury or leak.
- Pancreatic injury resulting in pancreatitis or pancreatic leak or fistula.
- Thrombocytosis.
  - Aspirin is prescribed if this occurs.
- Splenic vein thrombosis.
- Left lower lobe atelectasis or pneumonia.
- Superficial or deep space surgical site infection.
- Recurrence of disease (if splenectomy is performed for hematologic disease).

PEARLS AND TIPS

- Consider preoperative embolization in patients with severe hypersplenism.
  - This may reduce intraoperative blood loss.
- After a difficult or traumatic dissection, consider placement of a drain in the left upper quadrant at the conclusion of the operation.
  - Test the drain effluent for evidence of a pancreatic leak after the patient resumes a normal diet and before removing the drain.

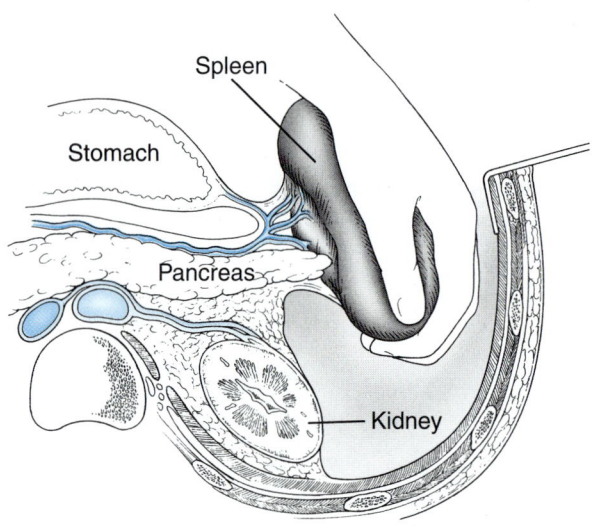

Figure 18–7

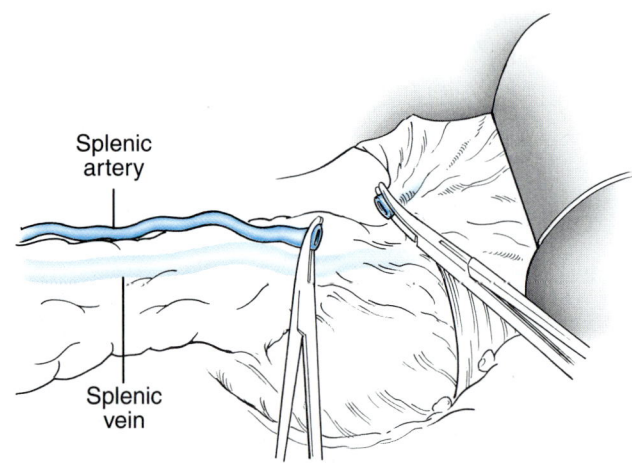

Figure 18–8

- Instruct patients to seek prompt medical evaluation for signs of infection, which may indicate post-splenectomy sepsis.

REFERENCES

Fraker DL. Splenic Disorders. In: Mulholland MW, Lillimoe KD, Doherty GM, et al, eds. *Greenfield's Surgery: Scientific Principles & Practice,* 4th ed. Philadelphia, PA: Lippincott Williams & Wilkins; 2006:1222–1250.

Mourtzoukou EG, Pappas G, Peppas G, Falagas ME. Vaccination of asplenic or hyposplenic adults. *Br J Surg.* 2008;95:273–280.

Poulin EC, Schlachta CM, Mamazza J. Splenectomy. In: Souba WW, Fink MP, Jurkovich GJ, et al, eds. *ACS Surgery: Principles and Practice.* WebMD Professional Publishing; 2007.

Rescorla FJ, West KW, Engum SA, Grosfeld JL. Laparoscopic splenic procedures in children: experience in 231 children. *Ann Surg.* 2007;246:683–688.

CHAPTER 19

Small Bowel Resection

Junewai L. Reoma, MD, and Daniel B. Hinshaw, MD

INDICATIONS

- Tumor.
- Ischemia or incarceration.
- Trauma or perforation.
- Fistula.
- Ulcer or bleeding.
- Obstruction.
- Stricture or Crohn's disease.

CONTRAINDICATIONS

Absolute

- Poor blood supply to bowel ends (ie, radiation-injured bowel).
- Unclear bowel viability after a revascularization procedure.
  - Both ends of the small bowel may be brought up to skin level as temporary ostomies if the distal small bowel is involved. A proximal small bowel ostomy will create a high-output fistula that is difficult to manage.
  - Alternatively, both ends can be stapled closed and a plan made for a second-look laparotomy in 24–48 hours.
  - In extreme situations (eg, acute mesenteric ischemia with gangrene extending from the ligament of Treitz to mid colon), the likelihood of survival is very small. This is an absolute contraindication to attempted resection and anastomosis.
- Inadequate tumor margins.
  - If a tumor is unresectable, and small bowel obstruction is likely to occur, a side-to-side anastomosis in uninvolved bowel proximal and distal to the obstruction may be performed as a bypass procedure, leaving the tumor in situ.

Relative

- Peritoneal sepsis.
- Hemodynamically precarious patient.

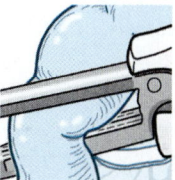 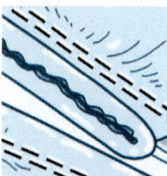 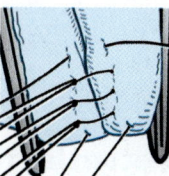
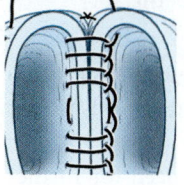 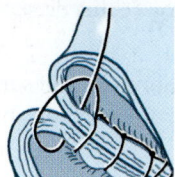 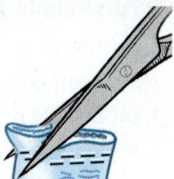
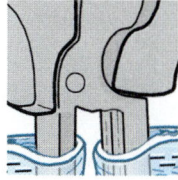 

- Extensive Crohn's disease.
  - Stricturoplasty should be considered to minimize the need for extensive resection and risk of short gut syndrome; 90 cm is the approximate shortest length of small bowel that might still support a viable oral nutrition program.

INFORMED CONSENT

Expected Benefits
- Relief of obstruction.
- Control of gastrointestinal hemorrhage.
- Treatment of gastrointestinal ischemia, necrosis, or perforation.

Potential Risks
- Common complications include:
  - Surgical site infection (either deep or superficial).
  - Bleeding.
  - Systemic complications of major surgery, including pneumonia, venous thromboembolism, and cardiovascular events.
- Small bowel obstruction, stricture, and need for further surgery are also potential risks of small bowel resection.
- Patients with extensive intra-abdominal sepsis or who are in a malnourished state are at increased risk for anastomotic leak and enteric fistula.

EQUIPMENT
- Self-retaining retractors are useful to help provide adequate exposure and access.
- Gastrointestinal anastomosis (GIA) stapler or thoracoabdominal (TA) stapler, or both (depending on surgeon's preference for anastomotic technique).

PATIENT PREPARATION

Preoperative Evaluation
- CT scan.
- Small bowel follow-through versus small bowel enteroclysis.
- As indicated for bleeding:
  - Esophagogastroduodenoscopy, push enteroscopy, or double balloon enteroscopy.
  - Capsule endoscopy.
  - Nuclear scan.
  - Angiography.

At the Time of the Procedure
- Nutritional status should be optimized preoperatively if possible.
- Treatment of systemic illness.
- Intravenous perioperative antibiotics.
- Nasogastric tube, in cases of obstruction.

PATIENT POSITIONING
- The patient should be supine.
- The abdomen is usually entered through a midline incision.

PROCEDURE

Hand-Sewn Anastomosis
- The abdomen is entered via a standard midline incision.
- A thorough four-quadrant examination should be performed, with lysis only of those adhesions necessary to gain access to the area of pathology.
- **Figure 19–1:** After the margins of resection have been determined (*dotted line*), electrocautery is used to score the mesentery to encompass only vessels and lymph nodes (if cancer operation) related to the section to be removed.
- The first step in resection is to make a window in the mesentery adjacent to the bowel that is free of blood vessels at the site of the planned margins. This can be done using gentle dissection with a right-angle or Coller clamp.
- **Figure 19–2A, B:** Creation of this window allows a GIA stapler to be passed through on either side of the segment of bowel to be divided (Figure 19–2A). Typically the blue load (3.8 mm) is used to divide the bowel, creating two staple lines and two ends (Figure 19–2B).

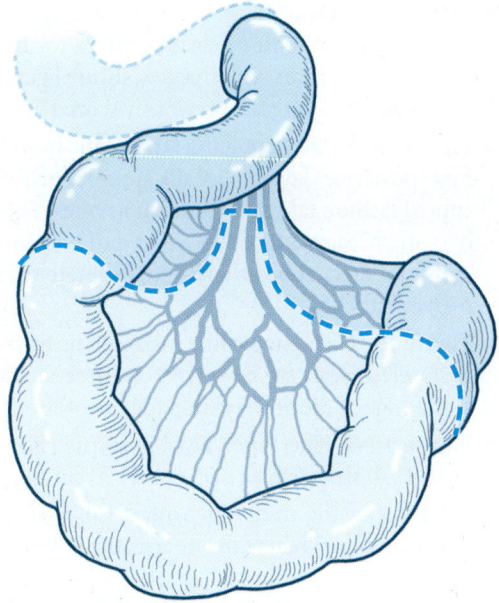

Figure 19–1

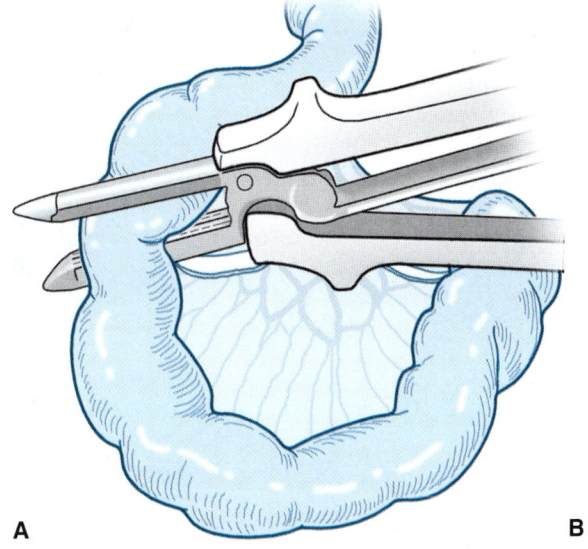

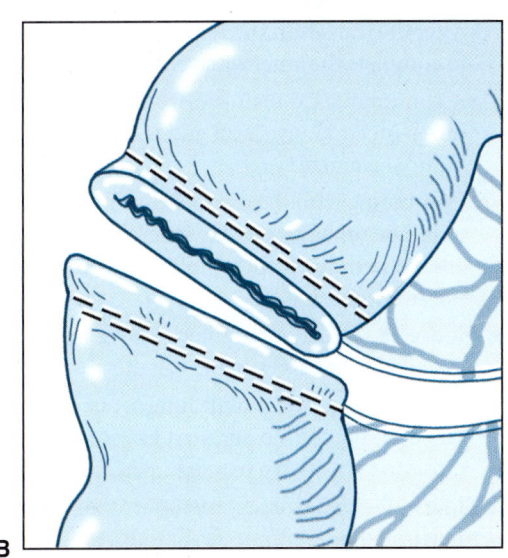

Figure 19–2A–B

- After the bowel is divided, the mesentery can be divided using a combination of electrocautery for further dissection plus hemostats with free ties, suture ligatures, or a harmonic scalpel along the previously scored line.
- **Figure 19–3:** After applying atraumatic bowel clamps, the first (posterior) layer of 3-0 silk suture is placed in an interrupted fashion taking seromuscular bites. This is the Lembert stitch. Stay sutures on either end help keep the bowel ends oriented appropriately to facilitate accurate placement of stitches.
- **Figure 19–4:** The staple line is excised using the cut setting of the electrocautery device. A 2-cm area should be allowed at the edge of the bowel clamp for a two-layer anastomosis.
- **Figure 19–5:** The inner layer is started using a double-armed 3-0 absorbable (PDS or Vicryl) suture.
  - Starting in the midpoint with a full-thickness bite, the suture is tied. Then with one arm, the posterior inner layer is closed by including full-thickness bites of mucosa, submucosa, and seromuscular tissue in continuous fashion.
  - Care should be taken to avoid inverting too much mucosa, which would narrow the anastomosis. Instead, just enough mucosa (1–2 mm), approximately half the thickness of the other layers, should be taken.
  - To reduce strangulation of tissues within the anastomosis, the posterior full-thickness sutures are often locked to prevent the purse-string effect. This is usually a matter of surgeon's preference.
- **Figure 19–6:** After the corner has been turned, a transition stitch from suturing inside the bowel to outside is taken to facilitate completion of the anterior layer.
  - Typically a narrow full-thickness horizontal mattress suture is used to end up with the suture on the outside.
  - This is repeated with the other arm of the continuous suture heading in the opposite direction.
  - After the transition stitch is completed, the suture is set up to complete the anterior layer.
  - A continuous Connell (horizontal mattress) stitch minimizes mucosal inversion and is another way to optimize luminal diameter.
  - Continuing with the over-and-over stitch is acceptable as well. The other arm of the suture can meet in the middle and be tied down to complete the full circumference of the anastomosis.
- **Figure 19–7:** The outer anterior layer of interrupted seromuscular (Lembert) stitches can then be placed easily.
  - Confirmation of a patent lumen can be made by gently pinching the thumb and first finger at the bowel anastomosis to verify that a patent lumen is present.
- **Figure 19–8:** The mesentery should then be closed with 3-0 interrupted or continuous silk sutures to prevent internal herniation.

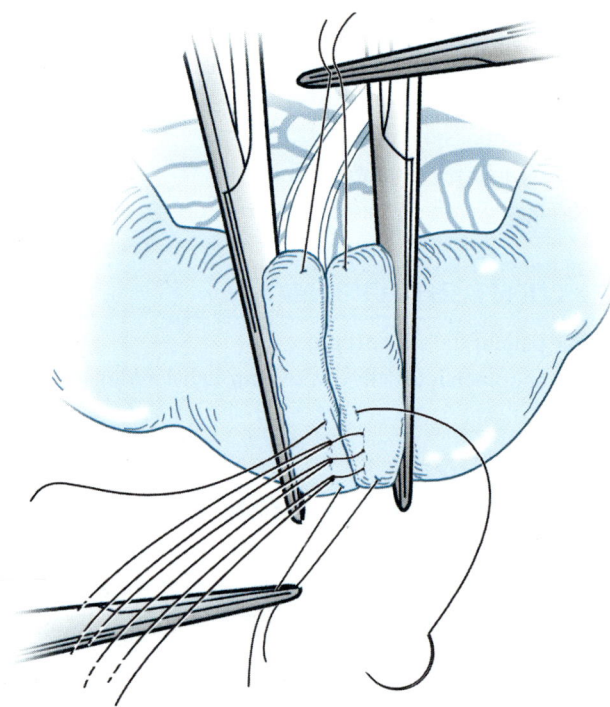

Figure 19–3

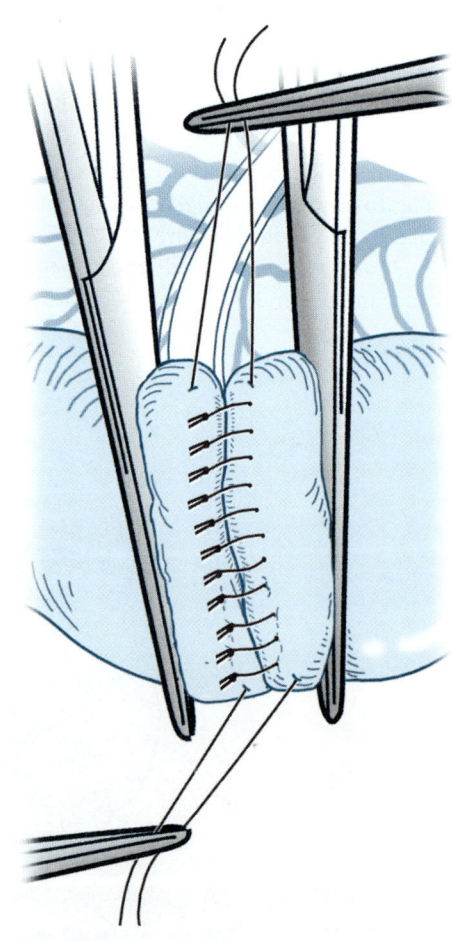

Figure 19–4

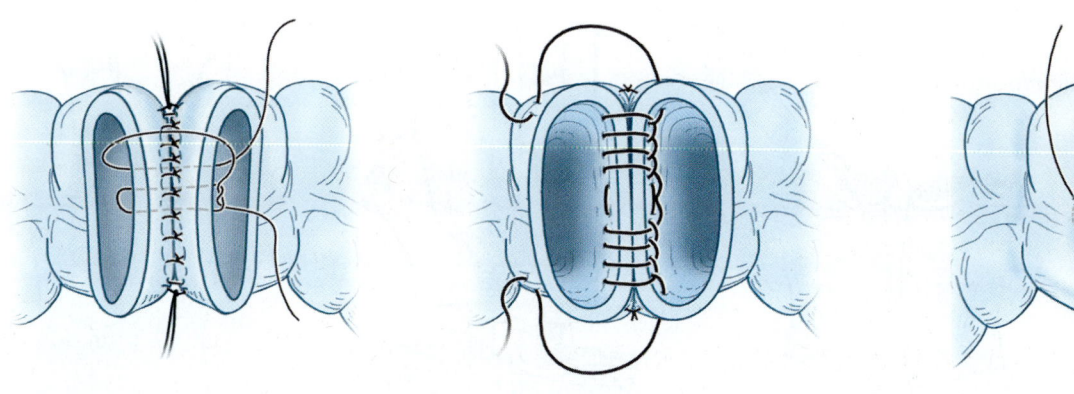

Figure 19–5

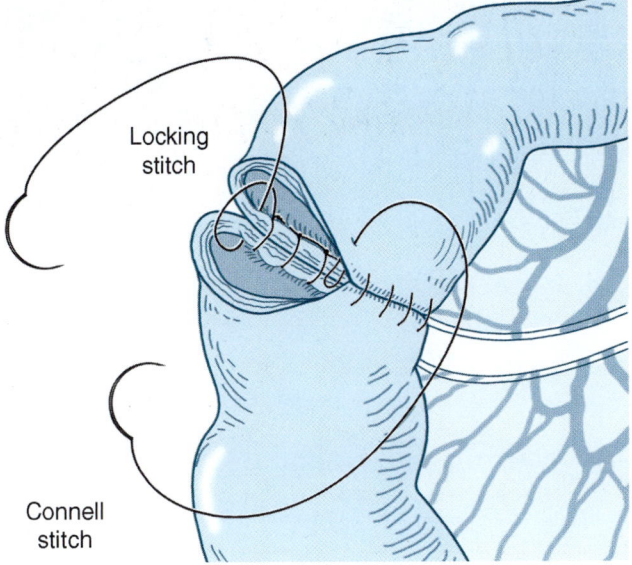

Figure 19–6

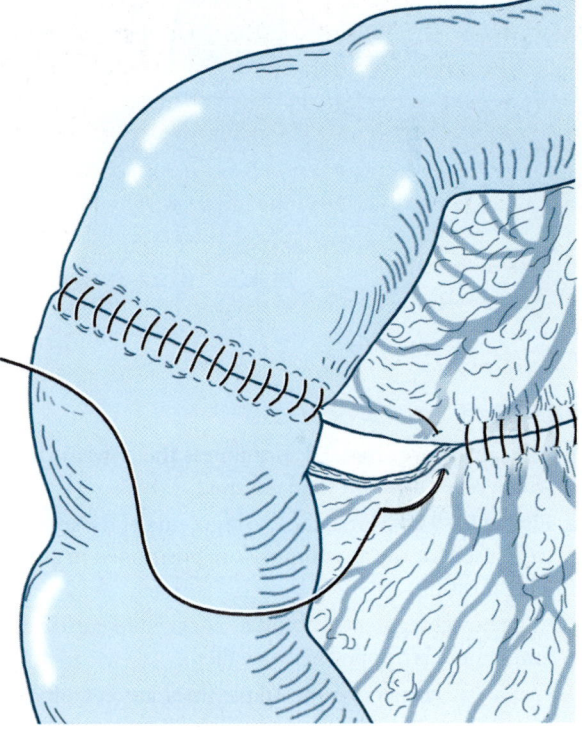

Figure 19–8

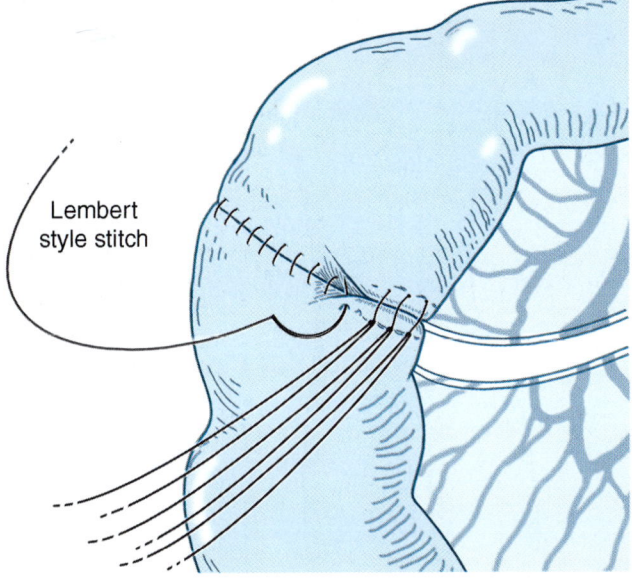

Figure 19–7

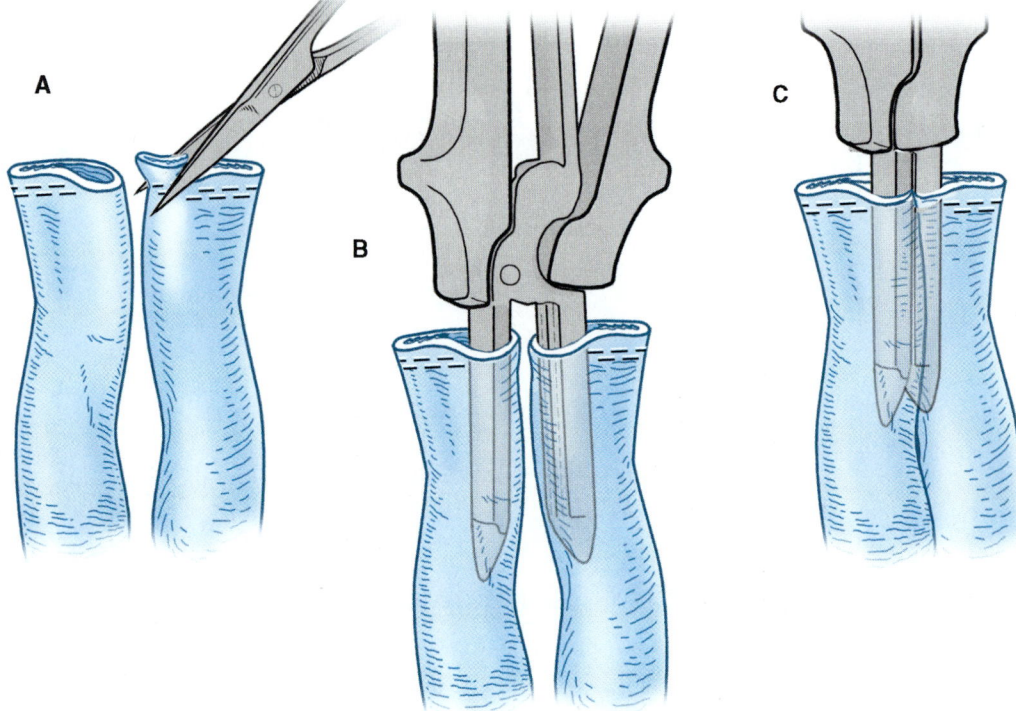

Figure 19–9A–C

Stapled Anastomosis

- All staplers are sized 3.8 mm unless the bowel is thick, in which case a 4.8-mm stapler is used.
- **Figure 19–9A-C:** First, the two segments of the small bowel to be used for the anastomosis are positioned in antiparallel apposition.
  - The bowel segments should be checked to ensure that no mesentery is trapped between them.
  - Adjacent corners of the staple lines are cut off (Figure 19–9A) and a GIA-60 mm or GIA-80 mm cutting stapler is inserted, with one limb of the stapler in the distal small bowel and the other limb in the proximal small bowel segment (Figure 19–9B).
  - The stapler is fired, which should make a connection with the length of the stapler between the two ends of the bowel, creating a side-to-side, functional, end-to-end anastomosis (Figure 19–9C).
  - The staple line is inspected by eversion to identify any sites of bleeding. Small interrupted 4-0 silk sutures can be placed to control any bleeding, or, alternatively, very light and controlled application of electrocautery may suffice.
- **Figure 19–10A, B:** The resultant enteroenterotomy is then closed using a TA stapler.
  - Firing of the stapler completes the anastomosis.
  - The staple line is often inverted by placing an outer layer of 3-0 silk interrupted Lembert sutures.

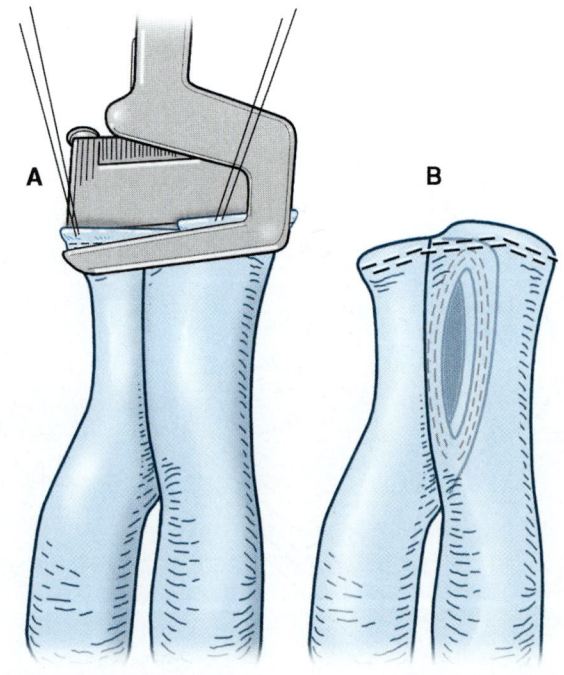

Figure 19–10A–B

POSTOPERATIVE CARE

- Epidural analgesia can decrease the amount of postoperative pain and ileus.
- The nasogastric tube should be left in place until resolution of postoperative ileus with nasogastric output < 200 mL per 8-hour shift. Diet should be advanced slowly after the passage of flatus.
- Perioperative antibiotics can be discontinued postoperatively if there has been no intraoperative contamination.
- Parenteral nutrition should be considered if the patient was malnourished preoperatively, if delayed resumption of oral intake is anticipated, or if prolonged postoperative ileus is expected.

POTENTIAL COMPLICATIONS

- Wound infection.
- Prolonged ileus.
- Mechanical obstruction.
- Anastomotic bleeding.
- Anastomotic leak.
- Enterocutaneous fistula.

PEARLS AND TIPS

- To determine adequacy of the blood supply, note the color of bowel ends and the presence of pulsatile flow in terminal arterial branches at bowel ends.
- Free up the bowel ends to ensure sufficient mobility to achieve a tension-free anastomosis.
- Accurate apposition of the layers of bowel is critical: submucosa to submucosa and seromuscular to seromuscular layers.
- There should be no fat, other tissues, or hematoma within the anastomosis. This can be a barrier to healing, and can increase the risk of leak.
- Clear no more than a 1-cm wide area of serosa for anastomosis to avoid devitalization.
- Avoid excessive force or tension when suturing the anastomosis to prevent strangulation and leak. Allow for some amount of postoperative edema.
- Avoid excessive manipulation of the bowel ends with forceps to prevent further injury and bruising.

REFERENCES

Irvin TT, Goligher JC. Aetiology of disruption of intestinal anastomosis. *Brit J Surg.* 1973;60:461–464.

Ravitch MM, Steichen FM. Techniques of staple suturing in the gastrointestinal tract. *Ann Surg.* 1972;175:815–837.

Scott-Conner CE, ed. *Chassin's Operative Strategy in General Surgery,* 3rd ed. New York, NY: Springer; 2001.

Souba WW, Fink MP, Jurkovich GJ, et al, eds. *ACS Surgery: Principles and Practice.* WebMD Professional Publishing; 2003.

CHAPTER 20

Appendectomy

Chandu Vemuri, MD, and Jonathan F. Finks, MD

INDICATIONS
- Clinical suspicion of appendicitis in an ill-appearing patient.

CONTRAINDICATIONS
Absolute
- None.

Relative
- Presence of large periappendiceal abscess, which may be treated best with initial drainage and interval appendectomy.
- Suspicion of Crohn's disease involving the cecum at the base of the appendix.

INFORMED CONSENT
Expected Benefits
- Treatment of acute appendicitis.

Potential Risks
- Bleeding requiring reoperation.
- Surgical site infection (deep or superficial).
- Fecal fistula.
- Conversion to open appendectomy.
- Need for midline laparotomy.
- Open wound.
- Need for additional tests or procedures.

EQUIPMENT
- The open procedure requires no special equipment.
- The laparoscopic procedure requires the following equipment:

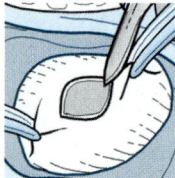
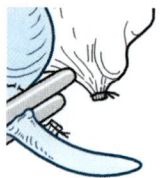
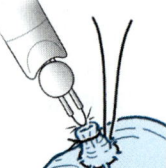
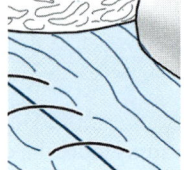

- 5-mm angled laparoscope.
- Veress needle or Hasson trocar.
- Endoscopic stapler.
- Endoscopic retrieval bag for removal of the appendix.

PATIENT PREPARATION

- No oral intake; maintenance intravenous fluids.
- Preoperative antibiotics to cover enteric flora.

PATIENT POSITIONING

Open Appendectomy

- The patient should be supine with both arms extended.
- The entire abdomen is prepared and draped in case a midline incision is needed (eg, unexpected disease is encountered or the operative course dictates it).

Laparoscopic Appendectomy

- **Figure 20–1:** The patient is supine with both arms tucked at the sides. The operating surgeon and assistant stand on the patient's left.
- A Foley catheter is placed to decompress the bladder.
- The patient's entire abdomen is prepared and draped.

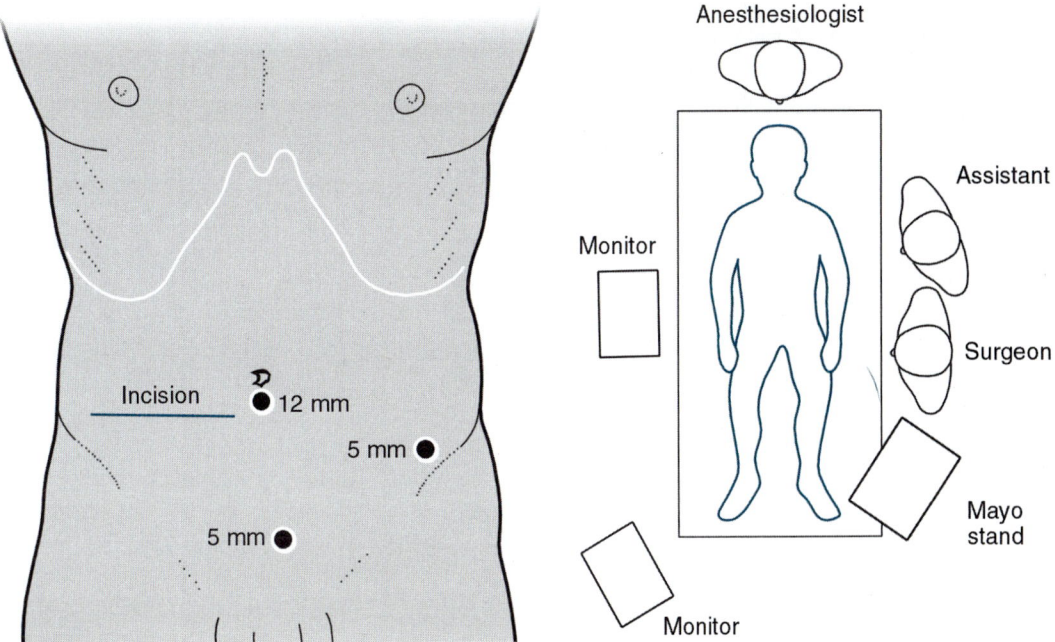

Figure 20–1

PROCEDURE

Open Appendectomy

- The classic transverse incision can be made with two thirds of the incision lateral to McBurney's point.
- Alternatively, the point of maximal tenderness or the location of the appendix based on preoperative imaging can be used to determine the location of the incision.
- **Figure 20–2:** A scalpel is used to incise the epidermis and the dermis. Bovie electrocautery is used to dissect down to the external oblique aponeurosis.
  - The aponeurosis is opened in a superolateral to inferomedial direction along the direction of its fibers to expose the internal oblique muscle.
  - The internal oblique muscle is bluntly divided perpendicular to the direction of its fibers.
  - The transverse abdominal muscle is similarly divided and the peritoneum is identified.
- **Figure 20–3:** The peritoneum is grasped with forceps and incised with a 15-blade knife.
- Attention is now focused on locating the appendix.
  - If the cecum is visualized, it can be used as a guide to help identify the appendix.
  - Babcock forceps can be used to grasp the taeniae coli and advanced until the appendix is externalized.
- Alternatively, a finger can be swept around the cecum, beginning superolaterally and continuing inferomedially to locate the appendix.
- **Figure 20–4:** Once identified, the mesoappendix is dissected and the appendiceal vessels are divided between clamps and ligated with silk sutures.
- **Figure 20–5:** A silk purse-string suture is placed around the base of the appendix. A right-angle clamp is applied to the base of the appendix and used to crush the tissue.
- The clamp is moved distally and an absorbable suture is used to ligate the appendix at the base at the site of the crushed tissue. A 15-blade is used to excise the appendix proximal to the level of the clamp.
- **Figure 20–6A, B:** The mucosa of the appendiceal stump may then be obliterated with electrocautery (Figure 20–6A). The purse-string suture is then used to invert the stump (Figure 20–6B).
- The wound is irrigated with warm saline to remove any inflammatory debris and hemostasis is achieved.
- **Figures 20–7 and 20–8.** The peritoneum and fascial layers are closed with running absorbable sutures.
- The skin is closed with monofilament absorbable suture.

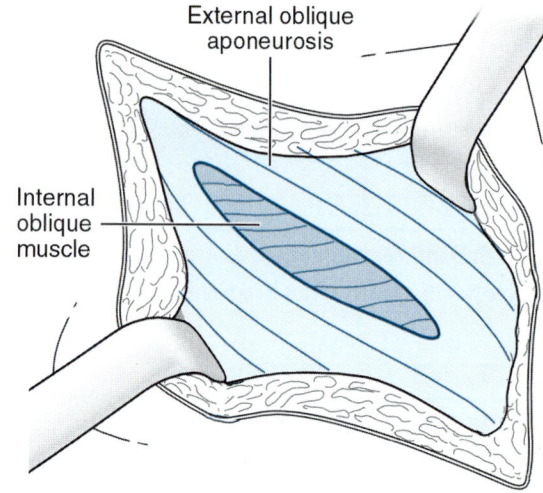

Figure 20–2

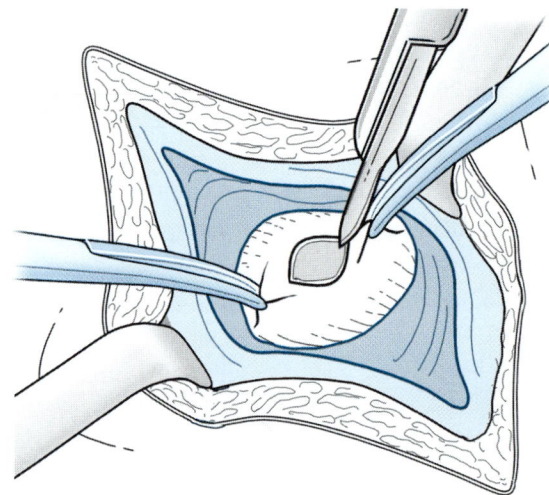

Figure 20–3

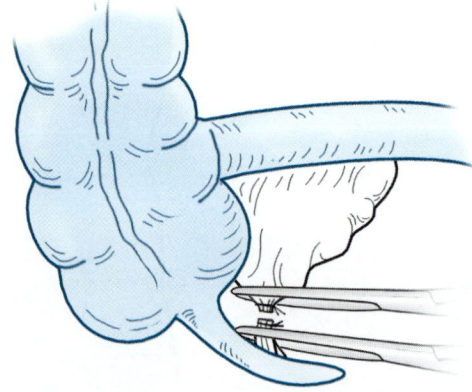

Figure 20–4

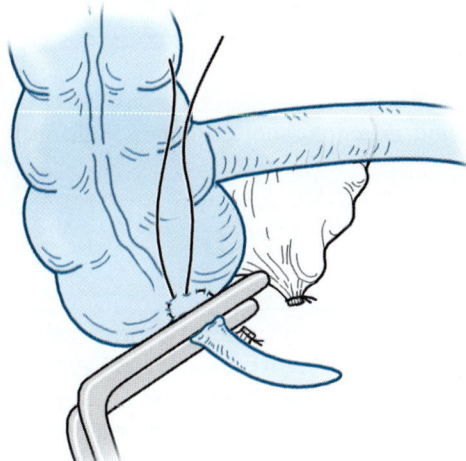

Figure 20-5

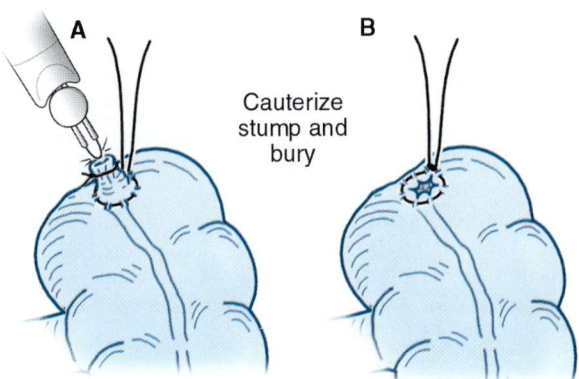

A B Cauterize stump and bury

Figure 20-6A-B

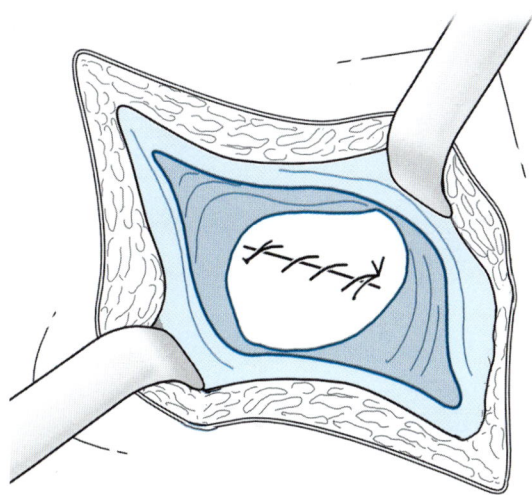

Figure 20-7

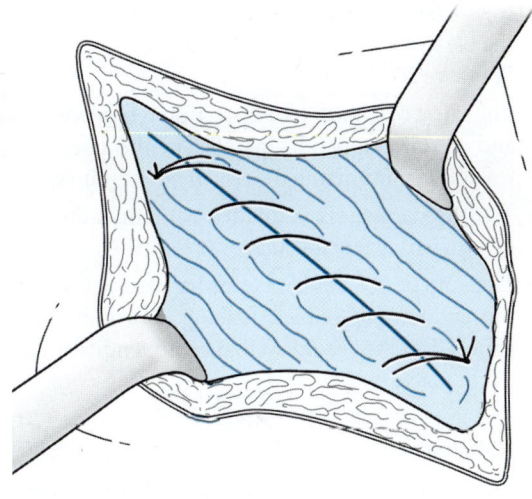

Figure 20-8

Laparoscopic Appendectomy

- A 12-mm infraumbilical incision is made and access to the abdomen is achieved using either a Veress needle or Hasson technique (see Figure 20–1). The peritoneal cavity is then insufflated with carbon dioxide gas and a 5-mm angled laparoscope is inserted.

- A 5-mm port is placed in the midline above the pubic bone and a second 5-mm port is placed laterally in the left lower quadrant (see Figure 20–1). The laparoscope is inserted through this lateral port, while the surgeon operates through the midline ports.

- Exploration of the abdomen is performed to rule out other disease. Attention then turns to the right lower quadrant.

- The patient is placed into steep Trendelenburg position with right side up to facilitate exposure.

- The omentum and small bowel are swept cephalad.

- The terminal ileum is identified by its antimesenteric fat (fold of Treves).

- The terminal ileum is then followed to the cecum. The appendix can usually be identified by following the teniae of the cecum.

- In the case of a retrocecal appendix, the cecum and ascending colon may need to be mobilized by division of the lateral retroperitoneal attachments.

- Inflammatory adhesions between small bowel, cecum, and appendix are often encountered and can usually be divided using blunt dissection, although sharp dissection may be required.

- Cautery should be avoided near the bowel.

- Once visualized, the tip of the appendix is grasped and elevated anteriorly off of the cecum.

- A Maryland dissector is used to create a window between the base of the appendix and the mesoappendix as shown in Figure 20–4.
- The safest orientation of dissection is to place the appendix and its mesoappendix parallel to the lateral abdominal wall, thus minimizing the risk of bowel injury.
- The mesoappendix is divided with an endoscopic stapler using a vascular staple load.
- The appendix is divided at its base using a second load of the endoscopic stapler, making sure that the stapler is apposed to the cecum so that an appendiceal stump is not left in place.
- The appendix is placed into an endoscopic retrieval bag and removed through the supraumbilical port.
- The appendiceal and mesoappendiceal staple lines are assessed for integrity and hemostasis.
- The abdomen is irrigated in all quadrants to prevent abscess formation.
- The small bowel is returned to the lower abdomen and the omentum is draped over the appendiceal stump.
- The laparoscope is placed back into one of the midline ports, and the remaining ports are removed under direct visualization to ensure hemostasis at the anterior abdominal wall.
- The 5-mm ports do not require fascial closure, but the fascia of the supraumbilical port should be closed with absorbable sutures.
- The skin is closed with monofilament suture or skin adhesive.

POSTOPERATIVE CARE

- Patients should be advanced to a regular diet as tolerated and discharged home when they can tolerate oral intake and manage pain with oral medication only.

POTENTIAL COMPLICATIONS

- Injury to bowel or other adjacent structures.
- Intra-abdominal abscess.
- Superficial wound infection (more common with open appendectomy).
- Colonic fistula.

PEARLS AND TIPS

- It is useful to place the incision where the patient's pain is the greatest or where preoperative imaging has identified the appendix. This is particularly important in pregnant patients, as the appendix may be in an atypical location.
- Conversion to an open procedure should be considered if visualization or dissection is difficult during laparoscopic appendectomy.

REFERENCES

Andersen BR, Kallehave FL, Andersen HK. Antibiotics versus placebo for prevention of postoperative infection after appendicectomy. *Cochrane Database Syst Rev.* 2005;3: CD001439.

Doria AS, Moineddin R, Kellenberger CJ, et al. US or CT for diagnosis of appendicitis in children and adults? A meta-analysis. *Radiology.* 2006;241:83–94.

Jones PF. Suspected acute appendicitis: trends in management over 30 years. *Br J Surg.* 2001;88:1570–1577.

Sauerland S, Lefering R, Neugebauer EA. Laparoscopic versus open surgery for suspected appendicitis. *Cochrane Database Syst Rev.* 2004;4:CD001546.

CHAPTER 21

Loop Colostomy, End Ileostomy, and Loop Ileostomy

Bedabrata Sarkar, MD, and Lisa M. Colletti, MD

INDICATIONS
- To defunctionalize bowel.
- Protection of distal anastomosis.
- Relief of obstruction.

CONTRAINDICATIONS
Absolute
- None.

Relative
- Carcinomatosis precluding mobilization of bowel.
- Morbid obesity such that mesentery or stoma cannot reach the skin surface.

INFORMED CONSENT
Expected Benefits
- Decompression of bowel obstruction.
- Protection of distal anastomosis to allow healing with decreased risk of intra-abdominal sepsis.

Relative Risks
- Bleeding.
- Intra-abdominal abscess.
- Wound infection.
- Parastomal hernia.
- Need for ostomy revision secondary to stenosis or ischemia.

EQUIPMENT
- Standard general surgery set for major gastrointestinal surgery.

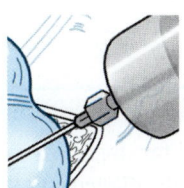 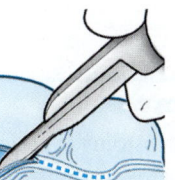 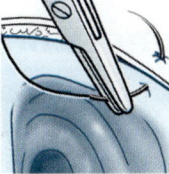
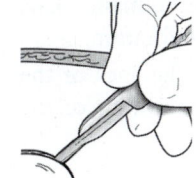 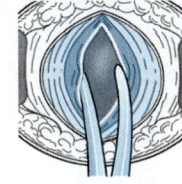 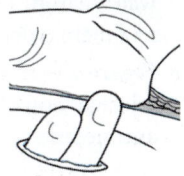
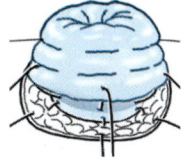 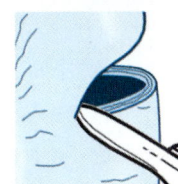 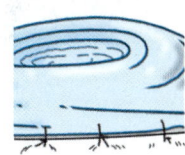

PATIENT PREPARATION

- Nasogastric tube in cases of perforation or obstruction.
- Resuscitation to correct any fluid and electrolyte abnormalities.
- Perioperative antibiotics and additional doses in the event operative time is prolonged.
- No bowel preparation is necessary for small bowel procedures.
- Preoperative evaluation and marking of optimal stoma position by an enterostomal therapist.

PATIENT POSITIONING

- The patient should be supine.

PROCEDURE

Loop Colostomy

- **Figure 21–1:** When ostomy is performed for diversion of the fecal stream due to distal obstruction, the dilated colon may be decompressed with a needle or catheter attached to wall suction. The collapsed bowel is easier to manipulate, and there is decreased risk of injury and perforation.
- **Figure 21–2:** An incision is made along the apex of the selected loop of bowel to prepare for stoma creation on the antimesenteric wall of the bowel.

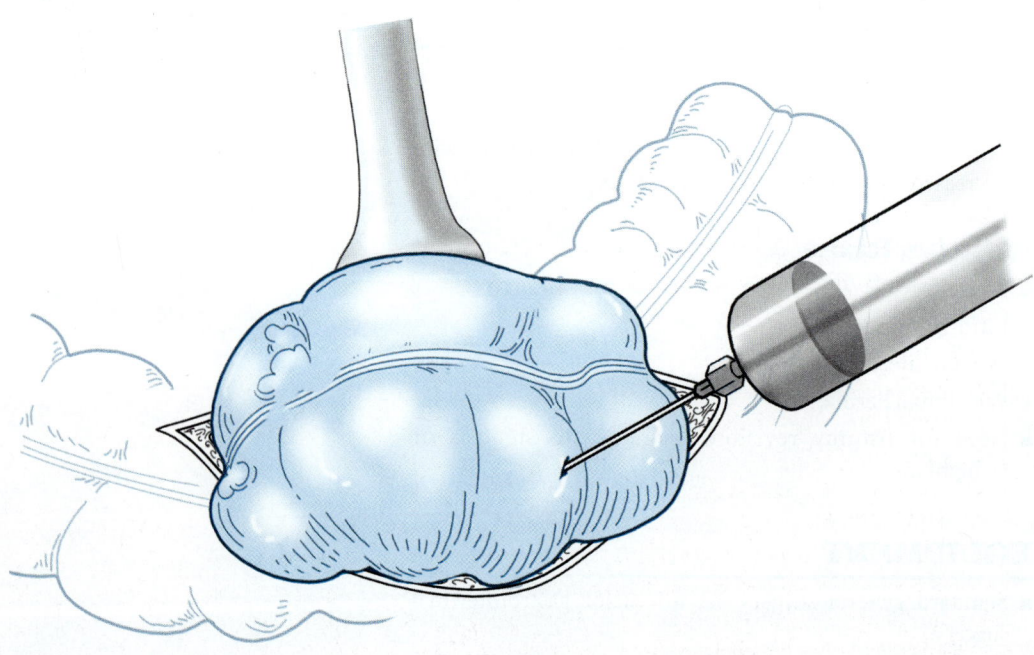

Figure 21-1

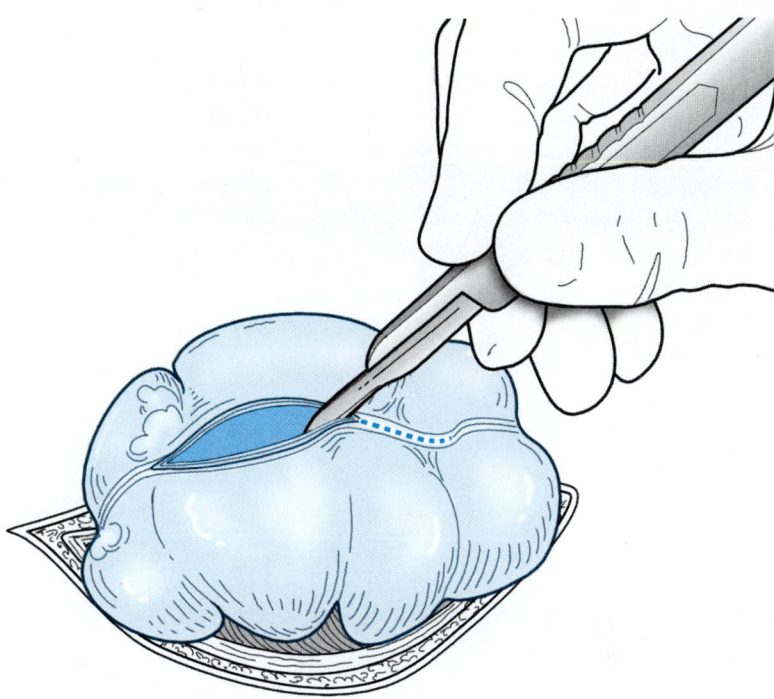

Figure 21–2

- **Figure 21–3:** The cut edges of the bowel are everted and interrupted sutures are placed using full-thickness bites of colon wall and subdermal bites of skin.
- A rod or red rubber catheter may be placed under the loop of colon being brought up; however, this step is not necessary and may interfere with placement of the ostomy appliance.

End Ileostomy

- **Figure 21–4A:** For creation of an end ileostomy, a circular incision approximately 2.5 cm in diameter is made overlying the rectus muscle.
- **Figure 21–4B:** Blunt dissection is used to divide the soft tissue to the level of the fascia.
  - A cruciate incision is made in the fascia and carried 2 cm in both directions.
  - The rectus muscle fibers are split using the clamps and retractors.
- **Figure 21–4C:** The posterior sheath is opened with a cruciate incision sufficient to permit passage of two fingers.
- **Figure 21–4D, E:** The small bowel is brought through this fascial opening using a Babcock clamp until 5 cm of ileum protrudes above the surface, with care taken to avoid twisting the mesentery.
  - Four Brooke-type sutures are then placed to evert the bowel. These are created by placing interrupted sutures through the full-thickness of the cut bowel edge, a seromuscular bite through the bowel wall at the level of the skin, and finally a subdermal skin bite.

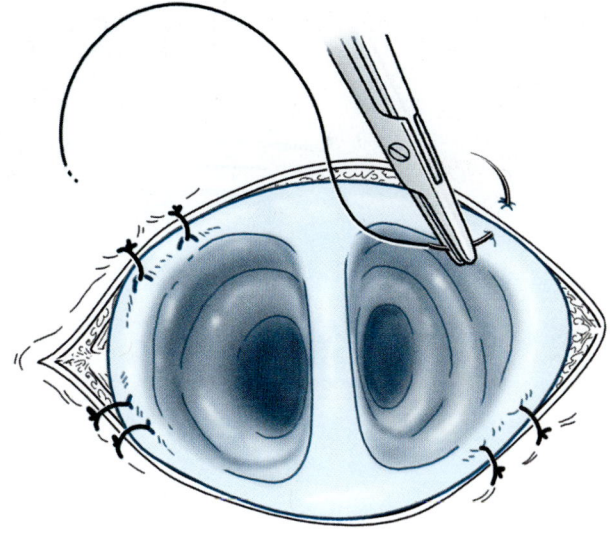

Figure 21–3

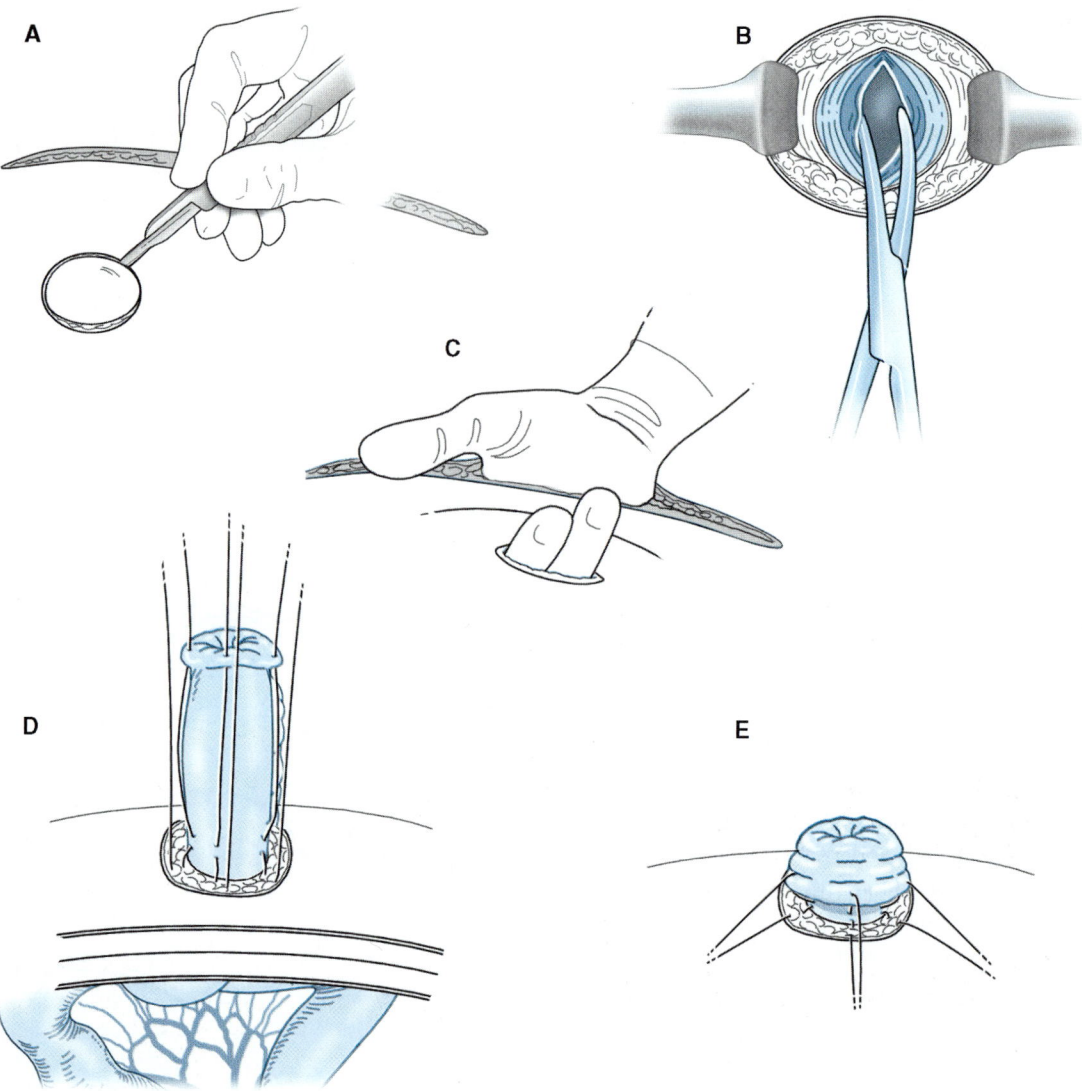

Figure 21-4A-E

- These sutures are placed in four quadrants avoiding the mesentery.
- The sutures are tied down, thus everting the bowel edges and elevating the lumen above the skin.
■ Additional interrupted sutures from the cut edge of the bowel to the dermis may be placed in between the four Brooke-type sutures.

Loop Ileostomy

■ **Figure 21-5A-D:** An ileal loop is brought out through the abdominal wall (Figure 21–5A) and an incision is extended to roughly 80% of the circumference of the distal limb (Figure 21–5B). The cut edge is everted over the proximal limb and secured with interrupted sutures (Figures 21–5C, D).

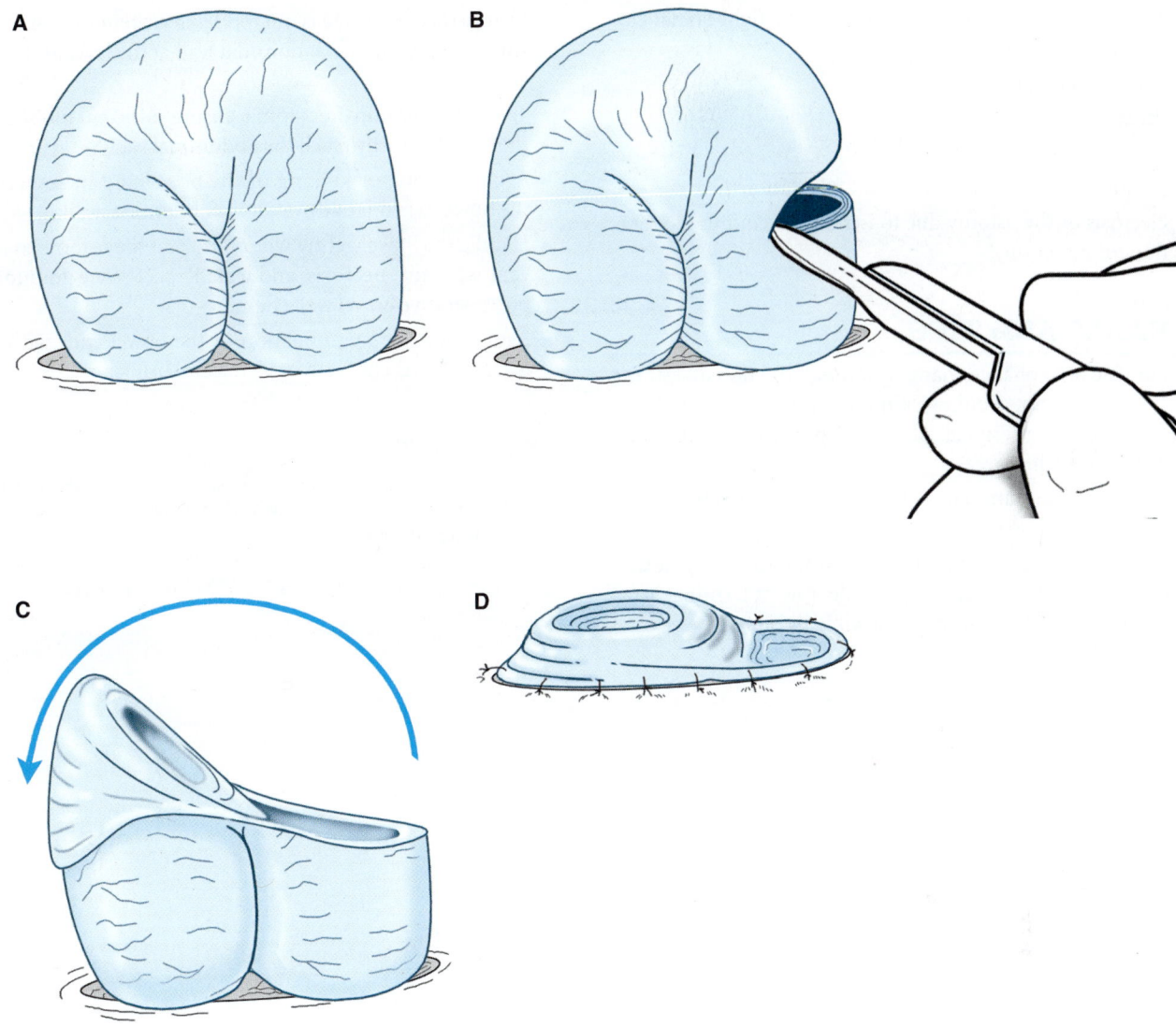

Figure 21–5A–D

- This results in elevation of the proximal limb of the stoma and leaves the defunctionalized or distal limb flush with the skin surface.

POSTOPERATIVE CARE

- Stoma may appear dusky with edema during the first postoperative week.
- Enterostomal therapists can assist with patient education about appliance care as well as treatment of any peristomal skin irritation.

POTENTIAL COMPLICATIONS

- Skin irritation from gastrointestinal contents.
- Ostomy retraction (common in obese patients).

- Mechanical obstruction due to an overly tight fascial closure around the stoma.
- Parastomal hernia.
- Prolapse.
- Fistula.
- Stenosis (may be treated with careful dilation).
- Necrosis of the ostomy due to ischemia (requires reoperation for resection).

PEARLS AND TIPS

- For ease of appliance changes, optimal selection of a stoma site on flat skin, avoiding skin folds, prior scars, and bony prominences, is critical. Also avoid placement in the "belt line" or waistline area.
- Avoid fecal contamination to prevent postoperative infection and incisional hernia.
- Ensure an adequate blood supply to the stoma by noting the color of the bowel and pulsatile flow of terminal arterial branches at bowel ends following division.
- Ensure that the stoma is not rendered ischemic by an overly small opening in the abdominal wall at the level of the fascia.
- To create a tension-free stoma, ensure sufficient mobility of the bowel to easily reach the abdominal wall.
- Avoid twisting or kinking of the bowel and mesentery as the bowel is brought through the abdominal wall.
- Handle the bowel gently when suturing the ostomy to prevent ischemia, necrosis, and leak. Expect some amount of postoperative bowel wall edema.
- Avoid excessive manipulation of the bowel ends with the forceps to prevent further edema and bruising.

REFERENCES

Souba WW, Fink MP, Jurkovich GJ, et al, eds. *ACS Surgery, Principles and Practice.* New York, NY: WebMD Professional Publishing; 2006.

Zollinger RM Jr, Zollinger RM Sr. *Zollinger's Atlas of Surgical Operations,* 8th ed. New York, NY: McGraw-Hill; 2002.

CHAPTER 22

Operative Management of Inflammatory Bowel Disease

Jennifer Cannon, MD, and Emina H. Huang, MD

COLECTOMY WITH ILEOSTOMY OR ILEAL POUCH ANAL ANASTOMOSIS

INDICATIONS

Emergency
- Total abdominal colectomy with end ileostomy is the only operation typically performed in the emergent setting for the following indications:
  - Ulcerative colitis: toxic megacolon, perforation, fulminant colitis, hemorrhage.
  - Crohn's disease: same indications, plus obstruction.

Elective

A. Ulcerative Colitis (Curative)
- Either total proctocolectomy with end ileostomy or ileal pouch anal anastomosis (IPAA) may be selected, depending on patient factors.
- Indications for proctocolectomy include:
  - Dysplasia or malignancy.
  - Condition refractory to medical management; intractability.
  - Growth retardation in children.
  - Complications secondary to adverse effects of medical treatment.

B. Crohn's Disease (Palliative)
- Total proctocolectomy with end ileostomy only; IPAA is not an option (see Contraindications later).
- Indications for proctocolectomy include:
  - Internal fistula.
  - Abscess.
  - Malignancy.
  - Intractability.

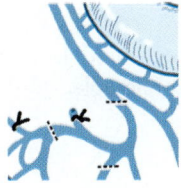
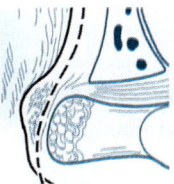
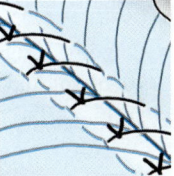
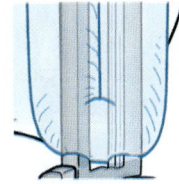
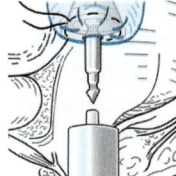
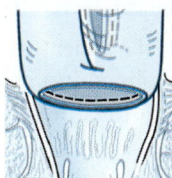
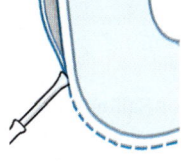
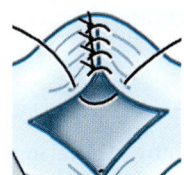

CONTRAINDICATIONS

Ileal Pouch Anal Anastomosis

A. Absolute
- Crohn's disease.
- Emergency procedure.
- Low rectal neoplasia.
- Disseminated carcinoma.
- Incontinence (fecal).
- Inability to tolerate a long period of general anesthesia (4–6 hours) due to comorbidities.

B. Relative
- Indeterminant colitis.
- Obesity (thick mesentery precludes adequate mobilization).
- Ongoing high-dose steroid therapy (eg, prednisone, 50–60 mg/day); a staged approach may be preferable.
- Malnutrition (serum albumin < 2 g/dL).

Total Proctocolectomy with End Ileostomy
- If a patient is extremely ill, as in the emergent setting, total abdominal colectomy with end ileostomy should be performed, leaving the rectum intact at that operative setting.

INFORMED CONSENT

Expected Benefits

A. Total Abdominal Colectomy with End Ileostomy (Emergent Surgery)
- Removal of the bulk of the diseased colon, allowing the patient to improve from a medical standpoint while enabling a restorative procedure to be performed at a later date.

B. Ileal Pouch Anal Anastomosis
- Restoration of gastrointestinal continuity precluding the need for permanent ostomy.
- Significantly reduces risk of developing colorectal malignancy secondary to chronic inflammatory bowel disease.

C. Total Proctocolectomy with End Ileostomy
- Prevents the development of colorectal malignancy secondary to chronic inflammatory bowel disease.
- Provides effective treatment for fistulous perineal disease.

Potential Risks

A. Men (All Procedures)
- Urinary retention.
- Erectile dysfunction.
- Retrograde ejaculation.

B. Women (All Procedures)
- Dyspareunia.
- Decreased fertility.
- Urinary dysfunction.
- Enlarged uterus may necessitate hysterectomy at the time of operation.

C. Both Men and Women
- Need for diverting ileostomy (IPAA).
- Anastomotic leak → abscess or sepsis → poor pouch function (IPAA).
- Anastomotic stricture (IPAA).
- Bowel obstruction (all procedures).
- Anal leakage (IPAA).
- Pouch failure requiring revision to end ileostomy (IPAA).
- Pouchitis (IPAA).

EQUIPMENT
- Lone-Star retractor (useful for exposure during the perineal dissection).
- Self-retaining retractor (helpful for the abdominal portions of the procedure to facilitate exposure of the operative field).
- Gastrointestinal anastomosis (GIA) stapler.
- End-to-end anastomosis (EEA) stapler (optional).

PATIENT PREPARATION
- Anesthesia consultation, as indicated by patient comorbidities.
- Preoperative consultation with enterostomal therapist for teaching and preoperative marking of the stoma site.
- Mechanical and antibiotic bowel preparation the day before surgery (although controversy exists in the current literature regarding the necessity of this practice).
- Nothing by mouth after midnight on the evening before surgery. (Again, there is some controversy in the literature as to the necessity of prolonged fasting. Current institutional practice dictates 6 hours without solid food.)
- Perioperative antibiotics with appropriate coverage (gram-negative bacilli, anaerobes, enterococci, etc), administered within 30 minutes of skin incision (by anesthesia personnel) and redosed as indicated during surgery.
- Deep vein thrombosis prophylaxis, initiated before induction of anesthesia.
- Foley catheter insertion after anesthetic induction.
- Consideration of stress-dose steroids, depending on the patient's current and past medication regimen.
- Consideration should also be given to placement of ureteral stents preoperatively.

PATIENT POSITIONING

- The patient should be in modified lithotomy position, with the legs supported in noncompressing stirrups.
  - This position allows easy access to both the abdomen and the perineum.
  - Arms may be tucked at the sides or extended on arm boards.
- During the operation, steep Trendelenburg position is helpful for obtaining access and exposure to the pelvis and perineum.

PROCEDURE

Total Abdominal Colectomy with End Ileostomy (Emergent Setting)

- In emergent cases, a two- or three-stage procedure is employed.
  - Total abdominal colectomy with management of the rectal stump and end ileostomy.
  - Either completion proctectomy with end ileostomy or IPAA with diverting loop ileostomy.
  - If IPAA is selected, then a third stage is required for reversal of the loop ileostomy.

A. Total Abdominal Colectomy with End Ileostomy

- Thorough abdominal exploration is performed through a midline incision, with special attention paid to the small intestine to detect any evidence of Crohn's disease.
- **Figure 22–1:** A standard abdominal colectomy is performed (see Chapter 23), dividing the small bowel as close

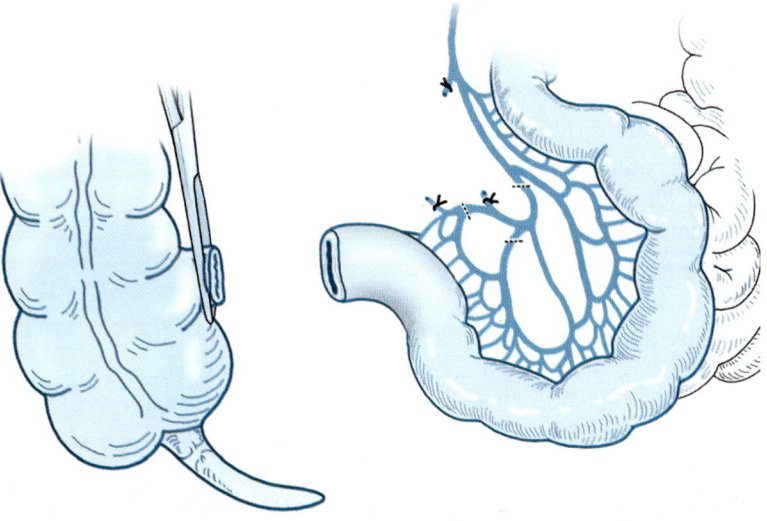

Figure 22–1

to the cecum as possible in order to preserve maximal length. The ileum is only mobilized sufficiently to reach the abdominal wall for ostomy creation. Oncologic principles do not apply, and wide mesenteric resection is not necessary.
- **Figure 22–2:** The inferior mesenteric vessels are preserved and ligated individually during removal of the sigmoid colon, which minimizes damage to pelvic autonomic nerves and reduces scar formation.
  - Preservation of the ileocecal artery is desired, although in most instances it is ligated if a subsequent restorative pouch procedure is performed, with the arterial supply maintained via the superior mesenteric artery.
- The rectal stump can be managed by a simple Hartmann pouch, either stapled or hand sewn, ideally at the level of the sacral promontory.
  - If the tissue is friable, a mucus fistula may be matured to the skin.
  - Alternatively, if there is insufficient length, the fistula may be brought through the fascia at the lower end of the midline incision and sutured in the subcutaneous space.
  - Transanal drainage of the rectal stump may further reduce the risk of pelvic sepsis.
- An end ileostomy is then constructed in standard Brooke fashion.

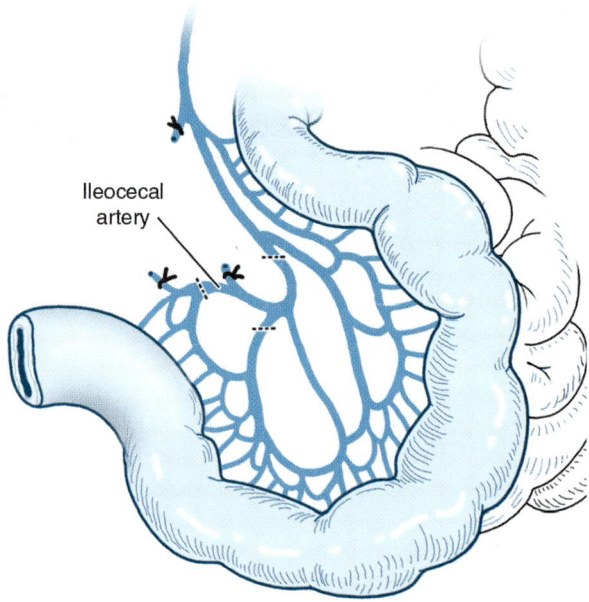

Figure 22–2

Total Proctocolectomy with End Ileostomy (Elective Setting)

- This is the conventional operative approach and gold standard against which other procedures are compared. It may be considered a first-line procedure in patients for whom IPAA is unsuitable.
- A midline incision is made and thorough abdominal exploration is performed.
- As earlier, a standard abdominal colectomy is performed (see Chapter 23 for additional details). If surgery is indicated for malignancy or dysplasia, oncologic principles should be followed (ie, wide excision of the mesentery and removal of the entire colon).
- The maximum length of small bowel should be preserved by dividing the terminal ileum immediately adjacent to the cecum.
- The ureters should be identified; the rectum is then carefully mobilized, preserving the pelvic nerves.
- **Figure 22–3:** Once the rectum is mobilized from the abdominal approach, an intersphincteric perineal dissection allows removal of the diseased organ, creating a smaller wound than that typically made for abdominoperineal resection.
- **Figure 22–4:** The resultant wound is closed in several layers. A drain may be placed according to surgeon preference.
- A standard Brooke ileostomy is matured.

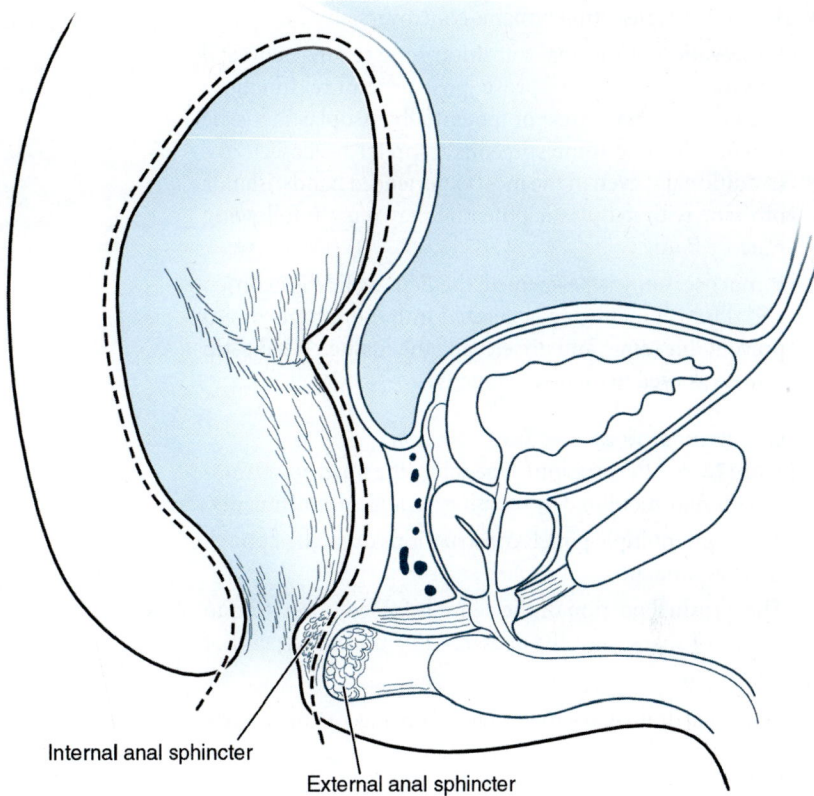

Figure 22-3

Ileal Pouch Anal Anastomosis (Elective Setting)

- The operation is best considered in four phases:
  - Excision of the intra-abdominal colon.
  - Dissection and removal of the rectum, taking care to spare pelvic nerves and preserve the anal sphincter mechanism.
  - Construction of the ileal pouch.
  - Anastomosis of the pouch to the anal canal.

A. Excision of the Intra-abdominal Colon

- Following midline incision and abdominal exploration, a standard abdominal colectomy is carried out as previously described.

B. Dissection and Removal of the Rectum

- As earlier, a close rectal dissection is performed. The rectum is mobilized first posteriorly, preserving the presacral nerves, and then moving anteriorly 1 cm above the peritoneal reflection.
- Anterior dissection proceeds posterior to Denonvilliers' fascia and is carried down to the lower one third of the vagina or the lower border of the prostate. This mobilizes the rectum fully to the level of the levators and the anorectal junction.
- The rectum is then transected.

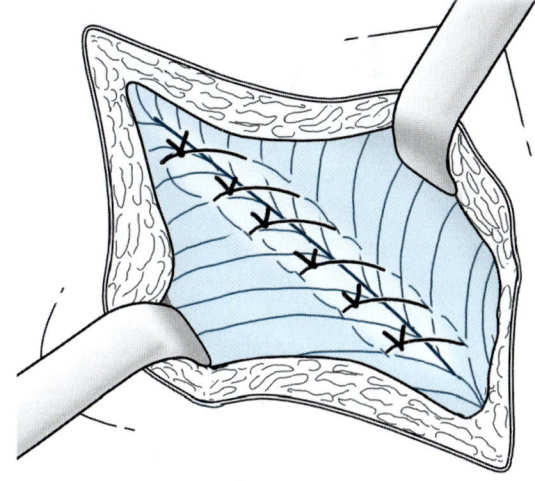

Figure 22-4

- The level of transection remains controversial:
  - Preservation of the anal transition zone retains neorectal sensation and may improve post-procedure function; however, a small area of potentially neoplastic tissue remains, leading some surgeons to prefer mucosectomy. (Additionally, even in the most experienced hands, islands of tissue with neoplastic potential may remain following mucosectomy.)
  - If mucosectomy is performed, the dentate line is exposed and dilute epinephrine is injected into the submucosa to prevent bleeding and to elevate the tissue. Needle-tip cautery is used to excise the mucosa.

C. Construction of the Ileal Pouch

- **Figure 22–5:** After excision of the colon, the small bowel mesentery is fully mobilized by releasing peritoneal attachments.
  - Although multiple pouch constructions exist, the J pouch is most popular.
  - The terminal portion of the ileum is folded upon itself to create a J shape with the apex 15–20 cm from the end of the ileum.

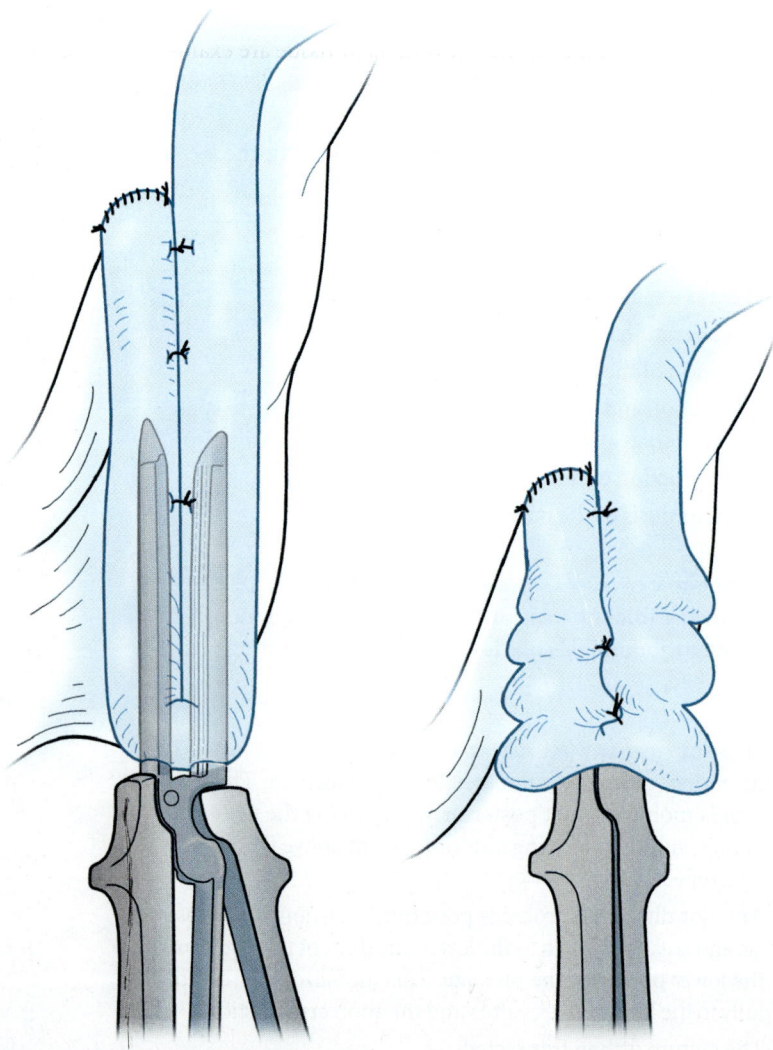

Figure 22–5

- An apical enterotomy is made and the pouch is created by serial firings of a linear GIA stapler (use of the GIA-80 mm stapler will allow fewer firings), taking care to keep the mesentery free as the bowel is accordioned onto the stapler.
- To estimate whether the created pouch will reach the anal canal, the apex of the pouch (or the segment of bowel destined to become the apex prior to construction) may be grasped and measured to ensure that it will reach approximately 4–6 cm beyond the pubic symphysis.

D. Anastomosis of the Pouch to the Anal Canal

- **Figure 22–6A, B:** Once the pouch is created, either a double-stapled or, if mucosectomy is performed, a hand-sewn ileoanal anastomosis (see Figure 22–7) is performed.
  - For a double-stapled anastomosis, the anvil of the circular EEA stapler is secured with a purse-string suture in the apical enterotomy of the J pouch (Figure 22–6A).
  - The stapler is passed transanally, and the pointed shaft is directed just posterior to the staple line on the anorectum.
  - The shaft is removed, stapler and anvil are joined and fired in customary fashion, and the donuts of tissue are examined for integrity (Figure 22–6B).

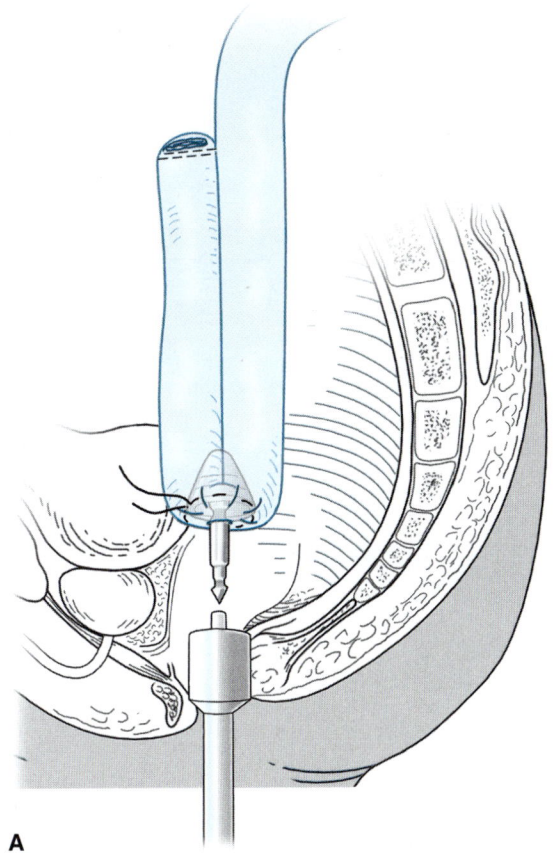
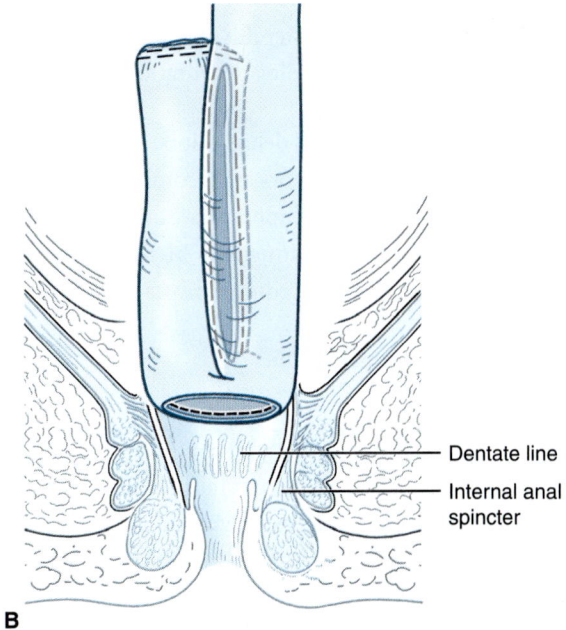

Figure 22–6A–B

- In women, particular care must be taken to avoid inclusion of the vagina in the staple line.
- The anastomosis is then tested via transanal insufflation with the staple lines submerged in saline and the small bowel occluded manually proximal to the anastomosis.

■ **Figure 22–7:** A hand-sewn IPAA entails radial placement of absorbable sutures at the dentate line, incorporating a small portion of the internal anal sphincter. The apex of the pouch is brought to the anal verge and the previously placed sutures are serially placed through the ileum (full thickness) and tied down.

E. Diverting Loop Ileostomy

■ A loop of ileum approximately 30–45 cm proximal to the pouch is brought up to the right lower quadrant (or previously marked location) and a standard loop ileostomy is created.

■ To provide maximal length for absorption, a too-proximal limb should be avoided.

■ Controversy exists over the need for diversion; the morbidity associated with both creation of an ostomy and subsequent ostomy reversal must be weighed against potentially increased anastomotic complications in the absence of diversion. Some surgeons forego ileostomy creation in favor of a single-stage procedure.

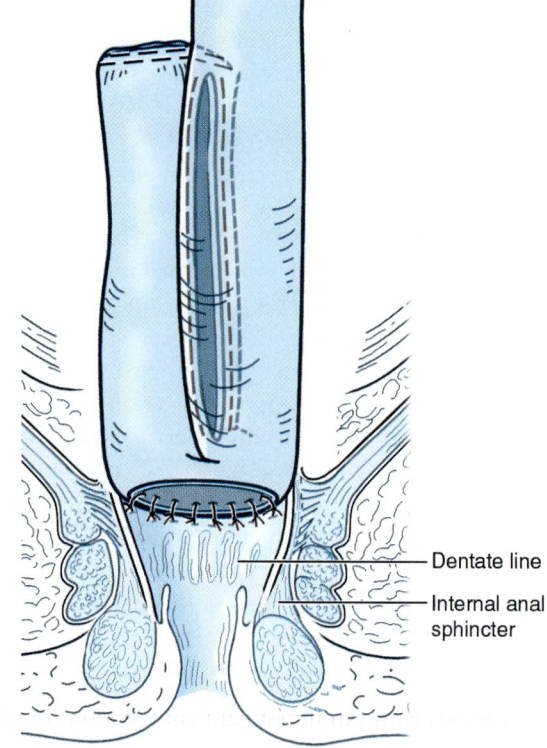

Figure 22-7

POSTOPERATIVE CARE

■ Await resolution of ileus.
■ For total proctocolectomy, vigilant care of the perineal wound and avoidance of pressure or weight bearing on the perineum.
■ Close monitoring for signs and symptoms of anastomotic leak and pelvic sepsis.
■ Tapering of stress-dose steroids, if appropriate.
■ Patient education regarding dehydration, including information on:
  - Signs and symptoms of dehydration.
  - Recognition of risk factors for becoming dehydrated.
  - Proper maintenance of appropriate oral fluid intake.
  - Recognition of and treatment for high ostomy output.
■ Enterostomal therapist education of patient and family regarding ostomy care.
■ Nutritional counseling.

POTENTIAL COMPLICATIONS

■ Dehydration and electrolyte abnormalities.
  - Although a diverting ostomy is in place, patients may require readmission to the hospital for hydration and correction of electrolyte derangements.
  - If this problem is recurring or severe, it may necessitate early reversal of ostomy.

- Small bowel obstruction occurs in 15% of patients (half require operative intervention).
  - Common causes include adhesions, internal hernia, and volvulus.
- Sepsis.
  - Pelvic abscess.
  - Anastomotic leak.
- Fistula.
  - Pouch-vagina.
  - Perineal.
  - Potentially indicative of Crohn's disease if it occurs after IPAA.
- Anastomotic stricture.
  - Usually resolves with digital or balloon dilation.
  - May require pouch revision.
- Pouchitis.
  - Poorly understood entity, occurring in 30–50% of pouch patients.
  - Generally responds to treatment with antimicrobial drugs (metronidazole, fluoroquinolones).
  - Patients with extraintestinal manifestations of ulcerative colitis, particularly primary sclerosing cholangitis, are at increased risk.
  - In 10–15% of patients with chronic pouchitis, pouch excision and end ileostomy is required.
- Malignancy.
  - May occur irrespective of whether mucosectomy was performed.
  - Continued screening is required for all patients.
- Pouch failure.
  - Occurs in 5–10% of patients.
  - Risk factors include tension on the anastomosis, compromised blood supply, hand-sewn anastomosis, unsuspected Crohn's disease, leak or sepsis, and use of a diverting ileostomy.
- Sexual dysfunction.
  - Men: occurs due to injury of the parasympathetic nerve trunks during rectal dissection in 1–3% of patients; may be transient or permanent. Problems include impotence, difficulty emptying the bladder, and retrograde ejaculation.
  - Women: problems include decreased fertility (sometimes due to adhesions), dyspareunia, and leaking during intercourse. Normal pregnancies and deliveries are possible, but patients may have increased incontinence or temporary stoma dysfunction. There is no specific contraindication to vaginal delivery unless indicated for obstetric reasons, although scarred perineum may be an indication for cesarean delivery.

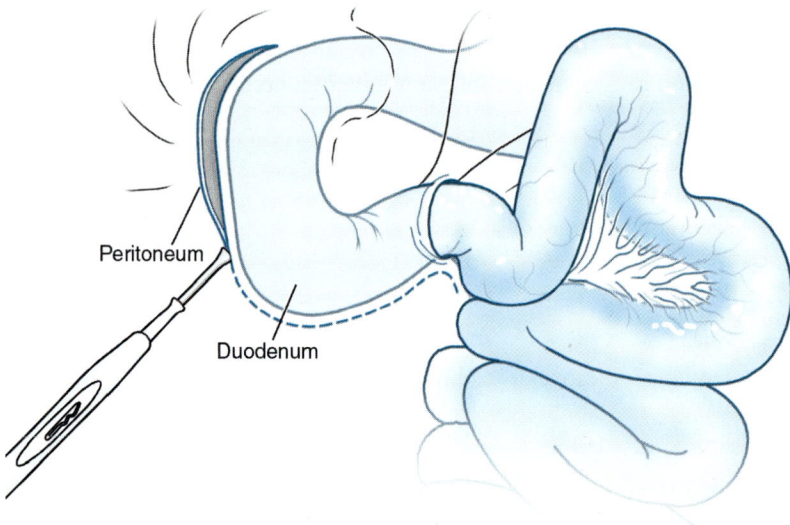

Figure 22–8

PEARLS AND TIPS

- If it is not clear that a tension-free anastomosis can be performed, various maneuvers can be used to increase length:
  - **Figure 22–8:** The small bowel mesentery can be mobilized to the third portion of the duodenum.
  - **Figure 22–9:** Peritoneal windows in the mesentery can be created over vessels causing tension and may provide additional length. This maneuver can be repeated on both sides of the mesentery.
- Transillumination and confirmation of adequate blood flow by Doppler ultrasound is useful to identify vessels that may be sacrificed.
- Elective operations may be completed via laparoscopic-assisted techniques.

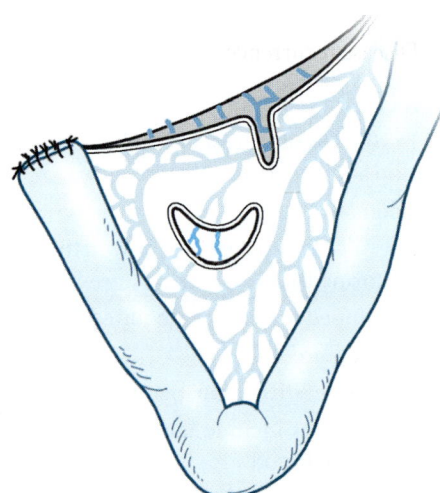

Figure 22–9

OPERATIVE MANAGEMENT OF CROHN'S DISEASE: STRICTUROPLASTY

INDICATIONS

- Jejunoileitis with single or multiple fibrotic strictures.
- History of multiple small bowel resections and risk for development of short-gut syndrome.
- Disease with history of rapid recurrence.
- Isolated duodenal strictures.

CONTRAINDICATIONS

- Abscess.
- Fistula.
- Generalized peritonitis.
- Phlegmon or acute inflammatory reaction.
- Long, high-grade strictures.
- Severe malnutrition (serum albumin < 2 g/dL).

INFORMED CONSENT

Expected Benefits

- Palliative measure to relieve obstructive symptoms.

Potential Risks

- Operation is not curative.
- Findings at operation may require abortion of the procedure or change of the planned procedure, including the need for an ostomy.
- Malignancy may be discovered at the site of the stricture.
- Surgical risks include:
  - Disease recurrence.
  - Bleeding at suture lines.
  - Leak or dehiscence at suture lines.
  - Need for a bowel resection if strictures are not amenable to stricturoplasty.

EQUIPMENT

- No special equipment is required.
- A self-retaining retractor is useful to facilitate exposure of the operative field.

PATIENT PREPARATION

- Contrast radiography prior to any surgical undertaking is essential to rule out surgical contraindications, and to define the indication for operation. CT enterography is preferred.
- Perioperative antibiotics with appropriate coverage (gram-negative bacilli, anaerobes, enterococci, etc), administered within 30 minutes of skin incision (by anesthesia personnel) and redosed as indicated during surgery.
- Deep vein thrombosis prophylaxis, initiated prior to incision.
- Consideration of stress-dose steroids, depending on the patient's current and past medication regimen.

PATIENT POSTIONING

- The patient should be supine on the operating table.
- The arms may be tucked at the sides or extended on arm boards.

PROCEDURE

Heineke-Mikulicz Stricturoplasty

- Suitable for strictures < 7–10 cm.
- A midline incision is made and the abdominal cavity is thoroughly explored to rule out unanticipated findings that would alter the planned operative approach.
- **Figure 22–10:** A longitudinal incision is made in the antimesenteric border of the stricture and carried 1–2 cm into normal-appearing bowel on either side.
  - The mucosa is carefully inspected and biopsy specimens are taken from any suspicious-looking areas to evaluate for possible occult malignancy.
  - Stay sutures are placed on either side of the midpoint of the enterotomy, traction is applied, and the longitudinal incision is closed horizontally in one or two layers.

Finney Stricturoplasty

- Used for strictures 10–15 cm in length.
- **Figure 22–11A-C:** A longitudinal incision is made on the antimesenteric side of the bowel, extending the enterotomy into normal bowel (Figure 22–11A).

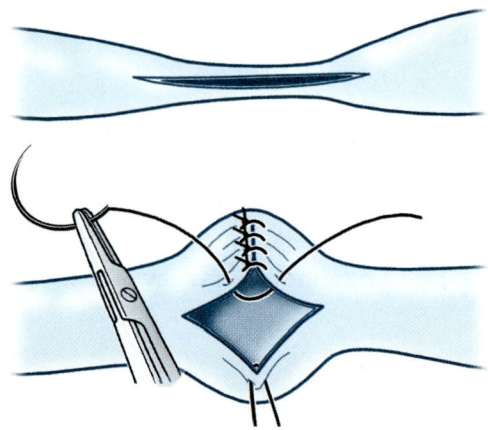

Figure 22–10

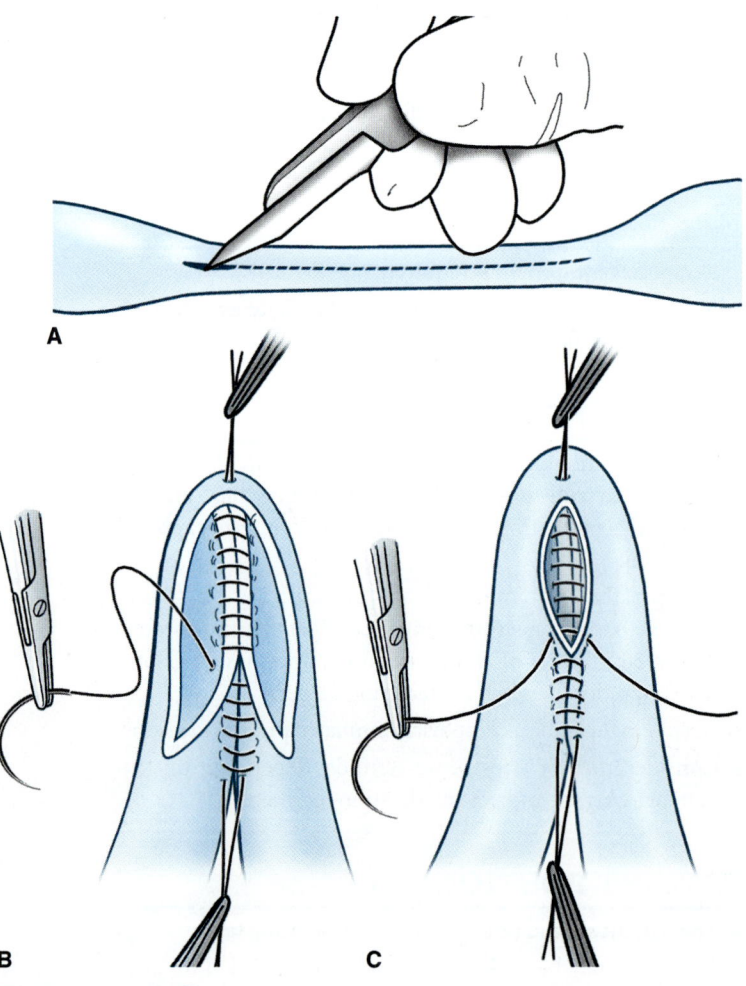

Figure 22–11A–C

- The mucosa is inspected and biopsy specimens are taken as indicated.
- Stay sutures are placed at each end of the incision and on the superior side of the midpoint of the incision.
- The bowel is then folded upon itself, creating an inverted U shape.
- A side-to-side anastomosis is performed with absorbable suture. The posterior wall is completed first, beginning at the apex and continuing anteriorly (Figure 22–11B, C).
- This suture line is then reinforced with nonabsorbable, interrupted, inverted Lembert sutures.

POSTOPERATIVE CARE

- Await resolution of ileus.
- Tapering of stress-dose steroids, if indicated.

POTENTIAL COMPLICATIONS

- Hemorrhage from the suture line.
- Dehiscence.
- Abscess.
- Long strictures treated with Finney stricturoplasty may result in functional intestinal bypass with bacterial overgrowth in the resultant diverticulum.
- Fistula formation.

PEARLS AND TIPS

- Areas of small bowel stricture too long to be treated with stricturoplasty should be resected.
- Frozen sections obtained from areas under consideration for stricturoplasty should be sent for pathologic evaluation to rule out malignancy.
- Consider marking sites of stricturoplasty with metal clips to enable radiographic tracking for recurrence.
- When short-gut syndrome is of significant concern, or a patient has multiple strictures in close proximity, a "side-to-side isoperistaltic" or Michelassi stricturoplasty (not described here) may be considered.

REFERENCES

Cima RR, Pemberton JH. Medical and surgical management of chronic ulcerative colitis. *Arch Surg.* 2005;140:300–310.

Cohen JL, Strong SA, Hyman NH, et al. Practice parameters for the surgical treatment of ulcerative colitis. *Dis Colon Rectum.* 2005;48:1997–2009.

Cohen Z, Senagore AJ, Dayton MT, et al. Prevention of postoperative abdominal adhesions by a novel, glycerol/sodium hyaluronate/carboxy-methylcellulose-based bioresorbable membrane: a prospective, randomized, evaluator-blinded multicenter study. *Dis Colon Rectum.* 2005;48:1130–1139.

Galandiuk S. Crohn's Disease. In: Souba WW, Fink MP, Jurkovich GJ, et al, eds. *ACS Surgery, Principles and Practice.* New York, NY: WebMD Professional Publishing; 2005:665–673.

Huang E. Ulcerative Colitis. In: Mulholland MW, Lillemoe KD, Doherty GM, et al, eds. *Greenfield's Surgery: Scientific Principles & Practice,* 4th ed. Philadelphia, PA: Lippincott Williams & Wilkins; 2006:1066–1080.

Hurst RD, Michelassi F. Fulminant Ulcerative Colitis. In: Souba WW, Fink MP, Jurkovich GJ, et al, eds. *ACS Surgery, Principles and Practice.* Online Edition. New York, NY: WebMD Professional Publishing; 2005.

Michelassi F, Hurst RD, Fichera A. Crohn's Disease. In: Mulholland MW, Lillemoe KD, Doherty GM, et al, eds. *Greenfield's Surgery: Scientific Principles & Practice,* 4th ed. Philadelphia, PA: Lippincott Williams & Wilkins; 2006:788–807.

CHAPTER 23

Colectomy

Barry L. Rosenberg, MD, MBA, and Arden M. Morris, MD, MPH

INDICATIONS
- Colon cancer.
- Colon polyps not amenable to colonoscopic polypectomy.
- Diverticular disease.
- Perforation of the colon for which ostomy is not needed.
- Inflammatory bowel disease.
- Volvulus.
- Stricture.
- Ischemia.
- Bleeding.
- Slow-transit constipation refractory to medical therapy.

CONTRAINDICATIONS
- Widely metastatic colon cancer that is nonoperative or requires a palliative ostomy.
- Severe peritonitis requiring diverting ostomy, in which primary anastomosis would have an unacceptable leak rate.
- Hemodynamic instability requiring expeditious ostomy, making primary anastomosis inappropriate.

INFORMED CONSENT

Expected Benefits
- Treatment of established colon cancer (or prevention of development).
- Relief of functional or mechanical colonic obstruction.
- Treatment (or prevention) of intra-abdominal sepsis secondary to colonic perforation.
- Treatment of colonic bleeding.

Potential Risks
- Bleeding.
- Infection.
- Damage to adjacent structures, including ureter, bowel, spleen, and others.

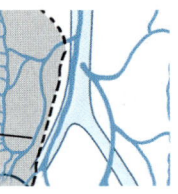
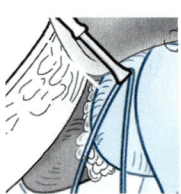
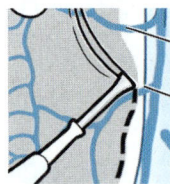
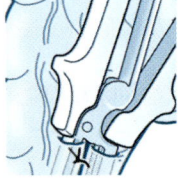
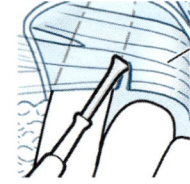
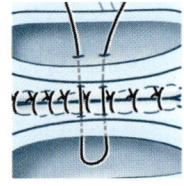
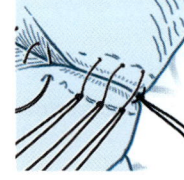
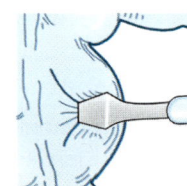
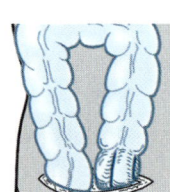

- Need for further operations.
- Anastomotic leak.
- Need for ostomy.
- Unresectability.
- Recurrence of cancer.
- Cardiopulmonary or other organ failure.
- Death.

EQUIPMENT

- Bookwalter or similar self-retaining abdominal retractor.
- Long instruments.
- Gastrointestinal anastomosis (GIA), linear cutting stapler.
- Linear thoracoabdominal (TA) stapler.
- Intraluminal circular end-to-end anastomosis (CEEA) stapler.
- Laparoscopic equipment if procedure will be performed using laparoscopic techniques, to include:
  - Angled laparoscope.
  - Atraumatic bowel graspers.
  - Laparoscopic GIA staplers.
  - Device for dividing mesenteric vasculature (ie, GIA vascular staple load, LigaSure device, etc).

PATIENT PREPARATION

- Preoperative blood work:
  - Complete blood count to rule out anemia.
  - Type and screen.
  - Carcinoembryonic antigen level.
- Examination of abdomen for prior incisions.
- Full colonoscopy to cecum before elective operation, and tattooing of lesions with permanent ink as appropriate.
- CT scan of abdomen and pelvis with oral and intravenous contrast to evaluate for liver metastasis in patients with cancer.
- Other diagnostic imaging as appropriate.
- Mechanical bowel preparation.
- Deep vein thrombosis prophylaxis with sequential compression devices and consideration of subcutaneous heparin dosing before induction of anesthesia, especially if the patient has been diagnosed with cancer.
- For patients older than 50 years, β-blockade before induction of anesthesia.
- General anesthesia.
- Foley catheter.
- Nasogastric tube.

- Preoperative antibiotics covering skin and bowel flora (eg, second- or third-generation cephalosporin or penicillin derivative).

PATIENT POSITIONING

- The patient should be supine, with the entire abdomen prepared and draped.
- Consider lithotomy position if splenic flexure mobilization may be necessary, and for sigmoid colectomy.

PROCEDURE

- Laparotomy is performed via a midline incision about the umbilicus.
- The abdomen is explored to palpate the liver for metastasis, visualize peritoneum, examine omentum and lymph nodes, and "run" the bowel. A Bookwalter retractor is placed.
- Figure 23–1: Vascular anatomy of the colon.

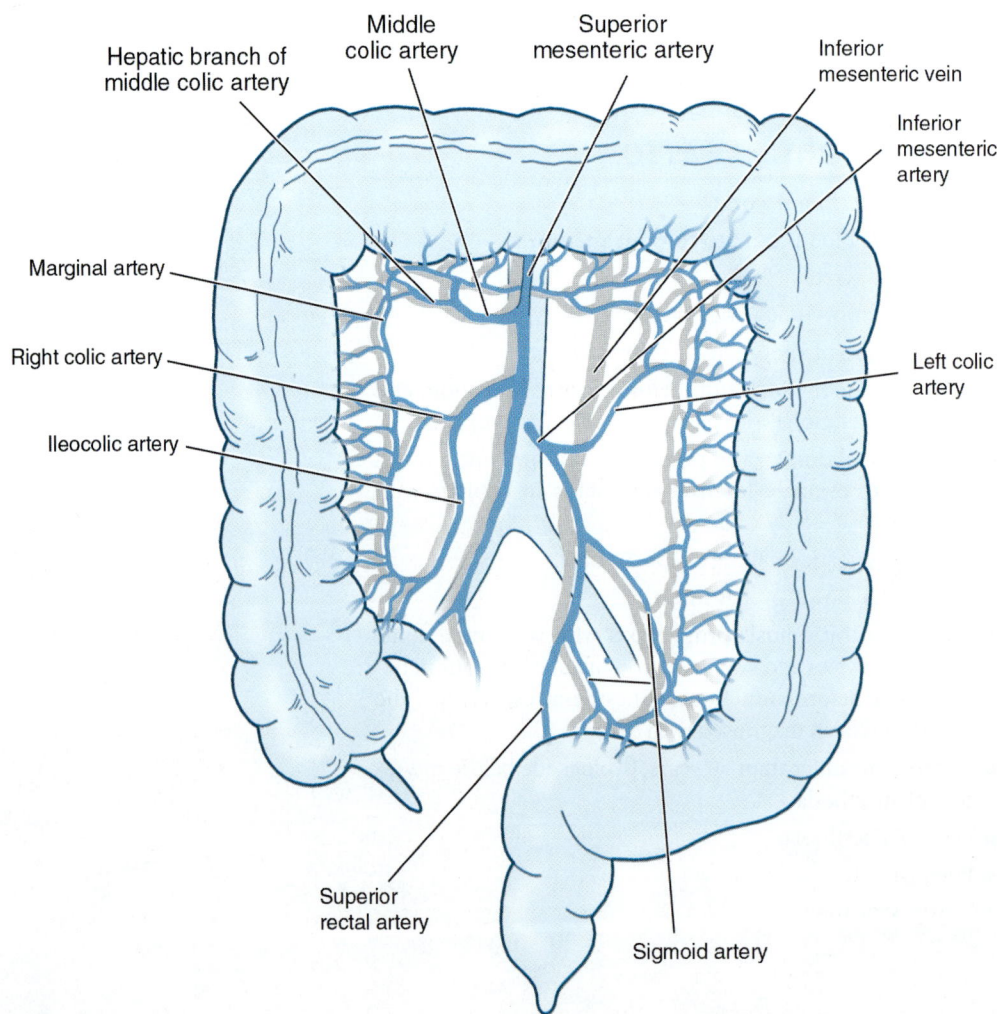

Figure 23–1

- The superior mesenteric artery (SMA) supplies the cecum, ascending colon, and proximal transverse colon. The SMA divides into the ileocolic artery (ICA), right colic artery (RCA), and middle colic artery (MCA). Note the hepatic (right) and left branches of the middle colic artery.
- The inferior mesenteric artery (IMA) supplies the distal transverse colon, splenic flexure, descending colon, sigmoid colon, and upper rectum. The IMA divides into the left colic artery (LCA) and the sigmoid artery (SA), and terminates in the superior hemorrhoidal artery.
- The marginal artery of Drummond provides collateral circulation along the colon.
- The inferior mesenteric vein (IMV) meets the splenic vein at the inferior border of the pancreas.

■ **Figure 23–2A-D:** Extent of resection for colon cancer.
- Cecal mass: right colectomy is indicated for a mass in the cecum or ascending colon (Figure 23–2A).
- Transverse colon mass: transverse colectomy or extended right colectomy is indicated for a mass in the transverse colon (Figure 23–2B).
- Splenic flexure mass: left colectomy is indicated for a mass in the splenic flexure or descending colon (Figure 23–2C).
- Sigmoid colon mass: sigmoid colectomy is indicated for a sigmoid colon mass (Figure 23–2D).

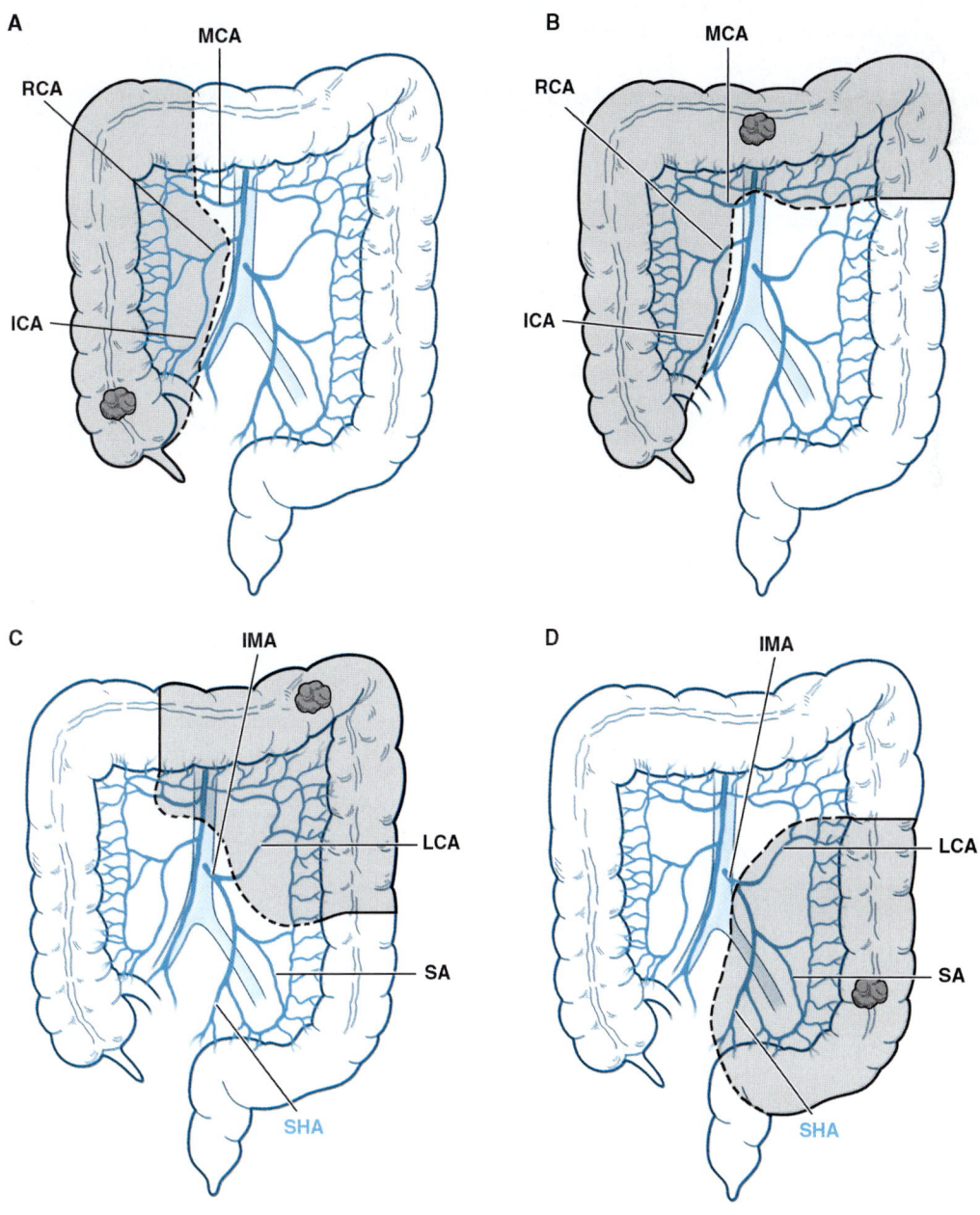

Figure 23–2A–D

Right Colectomy

- Indicated for a mass in the cecum or right colon.
- Resection will include distribution of the ileocolic and right colic arteries, and the hepatic branch of the middle colic artery.
- **Figure 23–3A, B:** Lateral peritoneal reflection of the right colon.
  - The right colon is mobilized along the retroperitoneal fold, which forms an avascular attachment of the right colon to the lateral peritoneal wall. A gauze sponge is used to dissect the underlying loose areolar tissue (Figure 23–3A).
  - The duodenum is identified, with care taken to avoid injury. When dissection is carried out in the correct plane, the duodenum should be visualized but not elevated. A soft sponge can be used to keep the duodenum down. Care should be taken to avoid injury to the kidney or Gerota's fascia (Figure 23–3B).
- **Figure 23–4:** Transection of the right colon mesentery and named vessels.
  - The right colon is now completely free, except for its mesentery. The right colon is elevated and the mesentery transilluminated to identify avascular tissue for cutting with Bovie electrocautery. As vessels are encountered, they should be clamped as proximally as possible, transected, and ligated.
  - The right colic artery (if present) is ligated at its origin.
  - If the right colic artery is absent and the ileocolic artery arises directly from the superior mesenteric artery, the ileocolic artery is ligated at its origin.
  - The right (hepatic) branch of the middle colic artery is also ligated, sparing the main middle colic artery.
  - Named vessels, including the ileocolic and right colic arteries, and the hepatic branch of the middle colic artery, should be tied twice on the patient's side to reduce bleeding risk.
  - If cancer is suspected, generous mesentery is removed with the goal of achieving a maximal lymphadenectomy.
- **Figure 23–5A-C:** Two-load GIA-stapled anastomosis for right colectomy.
  - The right colon is completely free of peritoneal and mesenteric attachments.

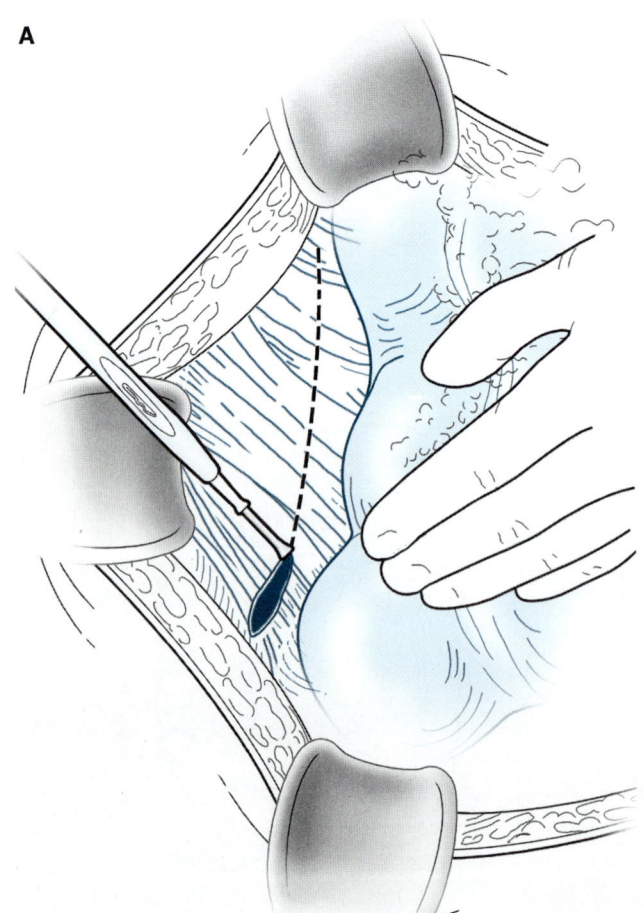

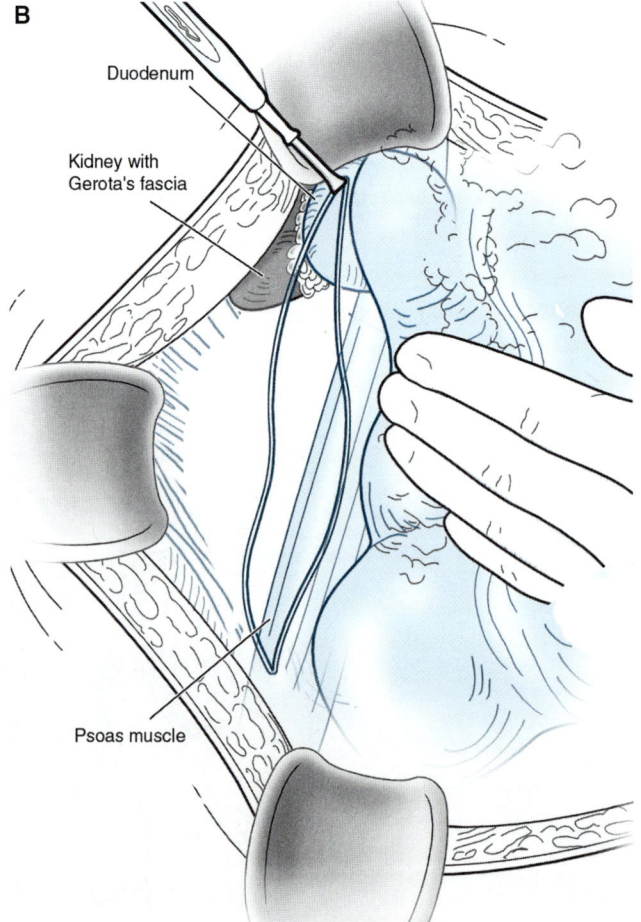

Figure 23–3A–B

- The planned anastomosis site is now identified by bringing together 5 cm of terminal ileum proximally and the hepatic branch of the middle colic artery distally.
- Atraumatic bowel clamps are placed 5 cm beyond the planned anastomotic site on each end to prevent spillage.
- The surgeon should verify that the planned anastomosis will not be under tension when bringing together the antimesenteric border of the two bowel loops.
- Stay sutures are placed (Figure 23–5A), and hemostats are attached to them.
- A small enterotomy is made in antimesenteric side of each bowel loop. One fork of the GIA-80 stapler is introduced into each enterotomy (Figure 23–5B).
- The GIA-80 stapler is fired along the antimesenteric border to anastomose the bowel.
- Next a second load of the GIA-80 stapler is used to amputate the specimen, including the two enterotomy sites, thereby simultaneously closing the end luminal defects (Figure 23–5C).

■ Alternatives to the two-load GIA-stapled anastomosis include a hand-sewn end-to-end anastomosis (see Figure 23–7), a hand-sewn side-to-side anastomosis, or a four-load GIA-stapled anastomosis.

■ Closure of the resultant mesenteric defect is optional.

■ The abdomen is irrigated with warm saline and closed in standard fashion.

Transverse Colectomy

■ Based on the right colectomy, the transverse colectomy or extended right colectomy for a mass in the transverse colon also includes resection of the right omentum, division of the hepatocolic ligaments, and inclusion of the entire middle colic artery in the resection.

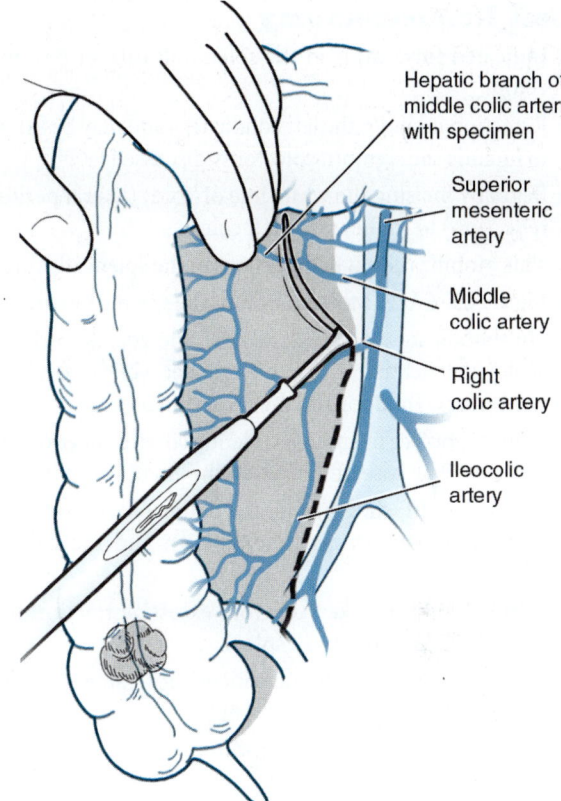

Figure 23–4

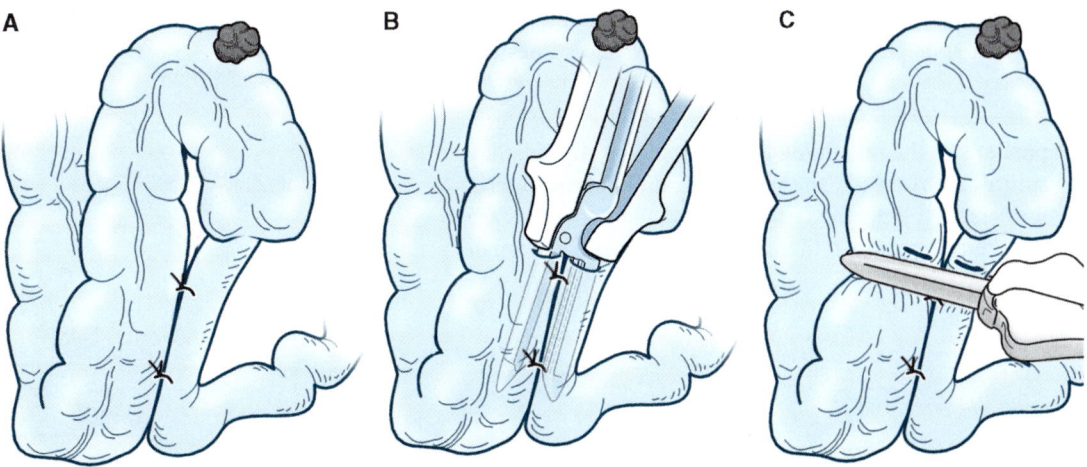

Figure 23–5A–C

Left Hemicolectomy

- Indicated for a mass in the splenic flexure or descending colon.
- Resection includes the left colic artery and may be extended to include the sigmoid colectomy discussed later.
- Begin by incising the white line of Toldt (lateral peritoneal reflection) to mobilize the left colon.
- This mobilization is extended up to the splenic flexure.
- **Figure 23–6A, B:** Mobilization of the splenic flexure.
  - In mobilizing the splenic flexure, the goal is to divide all colonic attachments in a safe manner while preserving the mesentery. Traditionally, the dissection proceeds retrograde.
  - The renocolic ligament is identified and incised (Figure 23–6A). The base of the spleen should now be visible.
  - Next the attachments between the omentum and the spleen, and between the omentum and the colon, are divided.
  - Care should be taken to avoid excessive traction on the colon, which can cause a splenic capsule tear.
  - The splenocolic and pancreaticocolic ligaments are identified and incised (Figure 23–6B).
  - Alternatively, the dissection can proceed anterograde, by elevating the omentum to access the lesser sac. The attending physician may stand between the patient's legs to facilitate this dissection. The splenic flexure is freed.
- Similar to Figure 23–4, the left colon is elevated and its mesentery transilluminated to identify avascular tissue to be divided with the electrocautery device.
- As they are encountered, large vessels are clamped and divided at their origin, and ligated twice on the patient side. If cancer is suspected a broad en bloc mesenteric resection is performed to remove as many lymph nodes as possible.
- **Figure 23–7A-E:** Hand-sewn, double-layer, end-to-end anastomosis for left colectomy.
  - The left colon specimen has been passed off the field.
  - End-to-end hand-sewn anastomosis begins by placing atraumatic bowel clamps 5 cm past the GIA staple line to prevent spillage of stool. Next, the GIA staple lines are excised.
  - *Alignment of bowel:* the mesenteric and antimesenteric portions of the remaining bowel should be aligned. Stay sutures are placed at the mesenteric and antimesenteric borders of the planned anastomosis, and hemostats are attached to them. If there is a size mismatch, a small

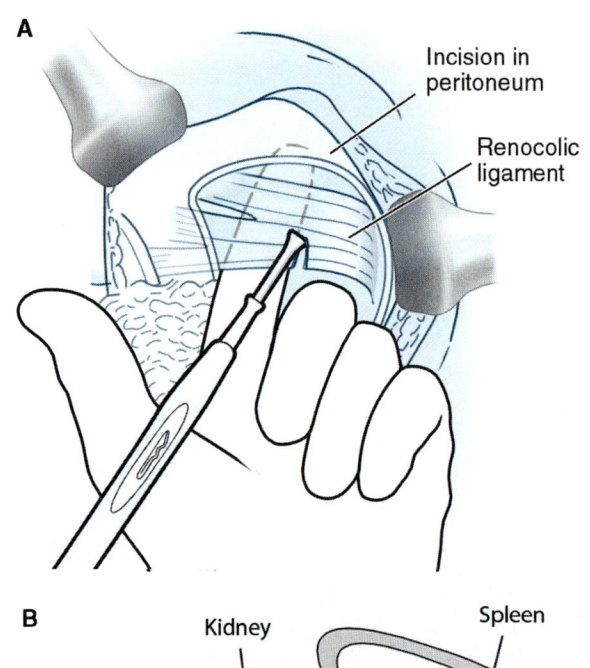

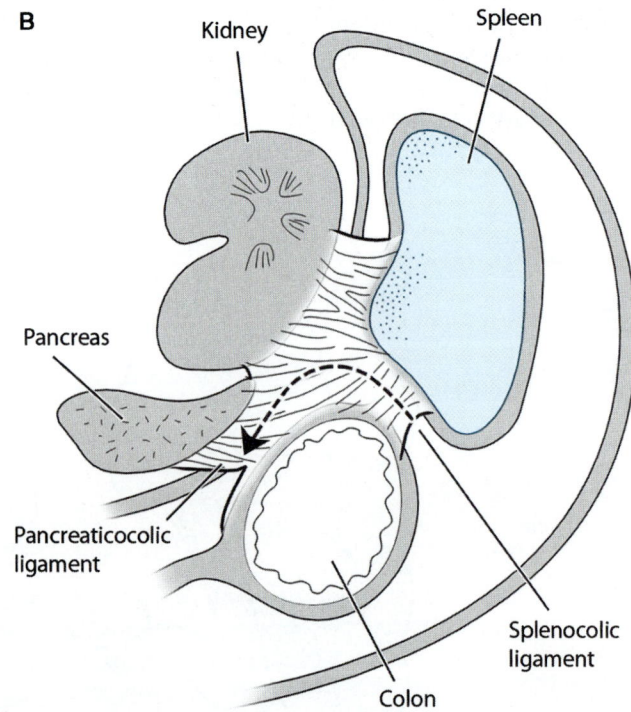

Figure 23–6A–B

Cheatle slit can be created in the antimesenteric border of the smaller diameter segment (Figure 23–7A).

- *Posterior outer layer Lembert stitches:* interrupted 3-0 Lembert sutures are placed in the posterior seromuscular layer to form the posterior outer layer of the anastomosis (Figure 23–7B).
- *Inner layer running stitch:* a double-armed 4-0 absorbable monofilament suture is used to create the inner layer of the anastomosis in a running fashion, with full-thickness bites. The submucosa provides the strength (Figure 23–7C, D).
- *Anterior outer layer Lembert stitches:* interrupted 3-0 Lembert sutures are placed in the seromuscular layer to form the anterior outer layer, which completes the two-layer anastomosis (Figure 23–7E).

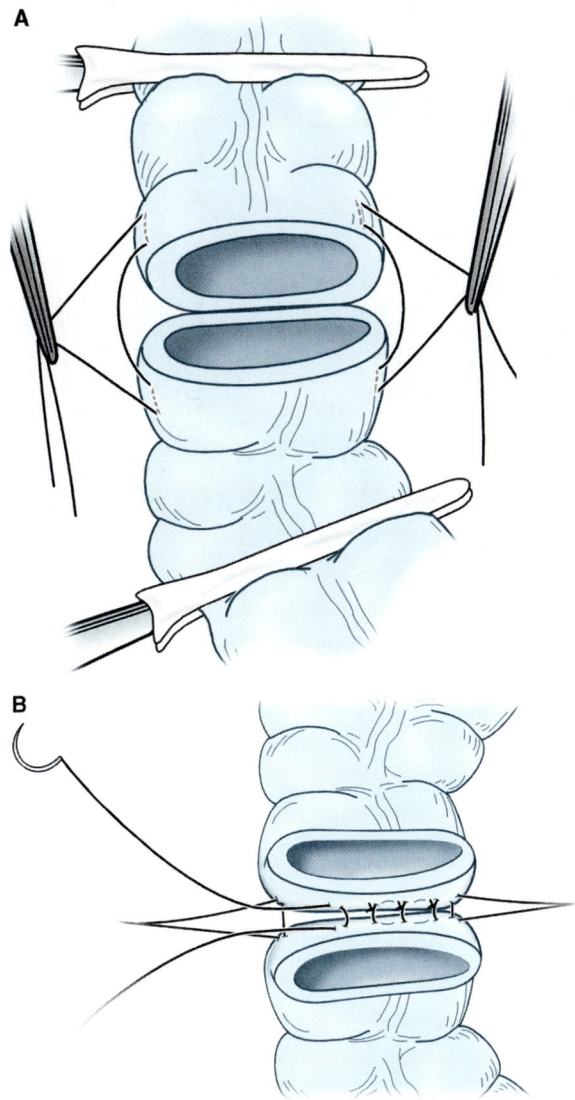
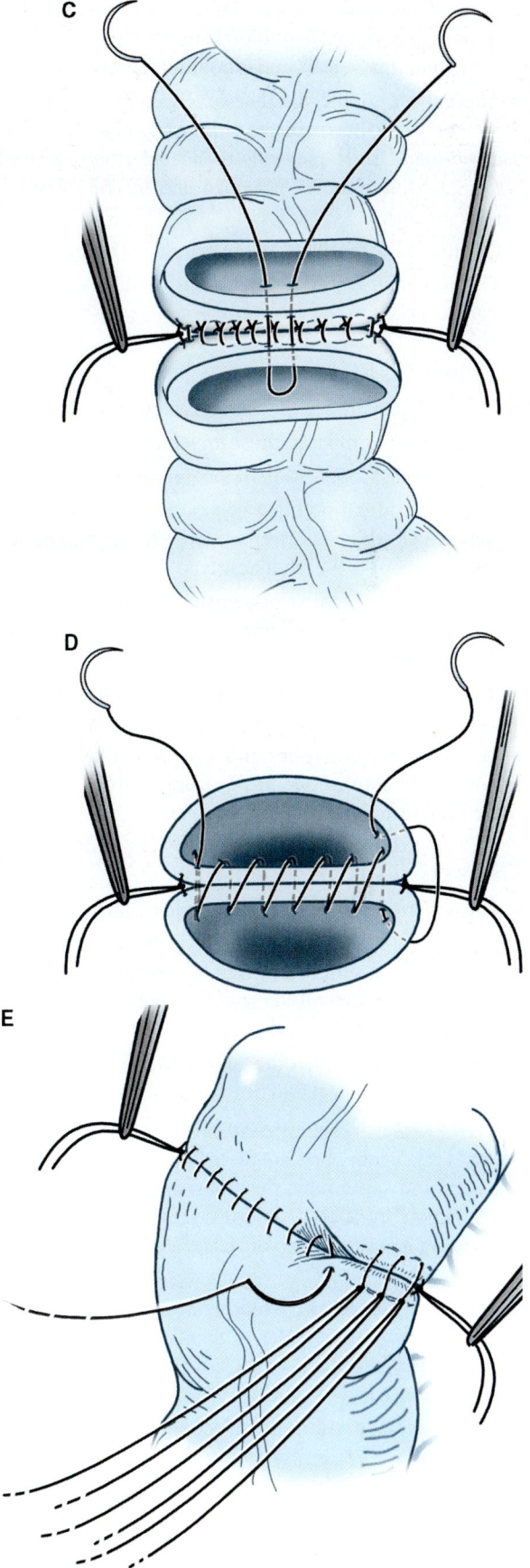

Figure 23–7A–E

- The anastomosis is examined to verify that it is widely patent, has an excellent blood supply, shows no evidence of hematoma or leak, and is not under tension.
■ Alternatives to the hand-sewn end-to-end anastomosis include a hand-sewn side-to-side anastomosis (not shown), a two-load GIA stapled side-to-side anastomosis (see Figure 23–5), and an EEA stapled end-to-end anastomosis (not shown).
■ Closure of the resultant mesenteric defect is optional.
■ The abdomen is irrigated with warm saline and closed in standard fashion.

Sigmoid Colectomy
■ Indicated for a mass in the sigmoid colon or for diverticulitis.
■ Principles are similar to those for left colectomy.
■ **Figure 23–8:** Mobilization of the sigmoid colon.
  - Particular attention must be paid to avoid damaging the left ureter, which is extremely close to the sigmoid colon as it passes over the left iliac artery.
  - Consider preoperative placement of a ureteral stent, especially if significant inflammation or scar tissue is anticipated in the area.
■ It may not be necessary to always mobilize the splenic flexure; however, a tension-free anastomosis must be achieved.
■ The anastomosis may be hand sewn end to end, hand sewn side to side, stapled side to side using a GIA stapler, or stapled end to end using an EEA stapler.

Laparoscopic Colectomy
■ The patient is placed in deep Trendelenburg position, and the right side of the table is then rotated up.
■ Consideration should be given to preoperative placement of an infrared ureteral stent, which can be seen using a special laparoscope.
■ We prefer to approach the colon medially, thereby letting the lateral peritoneal fold provide initial retraction.
■ **Figure 23–9A-D:** Laparoscopic assisted right colectomy.
■ Port sites: 5-mm ports are placed in the midline at the epigastric and suprapubic positions, and a 12-mm port and 5-mm port are offset to the left side of the umbilicus, maintaining a hand's breadth of space between each port (Figure 23–9A).
  - Avascular mesenteric windows are created with cautery. An endovascular stapler is then used to staple vessels, beginning with the ileocolic artery, and repeating for the right colic artery (Figure 23–9B).
  - The lateral peritoneal reflection is divided (Figure 23–9C).
  - Next, a 5-cm long incision is made on the right side of the abdomen. The rectus is swept medially for a rectus-sparing incision through the posterior rectus sheath. The right colon is then externalized (Figure 23–9D).

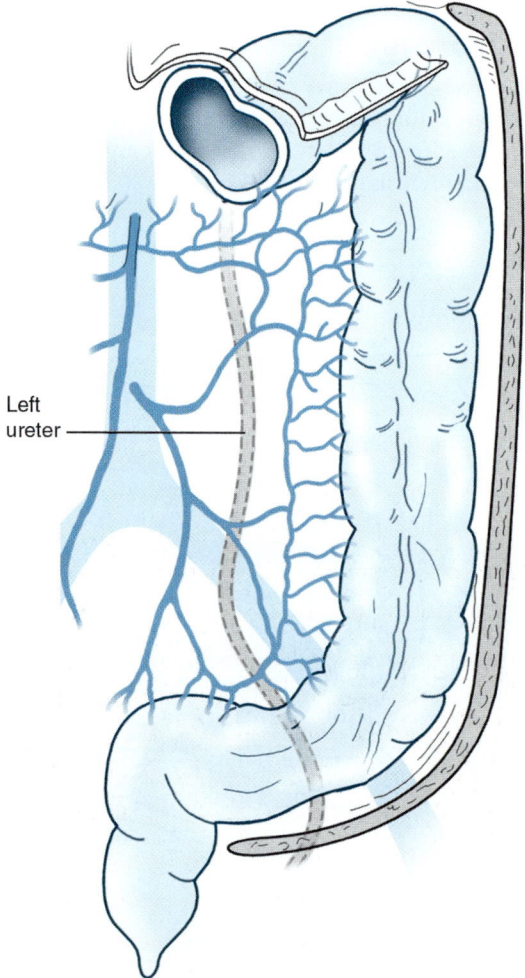

Figure 23–8

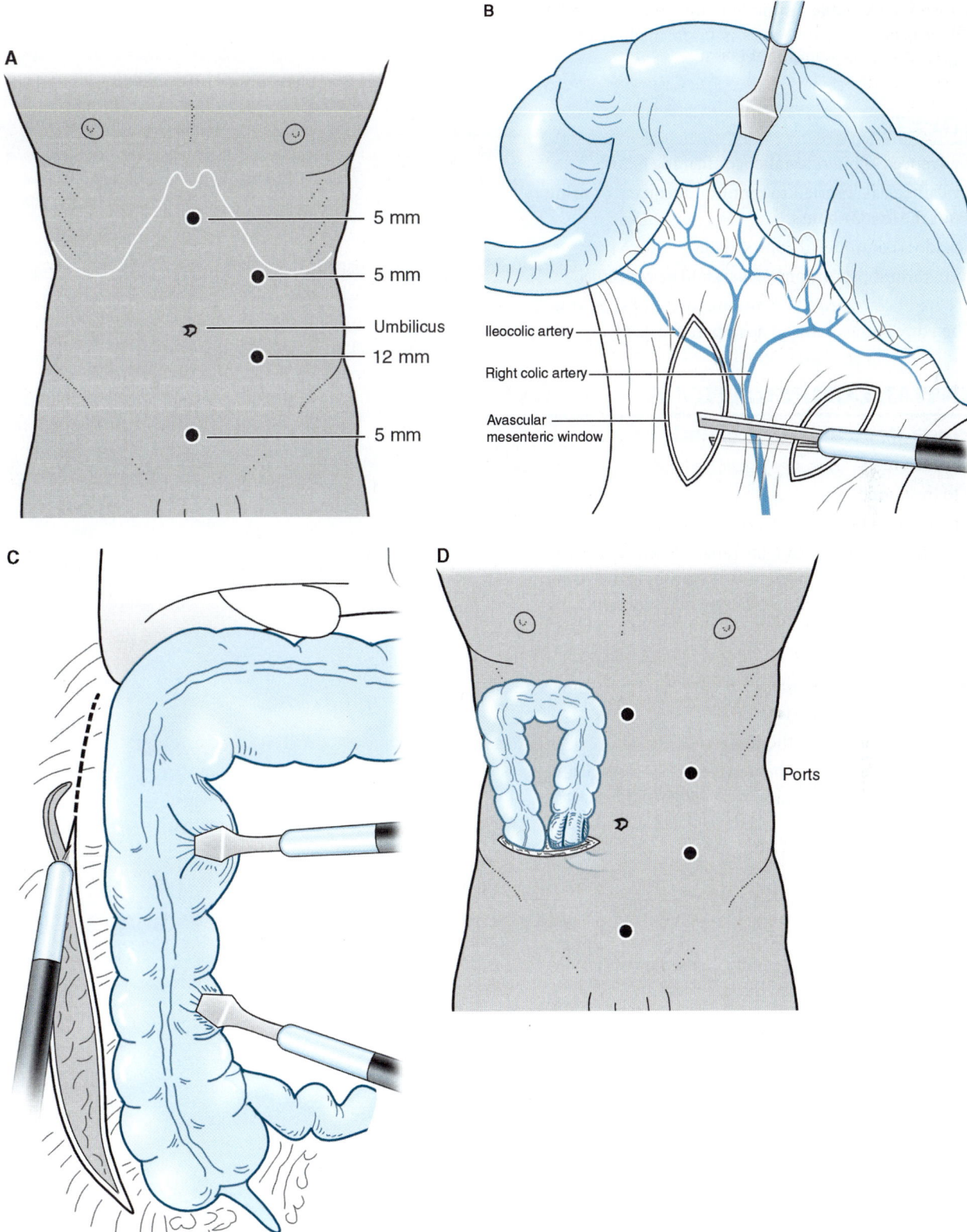

Figure 23-9A-D

- A two-load GIA-stapled simultaneous colon resection and extracorporeal anastomosis is performed, as previously described (see Figure 23–5).

POSTOPERATIVE CARE

- Diet is advanced as tolerated after confirming flatus.
- A Foley catheter is inserted to monitor adequacy of urine output for the first 24 hours.
- β-Blockade is continued if appropriate.
- Deep vein thrombosis prophylaxis should be continued.
- Patients are encouraged to be ambulatory and should be out of bed three times daily on postoperative day 1.

POTENTIAL COMPLICATIONS

Intraoperative and Technical

- Injury to the ureter.
- Injury to the duodenum.
- Injury to other bowel.
  - Small deserosalizations can be repaired with Lembert stitches. Care should be taken to avoid grasping the bowel during the operation. Epiploic appendages should be grasped instead.
- Injury to the spleen.
  - A topical hemostatic agent can be applied or splenorrhaphy or splenectomy performed.
- Inadequate blood supply at the anastomosis.
  - Additional bowel should be resected. Consider using Doppler ultrasound to evaluate blood flow to the anastomosis if concerned.
- Anastomosis under tension.
  - Additional bowel can be mobilized.
- Stool spillage and tumor cell spillage, creating the potential for abscess or "drop metastases."
  - Noncrushing bowel clamps should be used proximal and distal to the line of colonic division.

Early Postoperative Period

- Wound infection.
  - Staples should be removed as needed, followed by confirmation that fascia are intact. The wound should then be packed and allowed to heal by secondary intention.
- Anastomotic leak.
  - In some patients, tachycardia may be the only sign; others may have prolonged ileus or appear septic.
- Intra-abdominal abscess.
  - Typically diagnosed by CT scan on postoperative days 5–7.

- Can often be treated using a percutaneous drain placed by the radiology service.
- May be secondary to an anastomotic leak.
■ Colocutaneous fistula.

Late Postoperative Period
■ Anastomotic stricture.
■ Anastomotic recurrence of cancer.
■ Incisional hernia.
■ Internal hernia.
■ Ureteral stricture from ureteral devascularization.

PEARLS AND TIPS
■ Take no chances with the anastomosis. Ensure that the anastomosis is widely patent, has an excellent blood supply, shows no evidence of hematoma or leak, and is not under tension. Assess visually, tactilely, and via Doppler ultrasound if necessary. Do not leave the operating room if the viability of the anastomosis is questionable.
■ When mobilizing the splenic flexure, always avoid excessive traction on the colon to prevent tearing of the splenic capsule.
■ Suspect intra-abdominal abscess in patients with postoperative fever, tachycardia, or prolonged ileus. Diagnose with CT scan.

REFERENCES
Ballantyne GH. *Atlas of Laparoscopic Surgery.* Philadelphia, PA: WB Saunders; 2000.
Cameron JL. *Current Surgical Therapy.* Philadelphia, PA: Elsevier Mosby; 2004:211–216.
Scott-Conner CE. *Chassin's Operative Strategy in General Surgery.* New York, NY: Springer; 2002:359–418.
Zollinger RM Jr, Zollinger RM Sr. *Zollinger's Atlas of Surgical Operations.* New York, NY: McGraw-Hill; 2003:112–139.

CHAPTER 24

Operative Management of Rectal Tumors

David G. Heidt, MD, and Emina H. Huang, MD

INDICATIONS

Transanal Excision of Tumor

- Stage T1 tumors:
  - Mobile and < 4 cm in diameter.
  - Involving < 40% of the rectal wall circumference.
  - Located within 6 cm of the anal verge.
- Well or moderately differentiated histology only.
- Absence of vascular and lymphatic invasion.
- No evidence of nodal involvement on preoperative rectal ultrasound or MRI.

Low Anterior Resection (LAR) with Total Mesorectal Excision

- Malignant lesion of the rectum diagnosed by evaluation of a tissue biopsy specimen obtained within 2 cm of the anal sphincter in moderately or well-differentiated tumors or within 5 cm for poorly differentiated tumors.

Abdominoperineal Resection (APR) with Total Mesorectal Excision

- Malignant lesion of the rectum diagnosed by evaluation of a tissue biopsy specimen obtained < 2 cm from the anal sphincter for moderately or well-differentiated tumors or < 5 cm for poorly differentiated tumors.

CONTRAINDICATIONS

Transanal Excision of Tumor

- Tumors stage greater than T1N0M0.
- Fixed tumors.
- Tumors > 4 cm in diameter or involving > 40% of the circumference of the rectal wall.
- Tumors located > 6 cm from the anal verge.
- Tumors with poorly differentiated histology or angiolymphatic invasion, or those that show evidence of nodal involvement on preoperative rectal ultrasound or MRI.

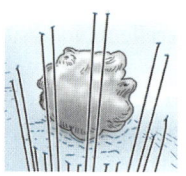 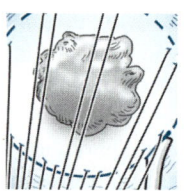 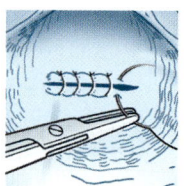
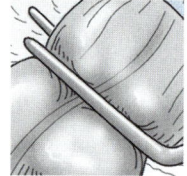 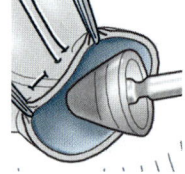 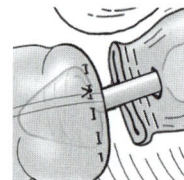
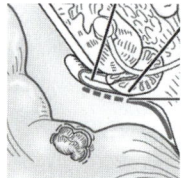 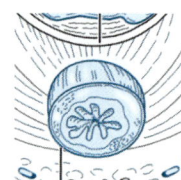 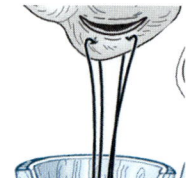

LAR with Total Mesorectal Excision

- Malignant lesion of the rectum diagnosed by evaluation of a tissue biopsy specimen obtained < 2 cm from the anal sphincter for moderately or well-differentiated tumors or < 5 cm for poorly differentiated tumors.

APR with Total Mesorectal Excision

- Malignant lesion of the lower rectum diagnosed by evaluation of a tissue biopsy specimen showing local invasion into the pelvic sidewall or pelvis that could benefit from neoadjuvant treatment to facilitate possible curative resection.

INFORMED CONSENT

Transanal Excision of Tumor

A. Expected Benefits
- Removal of tumor with preservation of anus.
- Avoidance of radical surgery.

B. Potential Risks
- Bleeding requiring reoperation.
- Rectal stricture.
- Need for further resection based on pathologic findings.
- Fistula to prostate or vagina.
- Injury to the urethra for distal anterior tumors in men.

LAR or APR with Total Mesorectal Excision

A. Expected Benefits
- Treatment of rectal cancer.
- Potential prevention of colonic obstruction, tenesmus, and invasion of adjacent pelvic structures.

B. Potential Risks
- Bleeding requiring reoperation from presacral or splenic injuries (LAR or APR) or from the anastomosis (LAR).
- Infection, including intra-abdominal or pelvic abscesses resulting from anastomotic leaks (LAR) or infected intra-abdominal or pelvic fluid collections (LAR or APR).
- Fistula formation from anastomotic leak (LAR).
- Postoperative ileus (LAR or APR).
- Ureteral injury (LAR or APR).
- Need for a permanent or temporary stoma (LAR).
- Bladder or sexual dysfunction (LAR or APR).
- Fecal incontinence (LAR).
- Clustering of bowel movements (LAR).

EQUIPMENT

Transanal Excision of Tumor
- Self-retaining (Ferguson) anoscope.
- Lone Star retractor (for more proximal lesions).

LAR or APR with Total Mesorectal Excision
- Self-retaining retractors.
- Bookwalter abdominal retractor with a lighted St. Mark's retractor.
- Lone Star retractor (for perineum).
- Handheld lighted St. Mark's retractor and long instruments (crucial for delicate dissection in the pelvis).
- Gastrointestinal anastomosis (GIA) stapler.
- End-to-end anastomosis (EEA) stapler (LAR).
- Thoracoabdominal (TA) stapler (LAR).

PATIENT PREPARATION

- Clearance of bowel for synchronous lesions by colonoscopy.
- CT scan of the chest, abdomen, and pelvis to evaluate for metastatic disease of the lungs, liver, or peritoneum.
- Endorectal ultrasound or endorectal MRI for local staging (T and N staging).
  - Patients with uT1N0 tumors may be appropriate candidates for transanal excision.
  - Patients with uT3NX or uTXN+ disease should be considered for possible neoadjuvant chemoradiation therapy.
- Consider preoperative tattooing of the lesion with permanent ink, especially if the lesion is small or the patient will receive neoadjuvant chemoradiotherapy.
- Preoperative carcinoembryonic antigen level.
- Nothing by mouth the evening before surgery.
- Mechanical bowel preparation according to surgeon's preference.
- Preoperative antibiotics and preoperative subcutaneous heparin.
- Anesthesiology consultation as needed.
- Stoma marking by an enterostomal therapist for patients undergoing LAR or APR.

PATIENT POSITIONING

Transanal Excision of Tumor
- For posterior lesions, the patient should be in a supine lithotomy position in gentle Trendelenburg using well-padded stirrups.
- For anterior lesions, the prone jackknife position is preferred.
- Sequential pneumatic compression devices should be applied.

LAR or APR with Total Mesorectal Excision

- The patient should be in a supine lithotomy position in gentle Trendelenburg using well-padded stirrups.
- Sequential pneumatic compression devices should be applied.
- A Foley catheter and nasogastric or orogastric tube should be placed, especially if mobilization of the splenic flexure is contemplated.
- Consideration should also be given to the placement of a left ureteral stent if a difficult pelvic dissection is anticipated.

PROCEDURE

Transanal Excision of Tumor

- Regional anesthesia may be adequate, although general anesthesia is sometimes required.
- A self-retaining retractor is placed and a 1:100,000 epinephrine solution is infiltrated into the submucosa to facilitate dissection.
- **Figure 24–1:** Stay sutures are placed circumferentially 1 cm from the gross margin of the lesion.
- **Figure 24–2:** Full-thickness excision of the lesion is performed down to the level of perirectal fat using electrocautery.
- The specimen is carefully marked to delineate the correct orientation for the pathologist.
- **Figure 24–3:** The defect in the rectal wall is closed transversely with absorbable suture.

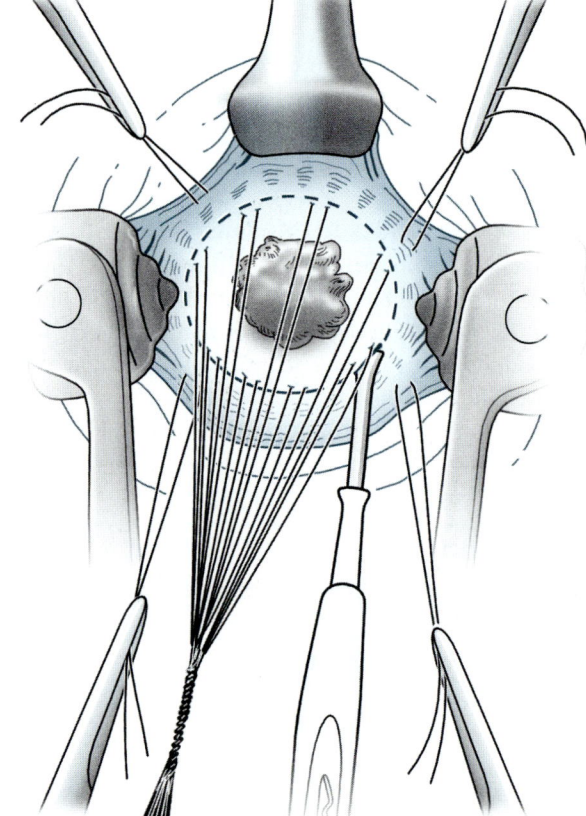

Figure 24–2

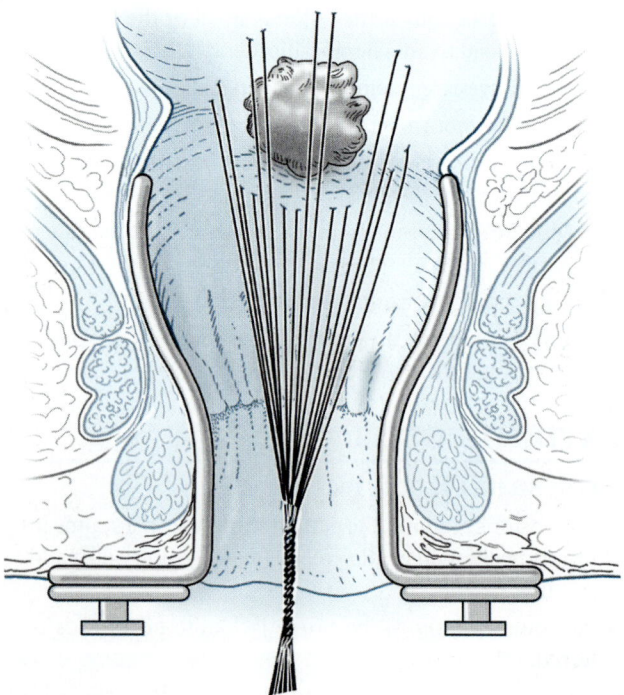

Figure 24–1

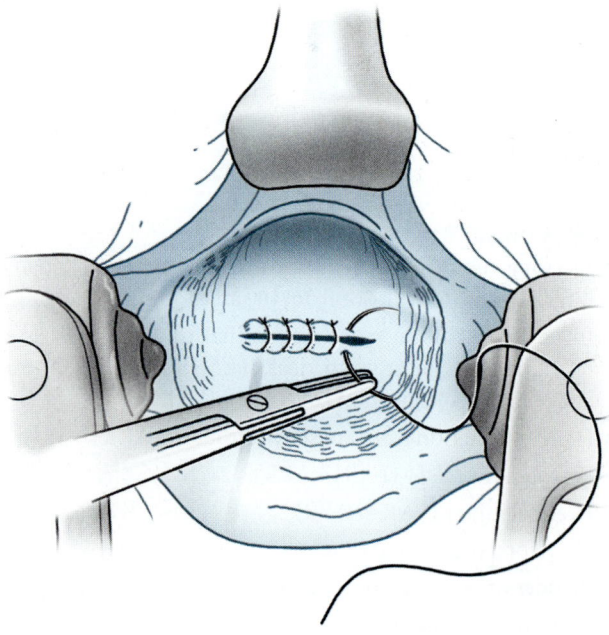

Figure 24–3

- Proctoscopic examination of the rectum is performed at the conclusion of the procedure to ensure patency of the rectum.

LAR or APR with Total Mesorectal Excision

- General anesthesia is required.
- The patient should be in the lithotomy position with the legs elevated at approximately 15 degrees and spread at 45 degrees. Positioning of the anus and buttocks at the end of the table is important for access.
- A median laparotomy incision from the pubis symphysis to above the umbilicus is performed.
- For an LAR or APR, a self-retaining retractor is placed and the small intestine is retracted superiorly and to the right under a moistened towel.
- The left colon is freed from its lateral peritoneal attachments along the avascular line of Toldt, and the splenic flexure is mobilized (see Chapter 23) as needed for a tension free anastomosis.
- The peritoneum of the pelvic colon is opened using electrocautery.
- Care must be taken to identify the ureters, on the left in particular.
  - The left ureter is identified as it crosses the pelvic brim over the left common iliac artery.
  - Especially in patients with a significant amount of adipose tissue, widely encircling the ureter with a vessel loop can aid in safe mobilization of the distal rectum.
- The inferior mesenteric artery is identified at its origin and suture-ligated.
- The distal descending colon is then divided with a GIA-60 stapling device at least 5 cm proximal to the tumor.
- **Figure 24–4:** The distal rectum is then sharply mobilized posteriorly to remove the mesorectum intact with its fascial envelope (see also Figures 24–7A and 24–7B).
- The bladder is retracted superiorly and the anterior rectal wall is separated from the seminal vesicles and the posterior capsule of the prostate in a man.
- The lateral dissection encompasses the lateral peritoneal reflections, and middle hemorrhoidal vessels are ligated and divided.
- **Figure 24–5:** The proximal rectum is then clamped and a linear stapling device is applied across the rectum at least 2 cm distal to the tumor.
- The proximal rectum is divided and the specimen is removed.

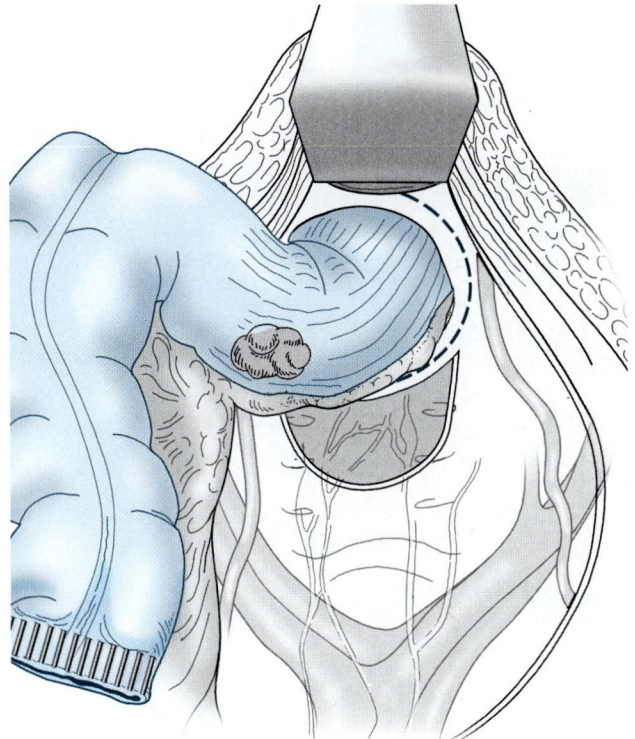

Figure 24–4

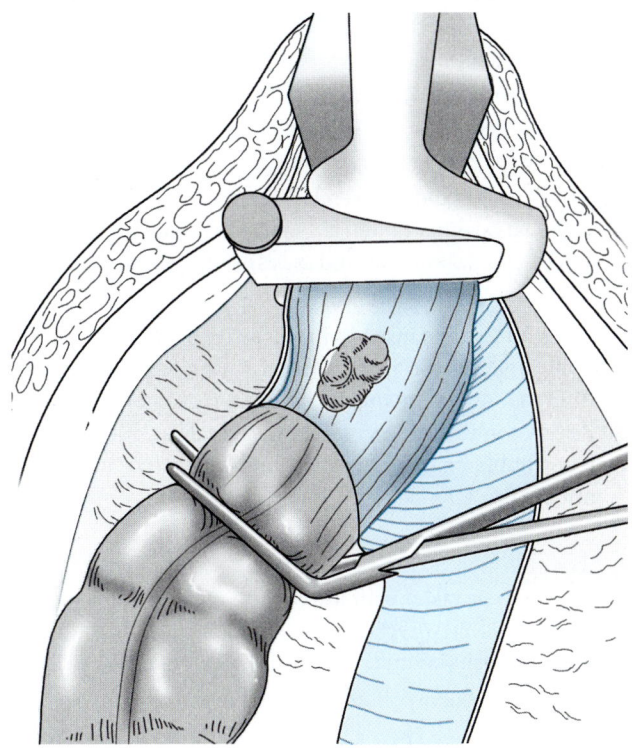

Figure 24–5

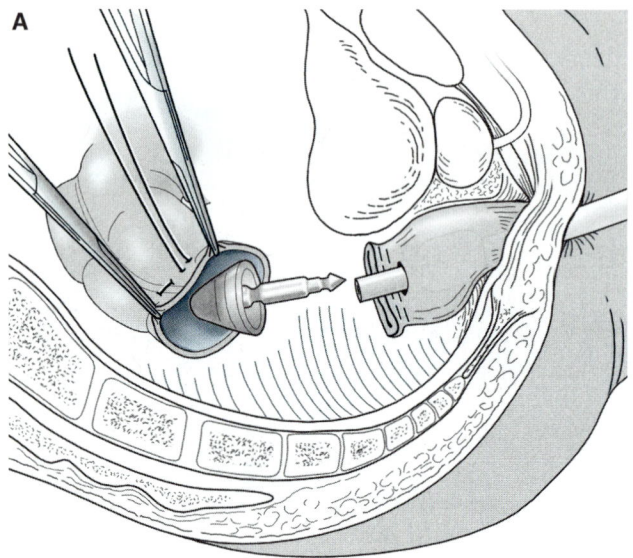 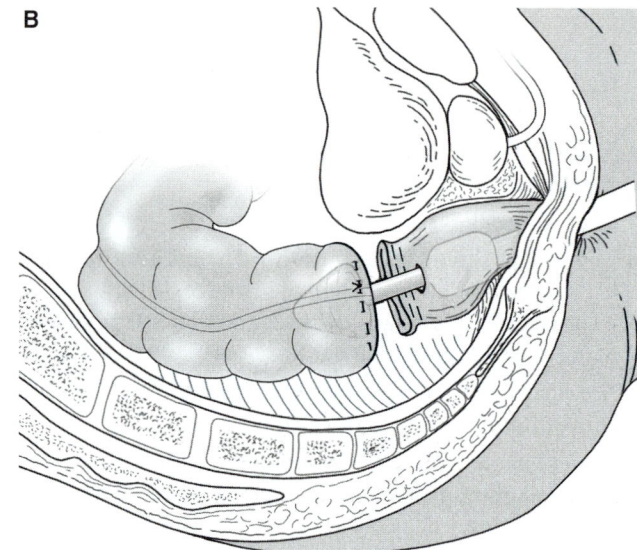

Figure 24–6A–B

- **Figure 24–6A, B:** Creation of the stapled LAR anastomosis.
  - The staple line of the descending colon is opened and a nonabsorbable purse-string suture is placed.
  - The anvil of a circular stapler is placed within the descending colon through the purse-string suture, and the suture is tied.
  - The assistant then passes the circular stapler through the anus, deploying the "spike" just anterior to the staple line on the rectum.
  - The anastomosis is completed as the surgeon marries the anvil placed in the end of the divided descending colon to the stapler exiting the rectum.
  - The surgeon guides the end of the stapler together, taking care that no other tissue (ie, bladder or vagina) is intervening in the anastomosis, and the assistant fires the stapler.
  - The rings of tissue ("donuts") are inspected for any defect.
- The assistant then inspects the integrity of the anastomosis by insufflating the rectum using a rigid sigmoidoscope, while the surgeon manually occludes the distal colon with the anastomosis submerged in sterile saline. The presence of any bubbling from the anastomosis suggests an anastomotic leak.

A. TOTAL MESORECTAL EXCISION
- Care must be taken with lower lying rectal cancers to perform a total mesorectal excision to prevent leaving nodal tumor deposits behind.
- The superior hemorrhoidal artery is identified and ligated.
- **Figure 24–7A-C:** There should be wide incision at the peritoneal reflection and sharp division of the Waldeyer's fascia posterior to the fascia propria of the rectum, as well as

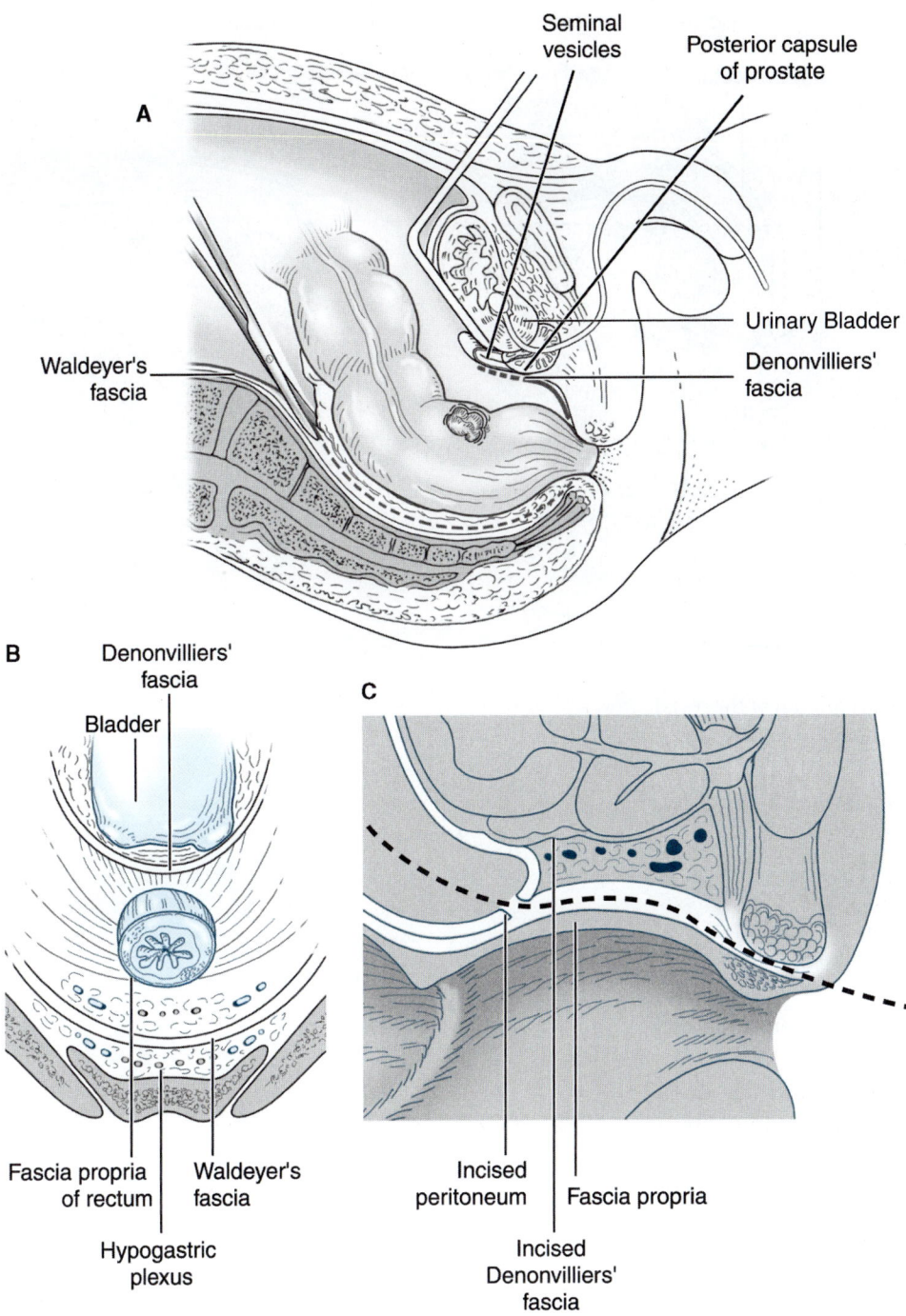

Figure 24–7A–C

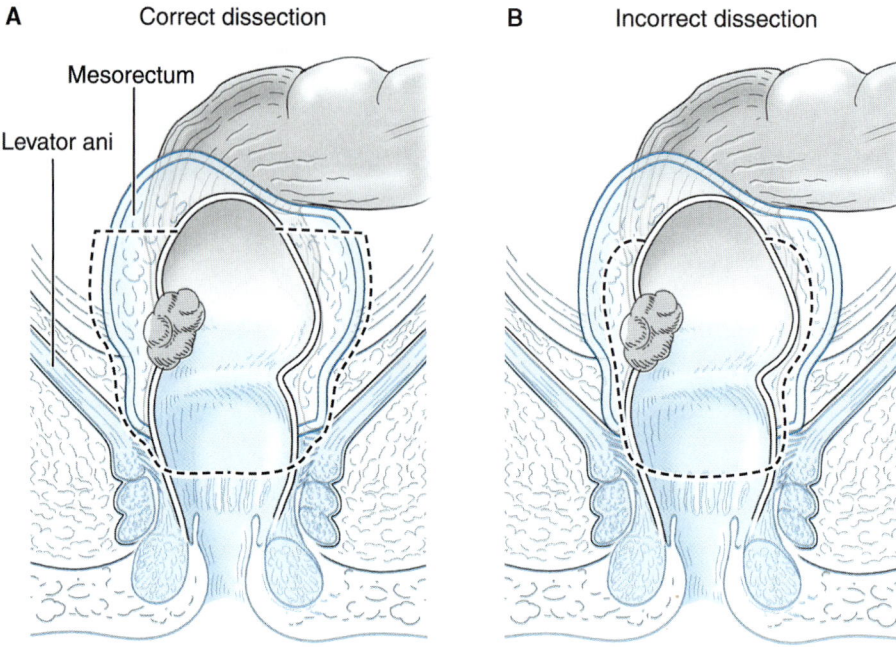

Figure 24–8A–B

incision of Denonvilliers' fascia and separation of the rectal wall from the seminal vesicles and the posterior capsule of the prostate anteriorly.

- **Figure 24–8A, B:** The correct and incorrect dissection planes for total mesorectal excision are depicted.

B. COLOANAL ANASTOMOSIS
- If it is not possible to obtain a distal rectal margin of at least 2 cm, a coloanal anastomosis may be contemplated.
- **Figure 24–9A-C:** The distal rectum is divided proximal to the dentate line following rectal dissection and total mesorectal incision.
  - A 5–6-cm colonic J pouch can be fashioned using a GIA stapler. The end-to-side J pouch coloanal anastomosis is then created by sewing the full-thickness colon to the mucosa and internal sphincter of the anus. Absorbable sutures are used to create this anastomosis, and the colotomy created to allow admission of the GIA stapler when creating the J pouch is used for the anastomosis (Figure 24–9A, C).
  - If there is insufficient length for a colonic J pouch, an end-to-end anastomosis can be fashioned using a circular stapler or hand-sewn anastomosis as outlined above (Figure 24–9B, C).

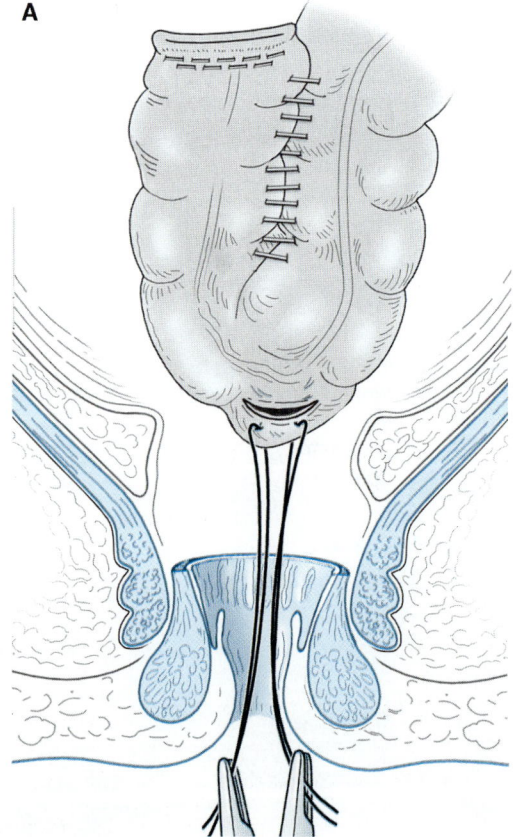

Figure 24–9A

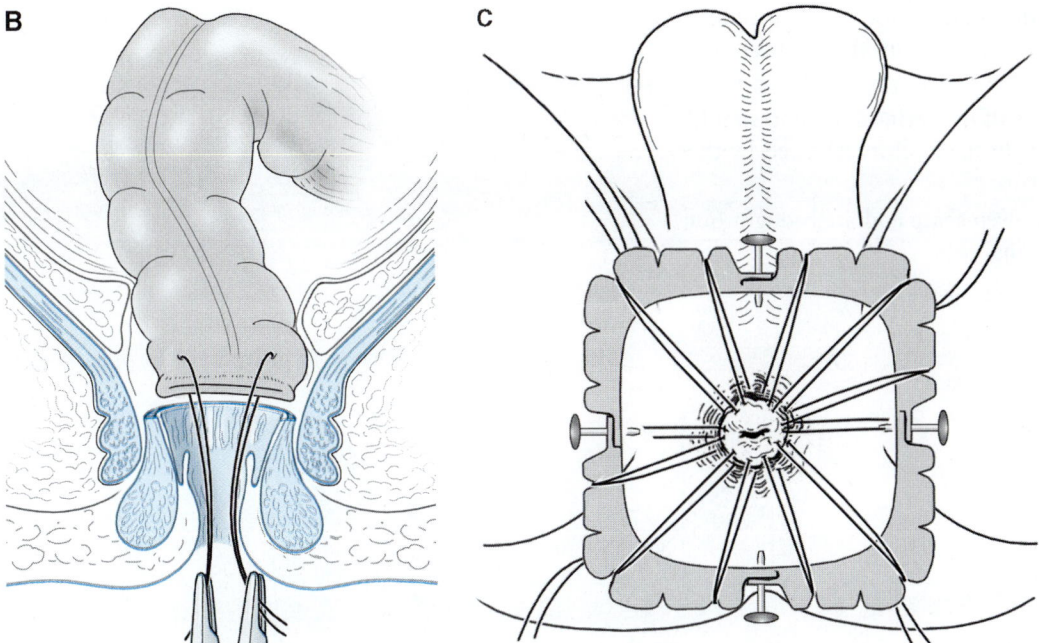

Figure 24–9B–C

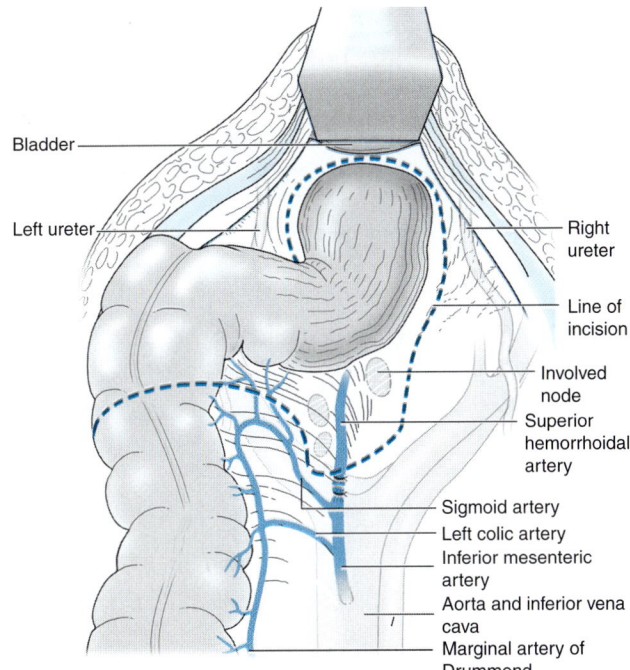

Figure 24–10

B. ABDOMINOPERINEAL RESECTION FOR LOW-LYING RECTAL CANCERS

- This procedure requires the same attention to obtaining adequate radial margins via total mesorectal excision.
- **Figure 24–10:** The sigmoid artery proximal to the takeoff of the superior hemorrhoidal artery is ligated.

- **Figure 24–11A, B:** The distal margin of resection should include the levators, as visualized from the perineal portion of the operation.
- **Figure 24–12:** The closure of the perineal incision should be in layers, beginning with the levators followed by the deep tissues and skin.
- Drains are placed in the deep space and are brought out through the lower abdominal wall.

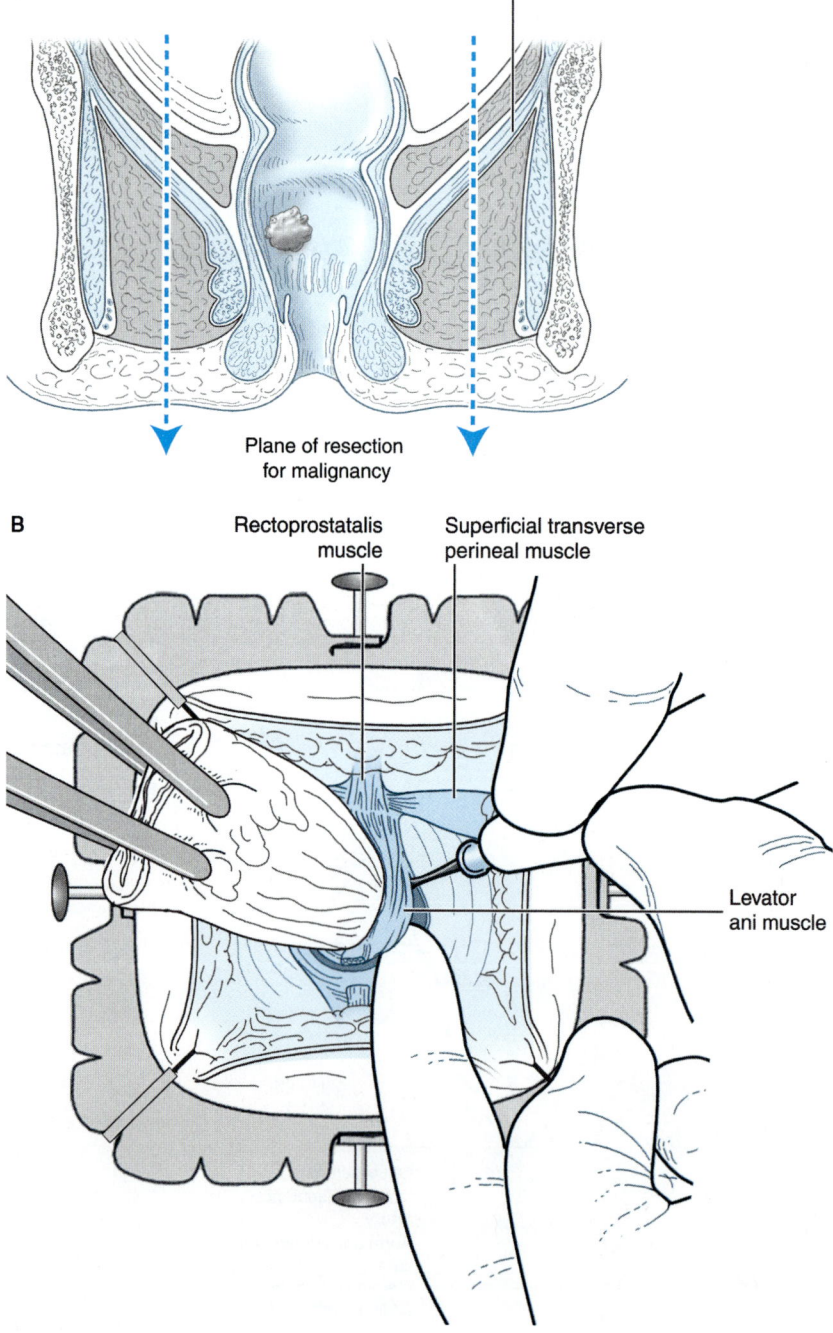

Figure 24–11A–B

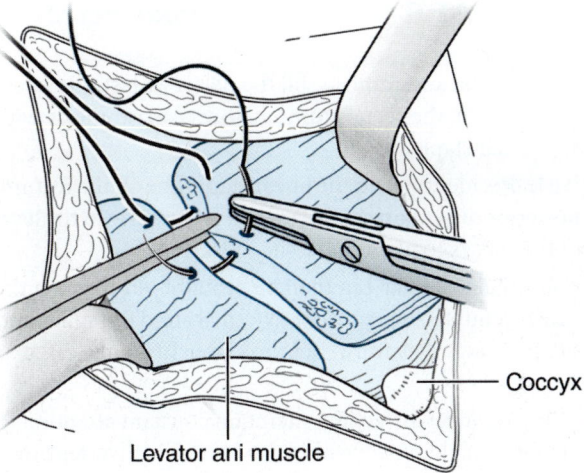

Figure 24–12

POSTOPERATIVE CARE

- Early ambulation is encouraged and diet is advanced as soon as tolerated.
- Patients requiring abdominal incision receive epidural analgesia and are transitioned to oral pain medications as soon as they can tolerate solids.
- Patients with ileostomies may require aggressive management of fluid status after the resumption of bowel function. We promote aggressive isotonic liquid consumption by the patient, with avoidance of caffeine and chocolate, and prefer first to use fiber bulking agents, followed by the addition of the antimotility agent loperamide.
- Daily examination of the perineal wound is mandatory following APR, and sitting should be discouraged for the first 5 postoperative days. Walking, however, should be aggressively encouraged.
- Pelvic drains are generally removed on postoperative day 5.

POTENTIAL COMPLICATIONS

Transanal Excision of Tumor
- As excision of the rectal wall is carried out below the peritoneal reflection, intra-abdominal leak is generally not a problem.
- Deep space infections can occur and should be treated by local drainage.
- More commonly, pathologic evaluation reveals more extensive disease than was appreciated preoperatively, necessitating further local or more radical resection.

LAR and APR with Total Mesorectal Excision
- Postoperative ileus is common, usually lasting 2–3 days and rarely requiring nasogastric decompression.
- Colonic ileus lasting longer than 2–3 days after LAR should prompt suspicion of an anastomotic hematoma, mechanical obstruction, or peritonitis associated with an anastomotic leak.
- Anastomotic leak is a potentially devastating complication following LAR and typically occurs 5–7 days following resection.
  - Fever, leukocytosis, ileus, and distention may be early signs of a leak.
  - Peritonitis mandates exploration with proximal diversion if a leak is discovered.
  - More subtle clinical presentations may require imaging with water-soluble contrast enema for identification.
- Intra-abdominal abscesses from breaks in surgical technique may require intravenous antibiotics, bowel rest, and percutaneous drain placement.

- Splenic injury can occur when mobilization of the splenic flexure is necessary to perform a tension-free anastomosis (LAR), or as necessary for the colon to be easily brought up for end colostomy (APR).
- Ureteral injury can result from altered rectosigmoid anatomy associated with malignancy, inflammation, and neo-adjuvant radiotherapy.
- Bladder or sexual dysfunction can occur due to injury of the sympathetic or parasympathetic nerves in the pelvis.

PEARLS AND TIPS

Transanal Excision of Tumor

- Pin the specimen out on suture card or cardboard and deliver it to the pathologist with correct orientation.
- Perform proctoscopy at the end of the procedure to ensure that the rectal lumen has not been sutured closed.
- Patients are usually hospitalized overnight for observation.
- Fever > 38.8°C is not uncommon in the immediate postoperative period, but if fever continues through the first postoperative night, blood and urine cultures as well as plain films of the chest should be ordered to evaluate for other, treatable sources of infection.

LAR and APR with Total Mesorectal Excision

- For low rectal anastomosis, fill the pelvis with sterile saline and insufflate the rectal stump before reanastomosis with the circular stapler.
  - If a leak is identified in the linear staple line on the rectum, posterior dissection should extend posteriorly to the level of the coccyx to identify the site of leakage.
  - The circular stapler can then be brought out through the defect, a purse-string suture placed around the spike, and the purse-string suture excluded after firing the circular stapler.
- During perineal dissection, maintain constant attention to palpation of the Foley catheter to avoid inadvertent urethral injury.

REFERENCES

Chang AE, Morris AM. Colorectal Cancer. In: Mulholland MW, Lillemoe KD, Doherty GM, et al, eds. *Greenfield's Surgery: Scientific Principles & Practice,* 4th ed. Philadelphia, PA: Lippincott Williams & Wilkins; 2006:1103–1128.

Huang EH. Complications of Appendectomy and Colon and Rectal Surgery. In: Mulholland MW, Doherty GM, eds. *Complications in Surgery.* Philadelphia, PA: Lippincott Williams & Wilkins; 2006:498–522.

CHAPTER 25

Operative Management of Rectal Prolapse

Brian S. Knipp, MD, and Richard E. Burney, MD

INDICATIONS
- Symptomatic rectal prolapse with or without fecal incontinence.

CONTRAINDICATIONS

Resection Rectopexy
- Elderly patients with limited life expectancy.
- Patients with severe comorbidities or those unable to tolerate general anesthesia or major abdominal surgery.

Perineal Rectosigmoidectomy (Altemeier Procedure)
- None.

INFORMED CONSENT

Resection Rectopexy

A. Expected Benefits
- Resection rectopexy is more durable than perineal rectosigmoidectomy and can often be performed via a laparoscopic approach.

B. Potential Risks
- Bleeding or hematoma development requiring reoperation.
- Wound infection.
- Injury to one or both ureters requiring repair.
- Sexual dysfunction, including impotence or retrograde ejaculation in men.
- Incisional hernia.
- Possible temporary or permanent colostomy.

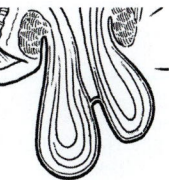
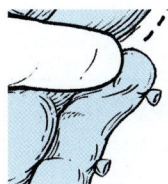
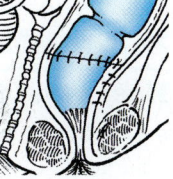
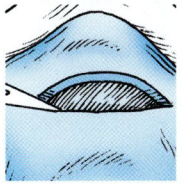
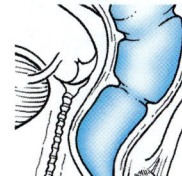
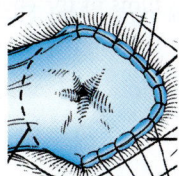
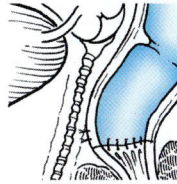

Perineal Rectosigmoidectomy (Altemeier Procedure)

A. Expected Benefits
- Preferred over an abdominal approach in high-risk patients.

B. Potential Risks
- Infection, most notably perirectal abscess.
- Bleeding, primarily from the sacral venous plexus but also potentially from the mesenteric vascular supply divided as part of the procedure.
- Anastomotic dehiscence.
- Recurrence of rectal prolapse.
- Loss of or failure to regain fecal continence.

EQUIPMENT

Resection Rectopexy
- Standard general surgery set used in gastrointestinal surgery.

Perineal Rectosigmoidectomy (Altemeier Procedure)
- Lone Star retractor.

PATIENT PREPARATION
- Complete colonoscopy (preferable) or barium enema and sigmoidoscopy to rule out malignancy or other colonic disease.
- Bowel preparation according to surgeon preference.

PATIENT POSITIONING

Resection Rectopexy
- The patient should be supine on the operating table.
- A Foley catheter is placed to decompress the bladder.
- Either a nasogastric or an orogastric tube is placed to decompress the stomach.

Perineal Rectosigmoidectomy (Altemeier Procedure)
- The patient may be positioned either in the lithotomy position or in the prone jackknife position.
- A Foley catheter is inserted to decompress the bladder.
- A Lone Star retractor is used for exposure.

PROCEDURE

Resection Rectopexy
- **Figure 25–1:** As the normal rectal attachments become lax, the rectum intussuscepts through the pelvic floor, telescoping through the anus.

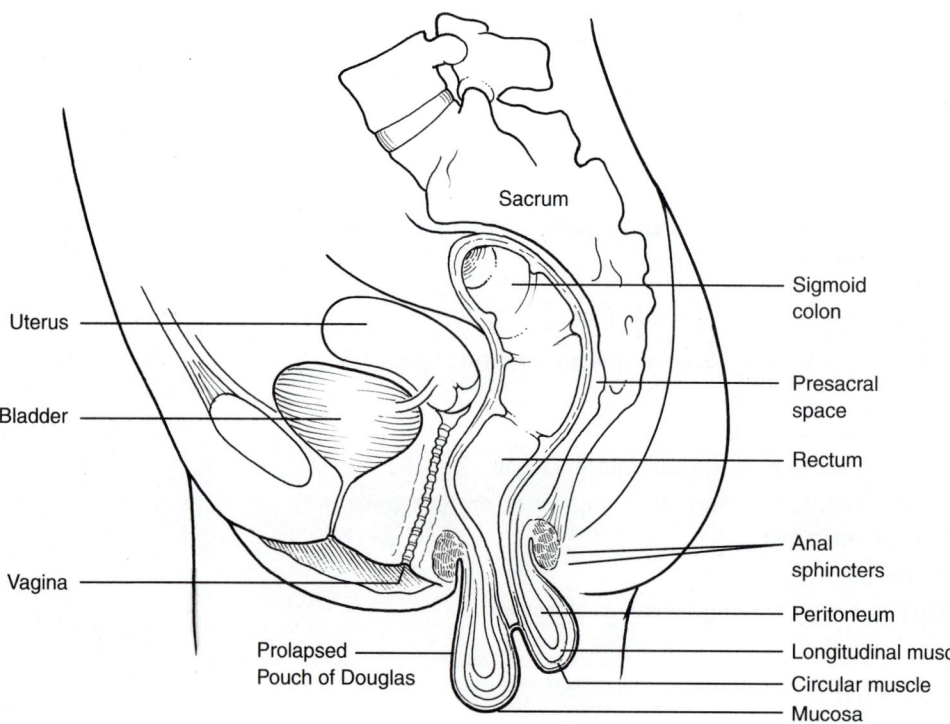

Figure 25–1

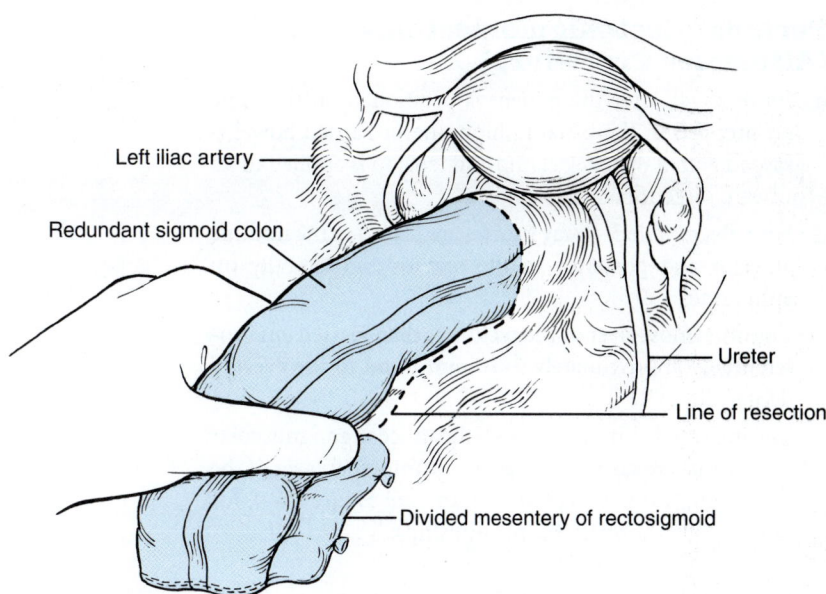

Figure 25–2

- **Figure 25–2:** The redundant sigmoid colon is resected in the usual manner, down to the peritoneal reflection.
  - The peritoneum is incised posteriorly and laterally to mobilize the rectosigmoid out of the pelvis, but the lateral attachments of the rectum are left intact.
  - Redundant rectosigmoid is resected.
  - The proximal colon is then anastomosed to the rectum to provide intestinal continuity and the rectum is sutured to the presacral fascia to fix it in place.
- **Figure 25–3:** The completed procedure is shown, with the anastomotic line at or below the peritoneal reflection and tacking sutures between the rectum and the presacral fascia fixing the colon in place.

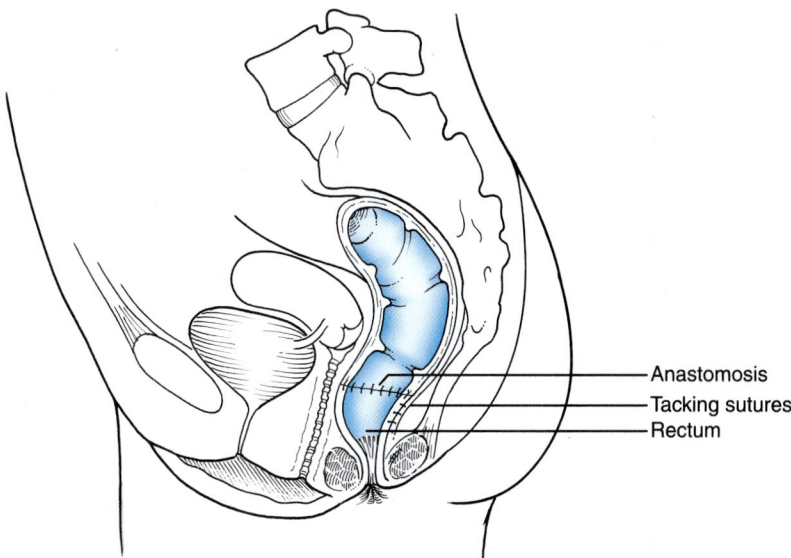

Figure 25–3

Perineal Rectosigmoidectomy (Altemeier Procedure)

■ **Figure 25–4:** After the patient is positioned on the table and prepped in the usual fashion, the prolapsed bowel is grasped with a Babcock clamp and tension is applied in an outward direction.

- Four absorbable 3–0 stay sutures are placed in the midline anterior and posterior to the rectum and laterally on either side.
- The outermost layer of the rectum is then incised circumferentially approximately 5–10 mm distal to the everted dentate line.
- The incision is carried through the mucosa and muscular layer, with care taken not to enter the muscular layer of the underlying intussuscepted rectum (see Figure 25–1 for further illustration of this relationship).

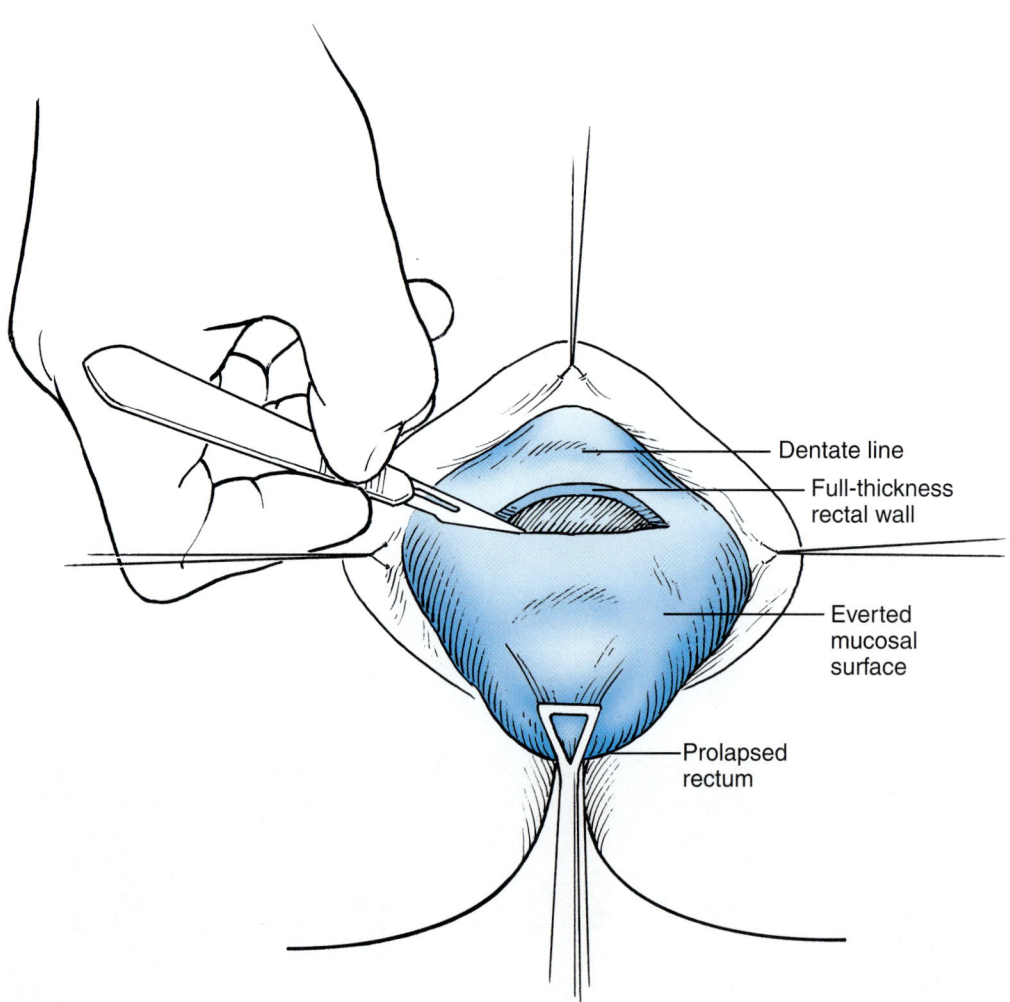

Figure 25–4

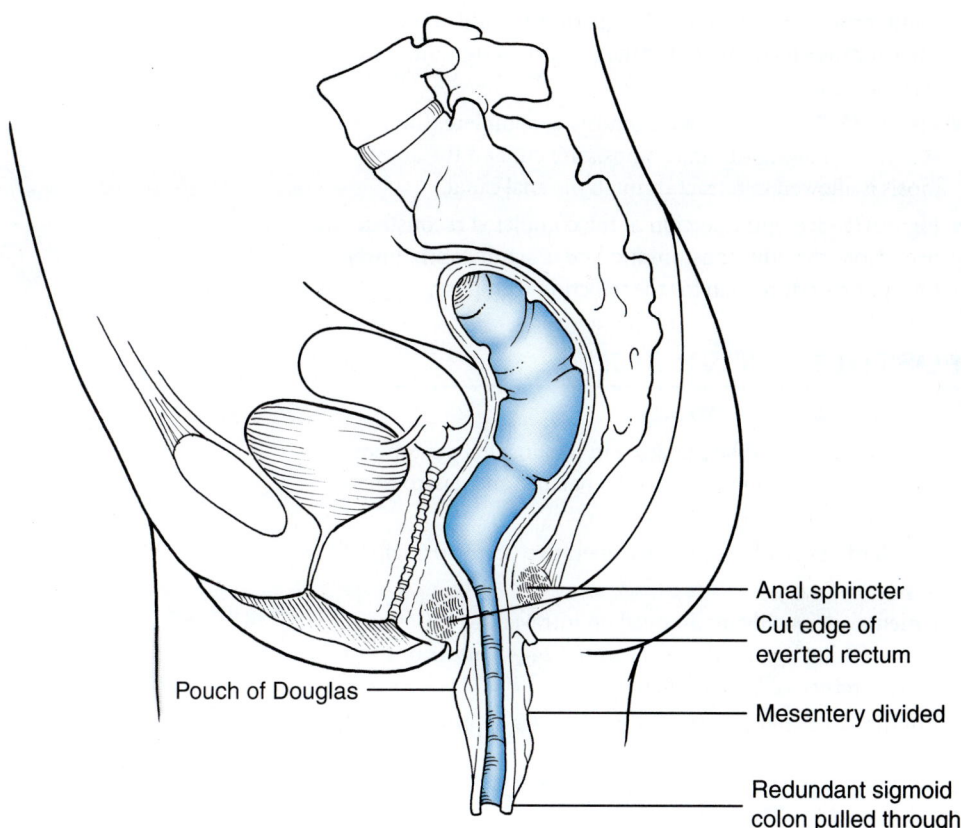

Figure 25-5

- **Figure 25–5:** Once the entire outer layer of intussuscepted rectum has been incised, it is folded outward and the mesenteric attachments to the intussusception are divided as they are encountered.
  - As mesenteric attachments are divided, more rectosigmoid colon can be pulled out.
  - The location for transection of the redundant rectosigmoid colon is identified when no more sigmoid can be pulled through and the anastomosis can be made with minimal tension.
- **Figure 25–6:** The redundant rectosigmoid colon is divided axially along the anterior and left lateral surfaces and stay sutures are placed through at the base of these cuts, through the mucosa and muscular wall, attaching them to the cut edge of the distal mucosa.
  - The redundant tissue between these stay sutures is resected and the first quadrant, from 12 o'clock to 3 o'clock, is closed with interrupted fine, absorbable sutures.
  - Another axial cut is made along the posterior surface of the redundant mucosa, a stay suture is placed at 6 o'clock and the second quadrant is closed with interrupted fine, absorbable sutures.

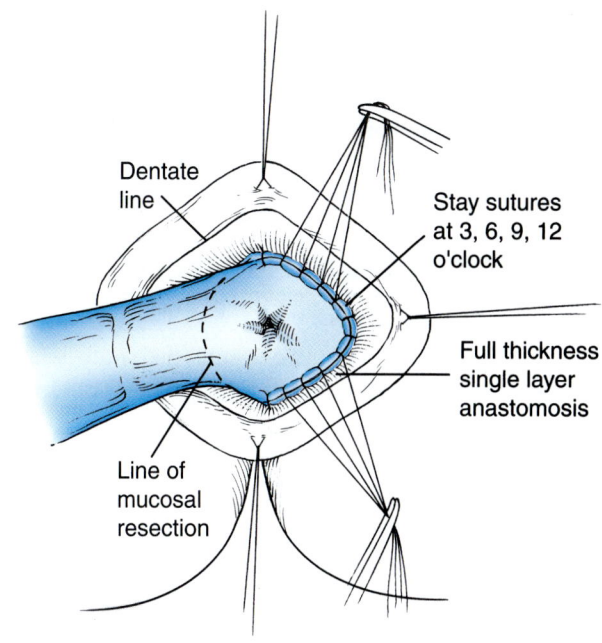

Figure 25-6

- This procedure continues by quadrants until the entire anastomosis is complete and the redundant sigmoid colon is removed.
- **Figure 25–7:** Once the anastomosis is complete, the four stay sutures along the anastomosis are cut and the anastomosis is allowed to retract through the anal canal.
- **Figure 25–8:** Sagittal section of the completed reconstruction. Note that the anastomotic line is significantly lower for this procedure than for the resection rectopexy.

POSTOPERATIVE CARE

Resection Rectopexy

- The patient should be managed in the hospital postoperatively, with attention paid to fluid balance and gastrointestinal function.
- Standard postcolectomy perioperative care principles apply.
- Patients are usually maintained on intravenous fluids only with nothing by mouth for the initial 24–48 hours or until there is return of bowel function.
- Epidural or patient-controlled analgesia is appropriate.

Perineal Rectosigmoidectomy (Altemeier Procedure)

- Patients should have minimal pain.
- The patient should be monitored in the hospital postoperatively with attention paid to bowel function.
- Nothing should be inserted per rectum.
- The diet is advanced as tolerated.
- The patient may use sitz baths three times daily and after all bowel movements.
- Stools softeners should be used to keep stools from becoming hard and disrupting the anastomotic suture line.
- Digital rectal examination should be deferred and no rectal suppositories should be given in the first 2–4 weeks postoperatively.

POTENTIAL COMPLICATIONS

Resection Rectopexy

- Mortality rate of 0% in all but one published study (which had one death in 15 patients for a 6.7% mortality rate).
- Recurrence rates range from 0–5%.
- Postoperative constipation rates range from 18–80% in reported surgical series.
- Incontinence may not improve with the procedure.

Perineal Rectosigmoidectomy (Altemeier Procedure)

- Mortality rate of 0% in all studies except one (which had one death in 20 patients for a 5% mortality rate).

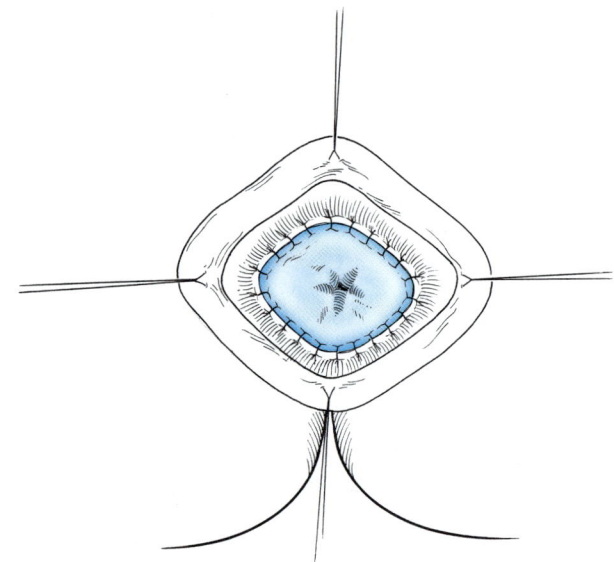

Figure 25–7

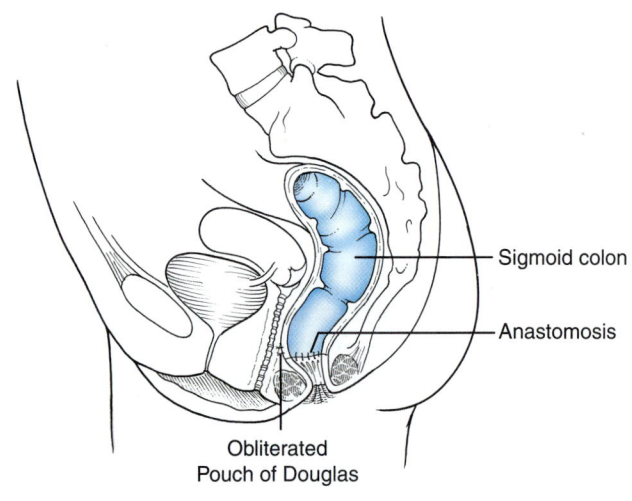

Figure 25–8

- Rectal prolapse recurrence rate is higher with the Altemeier procedure than with resection rectopexy, ranging from 0–16%.
- Bowel injury can occur upon entering the hernia sac in the anterior plane of dissection, particularly when the patient is in the lithotomy position.

PEARLS AND TIPS

Resection Rectopexy

- The recognition of full-thickness rectal prolapse as distinguished from redundant or prolapsed mucosa, severe hemorrhoidal disease, or skin tags is classically based on detecting circular mucosal layers rather than radially oriented folds on external examination.
- Examination of the patient after sitting and straining on a commode can facilitate visualization of the extent of prolapse.
- Defecography can be helpful if there is any question about the diagnosis.

Perineal Rectosigmoidectomy (Altemeier Procedure)

- Care must be taken when incising the anterior surface of the intussuscepted rectosigmoid, as intra-abdominal contents such as small intestine may be present in the pouch of Douglas.

REFERENCES

Altemeier WA, Culbertson WR, Schowengerdt C, Hunt J. Nineteen years' experience with the one-stage perineal repair of rectal prolapse. *Ann Surg.* 1971;173:993–1006.

Madiba TE, Baig MK, Wexner SD. Surgical management of rectal prolapse. *Arch Surg.* 2005;140:63–73.

CHAPTER 26

Benign Anorectal Procedures

Erica N. Proctor, MD, and Emily V.A. Finlayson, MD

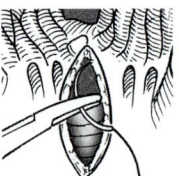 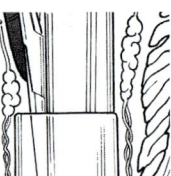 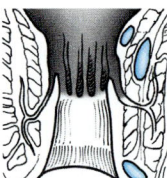
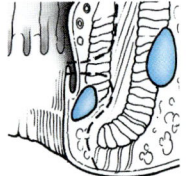  

INDICATIONS

Hemorrhoidectomy
- Internal hemorrhoids: grade III and IV hemorrhoids, symptomatic combined internal and external hemorrhoids, bleeding, incarceration, or failure of conservative management.
- External hemorrhoids: acute thrombosis < 72 hours postonset.

Pilonidal Cyst Excision and Marsupialization
- Recurrent acute pilonidal infections.
- Chronic pilonidal sinus.

Anorectal Abscess and Fistula
- Acute perirectal abscess.
- Anorectal fistula.

CONTRAINDICATIONS

Hemorrhoidectomy

A. Absolute
- Anorectal Crohn's disease or Crohn's proctitis.
- Acquired immunodeficiency syndrome.

B. Relative
- Portal hypertension.
- Pregnancy.
- Coagulopathy.

Pilonidal Cyst Excision and Marsupialization
- The presence of cancer requires additional treatment.

Anorectal Abscess and Fistula
- Multiple fistulous tracts in a patient with Crohn's disease may require additional studies of the colon and sphincter mechanism prior to definitive surgical treatment.

INFORMED CONSENT

Hemorrhoidectomy

A. Expected Benefits
- Resolution of hemorrhoids and symptoms.

B. Potential Risks
- Common complications include significant postoperative pain, urinary retention, bleeding, incontinence, infection, and anal stenosis.
- Risk of bleeding is increased with emergent hemorrhoidectomy, during pregnancy, and in patients with portal hypertension or coagulopathy.
- Rectal perforation, rectovaginal fistula, and retroperitoneal and pelvic sepsis are rare risks of circular stapled hemorrhoidopexy and may be avoided with proper technique.

Pilonidal Cyst Excision and Marsupialization

A. Expected Benefits
- Resolution of cyst and infection.
- Prevention of recurrence.

B. Potential Risks
- Primary cyst excision with marsupialization requires daily wound scrubbing and strict attention to shaving hair in wound proximity.
- Time to healing may be several months.
- Rate of recurrence is approximately 6%.
- Rate of wound breakdown is 2–3%.

Anorectal Abscess and Fistula

A. Expected Benefits
- Resolution of abscess or fistula.

B. Potential Risks
- Common complications of surgery include:
  - Fistula in ano.
  - Abscess.
  - Incontinence due to iatrogenic sphincter injury.

EQUIPMENT

- No special equipment is required for hemorrhoidectomy, pilonidal cyst excision, or the treatment of anorectal abscess and fistula.

Circular Stapled Hemorrhoidopexy
- 33-mm hemorrhoidal circular stapler.

PATIENT PREPARATION

Hemorrhoidectomy
- Thorough preoperative workup to confirm diagnosis, hemorrhoid grade, and symptomatic status is essential before recommending hemorrhoidectomy.
- If bleeding is the indication for hemorrhoidectomy, examination of the colon and rectum for other potential sources of bleeding may be indicated.
- In patients with portal hypertension, hemorrhoids must be distinguished from anorectal varices.
- The rectum may be evacuated with an enema immediately before the operation.

Pilonidal Cyst Excision and Marsupialization
- Digital rectal examination should be performed to evaluate for a presacral tumor.
- The patient is examined to identify the location of pits and presence of infection or abscess.
- Surrounding hair is shaved after patient positioning on the operative table.

Anorectal Abscess and Fistula
- A thorough preoperative workup is essential to confirm the diagnosis, evaluate the immune status of the patient, and determine the presence of an underlying disease process such as Crohn's disease that might require additional studies prior to surgical therapy.
- Preoperative anorectal examination to determine the complexity of the process may guide anesthetic choices and surgical planning.

PATIENT POSITIONING

Hemorrhoidectomy
- The patient should be in the prone jackknife position with buttocks taped aside.
- The procedure is performed under general anesthesia or intravenous sedation with local anesthesia.
- Left anterolateral positioning and local anesthesia are suggested for pregnant patients.

Pilonidal Cyst Excision and Marsupialization
- The patient should be in the prone jackknife position; lateral decubitus position may also be used.
- The procedure may be performed under general anesthesia or local anesthesia with intravenous sedation.

Anorectal Abscess and Fistula

- The patient should be in the prone jackknife position with buttocks taped aside.
- The procedure is performed under general anesthesia, regional anesthesia, or intravenous sedation with local anesthesia.

PROCEDURE

Surgical Hemorrhoidectomy

- A Hill-Ferguson retractor is inserted to obtain exposure.
- **Figure 26–1A:** The internal hemorrhoid is grasped with forceps and retracted outward. A suture ligature is placed at the proximal aspect of the vascular pedicle. This suture should not be cut.
- **Figure 26–1B:** The internal hemorrhoid and external component are grasped with a clamp.
  - Electrocautery is used to make a V-shaped incision in the mucosa around the hemorrhoidal bundle starting at the base of the internal hemorrhoid beyond the anal verge and continuing toward the ligated pedicle.
  - The hemorrhoid is then carefully dissected from the underlying anal sphincter.
  - Dissection should be continued cephalad in the avascular plane between the hemorrhoid and internal sphincter using Metzenbaum scissors or electrocautery.
  - When the internal portion of the hemorrhoid is elevated off the sphincter muscle to the level of the pedicle, the pedicle should again be suture-ligated followed by excision of the hemorrhoid.

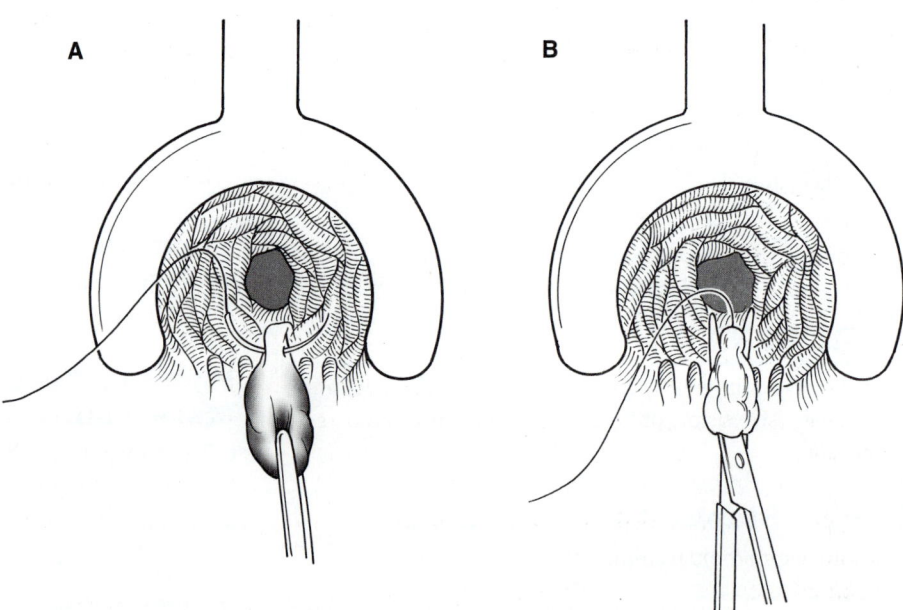

Figure 26–1A–B

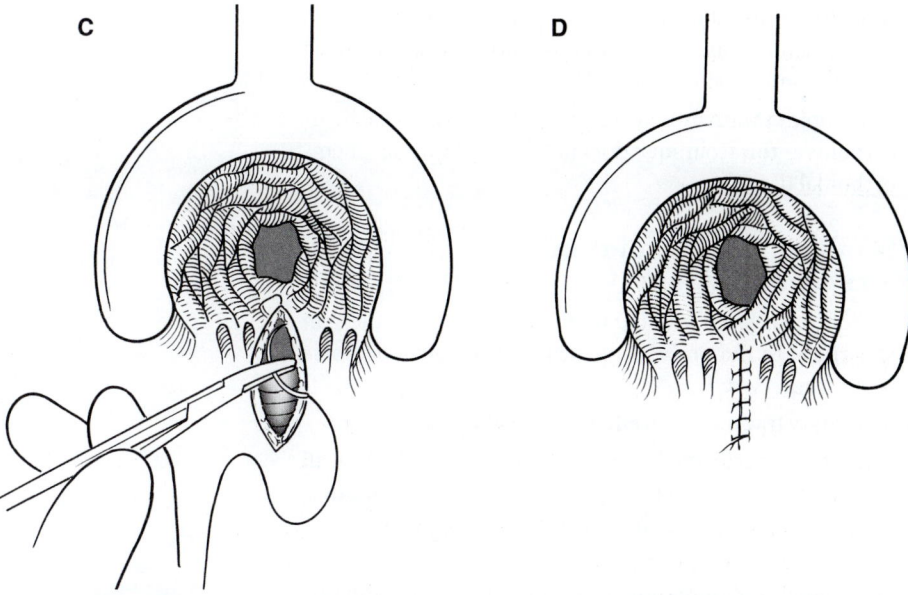

Figure 26–1C–D

- **Figure 26–1C:** After the hemorrhoid is excised, the mucosal defect should be reapproximated using running 3-0 Vicryl or other absorbable suture of adequate tensile strength starting proximally at a site immediately adjacent to the suture-ligated base of the hemorrhoid.
- **Figure 26–1D:** The completed hemorrhoidectomy, showing reapproximation of the mucosal defect with running absorbable suture.

Circular Stapled Hemorrhoidopexy

- A retracting anoscope and dilator is inserted and the obturator is removed. Upon removal of the obturator, prolapsed tissue should fall into the dilator lumen. The operating anoscope is then inserted and a purse-string suture is placed.
- **Figure 26–2:** A monofilament purse-string suture is placed 4–5 cm above the dentate line taking care to avoid suture gaps by starting the new stitch where the previous stitch exits.
- A circular stapler is carefully placed through the purse-string suture and the suture is tied down to the stapler rod. The suture ends are brought through the lateral openings in the stapler.
- The purse-string suture is retracted with moderate traction to pull the anorectal mucosa into the stapler and the stapler is closed.
  - Tissue around the stapler should be examined before firing the stapler to ensure that the dentate line is not incorporated into the staple line.
  - In women, a digital vaginal examination should be performed to ensure that the posterior vaginal wall is not tethered to the staple line.

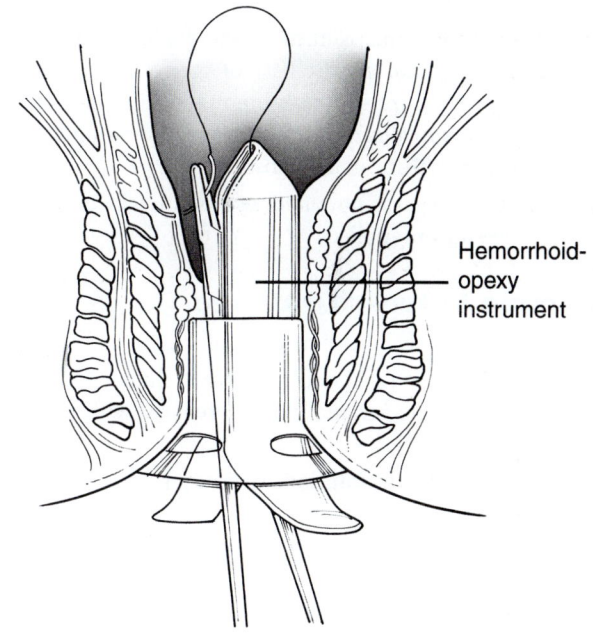

Figure 26–2

- After firing, the stapler is kept in place for 20 seconds to ensure hemostasis. The stapler should then be removed carefully and the site inspected.
- Anoscopic examination will reveal persistent internal hemorrhoids as this technique does not completely excise hemorrhoidal tissue.

Pilonidal Cyst Excision and Marsupialization

- A probe is inserted into the midline opening, and the skin superficial to the probe is opened with a scalpel or Bovie electrocautery.
- Secondary tracts are unroofed in an analogous manner.
- Curettage is performed at the base of the wound. Once all tract and pits have been exposed, a symmetric elliptical skin incision is marked that incorporates all openings.
- An en bloc excision of the cyst, pits, secondary openings, and areas of inflammation is performed with creation of a shallow funnel-shaped wound.
- Care should be taken to avoid undermining the wound edges.
- **Figure 26–3:** Marsupialization is performed by sewing the skin edges to the fibrotic base of the wound using a 2-0 absorbable suture in a continuous locking fashion. The goal of marsupialization is to minimize the wound size and prevent premature wound closure.
- After hemostasis is obtained, petroleum jelly gauze and a dry dressing are applied.

Simple Abscess Drainage

- **Figure 26–4:** Classification system for anorectal abscesses.
- After the area of maximal erythema or fluctuance, or both, is identified, the perianal skin is prepared with povidone-iodine.
- A local anesthetic solution, typically lidocaine with epinephrine, is administered.
- A cruciate or elliptical incision is made and the skin edges are trimmed to allow adequate drainage and prevent closure of the skin prior to adequate granulation of the abscess cavity.
- The site is inspected to ensure hemostasis and the cavity is then lightly packed with gauze.

Anorectal Fistula

- **Figure 26–5:** Classification of fistula in ano. **A,** Subcutaneous. **B,** Intersphincteric. **C,** Transsphincteric. **D,** Supralevator. **E,** Extrasphincteric.
- The perianal area is prepared with povidone-iodine.
- The external opening of the fistula is identified on the perianal skin.
  - An anoscope is inserted to evaluate the anal canal and rectum and identify the internal opening of the fistula.

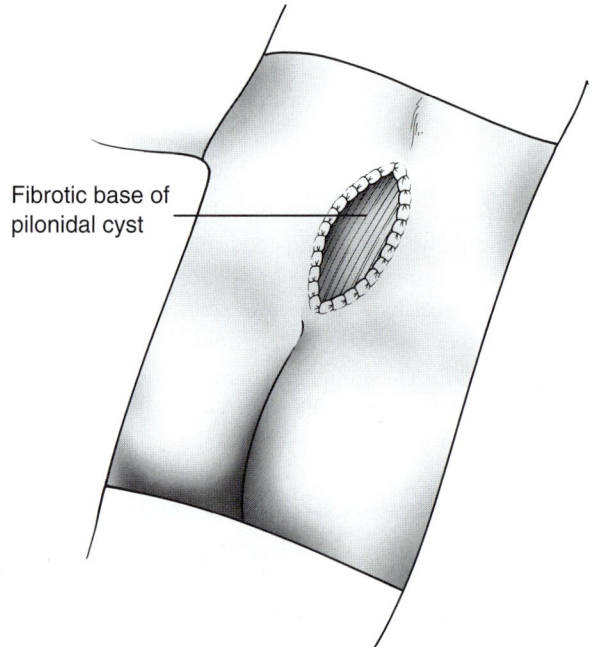

Fibrotic base of pilonidal cyst

Figure 26–3

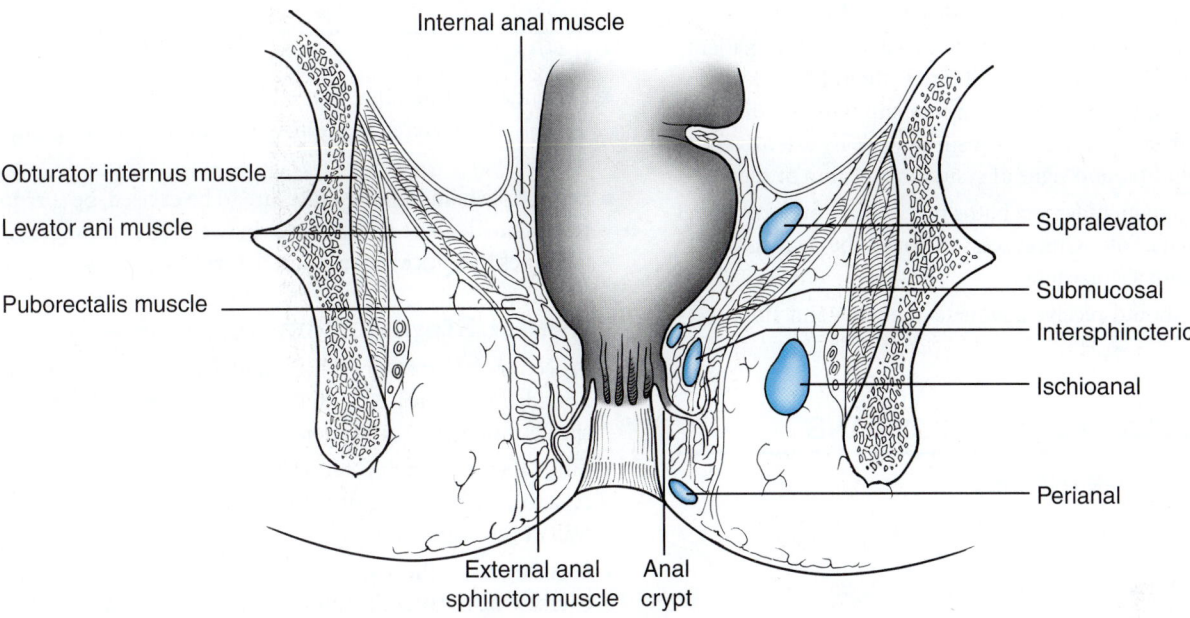

Figure 26-4

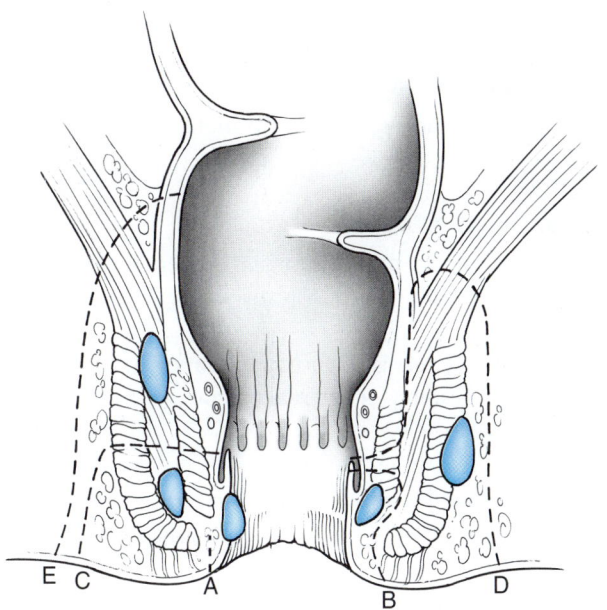

Figure 26-5

- A probe is gently passed from the internal opening of the fistula toward the external opening to determine the direction of the fistulous tract.
- If the internal opening is not easily identified, hydrogen peroxide can be injected through the external opening using a 10-mL syringe and an 18-gauge angiocatheter. If the injection is successful, the internal opening will be marked by the presence of bubbles.
- Careful palpation is performed to assess the involvement of the anal sphincter. If < 50% of the sphincter muscle is involved, a fistulotomy should be performed by passing the metal probe along the entire length of the fistula tract and dividing the tissue overlying the probe.
- Curettage is performed on the opened tract to remove epithelialized tissue.
- If > 50% of the sphincter is involved, a vessel loop should be attached to the probe, introduced through the fistula tract, and secured to form a seton around the sphincter.

POSTOPERATIVE CARE

Hemorrhoidectomy

- Postoperative care includes analgesia, stool softeners, fiber supplementation, and sitz baths.

Pilonidal Cyst Excision and Marsupialization

- Wound care includes daily showers or sitz baths, cleansing of wound, and removal of all hair within 3–4 cm of wound edges. The wound should be packed wet-to-dry with normal saline twice daily.

Anorectal Abscess and Fistula
- Antibiotics are generally not indicted in healthy patients with a simple abscess. Antibiotics should be given for abscesses in patients with immunosuppression, diabetes, valvular heart disease or prosthetic valves, extensive soft tissue cellulitis, and signs of systemic infection or sepsis.
- Wound care includes sitz baths twice daily and after bowel movements. Following abscess drainage, the cavity is lightly packed with a gauze tape.
- Patients should receive adequate analgesia and stool softeners.

POTENTIAL COMPLICATIONS
Hemorrhoidectomy
A. Early
- Pain.
- Urinary retention.
- Bleeding.
- Infection.
- Fecal impaction.

B. Late
- Anal stricture.
- Anal tags.
- Incontinence.
- Mucosal prolapse.
- Ectropion.

Pilonidal Cyst Excision and Marsupialization
- Recurrent pilonidal sinus formation.
- Infection.
- Bleeding.
- Delayed wound healing.

Anorectal Abscess Drainage
- Incomplete drainage may lead to recurrent anorectal abscesses, especially in patients with ischioanal and intersphincteric abscesses.
- Incontinence from iatrogenic injury to the sphincter.
- Necrotizing perineal infection occurs in < 1% of patients.
- Fistula in ano.
- Sepsis.

Anorectal Fistula
- Fecal incontinence.
- Bleeding.
- Recurrent fistula.

PEARLS AND TIPS
Surgical Hemorrhoidectomy
- Pudendal and perianal nerve block with local anesthetic may be administered to improve relaxation of anal sphincter muscles.
- If multiple hemorrhoidal piles are to be excised, be sure to retain an adequate tissue bridge between the various excision sites to reduce the risk of stricture.

Circular Stapled Hemorrhoidopexy
- Procedure is best reserved for grade II and III hemorrhoids not adequately treated with banding and grade IV hemorrhoids if reducible under general anesthesia.
- Limit the purse-string suture to the mucosa and submucosa to avoid incorporating the muscular layer of the rectal wall or the vaginal wall.
- Bleeding from the staple line may be easily controlled by oversewing the bleeding point.

Pilonidal Cyst Excision and Marsupialization
- To avoid sphincter injury, be aware of proximity to the anus.

Anorectal Abscess
- A modified Hanley procedure is indicated for horseshoe abscess.

Anorectal Fistula
- Avoid passing the probe through the external opening of a fistula to identify the tract as this may create a false passage.
- The Goodsall rule is often more accurate in women and may be misleading for external openings > 3 cm from the anal verge.
- The lay open fistulotomy technique may be used for intersphincteric and low transsphincteric fistulae. Seton placement is appropriate for high transsphincteric fistulae.

REFERENCES
Cintron JR, Abcarian H. Benign Anorectal Hemorrhoids. In: Wolff BD, Fleshman JW, Beck DE, et al, eds. *ASCRS Textbook of Colon and Rectal Surgery*. New York, NY: Springer; 2007:156–177.

Hull TL, Wu J. Pilonidal disease. *Surg Clin North Am.* 2002;82:1169–1185.

Vasilevsky CA, Gordon PH. Benign Anorectal Abscess and Fistula. In: Wolff BD, Fleshman JW, Beck DE, et al, eds. *ASCRS Textbook of Colon and Rectal Surgery*. New York, NY: Springer; 2007:192–214.

CHAPTER 27

Operative Management of Breast Cancer

Dawn M. Coleman, MD, and Kathleen M. Diehl, MD

INDICATIONS

Breast Lumpectomy
- Definitive therapy for a benign solid breast mass.
- Atypical cells or lobular carcinoma in situ on fine needle aspiration or core needle biopsy of a breast or mammographic abnormality.
- Stage I and II breast cancer (if combined with sentinel lymph node biopsy and adjuvant radiation therapy [XRT] to accomplish breast conservation therapy).
- Ductal carcinoma in situ.
- Nonpalpable mammographic abnormalities (eg, calcifications).

Modified Radical Mastectomy
- Local management of stage II breast cancer when breast conservation therapy is contraindicated or is not the patient's preference.
  - Residual large cancer after adjuvant therapy.
  - Multicentric cancer.
  - Patient preference.
  - Contraindication to subsequent radiation therapy.
- Local management of stage III breast cancer.
- Lymph node metastases discovered during sentinel lymph node biopsy or fine needle aspiration for a clinically palpable node.

Sentinel Lymph Node Biopsy
- Clinical stage I and II breast cancer.
  - May be performed in conjunction with breast-conserving therapy or simple mastectomy.
- Axillary nodal status is the most powerful prognostic feature available in stratifying the risk of breast cancer relapse.

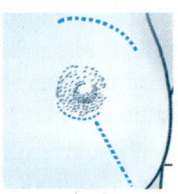
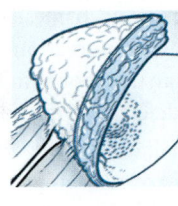
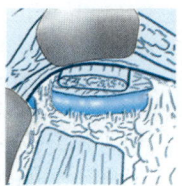
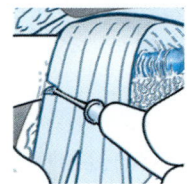
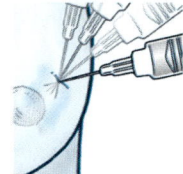
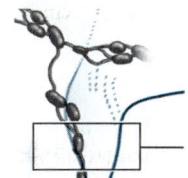
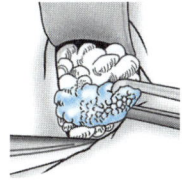
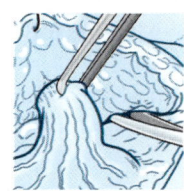
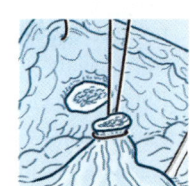

Areolar Duct Excision
- Lactiferous ductal dilation on imaging.
- Nipple discharge isolated to a single duct or quadrant of the nipple.
- Mass or mammographic abnormality underlying the nipple-areolar complex.

CONTRAINDICATIONS
Breast Lumpectomy
A. Absolute
- Multicentric disease (tumors in separate quadrants).
- Persistent positive margins after reasonable surgical attempts
- Pregnancy: first and second trimester (if XRT is intended with the goal of breast conservation therapy). Breast conservation therapy may be feasible in the third trimester if radiation therapy is deferred to the postpartum period.
- Prior therapeutic irradiation to the breast that would result in retreatment to an excessively high radiation dose (if XRT is intended with the goal of breast conservation therapy).
- Diffuse, malignant-appearing microcalcifications.
- Tumor size > 5 cm.

B. Relative
- History of collagen vascular disease (eg, scleroderma or systemic lupus erythematosus) especially if steroid dependent (if XRT is intended with the goal of breast conservation therapy; these patients may experience excessive radiation toxicity).
- Extensive gross multifocal disease in the same quadrant.
- Large tumor in a small breast that would offer suboptimal cosmetic results.
- Patient preference for mastectomy.
- Male breast cancer (rarely feasible).
- Skin cellulitis and open wounds.
- Stage IV disease.

Modified Radical Mastectomy
A. Absolute
- None.

B. Relative
- Stage IV disease.

Sentinel Lymph Node Biopsy
A. Absolute
- Clinically positive adenopathy on physical examination.
- Pregnancy, lactation.

B. Relative
- Previous regional breast surgery or radiation.
- Stage III or IV disease.
- Prior axillary surgery.
- Locally advanced primary cancer (> 5 cm).

Areolar Duct Excision
A. Absolute
- Inflammatory breast cancer.
- Stage III or IV invasive breast cancer.

B. Relative
- Skin cellulitis and open wounds.

INFORMED CONSENT
Breast Lumpectomy
A. Expected Benefits
- Complete removal of a breast mass with a margin of normal-appearing glandular tissue to achieve a tissue diagnosis.
- Definitive therapy for a benign breast mass.
- Local management of stage I and II breast cancer and ductal carcinoma in situ.

B. Potential Risks
- Common complications:
  - Surgical site infections (either deep or superficial).
  - Bleeding.
  - Hematoma.
  - Seroma.
- Less likely to occur:
  - Sampling error.
  - Recurrent breast edema and cellulitis.
  - Chronic incisional pain.
  - Brachial plexopathy from positioning.
  - Thrombosis of the thoracoepigastric vein.
- Pneumothorax (a rare complication for wire-localizing procedures).

Modified Radical Mastectomy
A. Expected Benefits
- Removal of any previous biopsy scar, skin, nipple-areola complex, breast tissue, and axillary lymph nodes (levels I, II, +/− level III) for local management of invasive breast cancer with lymph node metastases.

B. Potential Risks
- Common complications:
  - Surgical site infections (either deep or superficial).
  - Bleeding.

- Hematoma.
- Seroma.
■ Less likely to occur:
  - Chronic upper extremity edema with associated angiosarcoma.
  - Axillary webs.
  - Chyle leak.
  - Skin flap necrosis.
  - Axillary vein thrombosis.
  - Chronic incisional pain.
  - Brachial plexopathy from positioning.
■ Neurovascular injury resulting in axillary or upper arm sensory deficits and shoulder weakness.

Sentinel Lymph Node Biopsy
A. Expected Benefits
■ Identification, using lymphatic mapping with isosulfan blue dye (Lymphazurin) or colloids labeled with radioactive isotopes (usually technetium) with or without lymphoscintigraphy, of the first lymph node that receives drainage from a cancer in an effort to accurately stage invasive breast cancer and thus guide additional surgical and adjuvant therapy.

B. Potential Risks
■ Common complications:
  - Surgical site infections (either deep or superficial).
  - Bleeding.
  - Hematoma.
  - Seroma.
■ Less likely to occur:
  - Chronic upper extremity edema with associated angiosarcoma.
  - Axillary webs.
  - Chyle leak.
  - Axillary vein thrombosis.
  - Chronic incisional pain.
  - Brachial plexopathy from positioning.
■ Neurovascular injury resulting in axillary or upper arm sensory deficits and shoulder weakness.

Areolar Duct Excision
A. Expected Benefits
■ Excision of the lactiferous ducts en bloc for definitive management of benign breast disease and to establish tissue diagnosis.

B. Potential Risks
■ Common complications:
  - Surgical site infections (either deep or superficial).
  - Bleeding.
  - Hematoma and seroma.
  - Nipple-areolar necrosis and paraesthesia.
  - Difficulties with breast feeding.
■ Less likely to occur:
  - Recurrent breast edema and cellulitis.
  - Chronic incisional pain.
  - Brachial plexopathy from positioning.
  - Thrombosis of the thoracoepigastric vein.

EQUIPMENT
Breast Lumpectomy, Modified Radical Mastectomy, and Areolar Duct Excision
■ No special equipment is necessary.

Sentinel Lymph Node Biopsy
■ 5 mL of isosulfan blue dye for preoperative injection.
■ Gamma probe to detect radioactive colloid.
■ In instances where isosulfan blue dye is unavailable, methylene blue dye may be substituted. Care should be taken to avoid methylene blue dye injection into the dermis as it may cause skin necrosis.

PATIENT PREPARATION
Breast Lumpectomy
■ An appropriate history and physical examination should include risk stratification for breast cancer and a thorough bilateral breast examination.
■ Nodal disease and any evidence of inflammatory or T4 disease should be excluded on clinical examination.
■ Additionally, an appropriate preoperative workup for a breast lesion should include ultrasound, with or without fine needle aspiration, as well as mammogram if the patient is older than 40 years.
■ If a patient is undergoing wire-localized lumpectomy, a localization wire is placed preoperatively in radiology within 1 cm of the lesion. These patients should receive preoperative intravenous antibiotics before skin incision.

Modified Radical Mastectomy
■ All patients will have had prior biopsy of some variety to support the diagnosis of invasive breast cancer with lymph node metastases.
■ Ensure that a bilateral mammogram has been obtained.
■ A thorough history and physical examination preoperatively should assess for signs and symptoms of metastatic disease and gross axillary nodal involvement and should document a baseline neurologic examination.

- Additional studies (eg, CT scan, bone scan, chest radiograph, and liver function studies) are guided by clinical concern.

Sentinel Lymph Node Biopsy
- The morning of or the night before surgery, radioactive colloid (eg, technetium-99m–tagged sulfur colloid) is injected via three or four separate injections at the cancer site or retroareolar.
- Additionally, we suggest preoperative lymphoscintigraphy for further visual assistance in locating the sentinel lymph node.

Areolar Duct Excision
- +/– Ductography (well tolerated with local anesthesia).
- Retroareolar ultrasound and mammography should be obtained for all patients.

PATIENT POSITIONING

Breast Lumpectomy, Modified Radical Mastectomy, and Areolar Duct Excision
- The patient should be supine with the ipsilateral arm abducted 90 degrees.
- Attention should be paid to appropriately padding pressure points.

Modified Radical Mastectomy
- The patient should be supine with arms abducted 90 degrees.
- All pressure points should be padded appropriately.
- The axilla may be shaved.
- Preoperative antibiotics should be administered prior to skin incision.

PROCEDURE

Breast Lumpectomy
- **Figure 27–1:** Optimal cosmesis is considered when planning the incision.
  - Upper-inner quadrant incisions should be avoided when possible because of their greater visibility.
  - Circumareolar and inframammary incisions provide very good results.
  - Curvilinear incisions that parallel the Langerhans lines also offer acceptable scarring.
  - Some surgeons advocate a radial incision for lower breast lesions; this approach should be avoided in the upper half of the breast given the risk of scar contracture and resulting displacement of the nipple-areola complex.

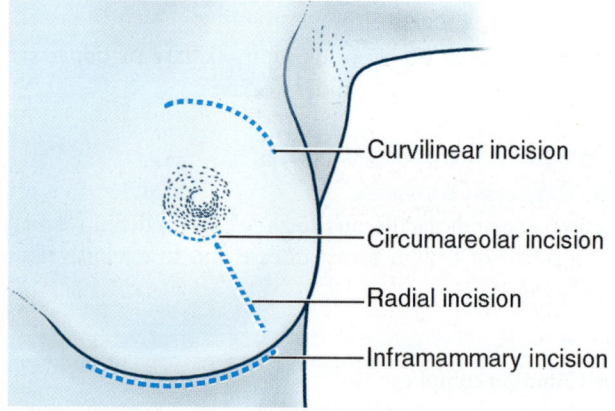

Figure 27–1

- Finally, the incision should be small and immediately overlying the mass.
- As further resection may be indicated, the incision should be placed within the appropriate boundaries of a mastectomy skin incision, while also allowing for a 1-cm skin margin around the scar.

■ **Figure 27–2:** Following sharp skin incision, skin flaps are raised on either side of the incision with electrocautery to ensure hemostasis.
- Thin flaps (< 7–10 mm) should be avoided to prevent skin flap ischemia and tissue necrosis.
- Allis forceps are used to grasp normal glandular tissue surrounding the palpable lesion, and this tissue is placed under gentle traction.
- The dissection proceeds around the lesion in an attempt to encompass the entire mass.
- Once excised, the specimen is oriented in three dimensions and sent for pathologic examination.
- With hemostasis obtained, the wound is irrigated.
- Deep dermal skin layers are approximated with interrupted 3-0 Vicryl sutures followed by skin approximation with a 4-0 Monocryl suture placed in a running subcuticular fashion or skin adhesive.

■ Needle-localized breast biopsy or lumpectomy.
- For nonpalpable mammographic lesions, wire localization is indicated.
- This requires the placement of a localization wire preoperatively in mammography within 1 cm of the lesion.
- The skin incision is placed directly over the lesion and dissection proceeds toward the wire.
- Once visible, the wire with surrounding normal tissue is grasped with an Allis clamp and placed under gentle traction to facilitate dissection around the angled distal tip of the wire.
- This approach should encompass the lesion in question. Following excision, the biopsy specimen is oriented and sent for radiographic or pathologic examination to confirm that the lesion of interest was in fact removed. Clips are placed in the lumpectomy bed.

Modified Radical Mastectomy

■ **Figure 27–3A:** A horizontal or an oblique elliptical incision is incised sharply with an axillary extension to facilitate the axillary dissection. This must encompass any previous biopsy scar in addition to the nipple-areola complex.

■ **Figure 27–3B:** This incision may be tailored if an immediate reconstructive procedure or skin-sparing mastectomy is intended.

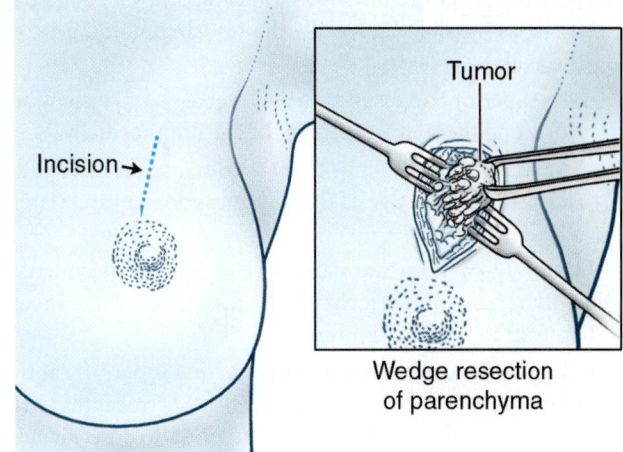

Figure 27–2

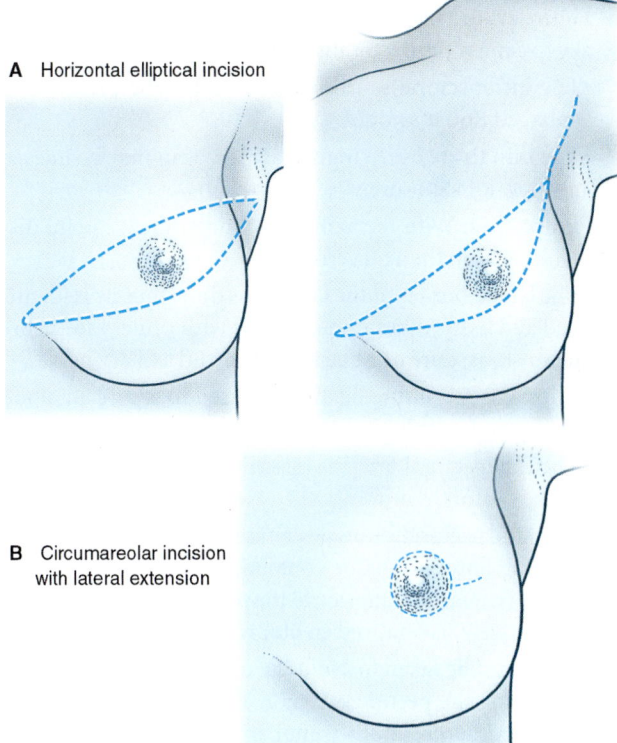

Figure 27–3A–B

- **Figure 27–4:** Superior and inferior skin flaps are raised with electrocautery to ensure hemostasis.
  - Gentle traction is applied to the specimen to facilitate the dissection.
  - Thin flaps (< 3 mm) should be avoided to prevent skin flap ischemia and tissue necrosis; however, this is balanced with the goal of removing as much fat and subcutaneous tissue as possible (especially the nodal-containing fat of the axilla).
  - The superior flap extends to the level of the clavicle superiorly and the lateral aspect of the sternum medially.
  - The inferior flap extends to the inframammary fold inferiorly and to the edge of the latissimus dorsi muscle laterally.
- **Figure 27–5:** With the flaps developed, the specimen is gently retracted inferiorly for the dissection of the breast tissue off the pectoralis muscles.
  - The glandular tissue is dissected starting superiorly at the level of the clavicle and proceeds with electrocautery parallel to the muscle fibers in a superior to inferior and medial to lateral direction.
  - Pectoralis major fascia is removed with the specimen.
  - Intercostal perforating arterial branches that supply the breast may require ligation.
- **Figure 27–6:** The pectoralis muscle is then retracted medially to expose the pectoralis minor muscle.
  - The intrapectoral space is explored for the presence of enlarged Rotter's nodes.
  - The thin tissue overlying the axillary vein may be incised to allow for exposure.
- **Figure 27–7:** With the axillary vein identified, careful dissection within the axilla ensues.
  - The lateral border of the latissimus dorsi muscle is identified and tissue dissection proceeds with cautery to ensure hemostasis. Care must be taken to avoid axillary nerves.
  - Clips and 3-0 suture ligation are used to secure all blood vessels and lymphatics encountered.
  - The clavipectoral fascia is incised along the lateral aspect of the pectoralis minor.
  - With the pectoralis muscles retracted superior and medially, the fibrofatty tissue containing level I and II lymph nodes (lateral and inferior to the pectoralis minor muscle, respectively) is removed en bloc with the specimen.
  - Care must be taken to avoid the medial and lateral nerves supplying the pectoralis major. The medial nerve passes through the pectoralis minor in approximately 70% of patients; in a minority of patients it passes lateral to the muscle. The lateral nerve passes medial to the pectoralis muscle and is typically found in close proximity to the thoracoacromial artery.

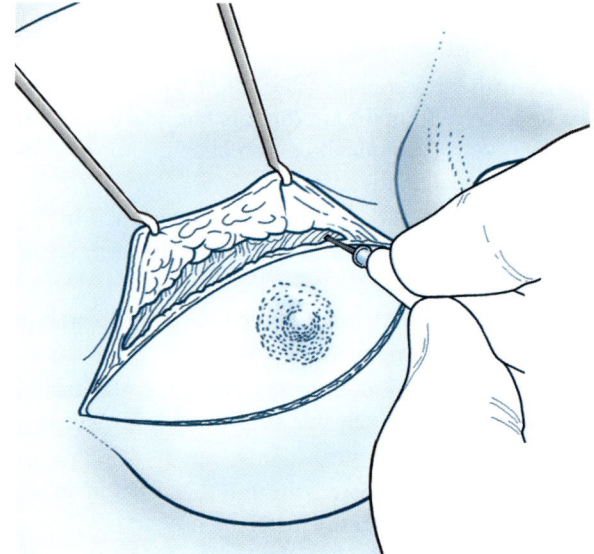

Figure 27-4

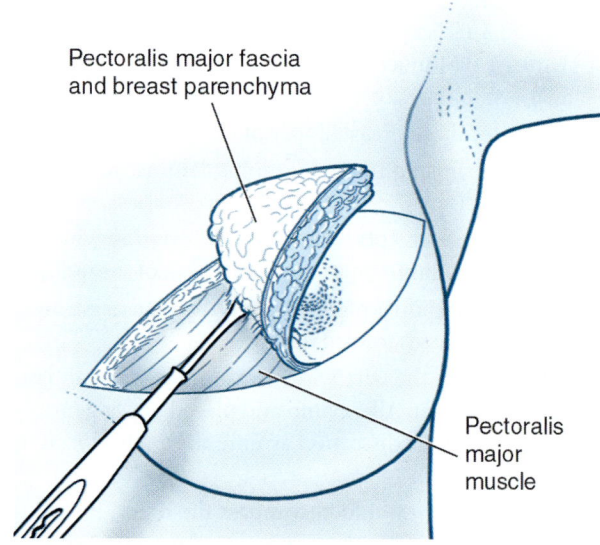

Figure 27-5

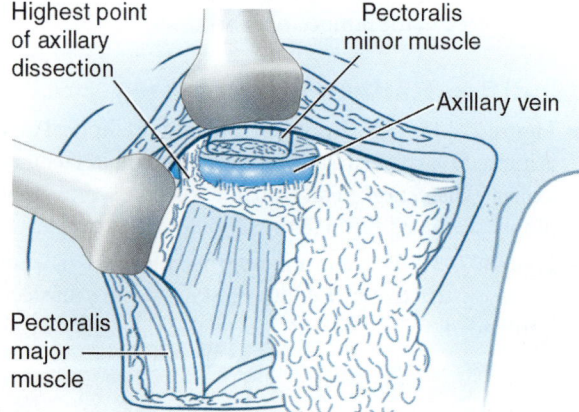

Figure 27-6

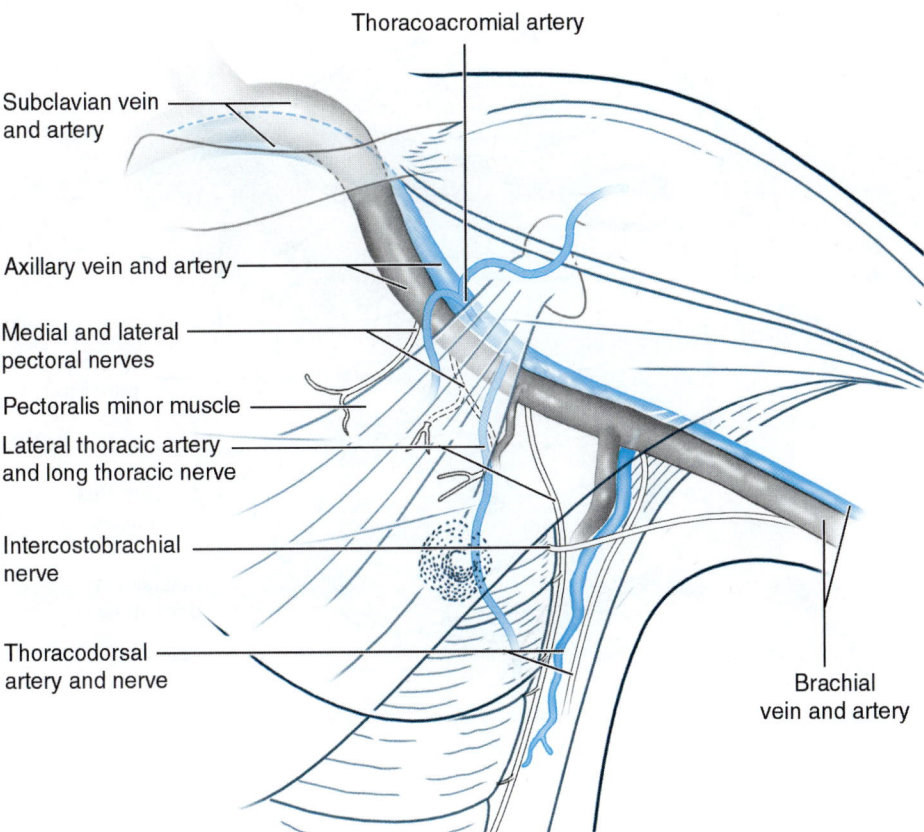

Figure 27–7

- The axillary dissection proceeds inferolaterally and progresses carefully with the identification of several important structures.
- The long thoracic nerve is identified and preserved deep to the axillary vein and extends inferiorly along the serratus anterior.
- The intercostobrachial nerve is identified originating beneath the second rib and extending transversely.
- Finally, the thoracodorsal vein is identified originating from the axillary vein and extending inferiorly, associated with the artery.
- The corresponding thoracodorsal nerve is located posteromedial to the vein; the entire bundle should be preserved.
- **Figure 27–8:** In the setting of grossly palpable apical axillary nodes, the axillary dissection is extended to include the level III lymph nodes medial to the pectoralis muscle.
  - This is termed a Patey modification and begins with the division of the pectoralis minor from its insertion on the coracoid process.
  - The operator's gloved finger protects the underlying brachial plexus.

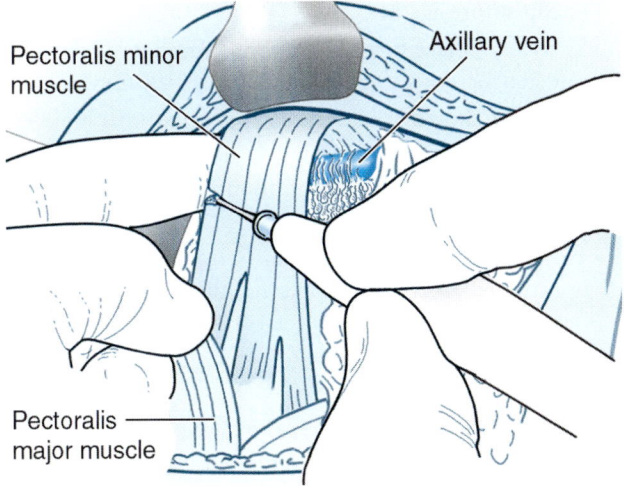

Figure 27–8

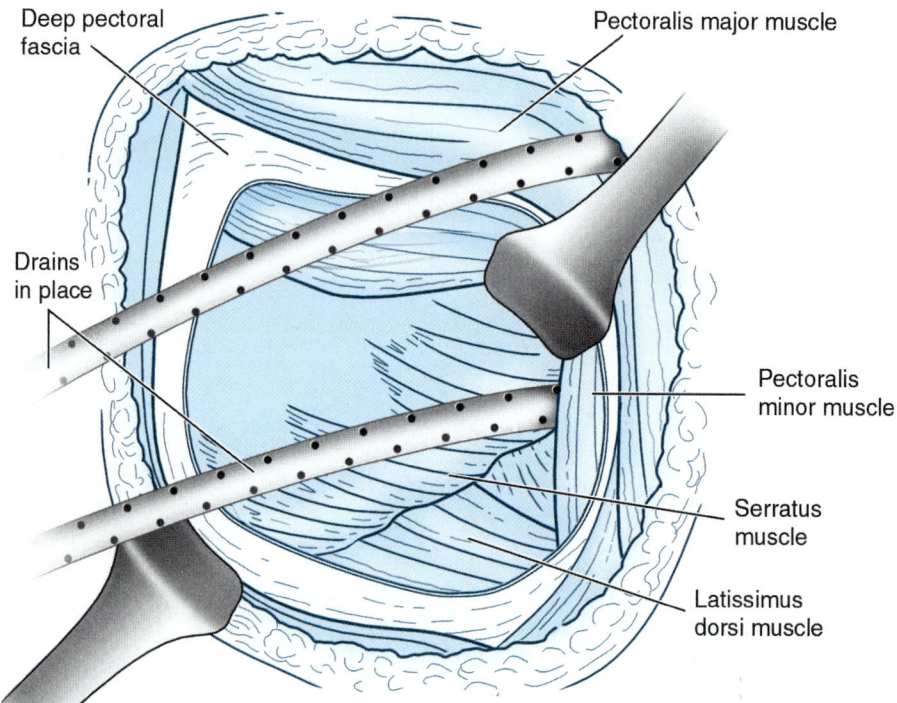

Figure 27–9

- **Figure 27–9:** With the critical vessels and nerves identified and preserved, the fibrofatty contents of the axilla are removed down to the level of the subscapularis muscle posteriorly and to the level of the latissimus dorsi muscle laterally with the breast tissue.
  - The specimen should be oriented and tagged for pathologic examination.
  - The surgical bed is inspected for hemostasis and all visible bleeding points should be controlled with electrocautery or clip/suture ligature.
  - Two No. 10 Blake surgical drains are placed through separate stab incisions after copious wound irrigation.
  - One drain should lie in the axillary bed; the other is placed along the inferior flap.
  - The drains are secured in position to the skin with 2-0 nylon suture.
  - The deep dermal layer of skin is reapproximated with interrupted 3-0 Vicryl sutures and the skin is reapproximated with skin adhesive or a 4-0 Monocryl suture in a running subcuticular fashion.

Sentinel Lymph Node Biopsy

- **Figure 27–10:** Approximately 5 mL of isosulfan blue dye is injected into the breast in a similar fashion to the previously injected radioactive colloid.

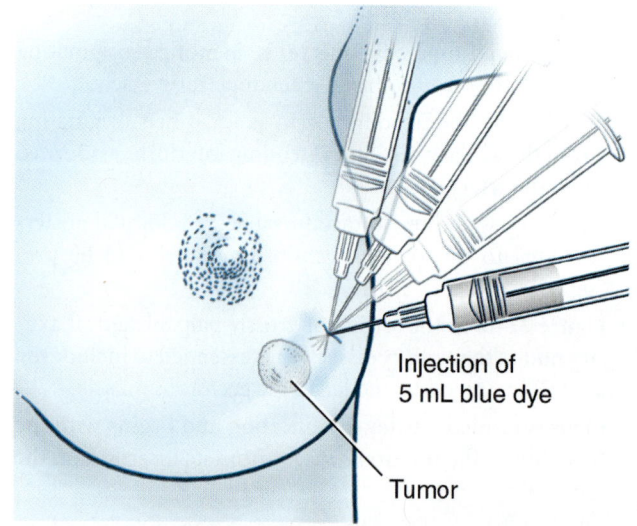

Figure 27–10

- The injection is placed deep to the tumor or biopsy cavity but not into the cavity, and may also be injected intradermally over the tumor or biopsy cavity, or retroareolar based on surgeon preference.
- The area is massaged for 5 minutes to encourage incorporation and flow into the dermal lymphatics.
- A gamma probe is waved over the axillary nodal basin scanning for the area with the highest focus of radioactivity.
- Once this area is localized, a limited skin incision is made sharply, directly over the area in a transverse fashion that will allow for scar incorporation if subsequent axillary lymph node dissection is indicated.
- Dissection then proceeds with electrocautery in an attempt to identify a blue node.

■ **Figure 27–11:** Visually tracing the blue lymphatics combined with gamma probe feedback will localize "hot" nodes.

- These sentinel nodes are typically blue in color and demonstrate notable radioactivity with the gamma probe.
- These nodes should be resected, minding hemostasis and lymphatic vessels.
- Once the nodes are removed, the wound should be scanned with the gamma probe to locate further radioactivity.
- All blue, grossly enlarged and firm nodes should be resected.
- All nodes that demonstrate ≥ 10% radioactivity on gamma probe of the "hottest" and theoretical sentinel node are resected as well.
- Resected nodes are sent for permanent pathology.
- Once hemostasis is ensured, the wound is irrigated.

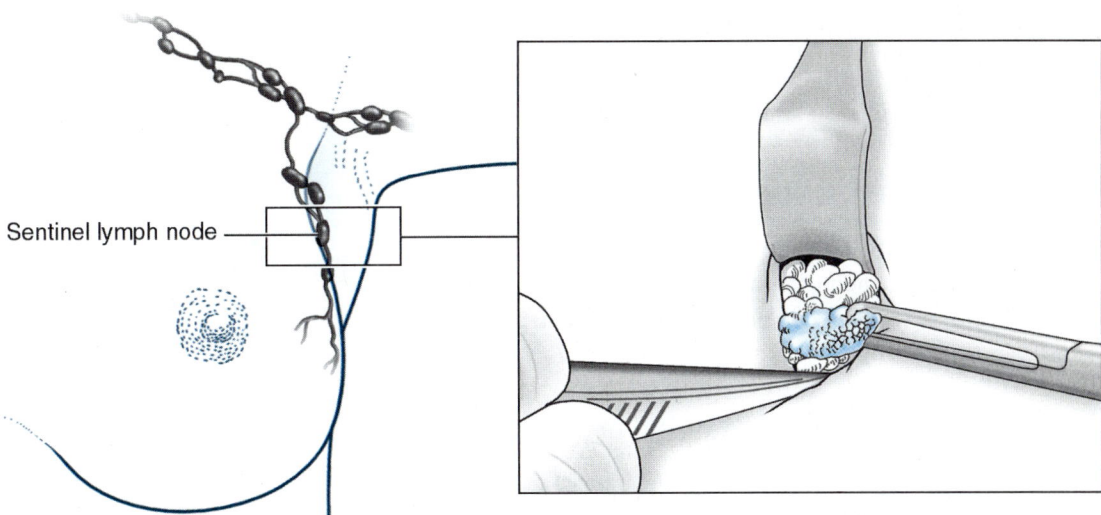

Figure 27–11

226 • CURRENT PROCEDURES: Surgery

- The subcutaneous tissue is reapproximated with interrupted 3-0 Vicryl sutures.
- The skin is reapproximated with skin adhesive or a 4-0 Monocryl suture placed in a running subcuticular fashion.

Areolar Duct Excision

■ **Figure 27–12:** If no palpable lesion is noted on clinical examination, a curvilinear skin incision is used as illustrated around the nipple-areolar complex.
■ If there is a palpable lesion, a conservative skin incision is made sharply in a curvilinear or radial fashion over the abnormality, allowing for future incorporation into a mastectomy incision if indicated.
■ **Figure 27–13:** Superior and inferior flaps are raised sharply with Metzenbaum scissors beneath the nipple-areolar complex.
- Suture or teethed forceps are used to place the areolar complex under gentle traction.
- Care is taken not to "buttonhole" the tissue.
- An Allis forceps is used to grasp the ductal tissue with any palpable abnormality and place this tissue under gentle traction.
- Dissection continues until the ductal system is isolated from surrounding breast parenchyma and the specimen encompasses the entire lesion, if palpable.
- Excision extends from the terminal duct proximally to approximately 2 cm into the breast parenchyma.
■ **Figure 27–14:** The proximal duct is ligated sharply flush with the nipple, while the remaining deeper dissection into the breast parenchyma is accomplished with electrocautery to ensure hemostasis.
- The specimen is tagged and sent for permanent pathology.
- Once hemostasis is ensured, the wound is irrigated.
- The underlying dermal layer is closed with interrupted 3-0 Vicryl sutures and the overlying skin is reapproximated with skin adhesive or a 4-0 Monocryl suture placed in a running subcuticular fashion.

POSTOPERATIVE CARE

Breast Lumpectomy

■ Patients typically go home the same day.
■ A supportive bra or breast binder and routine wound care instructions are advised.

Modified Radical Mastectomy

■ A supportive bra or binder is provided.
■ Routine drain care and wound care instructions are advised.

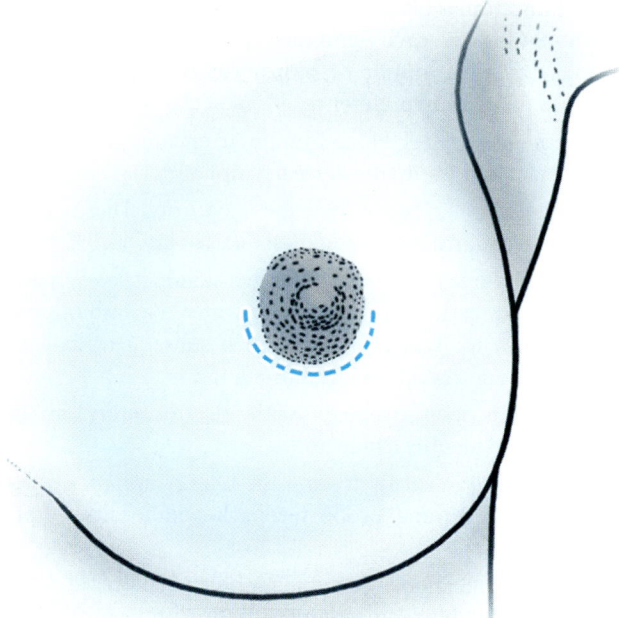

Figure 27-12

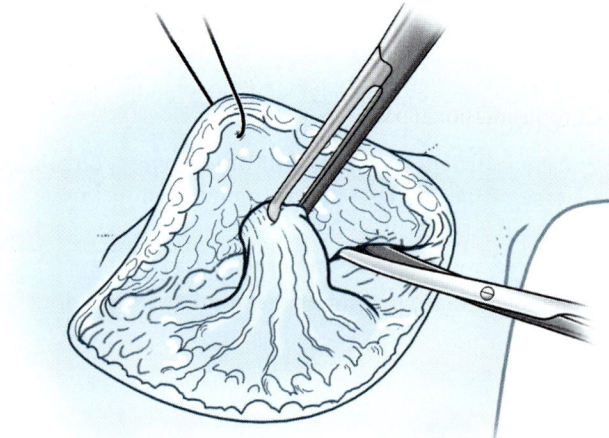

Figure 27-13

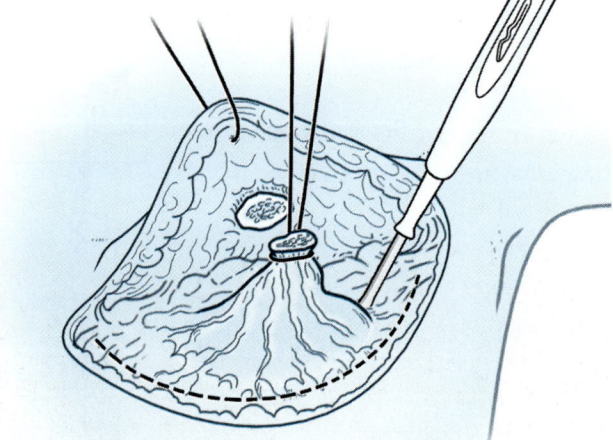

Figure 27-14

- The drains should remain in place until output is < 30 mL/day per drain.
- Outpatient and pathology follow-up should be ensured to promptly facilitate initiation of any indicated adjuvant therapy.

Sentinel Lymph Node Biopsy
- Routine wound care and judicious follow-up.
- Patients typically can be discharged the day of surgery with oral pain medication.

Areolar Duct Excision
- Routine wound care and judicious follow-up is advised.
- Patients typically may be discharged the day of surgery with oral pain medication and a supportive bra or breast binder.

POTENTIAL COMPLICATIONS

Breast Lumpectomy
- Bleeding and hematoma.
- Seroma.
- Recurrent breast edema and cellulitis.
- Wound infection, deep and superficial.
- Chronic incisional pain.
- Brachial plexopathy from positioning.
- Thrombosis of the thoracoepigastric vein.
- Sampling error (increased incidence with nonpalpable lesions).
- Pneumothorax (if wire localization is used).

Modified Radical Mastectomy
- Bleeding and hematoma.
- Seroma.
- Cellulitis and wound infection, deep and superficial.
- Chronic incisional pain.
- Brachial plexopathy from positioning.
- Thrombosis of the thoracoepigastric vein.
- Chronic upper extremity edema and associated angiosarcoma of the upper extremity (Stewart-Treves syndrome).
- Axillary webs.
- Chyle leak.
- Skin flap necrosis.
- Nerve and vascular injury.
  - Damage to the intercostobrachial nerve results in axillary and upper arm sensory deficits.
  - The axillary vein is susceptible to frank trauma with resulting injury and hemorrhage as well as retraction-associated thrombosis.
  - Damage to the thoracodorsal bundle denervates the latissimus dorsi and results in weakened internal rotation and shoulder abduction.
  - Damage to the long thoracic nerve denervates the serratus anterior and results in a "winged" scapula.
  - Damage to the medial and lateral pectoralis nerve results in atrophy of the pectoralis major.

Sentinel Lymph Node Biopsy
- Bleeding and hematoma.
- Seroma.
- Wound infection, deep and superficial.
- Chronic upper extremity edema and associated angiosarcoma of the upper extremity (Stewart-Treves syndrome); however, this risk is notably much lower than with a formal axillary lymph node dissection.
- Axillary webs.
- Chyle leak.
- Chronic incisional pain.
- Brachial plexopathy from positioning.
- Sampling error.

Areolar Duct Excision
- Bleeding and hematoma.
- Seroma.
- Nipple or areolar paresthesia and flap necrosis.
- Recurrent breast edema and cellulitis.
- Wound infection, deep and superficial.
- Chronic incisional pain.
- Brachial plexopathy from positioning.
- Thrombosis of the thoracoepigastric vein.
- Difficulties with future breast feeding.

PEARLS AND TIPS

Breast Lumpectomy
- Place clips around the circumference of the lumpectomy cavity at the base of the surgical bed to guide adjuvant radiation therapy.
- Consider protective Bovie tips and insulated retractors to prevent thermal injury to the skin edges.

Modified Radical Mastectomy
- Consider protective Bovie tips and insulated retractors to prevent thermal injury to the skin edges.
- The easiest way to identify the long thoracic nerve is to identify the crossing vein from the thoracodorsal vein passing laterally toward the chest wall.

Sentinel Lymph Node Biopsy

- Avoid rapid movements with the probe and allow counts to settle out.
- Direct the probe away from the site of breast injection to avoid "shine-through."

Areolar Duct Excision

- Taking > 50% of the subcutaneous tissue beneath the nipple risks nipple sloughing.
- Preoperative imaging can ensure identification of any abnormality distal in the duct that should be included in the surgical excision.

REFERENCES

Morrow M, Strom EA, Bassett LW, et al. Standard for breast conservation therapy in the management of invasive breast carcinoma. *CA Center J Clin.* 2002;52:277–300.

Newman L, Sabel M. Advances in breast cancer detection and management. *Med Clin North Am.* 2003;87:997–1028.

CHAPTER 28

Operative Management of Melanoma

Amir A. Ghaferi, MD, and Michael S. Sabel, MD

INDICATIONS

Wide Local Excision of Melanoma
- Biopsy-proven cutaneous melanoma.

Inguinal Lymph Node Dissection
- Documented metastatic disease in the inguinal lymph nodes with no evidence of distant metastases.
- Metastases detected in the inguinal nodes by sentinel lymph node (SLN) biopsy or by fine needle aspiration or excisional biopsy in a patient with a clinically evident lymph node metastasis.

Full-Thickness Skin Graft
- Coverage of large defects created by wide local excision of a melanoma that cannot be closed primarily or with a local flap.

CONTRAINDICATIONS
Absolute
- Inability to close donor site incision.

Relative
- Concern about incomplete resection (positive margins).
- Poor wound conditions (poor vascularization, exposed bone, open joint surfaces).

INFORMED CONSENT

Wide Local Excision of Melanoma
A. EXPECTED BENEFITS
- Removal of all melanoma cells at the primary site in order to provide durable local disease control for all patients, even when the likelihood for distant relapse is high, and to effect a cure in patients at low risk of harboring occult metastatic disease.

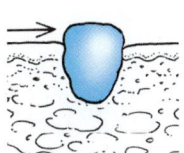
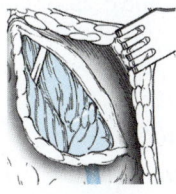
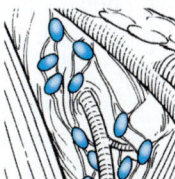
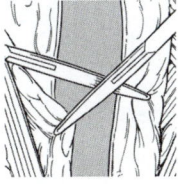
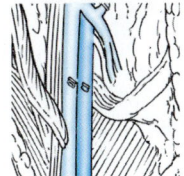
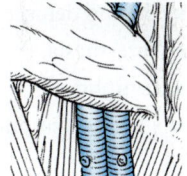
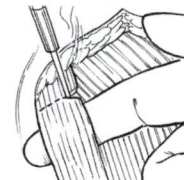

B. Potential Risks
- Surgical site infection.
- Bleeding or hematoma formation.
- Scarring.
- Return of melanoma at the surgical site or a distant site.
- Need for reexcision in the event of positive margins.

Inguinal Lymph Node Dissection
A. Expected Benefits
- Removal of all node-bearing tissue within the femoral triangle and suprainguinal location (superficial inguinal lymph node dissection) and possibly the iliac and obturator nodes (superficial and deep, or ilioinguinal lymph node dissection).

B. Potential Risks
- Surgical site infection.
- Bleeding or hematoma formation.
- Skin edge necrosis.
- Wound dehiscence.
- Paresthesia.
- Lymphocele.
- Chronic lymphedema.

Full-Thickness Skin Graft
A. Expected Benefits
- Autologous coverage of a large skin defect created by the excision of a melanoma.

B. Potential Risks
- Surgical site or donor site infection.
- Bleeding.
- Hematoma.
- Seroma.
- Partial or complete graft loss.

EQUIPMENT
- No special equipment is required.

PATIENT PREPARATION
Wide Local Excision of Melanoma
- A review of the histologic findings of the biopsied lesion should be undertaken before planning a local excision.
- The necessary surgical margins (in centimeters) for excision are determined by the Breslow depth (in millimeters) of the melanoma.
  - In situ lesions require a 0.5-cm margin.
  - Invasive melanomas < 1 mm require a 1-cm margin.
  - Melanomas > 2 mm in depth require a 2-cm margin.
  - Melanomas between 1 and 2 mm should be excised with 2-cm margins when possible, but 1.5-cm or even 1-cm margins are reasonable when 2-cm margins are not feasible without a skin graft or would require an excessively tight closure.
- SLN biopsy is typically performed in conjunction with wide local excision for melanomas ≥ 1.0 mm and for melanomas between 0.76 mm and 1.0 mm if other adverse factors are present (ulceration, high mitotic rate, angiolymphatic invasion). (See Chapter 27 for details of SLN biopsy.)

Inguinal Lymph Node Dissection
- When palpable adenopathy is present in the groin, a staging workup should be performed to rule out distant metastases and to evaluate the pelvic lymph nodes. CT scan of the chest, abdomen, and pelvis will accomplish this goal.
- If iliac or obturator adenopathy is observed, or metastasis to the deep inguinal nodes is established on SLN biopsy, a superficial and deep inguinal node dissection is indicated.
- Some surgeons also advocate the addition of a deep nodal dissection in patients with disease of Cloquet's node (the first node encountered in the femoral canal), three or more positive superficial nodes, or palpable superficial adenopathy.
- If the staging workup demonstrates evidence of stage IV disease, the decision to proceed with a palliative dissection should be based on the extent of both regional and distant disease and systemic therapy options.

Full-Thickness Skin Graft
- The anticipated site of coverage should be measured and an appropriate donor site selected.

PATIENT POSITIONING
Wide Local Excision of Melanoma
- Patient position depends on the location of the melanoma to be excised.
- Patients may need to be supine, prone, or in lateral decubitus position.

Inguinal Lymph Node Dissection
- The patient should be supine with the leg slightly flexed at the knee and externally rotated (frog leg position).
- A Foley catheter is placed.
- The abdominal wall, inguinal region, and proximal thigh are prepped and draped into the surgical field.

Full-Thickness Skin Graft
- Patient position depends on the location of the defect to be covered and the donor site.

PROCEDURE
Wide Local Excision of Melanoma
- If SLN biopsy is to be performed in conjunction with wide excision, the injection of the radionuclide tracer (technetium-99m–tagged colloid sulfur) and subsequent lymphoscintigraphy should take place prior to the patient's arrival in the operating room.
- After the induction of general anesthesia, the site of the melanoma is prepped with alcohol and isosulfan blue dye (Lymphazurin) is injected intradermally in four quadrants around the melanoma (or biopsy scar). The site is massaged for 5 minutes prior to prepping and draping.
- **Figure 28–1A:** The surgical incision should be carefully measured and marked using a ruler and a pen with water-soluble ink.
  - The margins are measured from the periphery of the lesion or the previous biopsy scar, not simply from the center of the scar.
  - An elliptical incision is made to facilitate closure.
  - The long axis should be oriented along the lymphatic drainage to the ipsilateral nodal basin.
  - On the extremities, the apices of the ellipse should be longitudinal with the extremity.
  - The long axis of the ellipse should ideally be 3.5–4 times the width of the excision, although a 3:1 ratio may be acceptable.
- **Figure 28–1B:** The cross-sectional view of the excision demonstrates the 2-cm margins as well as a 0.5-cm subcutaneous beveling of the margin to ensure capture of deep subdermal lymphatic channels.
  - Care is taken to avoid beveling toward the melanoma and compromising the margin.
  - The excision is carried down to the underlying fascia.
  - The fascia does not need to be excised with the specimen.
  - Orientation of the specimen should be indicated for the pathologist to enable designation of close or positive margins.
- Tension-free closure of the resulting defect is facilitated by elevation of the flaps just above the fascia, as much as twice the size of the excised skin margins.
- After assuring meticulous hemostasis, the wound is typically closed with deep dermal absorbable sutures followed by interrupted nylon sutures, typically vertical or horizontal mattress sutures.
- A subcuticular absorbable suture may be used if there is minimal tension.

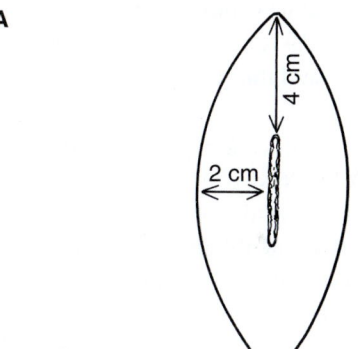

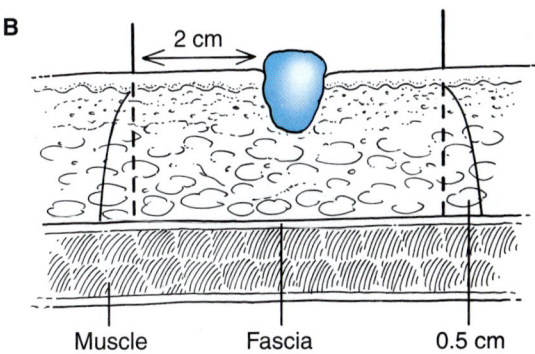

Figure 28–1A–B

- Closed-suction catheter drainage is rarely necessary.
- When the ratio of the length to width is < 3.5:1, excessive tissue ("dog ears") may be apparent. These can be excised using a V-plasty technique.

Inguinal Lymph Node Dissection

- **Figure 28–2A, B:** The classic incision for the inguinal lymph node dissection is the "lazy S" curvilinear incision.
  - This begins 3–4 cm medial to the anterior superior iliac spine, crosses the inguinal crease and then extends distally to the apex of the femoral triangle.
  - If a previous excisional (or SLN) biopsy was performed, the incision should include an ellipse of skin around the previous scar. Likewise, an ellipse of skin should be taken over any palpable adenopathy.
  - It is sometimes desirable to avoid an incision that crosses the inguinal crease. In this case, a dissection may be performed through a curvilinear incision beneath the inguinal crease with or without a second incision above the crease.
- **Figure 28–3:** The important anatomic borders of the superficial dissection include the sartorius muscle (lateral), inguinal ligament (superior), and adductor longus muscle (medial), which together comprise the femoral triangle.
  - There are contiguous superficial nodes superior to the inguinal ligament and this tissue must be included in the dissection.
  - The tissue to be included lies above the external oblique aponeurosis to the level of the umbilicus between the pubic tubercle and the anterior superior iliac spine.
  - If the incision is below the inguinal crease, a sufficient superior flap must be raised to include this tissue.
- **Figure 28–4:** Skin flaps are raised laterally to the sartorius muscle, medially to the adductor longus, and superiorly to the level of the umbilicus.
  - These flaps should not be too thin, as this increases the risk of wound complications.
  - The thickness of the skin flaps should be tapered so they gradually increase toward the base.
- **Figure 28–5:** Dissection of the nodal tissue usually begins with the suprainguinal tissue.
  - The superior boundary of the dissection is divided through the subcutaneous tissue and Scarpa's fascia down to the external oblique aponeurosis.
  - This tissue is dissected inferiorly off the aponeurosis and muscle to the level of the inguinal ligament.
  - The fascia over the medial sartorius is divided (to avoid injury to the lateral femoral cutaneous nerve) and the fibrofatty tissue is raised medially to expose the femoral vessels.
  - Likewise the lateral border of the fascia over the adductor longus is divided and the tissue raised laterally. The saphenous vein is encountered here.

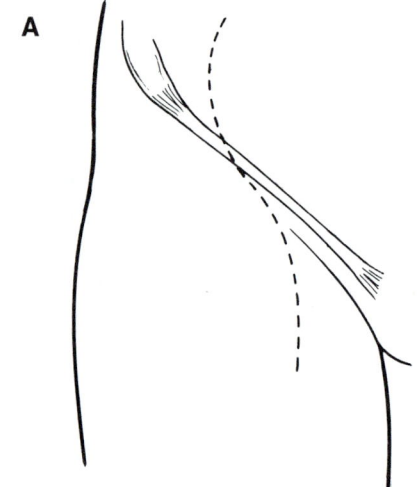

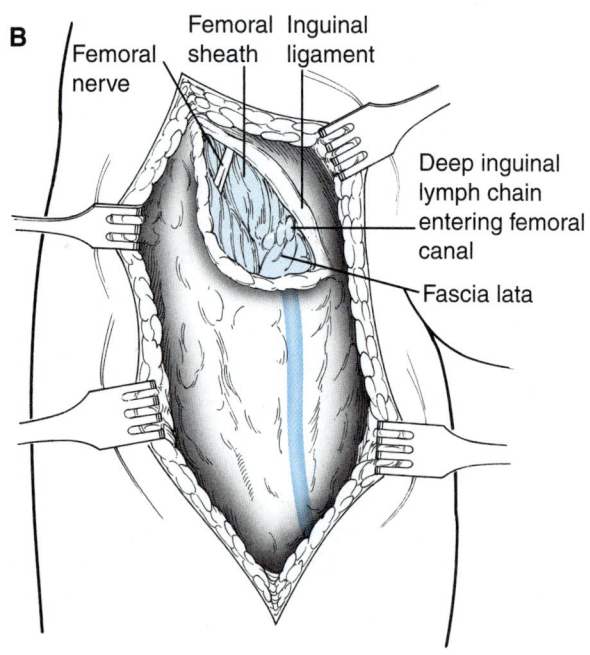

Figure 28–2A–B

Chapter 28 : Operative Management of Melanoma • 233

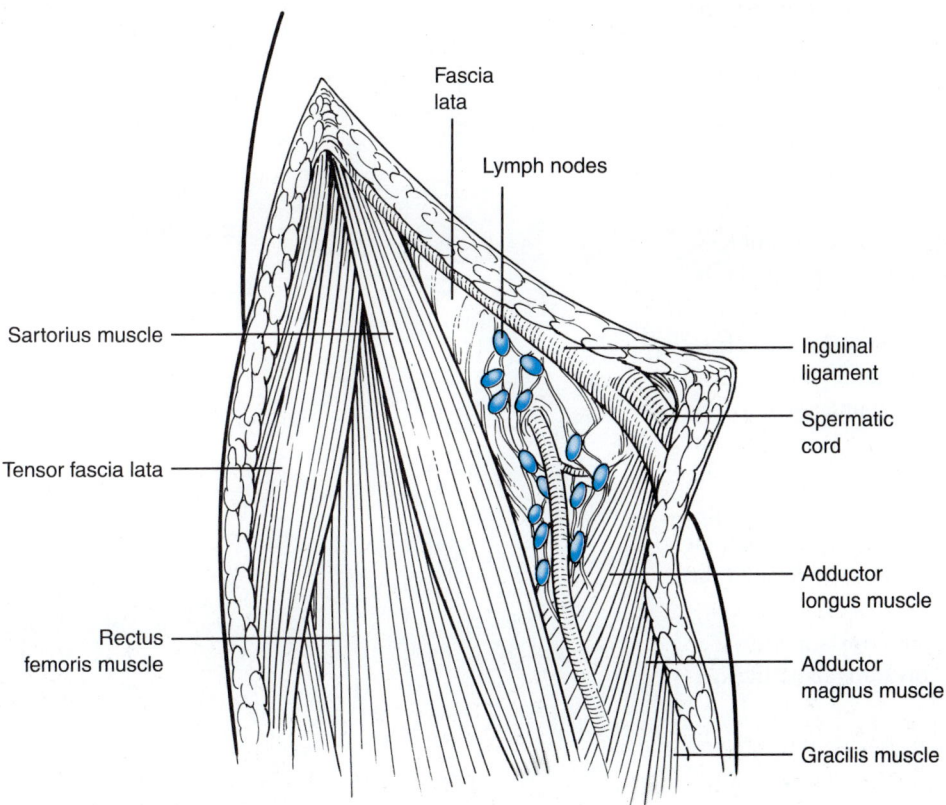

Figure 28-3

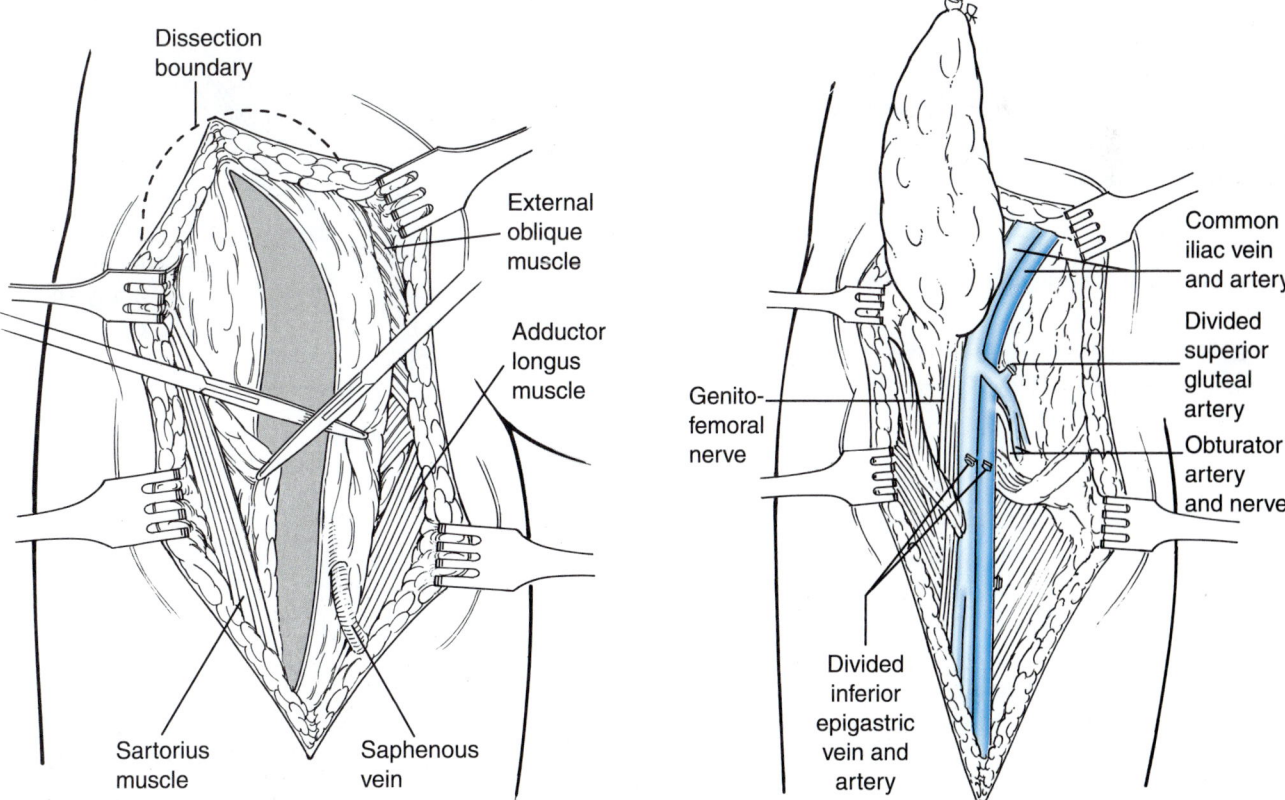

Figure 28-4

Figure 28-5

- Although many surgeons advocate routine sacrifice of the saphenous vein, we only recommend this when there is gross involvement or disease in close proximity to it. If it is to be included, it should be ligated at this point.
- The fibrofatty tissue can then be skeletonized off the femoral vessels from the femoral triangle to the inguinal ligament.
- If the saphenous vein was divided earlier, the saphenofemoral junction is identified and divided. The stump may be closed with a silk suture ligation or a vascular suture.
- The only remaining tissue at this point is the tissue running under the inguinal ligament; this represents the location where Cloquet's node is often encountered. If a deep dissection is not planned, the specimen is divided and Cloquet's node marked for the pathologist with a silk suture.
- If an iliac dissection is to be performed, the deep lymph nodes can be accessed by a separate incision through the external oblique aponeurosis.
  - This incision extends from the anterior superior iliac spine to the external ring, 2 fingerbreadths above the ligament.
  - The external oblique and internal oblique muscles and transversalis fascia are incised to allow for retroperitoneal dissection.
  - Alternatively, the inguinal ligament and external oblique muscle may be divided to allow access to the deep nodes. A vertical incision 3–4 cm medial to the anterior superior iliac spine is made in the external oblique and the inguinal ligament is divided medial to the femoral artery.
- The peritoneum is bluntly dissected and retracted cephalad and medially to expose the iliac vessels.
- The inferior epigastric vessels are ligated to avoid iatrogenic injury.
- Care is taken not to open the peritoneum, and in men care must be taken to avoid injury to the spermatic cord structures.
- **Figure 28–6:** The node-bearing tissue is dissected from the common iliac artery and vein and continued between the internal and external iliac artery.
  - The anterior surface of the external iliac vein is skeletonized down to the level of the inguinal ligament.
  - The ureter is identified as it courses over the iliac artery.
  - The fibrofatty tissue is dissected off the bladder wall. It is necessary to ligate the inferior epigastric vessels a second time at this point.
  - The obturator nerve is identified and the obturator nodes are resected en bloc with the specimen, clearing out the tissue between the nerve and the internal iliac artery.
- A drain may be placed in the pelvis through a separate stab incision.

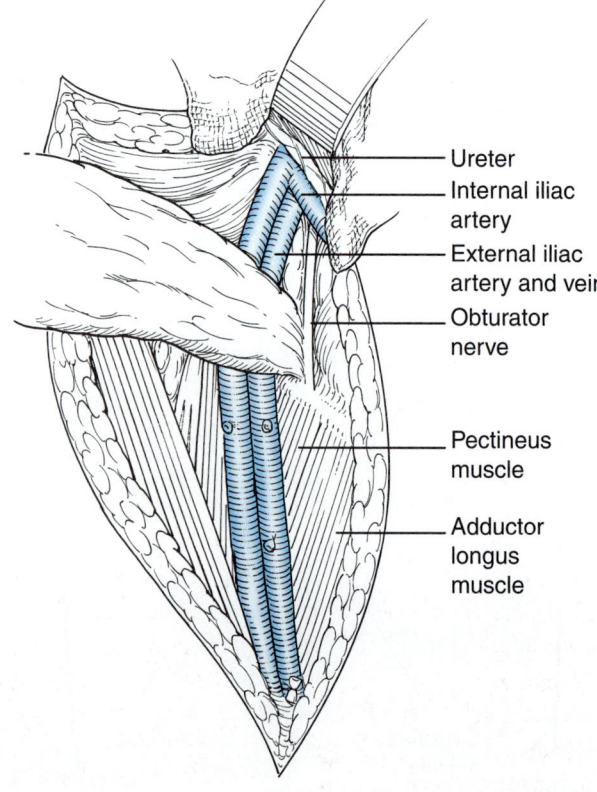

Figure 28–6

- The transversalis and internal and external obliques are reapproximated with nonabsorbable sutures.
- If the inguinal ligament was divided, it may be repaired directly with nonabsorbable suture.
- The defect in the femoral canal is closed by attaching the inguinal ligament to Cooper's ligaments.
- **Figure 28–7A, B:** Coverage of the exposed femoral vessels is achieved by dividing the attachments of the sartorius muscle at its origin (anterior superior iliac spine) and rotating it medially.
  - Be careful to preserve as much of the medial blood supply as possible.
  - The sartorius is secured to the inguinal ligament using absorbable U-type suture.
  - The sartorius is routinely transpositioned when a deep dissection is performed but may be used selectively for a superficial dissection, depending on the thickness and viability of the flaps and exposure of the vessels.
- A superficial drain is placed through a separate stab incision.
- The skin is reapproximated with interrupted absorbable deep dermal sutures followed by nylon sutures, staples, or a running subcuticular stitch.

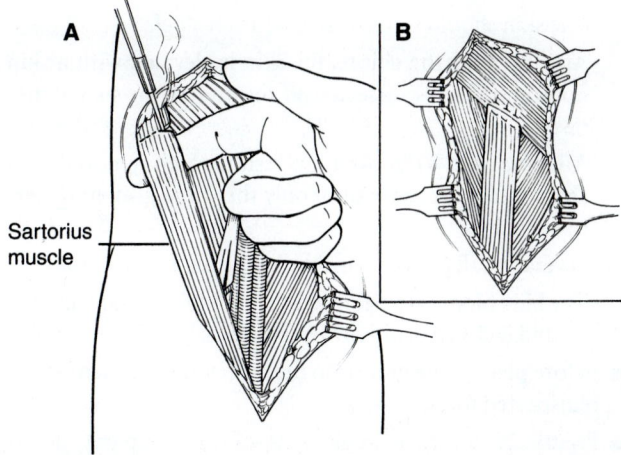

Figure 28–7A–B

Full-Thickness Skin Graft
- It was previously thought that a split-thickness skin graft was preferable for the closure of a defect left by a melanoma resection as it provided a better means for detecting local recurrences. However, it has subsequently been shown that the type of closure has no impact on risk for local recurrence or survival.
- Full-thickness skin grafts give a much better cosmetic result, as they develop a subcutaneous layer beneath the graft resulting in greater mobility. They are also less likely to contract and are more resistant to mechanical wear.
- Most patients undergoing melanoma resection are good candidates for a full-thickness skin graft.
- In patients for whom the margin status after wide excision is in question (particularly the deep margin), it is preferable to use a temporary graft (allograft or bioartificial graft) and defer a permanent skin graft until negative margins are assured.
- In patients for whom a suitable donor site for a full-thickness skin graft cannot be identified, a split-thickness skin graft should be performed.
- Typical donor sites for full-thickness graft harvest include the skin from natural body creases so that the donor site incision is well concealed.
- Thickness, texture, pigmentation and the presence or absence of hair should be matched as closely as possible.
- Outside of the head and neck, the most common melanoma resections that require skin grafting are on the distal extremities.

- When an SLN biopsy is planned in conjunction with a wide local excision, it is often useful to harvest the skin graft from the biopsy site.
  - The SLN biopsy incision is made in an elliptical fashion, large enough to accommodate the wide local excision defect and oriented in such a way that a subsequent lymph node dissection can be easily incorporated if necessary.
  - The skin should be harvested with a scalpel.
  - After incising the ellipse, the skin is elevated with a skin hook and sharply dissected off the underlying subcutaneous fat.
  - After the graft is removed, any residual fat is removed with sharp curved scissors until only the white glistening dermis remains.
  - Several small perforations should be made in the graft.
  - The SLN biopsy is performed through this incision and the wound is closed primarily with the excision of any dog ears.
- Before placing the graft into the defect, the recipient site is reinspected for hemostasis.
- **Figure 28–8:** Once hemostasis of the recipient site is assured, the graft is placed dermal side down and trimmed to fit the defect without excessive wrinkling or stretching.
  - Although many surgeons use staples to secure the graft, we prefer sutures as removal of staples is painful.
  - The graft can be secured with absorbable sutures, which do not need to be removed, or with silk sutures that can then be used to bolster the graft.
  - If absorbable sutures are used, a bolster made from foam rubber molded to the contour of the wound is secured radially around the wound with nonabsorbable sutures or staples.

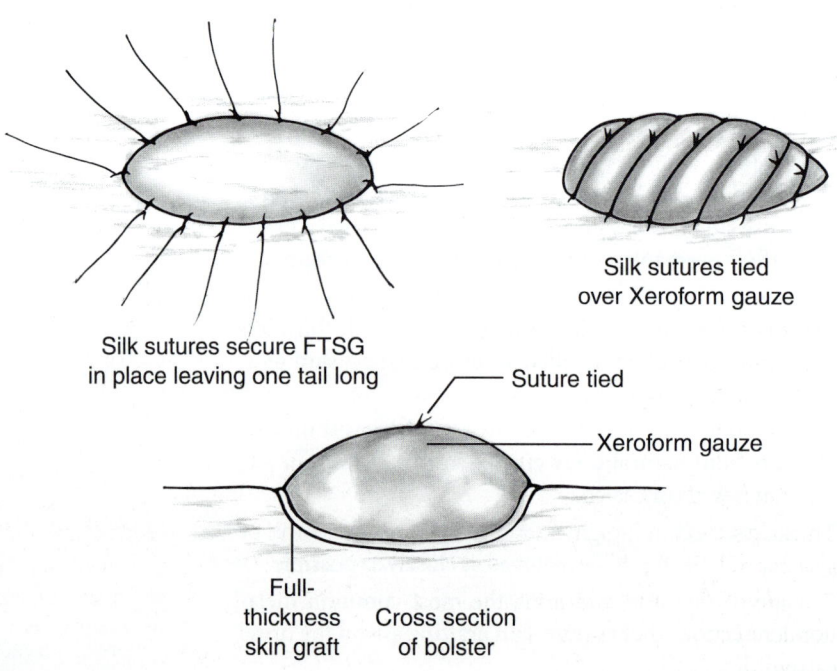

Figure 28–8

- We prefer to secure the graft with silk sutures left long and then tied over a bolster made from Xeroform folded over mineral oil–soaked cotton balls. These bolsters prevent shearing as well as seroma or hematoma formation beneath the graft.
- A splint is typically used to prevent excessive motion and shearing forces that can disrupt graft adherence.

POSTOPERATIVE CARE

Wide Local Excision of Melanoma

- Routine wound care.
- Removal of any external sutures at an interval of 7–14 days postoperatively, depending on wound tension and location (eg, shorter interval for facial sutures).
- Patients should protect the surgical site from excessive sun exposure during the first year to prevent darkening of the scar.

Inguinal Lymph Node Dissection

- Patients are admitted overnight with the Foley catheter left in place and the leg elevated.
- Antibiotics are maintained for 24 hours postoperatively.
- Patients may be discharged the next day.
- If the sartorius was transposed, we prefer to send the patient home with crutches and toe-touch weight bearing only.
- Patients are encouraged to wear compression stockings as soon as possible to minimize lymphedema.
- The drain to bulb suction is continued until output is < 30 mL per 24 hours for 2 consecutive days.
  - The drain should not remain in place longer than 3–4 weeks.
  - It may be better to accept a lymphocele than a wound infection.
- Sutures are removed after 10–14 days.
- Patients are followed closely for infection or other wound complications.

Full-Thickness Skin Graft

- Routine wound care for the donor or SLN biopsy site.
- The bolster is removed approximately 5 days after placement (sooner if there is evidence of bleeding or infection). For a tie-over bolster, after the silk sutures are cut, the bolster is moistened and carefully removed to avoid lifting the graft off the underlying wound bed.
- A nonadherent dressing can be placed over the graft.
- Immobilization, if needed, can be stopped 7–10 days after grafting.
- Any areas of graft loss heal by secondary intention with debridement of any sloughed graft and twice-daily wound care with "wet-to-dry" saline dressings.

POTENTIAL COMPLICATIONS

Wide Local Excision of Melanoma

- Wound infection.
- Need for reexcision if positive margins are encountered on final pathology examination.

Inguinal Lymph Node Dissection

- Wound infection.
- Wound necrosis or dehiscence.
- Hematoma.
- Lymphocele.
- Lymphedema.

Full-Thickness Skin Graft

- Graft failure.
  - The most likely reasons are hematoma beneath the graft, seroma formation, infection, shear forces, technical error, or a poor recipient site.
- Infection or wound separation of the donor site.
  - It is important to verify that enough skin can be harvested without leading to overly tight closure of the donor site.

PEARLS AND TIPS

Wide Local Excision of Melanoma

- Attempt to maintain the surgical scar within the natural creases of the skin for a cosmetically acceptable result.

Inguinal Lymph Node Dissection

- A common mistake while skeletonizing the vessels is to consider the proximal femoral vein as the medial boundary of the dissection. This ignores the medial node-bearing tissue at the level of the femoral canal between the pubic tubercle and vein (Remember NAVEL: nerve, artery, vein, empty space, lymphatics). This fibrofatty tissue should be excised down to the underlying pectineus muscle and included in the dissection. Retraction of the vein laterally with a vein retractor will help.
- If the inguinal ligament is divided, it is helpful to place two long sutures on each side to facilitate reapproximation.
- Wound complications are often secondary to vascular compromise. Prior to closure, trim any flaps that appear too thin (without causing too much tension) and avoid tying skin sutures too tight.

REFERENCES

Sabel MS. Oncology. In Doherty GM, ed. *Current Diagnosis and Treatment: Surgery*. New York, NY: McGraw-Hill; 2010: 1209–1232.

CHAPTER 29

Operative Management of Soft Tissue Sarcoma

Dan G. Blazer, III, MD, and Alfred E. Chang, MD

INDICATIONS

- Any soft tissue mass that is large or growing should be evaluated by biopsy using the techniques described later.
- When the diagnosis of sarcoma is established, surgery remains the mainstay of therapy.

CONTRAINDICATIONS

- Medical comorbidities such as severe cardiopulmonary compromise may preclude safe surgery.

INFORMED CONSENT

Expected Benefits
- Limb preservation for soft tissue sarcomas of the extremity.

Potential Risks
- Major neurovascular structures may need to be sacrificed to achieve oncologic goals, but management strategies designed to preserve these structures are preferable.
- Risk of recurrent disease.

EQUIPMENT

- No special equipment is needed.
- Occasionally, for deep lesions or lesions that have dramatically decreased in size with neoadjuvant therapy, intraoperative ultrasound may be useful to identify the lesion and to plan the incision.
- A self-retaining retractor can assist with exposure.

PATIENT PREPARATION

- Optimal management of soft tissue sarcomas requires a multidisciplinary approach at a high-volume center.
- Input from medical and radiation oncologists experienced in managing this disease is critical.

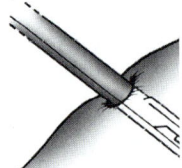
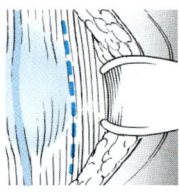
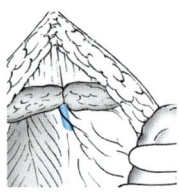
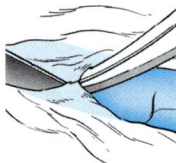
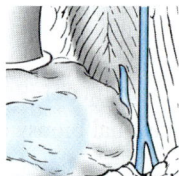
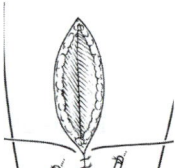

- Biopsy results should be evaluated by pathologists experienced with sarcoma.
- MRI, ultrasound, and CT scanning are all routinely used to evaluate soft tissue sarcomas of the extremity.
- Quite often, patients undergo extensive preoperative radiation therapy and chemotherapy before surgery.
- Plastic surgical assistance for reconstruction can be necessary for wound closure.

PATIENT POSITIONING

- The patient may be placed supine, prone, or in lateral position depending on the location of the lesion.
- If a soft tissue flap reconstruction is planned, communication with the plastic surgery team is essential when positioning the patient.

PROCEDURE

- **Figure 29–1:** Core needle biopsy.
  - For any soft tissue mass that is enlarging, symptomatic, or > 3–5 cm, biopsy should be performed.
  - Core needle biopsy is a reliable method to obtain sufficient material for accurate pathologic diagnosis.
  - Biopsy with ultrasound or CT guidance may be useful.
- **Figure 29–2:** Incisional biopsy and placement of incision for resection.
  - For lesions > 5 cm, incisional biopsy may be appropriate.
  - Proper orientation of the incision is critical.
  - The incision must be in a plane parallel to the long axis of the limb and one that can be subsequently excised by a more definitive surgical procedure, if necessary.
  - Hemostasis is important to avoid development of hematomas that can expand along fascial planes and compromise a more definitive wide excision of the lesion at a later date.
  - Radical resection of soft tissue sarcomas involves careful operative planning.
  - Similar to incisional biopsy principles, the operative incision should be in a plane parallel to the long axis of the limb.
  - The skin incision should be oriented such that any previous biopsy sites are included en bloc with the specimen.

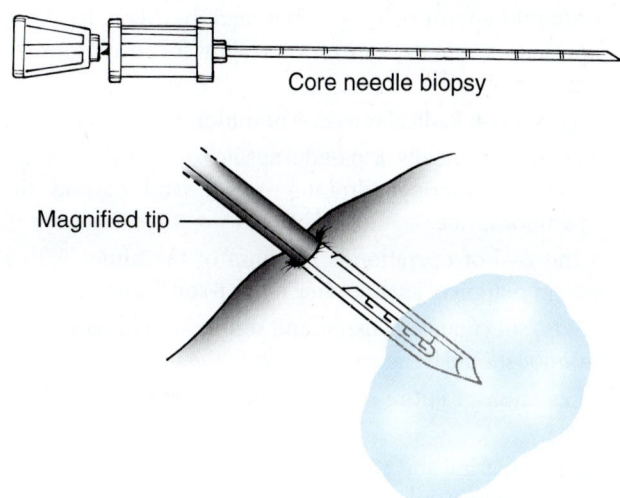

Figure 29–1

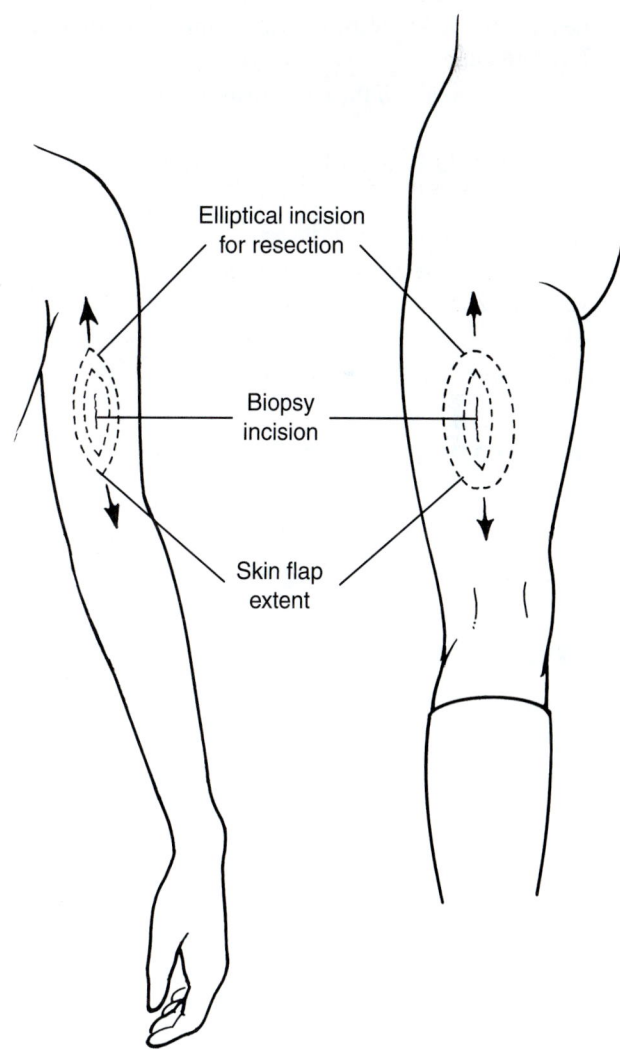

Figure 29–2

- **Figure 29–3:** Skin flaps.
  - After the appropriate incision is made based on the above principles, skin flaps are raised to allow for an appropriate margin of excision.
- **Figure 29–4:** Radical resection of tumor.
  - There is generally a pseudocapsule around the tumor; however, tumor infiltration may extend beyond the pseudocapsule.
  - The goal of operation is resection of the tumor with a 2-cm margin of surrounding normal soft tissue.
  - Skin, subcutaneous tissue, and soft tissue adjacent to the tumor should be taken en bloc with the specimen.
  - Resection of entire muscle compartments is not necessary.
  - Limb-sparing and preservation of limb function are cornerstone principles.
- **Figure 29–5A, B:** Preservation of the neurovascular bundle.
  - In most circumstances, identification and preservation of the neurovascular bundle in an extremity is a key component of the operation and does not compromise the oncologic outcome.
  - Careful dissection of the perineurium from a nerve (Figure 29–5A).
  - Completed dissection with nerve preservation (Figure 29–5B).
- **Figure 29–6:** Closure of the incision.
  - The skin is generally closed with staples or interrupted vertical mattress sutures over closed suction drains.
  - Closed suction drains are generally left in place for a few days to prevent seroma accumulation.

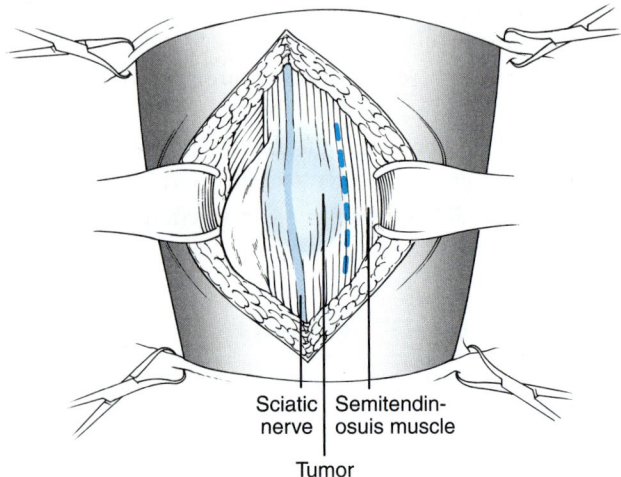

Figure 29–3

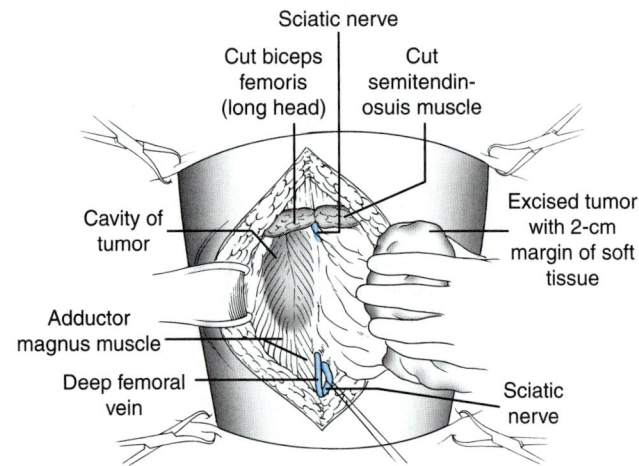

Figure 29–4

POSTOPERATIVE CARE

- Patients are quickly advanced to a regular diet.
- Activity restrictions vary and depend on the location of surgery and type of plastic surgical reconstruction, if any.

POTENTIAL COMPLICATIONS

- Common complications include surgical site infection, hematoma, seroma, and wound breakdown (especially in previously irradiated tissue).
- Sarcomas may lie in proximity to major neurovascular structures that may be inadvertently damaged or taken purposefully en bloc with the specimen.
- Other systemic complications of major surgery (pneumonia, venous thromboembolism, and cardiovascular events) can also occur.

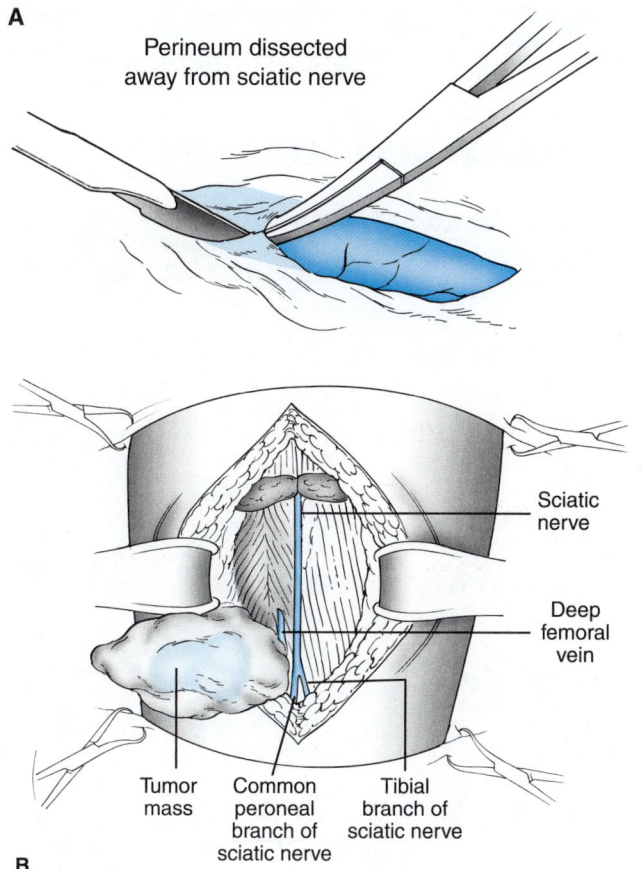

Figure 29–5A–B

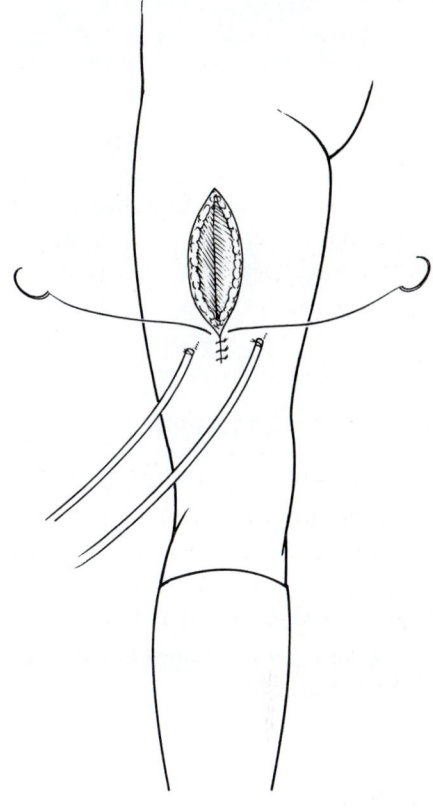

Figure 29–6

PEARLS AND TIPS

- A multimodality treatment approach is the rule.
- Soft tissue sarcomas are rare and should be referred to high-volume centers with the expertise necessary to properly manage this disease.
- In addition to surgical expertise, proper management requires input from medical oncology, radiation oncology, pathology, and radiology services.

REFERENCES

Brennan MF, Lewis JJ. *Diagnosis and Management of Soft Tissue Sarcoma.* London: Martin Dunitz; 2002.

Delman KA, Cormier JN. Soft-Tissue and Bone Sarcoma. In: Feig B, Berger D, Fuhrman G, eds. *The MD Anderson Surgical Oncology Handbook,* 4th ed. Philadelphia, PA: Lippincott Williams & Wilkins; 2006:121–144.

Pollock RE. *Soft Tissue Sarcomas.* Hamilton, ON: BC Decker; 2002.

CHAPTER 30

Renal Transplantation

Constance M. Mobley, MD, PhD, and Shawn J. Pelletier, MD

INDICATIONS

Donor Nephrectomy
- Appropriate volunteer to donate to a person with renal failure.

Renal Transplantation
- All causes of impending or established end-stage renal disease.

CONTRAINDICATIONS

Donor Nephrectomy

A. ABSOLUTE
- Impaired renal function (generally considered to be a glomerular filtration rate < 80 mL/min per 1.73 m^2).
- Active infection.
- Diabetes.
- Pregnancy.
- Age younger than 18 years.
- Poorly controlled psychosis.

B. RELATIVE (OPEN OR LAPAROSCOPIC)
- Proteinuria or hematuria.
- History of malignancy.
- Kidney stones.
- Disorder requiring anticoagulation.
- Active substance abuse.
- Cardiovascular disease.
- Chronic illness.
- Hypertension.
- Abnormal urologic anatomy.
- Family history of diabetes.
- History of kidney stones.
- Obesity.

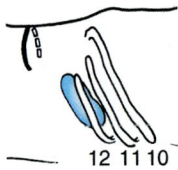
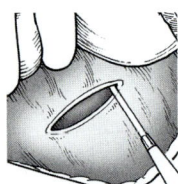
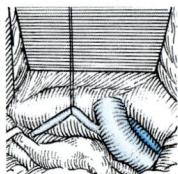
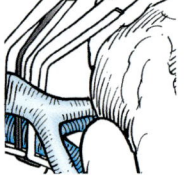
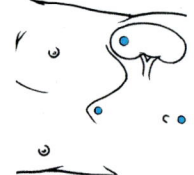
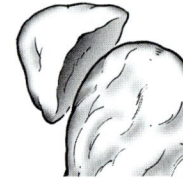
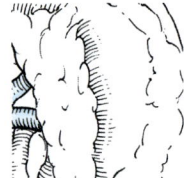
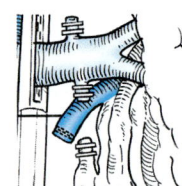
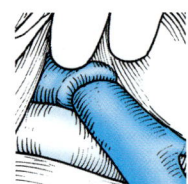

C. Relative (Laparoscopic)
- Previous laparotomies.
- History of pyelonephritis.
- Horseshoe kidney.
- Short right renal vein.
- Multiple renal arteries.

Renal Transplantation
A. Absolute
- Untreated ongoing infection.
- Active malignancy with short life expectancy.
- Chronic illness (with life expectancy < 1 year).
- Poorly controlled psychosis.

B. Relative
- Cardiovascular disease.
- Infection.
- Active substance abuse.
- Cerebrovascular disease.
- Obesity.
- Proven habitual noncompliance with medical recommendations.

INFORMED CONSENT
Donor Nephrectomy
- This procedure is unique in that it involves operating on a patient who has no chance for medical benefit from surgical intervention. For this reason, an extensive psychosocial evaluation is required prior to surgery.
- The motivation of the volunteer must be established as genuinely altruistic and the patient must be aware that he or she can opt out at any time.
- Postoperative pain, transient urinary retention, and superficial surgical site infections are common minor complications.
- Compared with an open approach, laparoscopic donor nephrectomy is associated with a quicker convalescence.
- Operative mortality and major complications are infrequent, but not nonexistent.
  - Major complications include systemic complications of major surgery (pulmonary emboli, cardiovascular events, pneumonia, sepsis, infection, and bleeding).
  - Other risks include pancreatitis; injury to bowel, spleen, or adrenal gland; small bowel obstruction; and conversion to an open procedure when a laparoscopic approach is planned.
- Importantly, there is no increased risk of renal failure after donor nephrectomy.

Renal Transplantation
A. Expected Benefits
- For most patients with end-stage renal disease, renal transplantation is superior to dialysis in terms of long-term mortality risk. Therefore, candidates commonly undergo transplantation once a suitable donor is identified and appropriately allocated.

B. Potential Risks
- Systemic complications associated with any major surgery (cardiovascular events, pneumonia, pulmonary emboli, and venous thromboemboli).
- Other operative risks include:
  - Acute rejection.
  - Arterial or venous thrombosis.
  - Post-transplantation renal dysfunction.
  - Urine leaks.
  - Ureteral obstruction.
  - Wound infection.
  - Abscess.
  - Seroma.
  - Allograft fracture.
  - Lymphocele and hemorrhage.
- Late complications include:
  - Acute or chronic rejection episodes.
  - Renal artery stenosis.
  - Infection.
  - Malignancy.

EQUIPMENT
Donor Nephrectomy
A. Open Nephrectomy
- No special equipment is required.

B. Laparoscopic Transperitoneal Donor Nephrectomy
- Laparoscope with 30-degree lens.
- Standard laparoscopic surgical instruments.
- Standard open vascular surgical instruments.

Renal Transplantation
- No special equipment is required.
- A self-retaining retractor allows the procedure to be performed by the surgeon and one assistant.

PATIENT PREPARATION

Donor Nephrectomy

- Comprehensive evaluation of potential donors is essential to establish donor suitability. This entails thorough assessment of the donor's physical and psychological condition and confirmation of normal kidney function prior to surgery.
- The first steps in the initial screening process include:
  - Brief history and physical examination to rule out medical conditions that would preclude donation.
  - ABO determination.
  - Cross-matching.
- The subsequent complete evaluation should include:
  - Psychosocial history.
  - Chest radiograph.
  - Electrocardiogram.
  - Urinalysis.
  - Comprehensive blood work.
- Laboratory screening should include:
  - Complete blood count.
  - Chemistry panel.
  - Liver function tests.
  - Creatinine clearance.
  - Serology for hepatitis B and C, HIV, cytomegalovirus, and Epstein-Barr virus.
  - Rapid plasma reagin (RPR) or VDRL tests.
  - Possibly glucose tolerance test (for diabetic families).
- As a final step, the renal anatomy of the donor is defined to determine which kidney will be removed and to rule out any anatomic abnormalities.
  - In general, the left kidney is easier to remove and transplant than the right kidney because of the longer length of the renal vein.
  - Evaluation of the renal anatomy can be done with an intravenous pyelogram and renal arteriogram in combination, or with a CT angiogram alone.

Renal Transplantation

- Extensive pretransplantation assessment focuses on evaluating the recipient's cardiovascular status, excluding malignancies and infections that would contraindicate transplantation, and clearly defining the renal disease.
- Initial routine screening laboratory tests include:
  - Complete blood count.
  - Chemistry panel.
  - Coagulation assays.
  - Liver function tests.
  - ABO blood typing.
  - HLA tissue typing.
  - Standard panel reactive antibody (PRA) testing.
- Virology screening tests for cytomegalovirus, HIV, Epstein-Barr virus, and hepatitis B and C and the tuberculum skin test are routinely ordered.
- An ECG in conjunction with a pharmacologic or exercise stress test is obtained to evaluate cardiovascular status (particularly in diabetic patients).
- Patients with ischemic heart disease should undergo angiography or a revascularization procedure as deemed appropriate with follow-up angiograms or stress tests repeated within 1 year of the actual transplantation.
- A baseline chest radiograph should be obtained.
- Screening colonoscopy, mammography, and Pap smear should be performed as indicated by standard guidelines.
- A complete genitourinary workup is probably only necessary for patients with recurrent infections, bladder dysfunction, or congenital abnormalities as the cause of renal failure. For these patients, urodynamics and a voiding cystourethrogram are indicated.
  - Some centers advise that all patients undergo screening renal ultrasonography prior to transplantation.
- Vaccination status of the recipient should be reviewed and influenza, hepatitis B, and pneumococcus vaccinations administered as necessary.
- Once an organ is procured for the recipient, the immediate preoperative care includes:
  - Urinalysis.
  - Coagulation assay.
  - Complete blood count.
  - Comprehensive metabolic panel.
  - Type and screen.
  - Repeat chest radiograph.
  - Electrocardiogram.
- If needed, arrangements for dialysis should be made, especially if potassium levels are elevated.
  - There is no consensus for induction therapy after renal transplantation.
  - Typical regimens use a combination of three or four drugs (corticosteroids, cyclosporine or tacrolimus, mycophenolate, and antibodies).

PATIENT POSITIONING

Donor Nephrectomy

- **Figure 30–1:** The patient should be in the right lateral decubitus position (for left nephrectomy) and carefully padded.

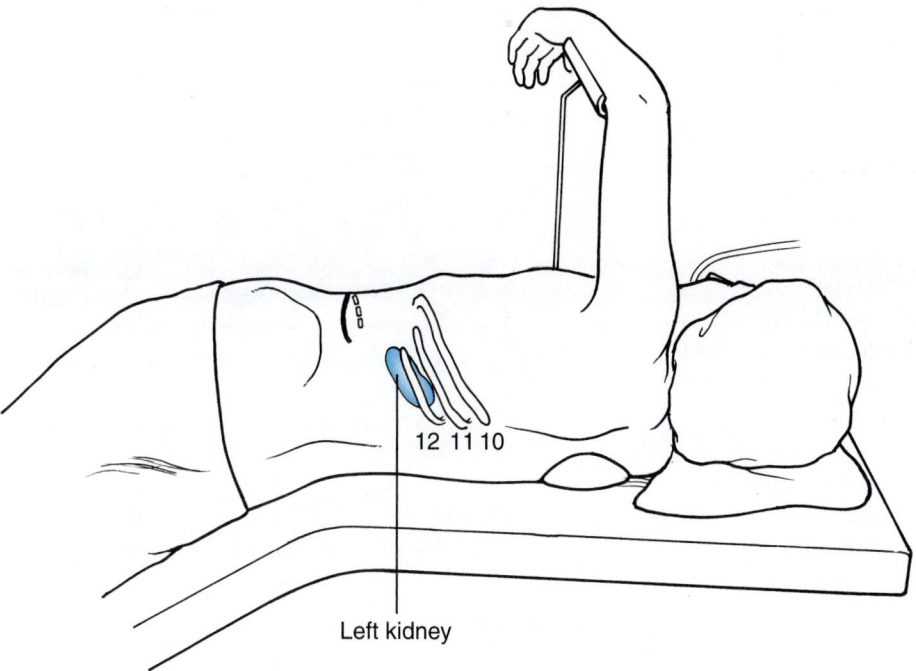

Figure 30–1

- The operating table is flexed to extend the left flank and maximize exposure.
- For open procedures, an oblique incision is made from a point just lateral to the lateral border of the rectus abdominus muscle and continued below the 12th rib to the paraspinous muscles posteriorly.

Renal Transplantation

- The patient should be supine on the operating table (for orientation see Figure 30–9, later).
- The abdomen is prepared and draped in standard sterile surgical fashion.
- A curvilinear incision is made in the left lower quadrant extending from 1 cm above the pubic symphysis to 2–4 cm lateral to the anterior superior iliac spine.

PROCEDURE

Open Donor Nephrectomy

- **Figure 30–2:** Extraperitoneal exposure of the kidney is achieved by first dividing the muscle with electrocautery and then mobilizing the peritoneum medially.
- Gerota's fascia is incised longitudinally and the kidney is mobilized using electrocautery and sharp dissection.

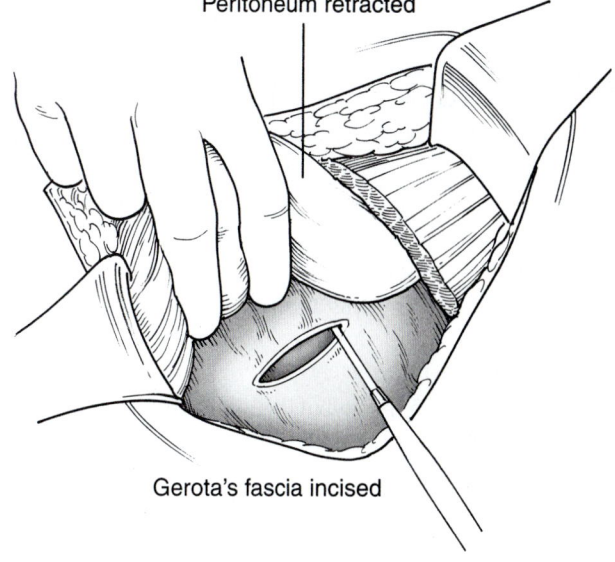

Figure 30–2

- **Figure 30–3:** The renal vessels and ureter are dissected free from surrounding tissues along a plane as close as possible to the aorta and below the adrenal and gonadal venous branches.
  - The gonadal, adrenal, and any lumbar veins are ligated and divided during the dissection as required.
  - The ureter is mobilized distally to the common iliac artery, ligated, and divided.
  - After transection of the ureter, diuresis is confirmed.
- After the renal hilum is completely dissected, the patient receives mannitol and furosemide to aid in diuresis. Arterial vasospasm is treated with a topical solution of papaverine (30 mg/mL).
- **Figure 30–4:** Once adequate lengths of renal artery and vein have been mobilized, a vascular clamp is placed on the renal artery, a Satinsky clamp is placed on the left renal vein below the gonadal and adrenal branches, and the vessels are transected. The renal vessels are doubly ligated or oversewn.
- The kidney is delivered from the operative field and immersed in ice-cold saline.
- The vein is opened and the kidney is immediately perfused with cold kidney preservation solution through the renal artery or arteries. Perfusion is complete once the entire kidney blanches (usually after perfusion of 200–300 mL of solution).
- The kidney is packaged for transport to the recipient operating room. The incision is closed in layers with absorbable sutures. If needed, a chest radiograph is obtained in the recovery room to evaluate for a pneumothorax.

Laparoscopic Transperitoneal Donor Nephrectomy

- **Figure 30–5A, B:** A small midline incision is made and a pneumoperitoneum is established. Once the operative field is expanded, the scope is inserted and additional ports are placed under direct visualization.
  - Typically, four ports are placed in the abdomen and the kidney is ultimately extracted through a 6–8-cm incision.
  - The small intestines and omentum are allowed to fall into the contralateral half of the abdominal cavity.
  - Alternatively, a hand port may be used. A minilaparotomy is made at the umbilicus and 10-mm and 12-mm trocars are placed below the left costal margin and in the left lateral abdomen, respectively.
- **Figure 30–6:** Mobilization of the colon is achieved by incising the lateral peritoneal reflection and dissecting along the line of Toldt from the splenic flexure to the level of the iliac vessels. The colorenal and splenorenal ligaments are divided.
- **Figure 30–7:** Retraction of the colon and its mesentery allows visualization of the renal hilum.

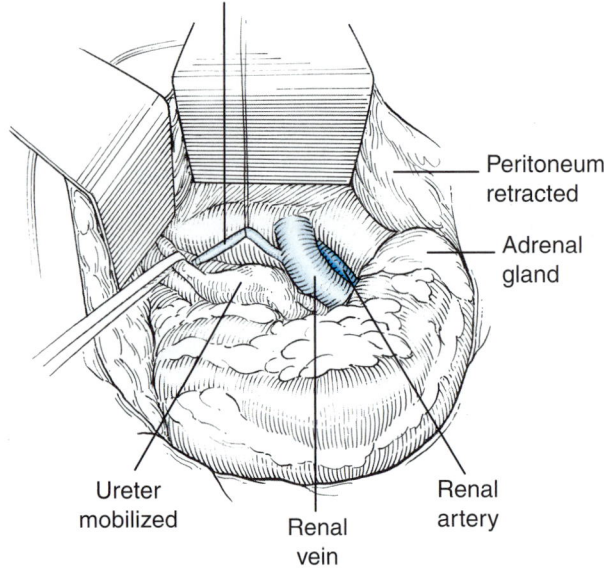

Figure 30–3

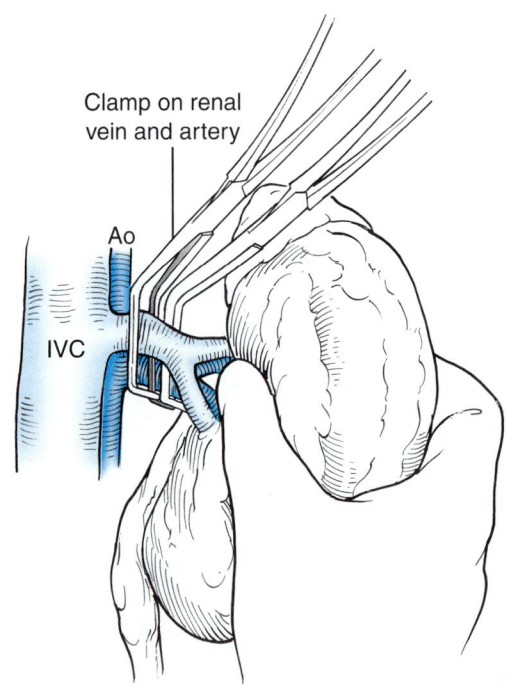

Figure 30–4

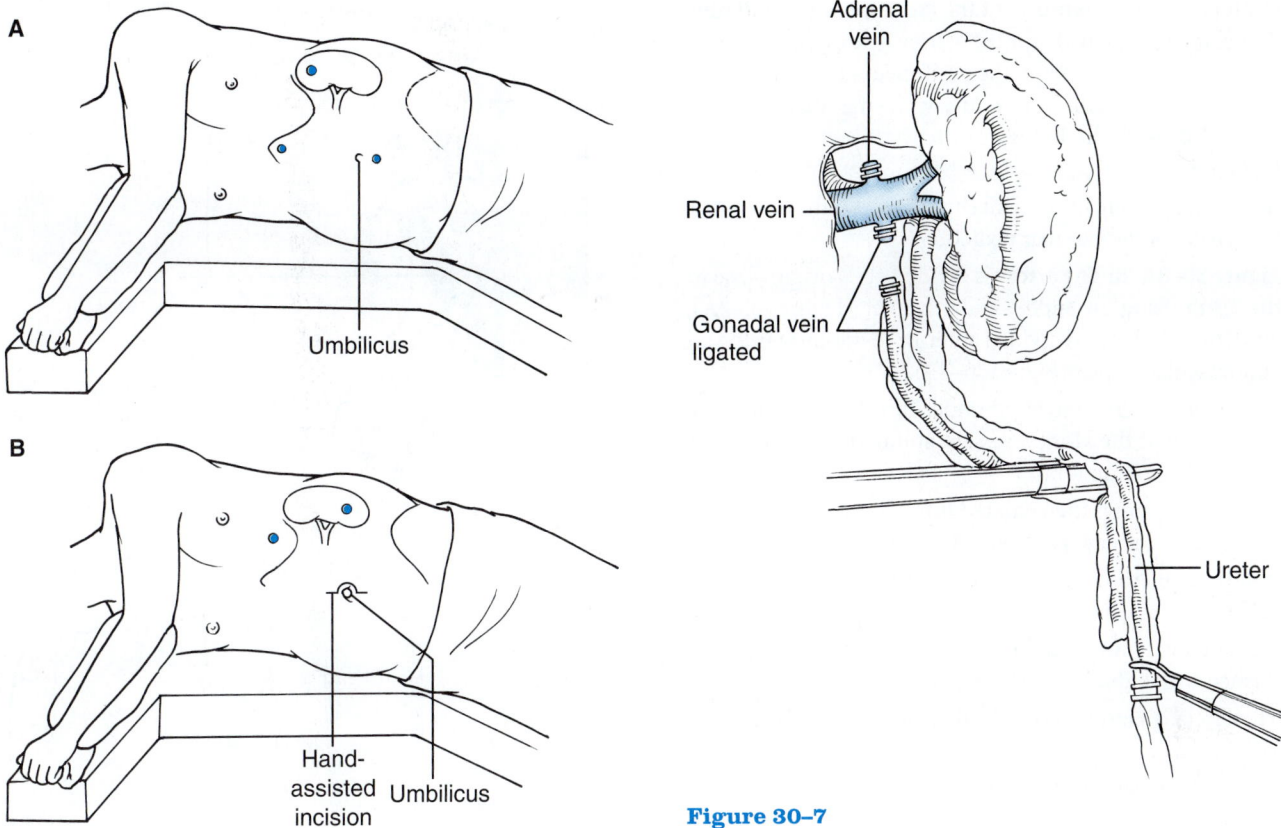

Figure 30–5A–B

Figure 30–7

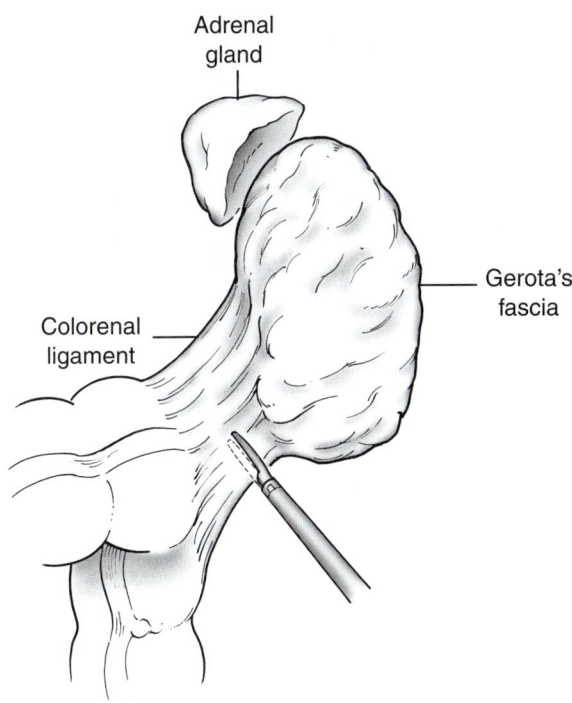

Figure 30–6

- The gonadal, adrenal, and lumbar veins are identified, clipped, and divided during the dissection.
- After the renal hilum is completely dissected, the patient receives mannitol and furosemide to aid in diuresis.
- Elevation of the lower pole of the kidney allows identification of the ureter.
- The ureter is dissected free to the level of the iliac bifurcation.
- Dissection proceeds from the renal hilum caudally along a plane medial to the gonadal vein in order to preserve the ureteral blood supply.
- The distal ureter is clipped at the level of the iliac vessels and divided.
- The renal vein is dissected medially away from surrounding tissues.
- The renal artery, which lies posterior to the vein, is identified.
- The renal artery is dissected medially to a point as close to the aorta as possible.
- Arterial vasospasm is treated with a topical solution of papaverine (30 mg/mL).

- In preparation for removal of the kidney, a 6–8-cm Pfannenstiel incision is made for the retrieval device and carried down to, but not through, the peritoneum to maintain the pneumoperitoneum. Alternatively, if the hand-assisted method is used, the kidney can be retrieved through the hand port.
- If heparin is given, the patient should receive the dose prior to division of the vascular pedicle.
- **Figure 30–8A, B:** The artery is divided at its origin close to the aorta using an endovascular stapler (Figure 30–8A). Next, the renal vein is divided anterior to the aorta using an endovascular stapler (Figure 30–8B).
- The kidney is then retrieved under direct vision with care to ensure that the kidney, vessels, and ureter are not damaged during extraction.
- The peritoneum is then entered through the previous incision and the kidney is delivered from the abdomen.
- If anticoagulation was used, it is reversed with protamine sulfate.
- The kidney is immersed in ice-cold saline and immediately flushed with kidney preservation solution.
- The fascia is closed and a pneumoperitoneum is reestablished.
- The field is carefully inspected for hemostasis.
- The instruments are removed and the port sites and abdominal incisions are closed.

Renal Transplantation

- **Figure 30–9:** Following patient positioning, as outlined earlier, the incision is carried down through the subcutaneous tissue and fascia with care taken not to enter the peritoneum.

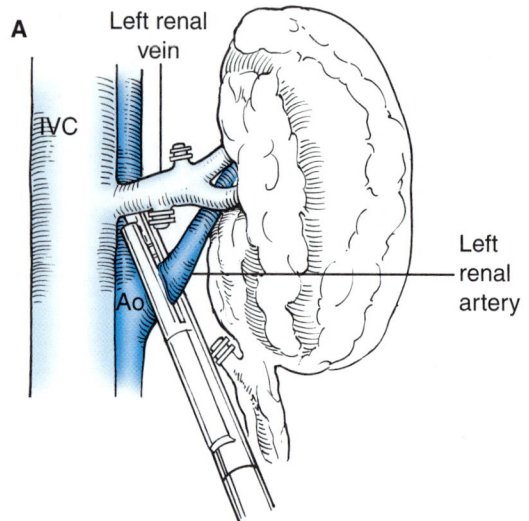
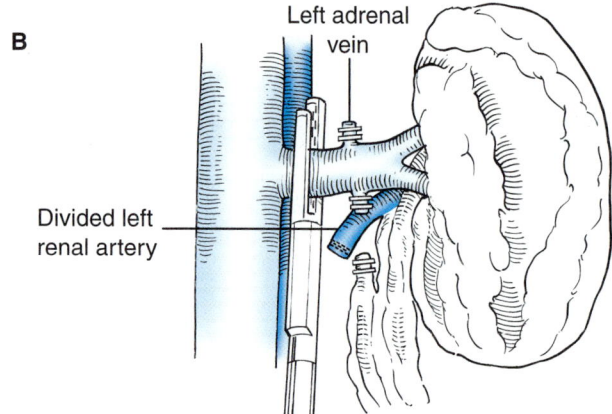

Figure 30–8A–B

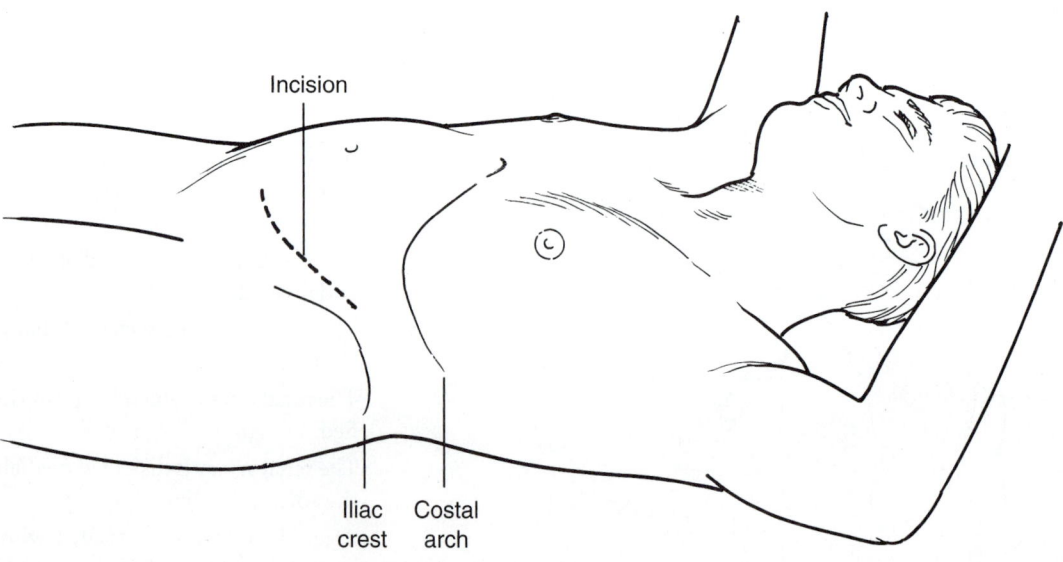

Figure 30–9

- The contents of the peritoneum are retracted medially to expose the retroperitoneum.
- **Figure 30–10:** The retroperitoneum is entered and the external iliac artery and vein are mobilized free from surrounding connective tissue, taking care to ligate all lymphatics to prevent lymphocele formation.
  - In men, the spermatic cord is secured with a vessel loop and retracted away from the operative field.
  - In women, the round ligament is identified, ligated, and divided.
- **Figure 30–11:** Once the external iliac artery and vein are completely skeletonized, the donor kidney is brought into the operative field.
  - The iliac vein is occluded with a single Satinsky clamp.
  - An appropriately sized venotomy is made and the renal vein is anastomosed to the external iliac vein in an end-to-side fashion.
- **Figure 30–12:** Typically the external iliac artery is anastomosed to the renal artery in an end-to-side fashion.
- The external iliac artery is clamped proximally and distally, and an arteriotomy is made on the anterolateral aspect of the artery.

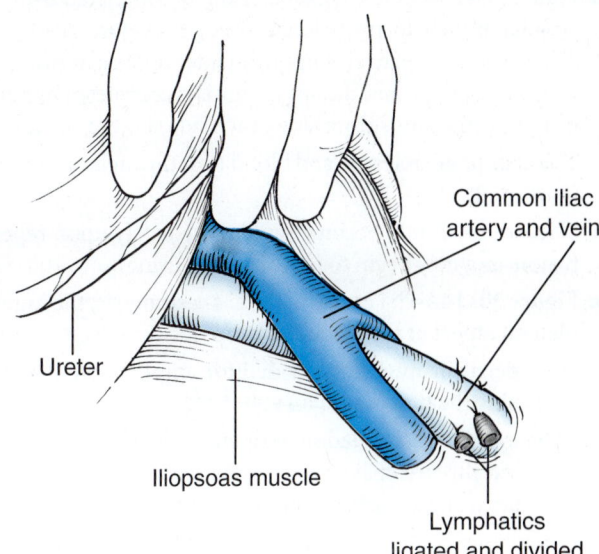

Figure 30–10

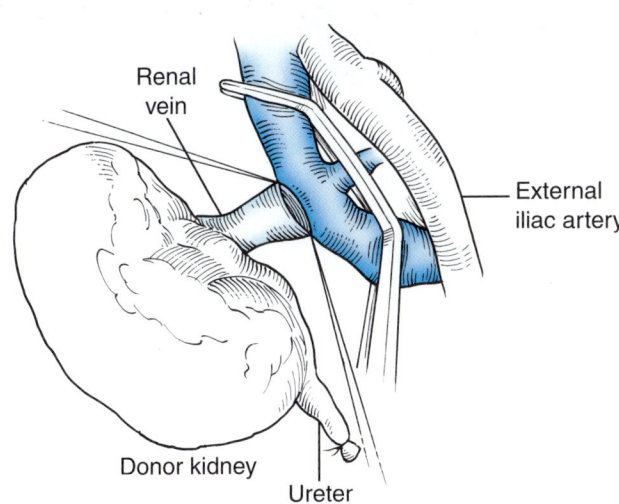

Figure 30–11

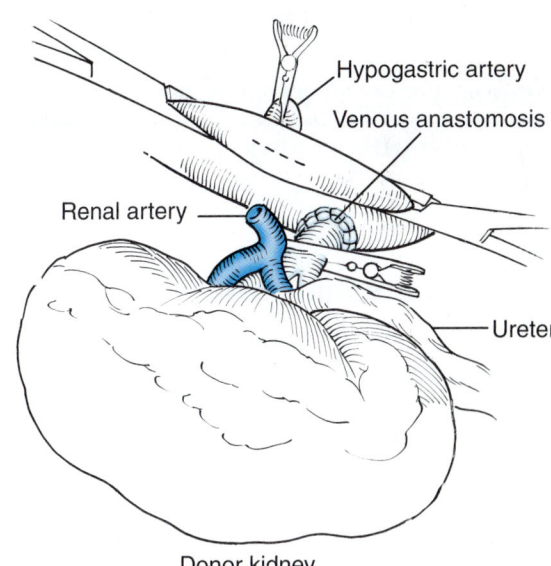

Figure 30–12

- **Figure 30–13A-C:** The small incision is completed using a circular punch to provide clean edges (Figure 30–13A). Two sutures are placed at opposite sides of the arteriotomy (Figure 30–13B), and the anastomosis is completed by running a continuous suture along each side (Figure 30–13C).
- The clamps are released and blood flow through the vessels is assessed.
- The kidney should become pink immediately upon reperfusion, and may begin to produce clear urine.
- **Figure 30–14A-C:** For the ureteral anastomosis, the anterolateral aspect of the bladder is exposed.
  - The detrusor muscle is divided for approximately 3 cm, exposing the mucosa (Figure 30–14A).
  - The mucosa of the bladder is opened for approximately 1 cm and the ureter is anastomosed to the mucosa of the bladder using absorbable suture (Figure 30–14B).
  - Interrupted sutures are used to close the muscle layer of the bladder over the distal portion of the ureter to limit reflux (Figure 30–14C).
  - Hemostasis is achieved, and the condition of the kidney is noted prior to closing.
- The abdominal wound is irrigated and closed in layers.
- Ureteral stents can be used if there is concern for the integrity of the bladder and the ureter.
- Alternative methods for reimplantation of the ureter include ureteroureterostomy over a double JJ stent, extravesical single-stitch (U-stitch) technique, and Politano-Leadbetter transvesical ureteroneocystostomy.

POSTOPERATIVE CARE

Donor Nephrectomy
- Analgesia.
- Oral intake when tolerated.

Renal Transplantation
- Appropriate immunosuppression.
- Fluid management should be adequate to ensure good diuresis without fluid overloading. Hourly urine output should be replaced with 0.45% normal saline at 1.0 mL saline per milliliter urine.
- Monitoring of electrolytes.
- Nothing by mouth.
- Await resolution of ileus.
- Kayexalate should not be given as this may cause colonic necrosis.

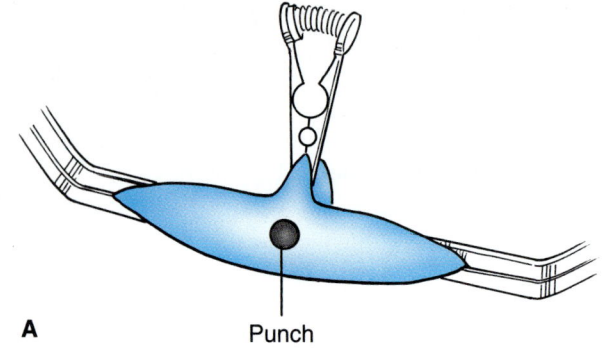

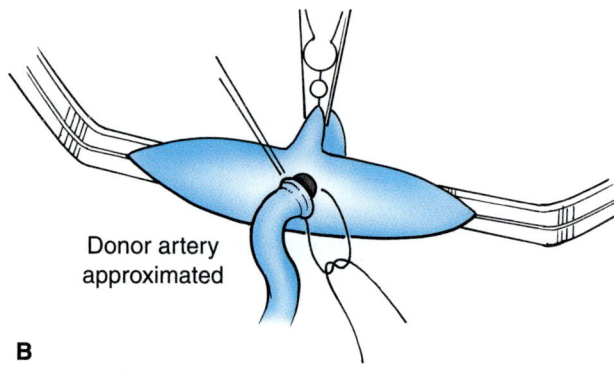

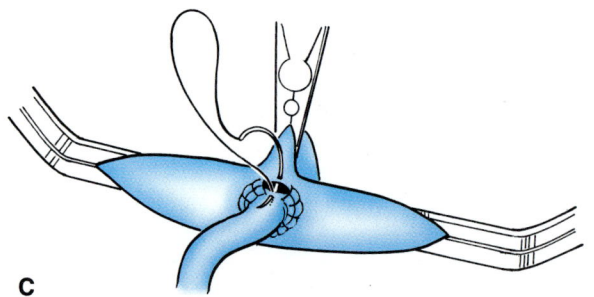

Figure 30–13A–C

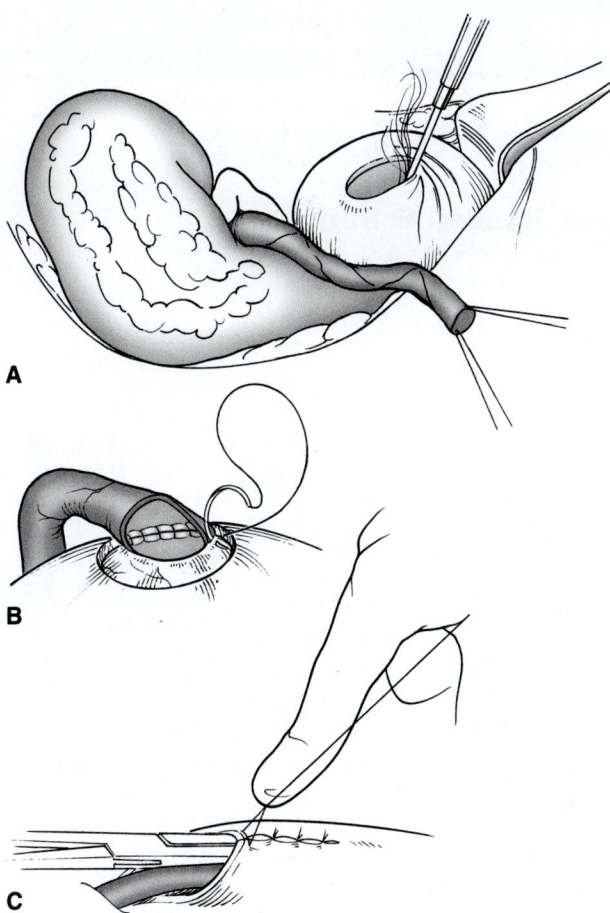

Figure 30–14A–C

POTENTIAL COMPLICATIONS

Donor Nephrectomy
- Pneumothorax.
- Infection.
- Bleeding.

Renal Transplantation
- Urinary obstruction.
- Arterial or venous thrombosis.
- Infection.
- Ureteral anastomotic leak.
- Bleeding.

PEARLS AND TIPS

Donor Nephrectomy
- Mobilizing the ureter before extensive dissection of the vessels allows quicker removal of the kidney if bleeding is encountered.
- Small accessory arteries to the superior pole can be sacrificed with minimal deleterious effect. However, small accessory arteries to the inferior pole may supply the ureter and need to be preserved or reconstructed.
- The right renal vein is thin and delicate and must be handled carefully.
- Staple the renal artery with an endovascular stapler. Clips, including locking clips, are more likely to fall off (laparoscopic donor nephrectomy).
- A hand port allows manual compression and control of bleeding and may increase safety of the laparoscopic approach (laparoscopic donor nephrectomy).

Renal Transplantation
- In type 1 diabetic patients, consider placing the kidney on the left to enable a future pancreatic transplantation procedure on the right side.
- Keeping the dissection extraperitoneal aids exposure by sequestering the bowel out of the surgical field and keeping the kidney in a smaller compartment, which helps to prevent intraperitoneal bleeding.

REFERENCES

Fabrizio, MD, Ratner, LE, Montgomery, RA, Kavoussi LR. Laparoscopic live donor nephrectomy. *Urol Clin North Am.* 1999;26:247–256.

Kasiske BL, Cangro CB, Harihan S, et al. The evaluation of renal transplant candidates: clinical practice guidelines. *Am J Transplantation.* 2001;1(Suppl 2):7–95.

Ratner LE, Ciseck LJ, Moore RG, et al. Laparoscopic live donor nephrectomy. *Transplantation.* 1995;60:1047–1049.

CHAPTER 31

Pancreas Transplantation

Raymond J. Lynch, MD, and Randall S. Sung, MD

INDICATIONS

- May be performed in diabetic patients with end-stage renal disease either as simultaneous pancreas-kidney (SPK) transplantation, or as pancreas-after-kidney (PAK) transplantation.
  - Pancreas transplantation has minimal impact on immunosuppression.
- Nonuremic patients with type 1 diabetes usually receive pancreas transplantation alone (PTA).
  - Risk of immunosuppression is added to the surgical risk.

CONTRAINDICATIONS

Absolute

- Untreated or recent malignancy.
- Active or chronic infection.
- Inability to comply with postoperative immunosuppression and follow-up.

Relative

- Advanced extrarenal complications of diabetes (coronary artery disease).
- Evidence of insulin resistance (type 2 diabetes, insulin requirements > 1 unit/kg, BMI > 30).

INFORMED CONSENT

Expected Benefits

- Improved quality of life.
  - Provides optimum glucose control.
  - Improves or minimizes complications of diabetes.
  - Reverses early diabetic nephropathy in both native and graft kidneys.
  - Results in euglycemia without hypoglycemia.
  - Conveys a survival benefit for type 1 diabetic patients with end-stage renal disease.
- 5-year graft survival is 57–71%.

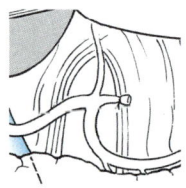
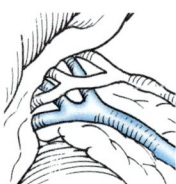
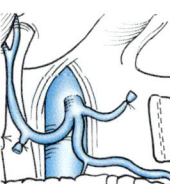
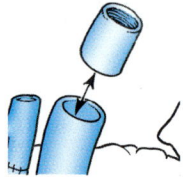
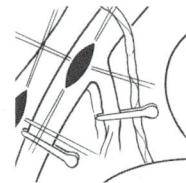
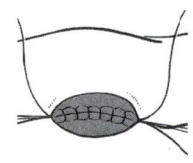
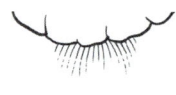
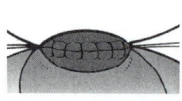
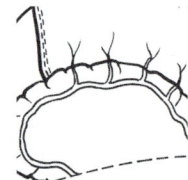

Potential Risks
- Inherent risks of postoperative immunosuppression.
- Venous thrombosis (affects 3–5% of grafts in the first 24–48 hours).
- Complications of exocrine drainage:
  - Cystitis and balanitis in bladder-drained grafts.
  - Abscess or leak in enteric drainage.
- Bleeding.
- Pancreatitis.

EQUIPMENT
- Sterile ice for back-table preparation and surface cooling of the graft.
- Fixed retractor for optimal exposure.

PATIENT PREPARATION
Donor
- Freedom from malignancy and infectious disease.
- Donor age, mechanism of death, medical history, and perimortem hyperglycemia or hyperamylasemia affect suitability of the pancreatic graft.
- Inspection at the time of donation.

Recipient
- Eligibility is based on utility of a pancreatic graft as well as individual fitness for operation, with emphasis given to preoperative weight loss as necessary.
- Preoperative evaluation is directed toward identification and treatment of diabetic complications, most importantly coronary artery disease, and includes:
  - Stratified cardiac evaluation (all recipients).
  - Assessment for coexistent pulmonary vascular obstructive disease in the absence of a femoral pulse.
  - Investigation of aortoiliac occlusive disease with noninvasive flow studies, MR angiogram, CT angiogram, or standard angiography.
- Preoperative preparation includes placement of arterial and central venous lines, nasogastric tube, and Foley catheter, as well as sequential compression devices. Patients should also receive preoperative antibiotic prophylaxis.

PATIENT POSITIONING
- For both donor and recipient procedures:
  - The patient should be supine.
  - The abdomen is entered through a midline incision.

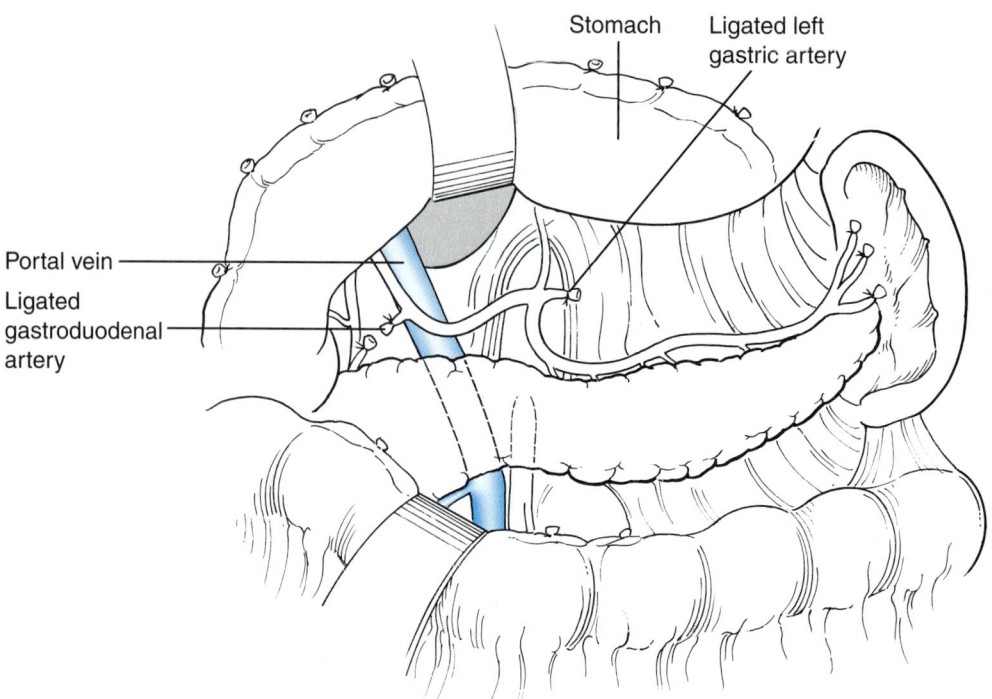

Figure 31-1

PROCEDURE

Donor Pancreatectomy

- **Figure 31–1:** The lesser sac is entered by dividing the gastrocolic ligament.
  - The stomach is retracted superiorly and the transverse colon inferiorly to expose the pancreatic body and tail.
  - Careful palpation of the pancreas to detect masses or abnormalities is followed by careful dissection of the gastrohepatic and hepatoduodenal ligaments.
  - The common bile duct, gastroduodenal artery, right gastric artery, and coronary vein are sequentially divided.
  - The celiac axis is exposed, the left gastric artery ligated, and the supraceliac aorta controlled.
  - The posterior aspect of the pancreas is inspected using a Kocher maneuver, with division of the gastroepiploic vessels to facilitate mobilization.
- **Figure 31–2:** The short gastric vessels, splenophrenic, splenocolic, and splenorenal ligaments are divided, freeing up the spleen.
  - The spleen is used as a handle for further mobilization of the pancreas.
  - Dissection is extended back toward the midline.
- **Figure 31–3:** The nasogastric tube is advanced into the duodenum and flushed with 200 mL of an antimicrobial solution.

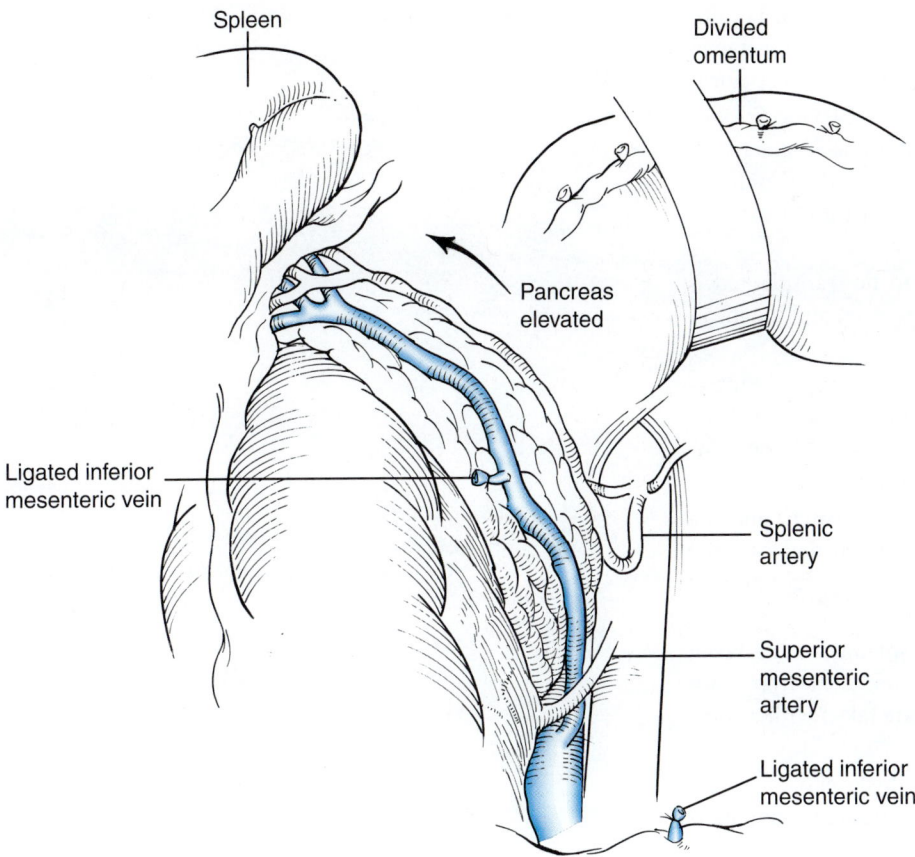

Figure 31–2

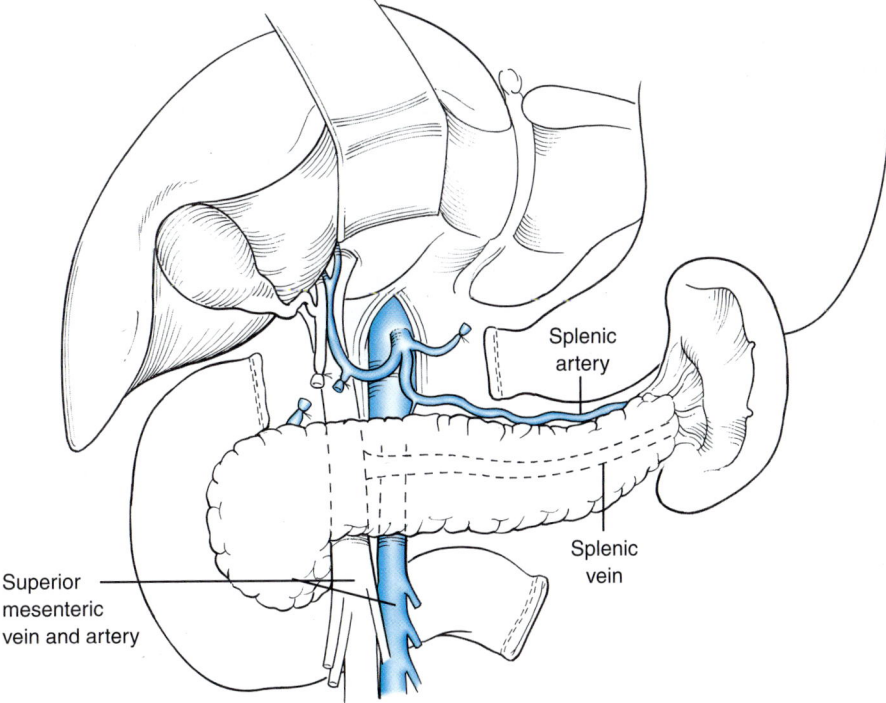

Figure 31–3

- The tube is then withdrawn into the stomach and a multi-row cutting (gastrointestinal anastomosis [GIA]) stapler is used to divide the duodenum just distal to the pylorus and again just proximal to the ligament of Treitz.
- A multirow noncutting (thoracoabdominal) stapler with a vascular load is used to divide the root of the mesentery, including the superior mesenteric artery (SMA) and vein (SMV).
- When dissection of other organs to be transplanted is complete, heparin anticoagulation is given and the infrarenal aorta is cannulated.
- Chilled preservation solution is infused through the infrarenal aorta, and the pancreas is bathed in sterile slush. After infusion of approximately 3 L of preservation solution, the organs are removed from the donor.

■ The SMA is removed with a small aortic patch, unless a replaced right hepatic artery is present. In that case the SMA is transected distal to the origin of the right hepatic artery.

■ If the patient is also a liver donor, the splenic artery is taken close to its origin for later reconstruction. If the liver is not to be procured, the celiac and SMA are taken with a common aortic patch.

■ The portal vein is usually divided at the level of the coronary vein to allow adequate length for both liver and pancreas grafts.

■ The pancreas is generally removed after the liver and placed in sterile, 4°C preservation solution for transport. The liver and pancreas may also be removed en bloc and separated on ice on the back table.

■ Segments of donor vessels, including the right iliac arterial bifurcation and common iliac vein, are explanted and stored in preservation solution.

Pancreas Transplantation

■ **Figure 31–4A, B:** Back-table preparation of the pancreatic graft is carried out in a pool of chilled preservation solution.
- The spleen is first removed by ligation of its vascular supply, and the distal duodenum is trimmed off to the level of the uncinate process. The proximal and distal staple lines, as well as the staple line across the mesenteric root, may be reinforced with running sutures (Figure 31–4A).
- For the recipient operation, the graft SMA and splenic artery must be joined into one conduit (Figure 31–4B).
- If a common aortic patch was taken, no reconstruction is necessary.
- If the two arteries are separate, however, a Y-graft is formed from donor iliac bifurcation, with vascular anastomosis of the internal iliac to the splenic artery, and external iliac to the SMA.

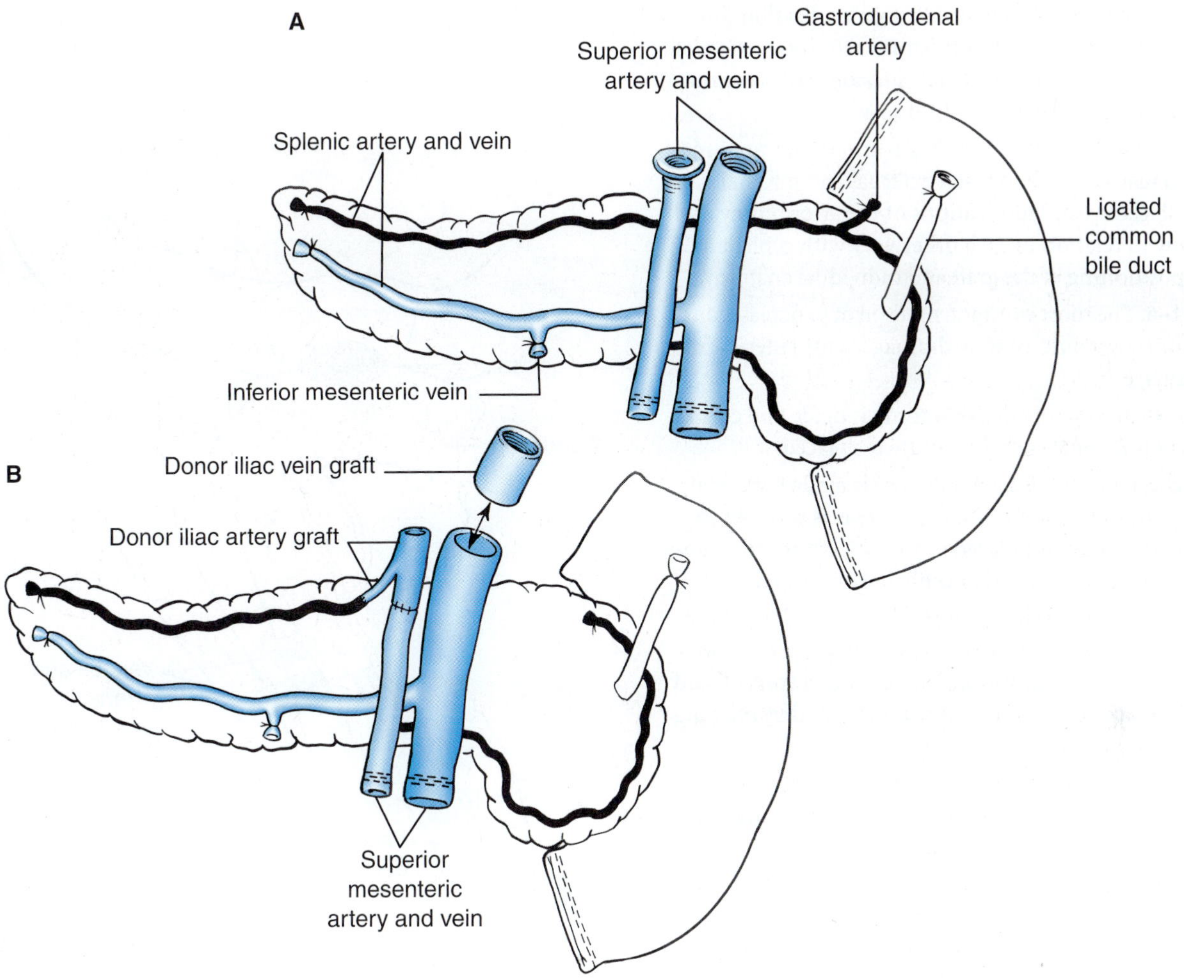

Chapter 31 : Pancreas Transplantation • 257

Figure 31–4A–B

- Each leg of the Y-graft should be 1–2 cm long, with adjustments to allow for suture lines that are tension and torsion free.
- Should the donor's iliac vessels be unsuitable for a Y-graft, another option is the donor brachiocephalic trunk. End-to-side tube interposition segments between splenic artery and SMA may be employed if needed.
- The portal vein is next mobilized with minimal dissection. If the donor portal vein segment is too short to allow implantation, a length of donor iliac vein may be attached end to end.
- **Figure 31–5:** The recipient procedure is preferentially performed on the right side, as the iliac vessels are more superficial and the vein lies lateral to the artery in the neutral position.
- The operation is begun with a low midline laparotomy, and dissection is carried down in the plane between the cecum and retroperitoneum. The right ureter is isolated and gently mobilized from the iliac vessels.

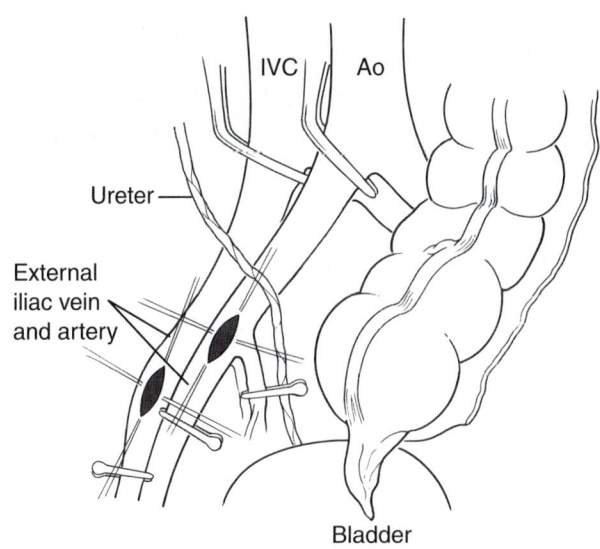

Figure 31–5

- The arterial supply usually needs no mobilization, but a tension-free venous anastomosis may require ligation of the hypogastric veins. The distal inferior vena cava may also be used for the venous anastomosis.
- With the patient systemically heparinized, the proximal common iliac vessels and distal external and internal vessels are all clamped. The locations of the arteriotomy and venotomy in relation to each other vary with cephalad or caudal positioning of the graft and individual anatomy.

■ **Figure 31–6:** The most common method of pancreas transplantation is systemic venous drainage with enteric exocrine drainage.
- With the vessels clamped, a venotomy is made and corner stitches of 6-0 nonabsorbable suture are placed.
- A final check of the vascular anatomy is made before taking the graft out of the ice. The pancreas is brought into the operative field and placed in the pelvis with the duodenal segment directed either cephalad or caudad.
- Excess donor portal vein is trimmed off to minimize kinking, and corner sutures are carried through corresponding points on the donor vessel. These sutures are tied, and the end-to-side venous anastomosis is secured by running the corner stitches to each other.
- The arteriotomy is made next and 6-0 corner sutures are placed. The arterial anastomosis is similarly secured and the vascular clamps are removed. The anastomosis, ligated donor vessels, mesenteric root, and duodenal staple lines are all meticulously inspected for hemostasis.
- A loop of mid-jejunum is brought down and laid flat to identify a good point for the side-to-side enteric anastomosis. Ideally, the exocrine secretions are directed into the jejunum approximately 50–60 cm past the ligament of Treitz to minimize postoperative diarrhea.
- Enterotomies are made in the antimesenteric borders of the two segments, each about 4 cm in length, and an inner layer of running 4-0 absorbable suture is used to approximate the edges. This is reinforced with an outer layer of interrupted 4-0 nonabsorbable sutures. Caution is used around the area of the ampulla of Vater to avoid impingement.
- Alternatively, the anastomosis may be made with a GIA or an end-to-end anastomosis (EEA) stapler, and backed with a layer of nonabsorbable sutures.

■ **Figure 31–7:** Systemic venous drainage with bladder exocrine drainage was the most popular technique for pancreas transplantation in the 1990s but has fallen from favor due to the associated risk of severe dehydration and urologic complications.
- Initial dissection includes mobilization of the anterior and lateral attachments of the bladder, taking care to avoid injury to the ureter.

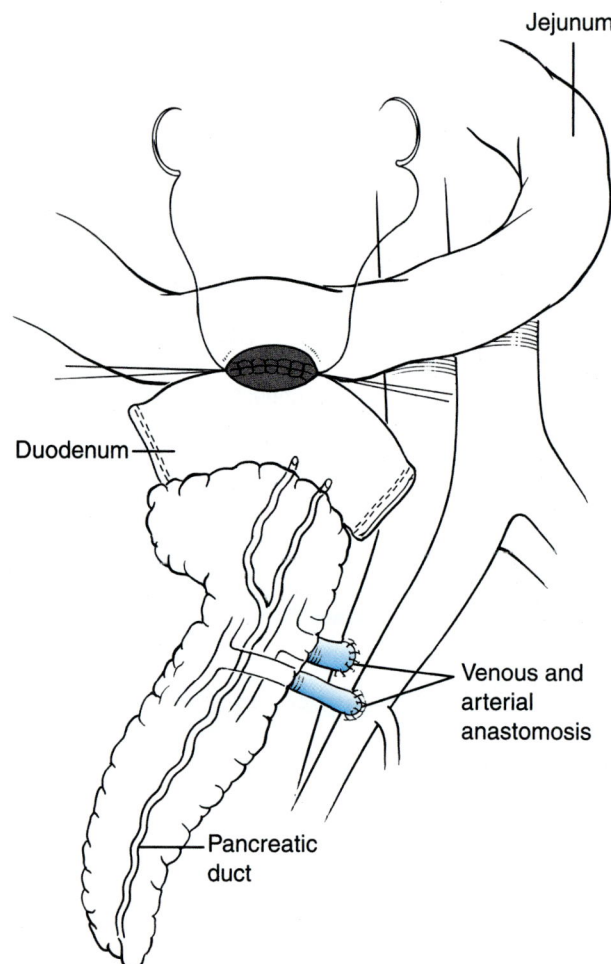

Figure 31–6

- Revascularization of the graft is performed just as in enteric drainage, but the pancreas is directed caudad.
- A horizontal posterior cystostomy is made, about 4 cm in length, with a matching enterotomy made in the antimesenteric aspect of the duodenum.
- The duodenocystostomy is closed with a running 4-0 absorbable suture line and an exterior layer of interrupted nonabsorbable stitches.

■ **Figure 31–8:** Enteric drainage of exocrine secretions may be combined with portal venous drainage for more physiologic insulin release and metabolism.

- In this variant, the arterial supply is through the common iliac artery, and venous drainage is accomplished by end-to-side anastomosis of the donor portal vein to the recipient SMV.
- The graft lies above the small bowel mesentery, with the arterial Y-graft traversing the mesentery.
- While the pancreatic graft is on the back table, an extension onto the single limb of the Y-graft is made by placing excess external iliac end to end onto the proximal common iliac segment. Of note, portal drainage does not allow use of a common Carrel patch due to the short length of this conduit.
- The recipient operation is performed through a midline laparotomy, and the transverse colon is retracted superiorly.

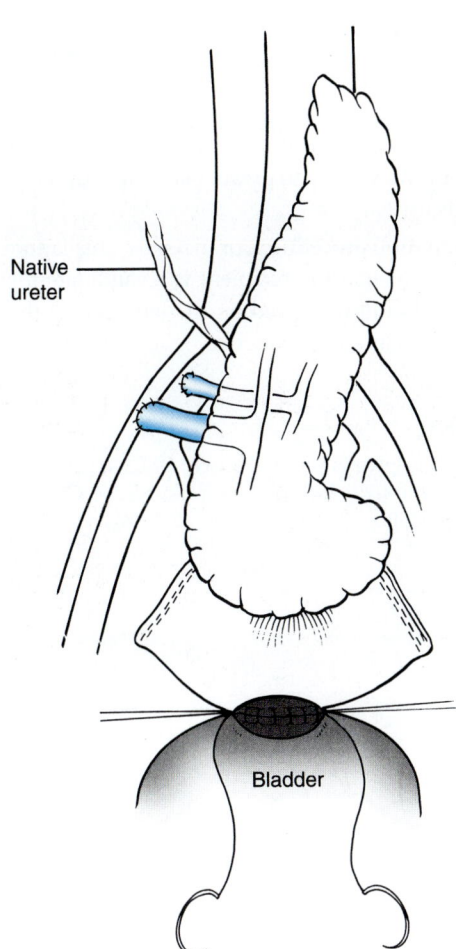

Figure 31–7

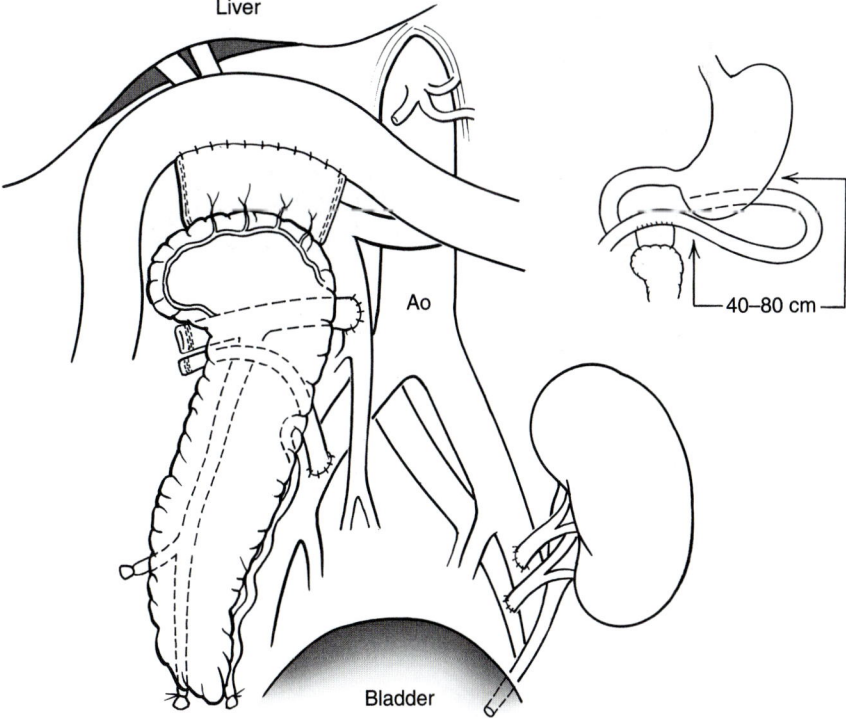

Figure 31–8

- The small bowel mesentery is stretched out horizontally, and the SMA is palpated. The SMV lies to the right and is dissected out with careful ligation of surrounding lymphatics.
- A 1–2-cm window is made through an avascular section of mesentery to allow tunneling of the Y-graft down to the common iliac artery.
- The patient is heparinized, clamps are applied to the vessels, and revascularization is performed as in systemic venous drainage.
- Following revascularization, a duodenojejunostomy is created for management of exocrine secretions.

POSTOPERATIVE CARE

- Nothing by mouth until return of bowel function.
- Exogenous insulin should not be necessary.
  - Exceptions: cases of delayed graft function or use of high-dose steroids for treatment of rejection.

POTENTIAL COMPLICATIONS

- Refer to Informed Consent, earlier.
- Enteric drainage is associated with leak, peritonitis, and abscess.
- Bladder drainage is associated with urethritis or cystitis, and dehydration.

PEARLS AND TIPS

- Direct handling of the pancreas should be kept to a minimum.
- During back-table preparation, avoid mass ligation of small vessels in the mesentery to prevent later development of arteriovenous fistula.
- In SPK transplantation procedures, or in renal transplantation procedures in which the recipient is a candidate for PAK, the kidney should be placed on the left, leaving the right side for placement of the pancreas.

REFERENCES

Punch JD. Organ Transplantation. In Doherty GM, ed. *Current Diagnosis and Treatment: Surgery.* New York, NY: McGraw-Hill; 2010:1233–1250.

CHAPTER 32

Liver Transplantation

Derek A. DuBay, MD, and Randall S. Sung, MD

INDICATIONS

- End-stage liver disease in patients who meet the minimal criteria for placement on the liver transplantation list as defined by the American Association for the Study of Liver Diseases.
- Fulminant acute liver failure.
- Hepatocellular carcinoma fulfilling Milan criteria (tumor > 2 cm but < 5 cm or up to three tumors each < 3 cm).
- Some pediatric metabolic liver diseases as defined by the United Network for Organ Sharing (UNOS).

CONTRAINDICATIONS

Absolute

- Recidivism to alcohol and drug abuse (6-month abstinence-free period essential).
- Significant portal venous thrombosis that precludes venous reconstruction.
- Extrahepatic malignancies.
- Systemic sepsis and certain untreated chronic infections (eg, tuberculosis, *Mycobacterium avium-intracellulare*).
- In the case of hepatocellular carcinoma:
  - Vascular or biliary tree invasion.
  - Tumors outside Milan criteria.

Relative

- Significant cardiopulmonary disease or other medical illnesses, with the exception of liver or biliary tree specific disease and renal disease.
- Certain chronic infections (eg, HIV infection).
- Profound physical deconditioning.
- Advanced age (older than 70 years).
- Poor psychosocial support (eg, homeless).
- Inability to obtain immunosuppressive medications.

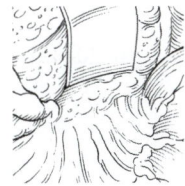
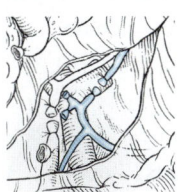
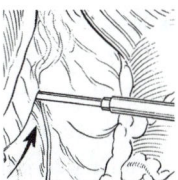
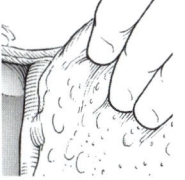
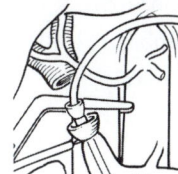
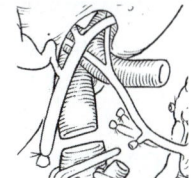
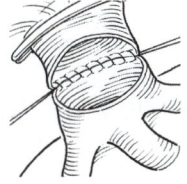
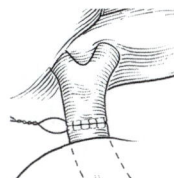
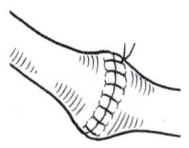

INFORMED CONSENT

- The 1-year survival following liver transplantation is 86–90% in the United States, with a death rate of approximately 5% per year death thereafter.
- Approximately 20% of patients will require retransplantation.

Expected Benefits
- Restoration of hepatic function.

Potential Risks
- Potential complications in the perioperative period are numerous given the magnitude of the procedure.
- Specific complications include:
  - Infection: 66% total (bacterial, 35–70%; fungal, 20–42%; viral, 5–26%).
  - Rejection (40–70%).
  - Biliary complications (7–29%).
  - Bleeding (10–25%).
  - Primary nonfunction (7%).
  - Hepatic artery thrombosis (2–10%).
  - Portal vein thrombosis (1–2%).

EQUIPMENT

- Rigorous fixed retractor (mandatory to facilitate exposure of the operative field).
- Argon beam coagulator (useful in patients with severe coagulopathy or in retransplantation).
- Cell saver (reduces allogenic packed red blood cell transfusion but should not be used in patients with hepatic malignancy).

PATIENT PREPARATION

- Patients are typically evaluated and deemed appropriate candidates for transplantation based on their preoperative transplant clinic evaluation.
- On the day of transplantation, laboratory values, ECG, and chest radiograph should be obtained and reviewed for potential contraindications soon after the patient is called to the hospital.
- Radiographic verification of portal vein patency should be up to date (within 6 months).
- Patients with known hepatoma should have up-to-date imaging of the chest, abdomen, and pelvis. The admission chest radiograph should be closely examined for evidence of metastatic disease.

- History and physical examination should specifically assess for potential contraindications to liver transplantation (eg, active infections, evidence of active alcohol or drug use).

PATIENT POSITIONING

- The patient should be supine.
- The left arm is extended and the axilla prepped in the sterile field (to provide access to the left axillary vein should venovenous bypass be required).
- The right arm can be tucked or extended.

PROCEDURE

- **Figure 32–1:** Incision and retractor placement.
  - The chest and abdomen are prepped from the nipples to the pubis.
  - A bilateral subcostal incision is made 2 fingerbreadths below the costal margin, or lower if the patient has significant ascites.
  - The incision should extend from the lateral border of the left rectus muscle to the right anterior axillary line.
  - In patients with a high costal margin, exposure of the suprahepatic vena cava is facilitated by a paraxiphoid midline extension.
  - Bilateral anchoring retractor posts are placed at the level of the nipples; the angle of the cephalad retractors is anterolateral to maximize cephalad exposure.
  - A separate anchoring post may be placed at either hip to support a lower bar to retract the viscera away from the portal structures.
- **Figure 32–2:** Recipient hepatectomy—hilar dissection.
  - The falciform ligament is divided and retractor blades are positioned to expose the porta hepatis.
  - The cystic artery and duct are divided and ligated.
  - The right and left hepatic arteries are divided high in the porta hepatis to maximize length.
  - The bile duct is dissected free with a generous amount of surrounding tissue to minimize devascularization to this structure.
  - The ties on the arteries and bile duct are left long to enable them to be identified easily during the reconstruction.
  - The portal vein is dissected free circumferentially but is not divided until just prior to the hepatectomy.
  - The region posterior to the bile duct and lateral to the portal vein is examined for the presence of a replaced or accessory right hepatic artery (arising from the superior mesenteric artery), which is encountered in 15% of patients.

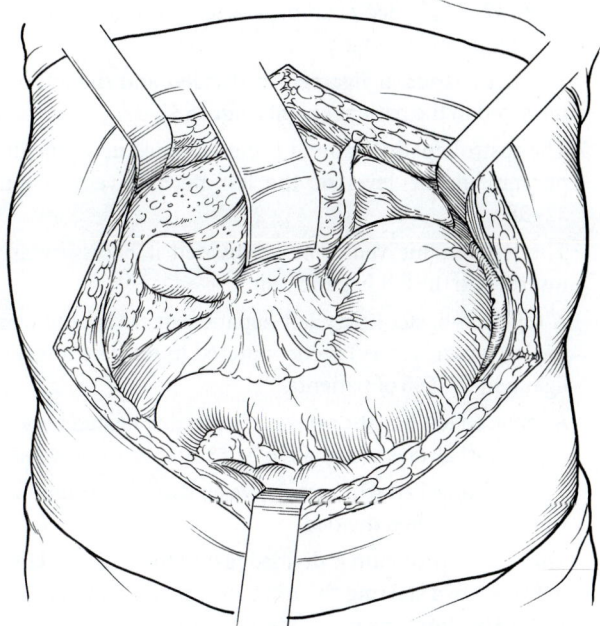

Figure 32–1

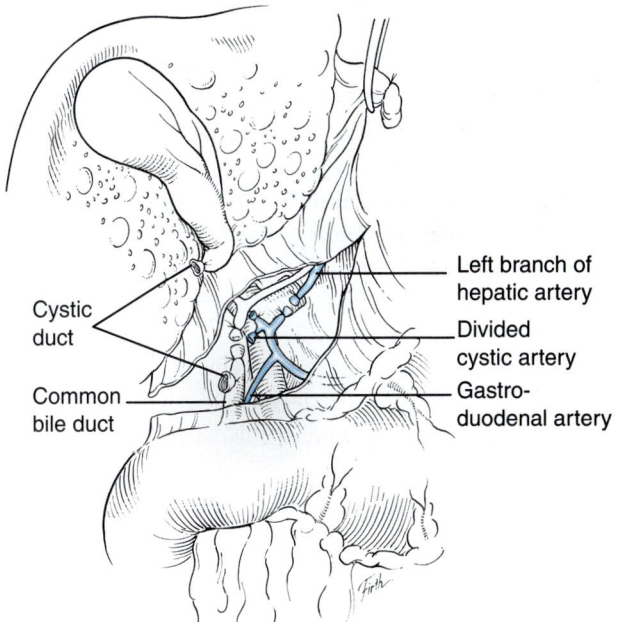

Figure 32–2

- **Figure 32–3A, B:** Recipient hepatectomy—mobilization of the left lobe and caudate.
  - The left triangular ligament is divided and the left lobe retracted to the patient's right (Figure 32–3A).
  - The gastrohepatic ligament is then divided up to the diaphragm at the level of the left hepatic vein (Figure 32–3B).
  - The left phrenic vein may be divided if necessary as it inserts into the left hepatic vein.
  - A replaced or accessory left hepatic artery (arising from the left gastric artery) is encountered in the gastrohepatic ligament in 10% of patients.
  - A replaced left hepatic artery is invariably ligated because it is almost always too small to be a suitable inflow vessel.
  - The peritoneal attachments between the caudate lobe and vena cava are then divided.
  - The retroperitoneum is divided just to the patient's left of the vena cava starting the retrocaval plane, which is later completed from the right side of the vena cava.
- **Figure 32–4:** Recipient hepatectomy—mobilization of the right lobe and recipient explant.
  - Mesenteric attachments to the gallbladder and retroperitoneal attachments to the inferior border of the liver are divided.
  - The right hepatic lobe is then mobilized from the diaphragm exposing the bare area of the liver.
  - The right adrenal gland is dissected off the liver and the adrenal vein is divided.
  - The mobilization is continued posterior to the vena cava and the retrocaval plane is completed from right to left.
  - The retrocaval plane is extended cephalad and caudal. There is a posterior phrenic vein at the most cephalad aspect (behind the hepatic veins) and rarely a lumbar vein near the position of the adrenal vein.
  - The suprahepatic and infrahepatic vena cava are sufficiently dissected to permit vascular clamps to be placed in these positions.
  - The portal vein is divided just proximal to the right-left bifurcation.
  - The suprahepatic and infrahepatic vena cava clamps are applied and the liver is dissected a short distance off the vena cava to facilitate production of adequate length vascular cuffs for anastomosis.
  - The vena cava is divided and the liver is removed from the field.
  - The retroperitoneum is made hemostatic prior to reconstruction.
- **Figure 32–5:** Venovenous bypass.
  - This technique is rarely required with contemporary liver transplantation techniques.

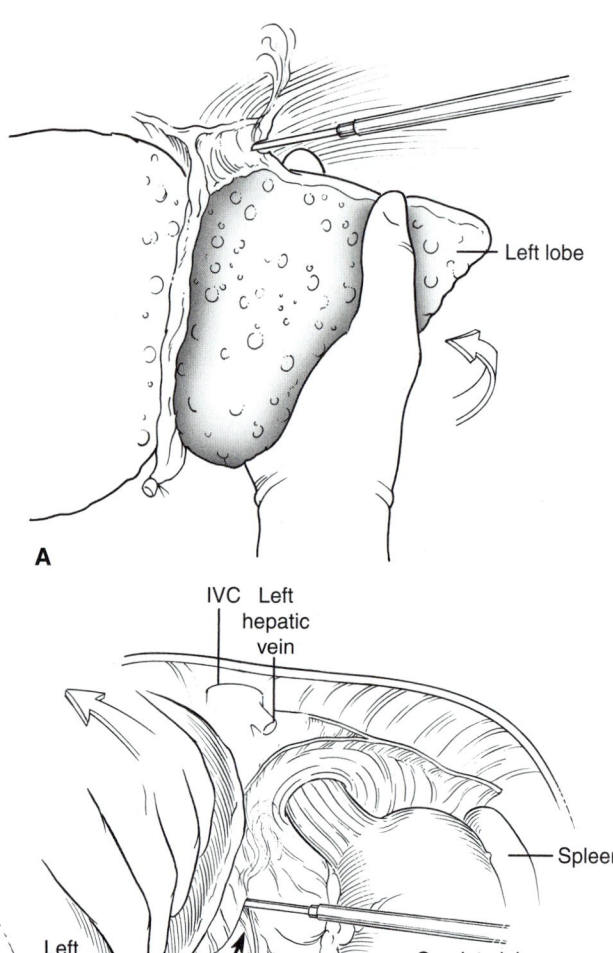

Figure 32–3A–B

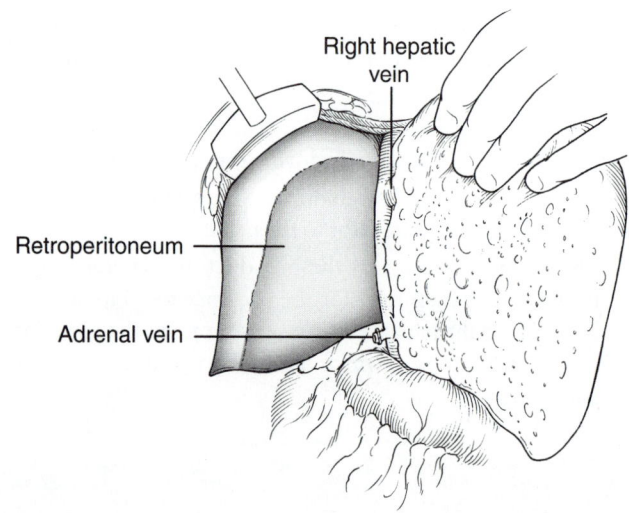

Figure 32–4

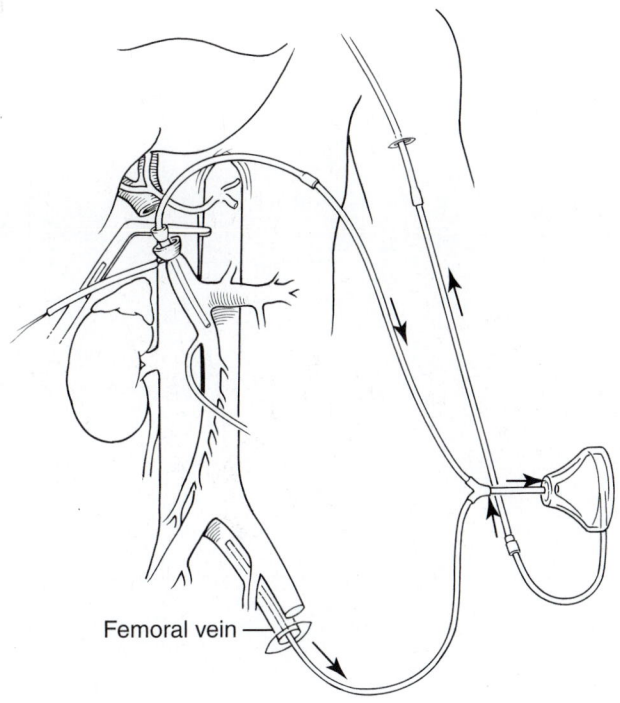

Figure 32–5

- Venovenous bypass is employed most commonly in patients without portal hypertension (ie, fulminate acute liver failure) who experience massive intestinal swelling with portal vein clamping or, in the other extreme, if exsanguinating portal hypertensive bleeding limits the ability to perform the recipient hepatectomy.
- In either case, the goal is to decompress the portal venous system.
- In rare cases, bypass may be necessary to maintain systemic blood pressure during caval occlusion. Inflow is provided via the portal vein and the femoral vein.
- Outflow is provided in an upper extremity vein.
- The left axilla is typically prepared into the surgical field specifically for this purpose.
- Alternatively, the anesthetist can exchange an internal jugular line with a bypass cannula for outflow.

■ **Figure 32–6:** Liver transplantation—suprahepatic and infrahepatic "bicaval" anastomosis.
- The supracaval anastomosis is performed first with a running 3-0 Prolene suture.

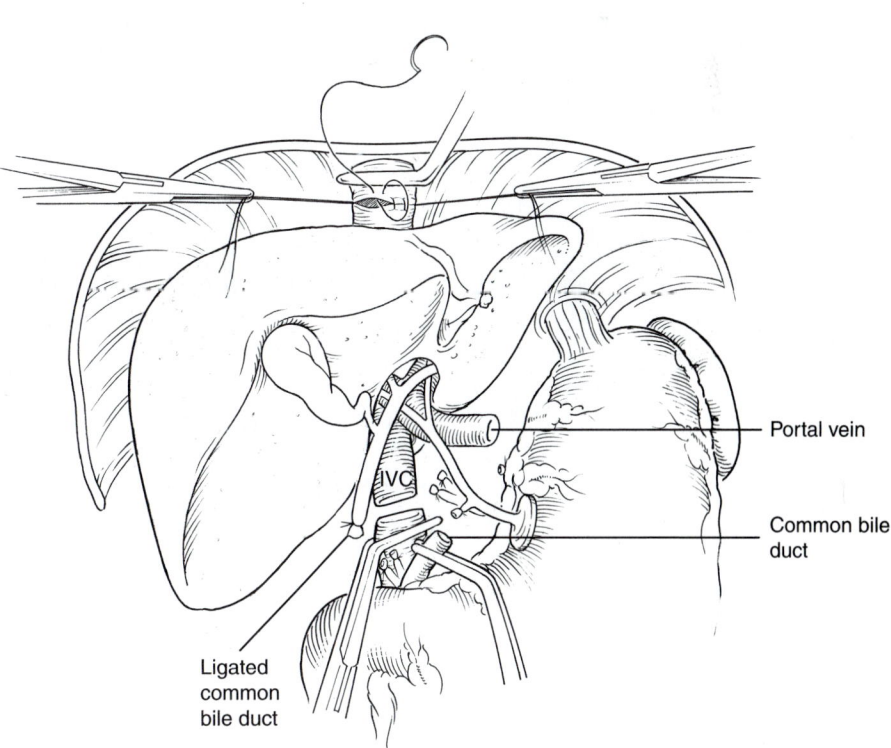

Figure 32–6

- Stay sutures are placed on each side of the vena cava (recipient to donor) and the back wall is run (from the inside of the vena cava), followed by the front wall.
- The infrahepatic caval anastomosis is performed next with a running 4-0 Prolene suture in a similar fashion.
- A small flexible chest tube or red rubber catheter may be placed through the infrahepatic inferior vena caval anastomosis at this time and used later for venting the first-pass circulation through the liver after reperfusion.

■ **Figure 32–7A-C:** Piggyback technique.
- Instead of replacing the vena cava with a typical bicaval approach, the recipient cava is preserved, and an anastomosis is created between the donor suprahepatic cava and a cuff of the recipient hepatic veins.
- The infrahepatic donor vena cava is stapled or tied off.
- This technique has the advantages of partial vena cava return from the lower extremities during liver transplantation, which minimizes the hemodynamic changes encountered with complete caval occlusion.
- The piggyback technique requires dissection of segments 6 and 7 and the caudate lobe from the vena cava with ligation of the venous branches that drain directly into the vena cava.

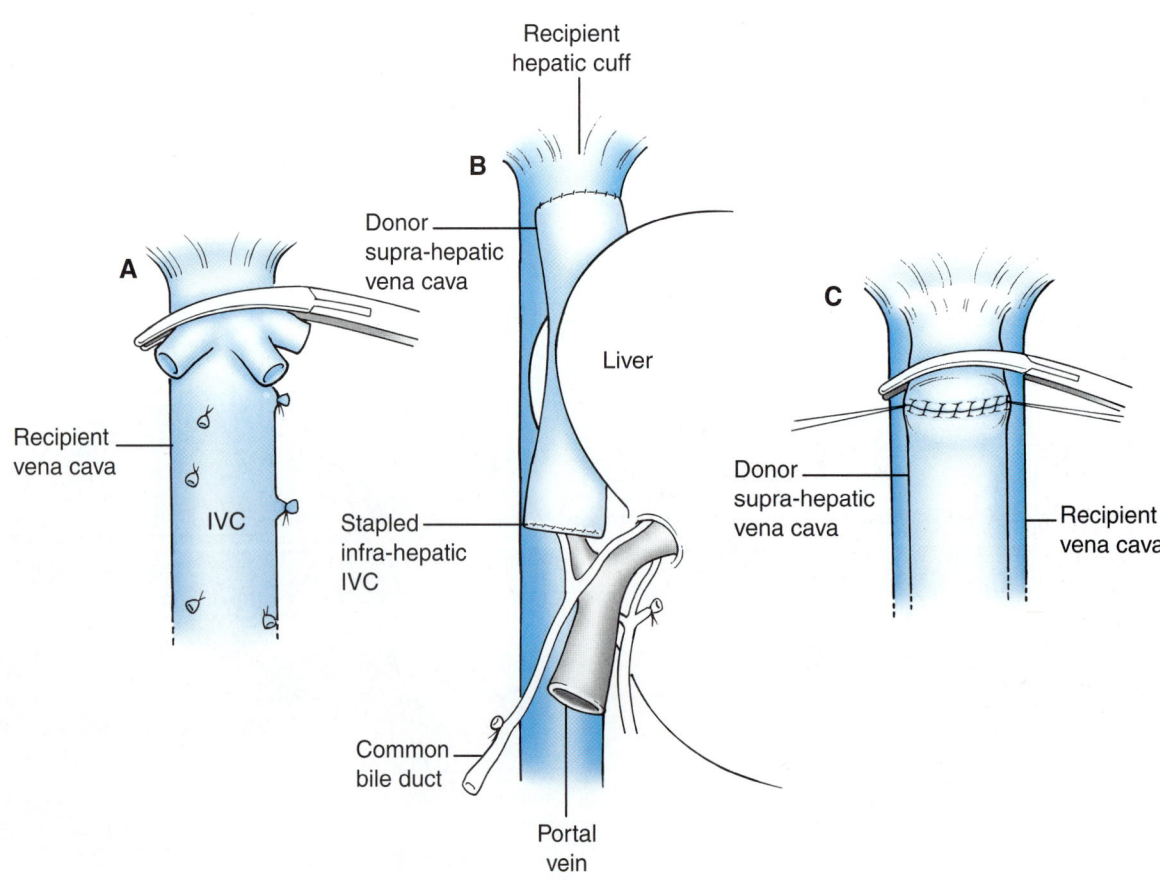

Figure 32–7A–C

- The potential disadvantages are the extra time required to dissect the liver from the vena cava and typically increased blood loss encountered during this maneuver.
- **Figure 32–8:** Liver transplantation—portal venous anastomosis.
  - The portal venous anastomosis is performed after the vena cava is reconstructed.
  - The donor portal vein is shortened such that the reconstructed portal vein will not have excessive length.
  - Care is taken to correctly align the donor and recipient portal veins to avoid twists or kinks.
  - The anastomosis is performed in a running fashion with a 5-0 Prolene suture.
  - Stay sutures are placed bilaterally and the back wall is run (from the inside of the portal vein), followed by the front wall.
  - A "growth factor" is created before tying the suture to allow the anastomosis to expand following reperfusion.
  - A rule of thumb is to make the growth factor approximately one-third to one-half the diameter of the anastomosis.
  - The liver is then reperfused.
  - During the portal vein anastomosis, the anesthetist prepares for reperfusion.
  - During reperfusion the heart becomes bathed with potassium-rich, cold perfusate from the donor liver that contains many metabolic byproducts of liver preservation. The patient is therefore loaded with calcium and bicarbonate, and given volume, and a cardiogenic vasopressor such as epinephrine is prepared.
  - The portal venous clamps are released and approximately 250 mL of first-pass blood is allowed to "vent" out of the infrahepatic anastomosis catheter.
  - This blood is discarded, and the infrahepatic anastomosis is tied down (or in the case of piggyback transplantation, the infrahepatic vena cava is ligated).
  - The caval clamps are then released and the liver is reperfused into the systemic circulation.
  - It is not uncommon for the patient to experience bradycardia and hypotension or even a short period of asystole during this phase.
  - The caval and portal venous anastomoses are inspected for hemostasis.
  - There often is bleeding from the donor portal structures requiring ligation.

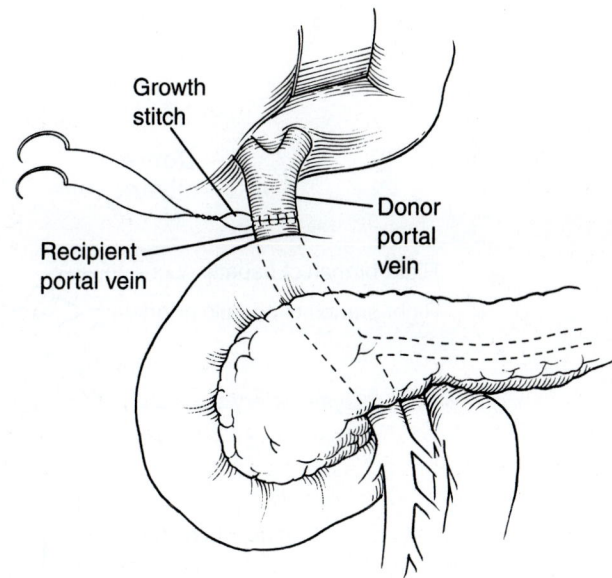

Figure 32–8

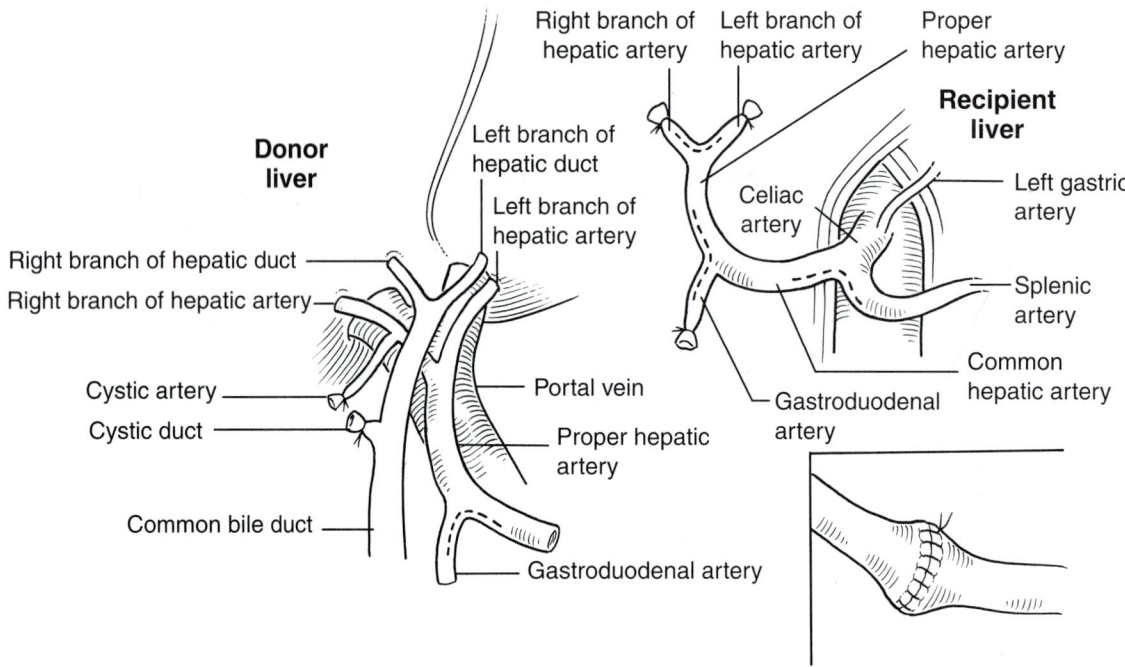

Figure 32–9

- **Figure 32–9:** Liver transplantation—hepatic arterial anastomosis.
  - After the patient is deemed hemodynamically stable and the caval and portal venous anastomoses are made hemostatic, the hepatic arterial anastomosis is performed.
  - Alternatively, the arterial anastomosis may be done prior to reperfusion if time allows.
  - There are many anatomic approaches to this anastomosis. Some surgeons prefer a simple end-to-end anastomosis while others advocate a branch patch technique.
  - The recipient branch patch can originate from the bifurcation of the right and left hepatic arteries, the gastroduodenal and proper hepatic arteries, or the common hepatic and splenic arteries (shown as dotted lines in the figure).
  - The donor branch patch can similarly arise from any of these arterial bifurcations.
  - The anastomosis is performed in a running fashion with a 6-0 Prolene suture.
  - The length of the reconstructed hepatic artery should be either perfect or excessively redundant.
- **Figure 32–10A, B:** Liver transplantation—biliary anastomosis.
  - The basic tenets of the biliary reconstruction are to create an anastomosis between healthy, viable donor and recipient bile duct ends (Figure 32–10A) with good blood supply, and to shorten the donor bile duct as much as possible.

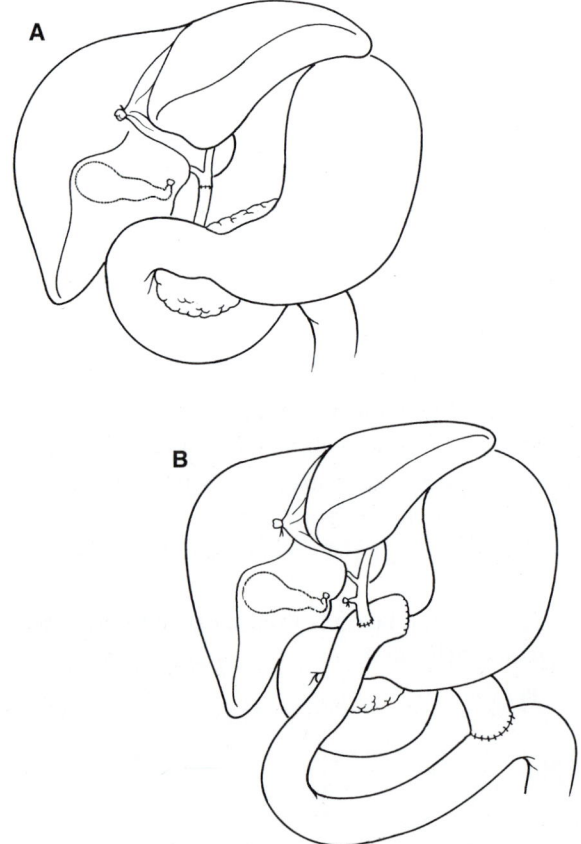

Figure 32–10A–B

- The bile duct anastomosis is usually performed with 5-0 or 6-0 PDS sutures in either an interrupted or running fashion.
- Placement of a T-tube across the anastomosis has fallen out of favor because immunosuppressed patients often do not form a good fibrotic tract around the transperitoneal portion of the tube.
- An internal biliary stent may be placed instead after blindly dilating the ampulla of Vater via the recipient common bile duct.
- Alternatively, a Roux-en-Y hepaticojejunostomy can be created (Figure 32–10B) when the recipient bile duct is ischemic, nonviable, or diseased (ie, primary biliary sclerosis or primary sclerosing cholangitis), when a replacement liver transplantation is being performed, or when there is more than one donor bile duct.
- A 40–60-cm retrocolic limb is fashioned with a stapled or hand-sewn enteroenterostomy.
- The biliary-enteric anastomosis is typically performed in an interrupted or running fashion with 5-0 or 6-0 PDS suture.
■ All anastomoses are then reinspected to ensure that they are hemostatic and lying in an appropriate anatomic position without twisting, or excessive tension or redundancy.
- The right upper quadrant is irrigated and the abdominal wall fascia is closed in layers with a running No. 1 PDS suture.
- The skin is closed with staples.
- Intraperitoneal drains are not typically employed.

POSTOPERATIVE CARE

■ All patients are admitted to the ICU. The majority of patients remain intubated with the anticipation of extubation on postoperative day 1.
■ Serial laboratory values are obtained (complete blood count, coagulation function, liver function tests).
■ Immunosuppression.
■ Oral medications (especially immunosuppression) are provided via nasogastric tube.
■ Infections and other postoperative complications are treated in a similar manner to all other ill patients (ie, do not overtreat because the patient has undergone transplantation).
■ Adequate nutritional support is of paramount importance in chronically malnourished patients with liver failure.
■ Volume overload should be avoided.

POTENTIAL COMPLICATIONS

■ Potential complications are numerous.
- Acute renal insufficiency is common.
- Other specific complications include infections (bacterial, fungal, and viral), rejection, biliary complications, bleeding, primary nonfunction, hepatic artery thrombosis, and portal vein thrombosis.

PEARLS AND TIPS

■ In the case of acute renal insufficiency, consider lowering the dose of calcineurin inhibitors or going to a calcineurin-free regimen in the early postoperative period.
■ Abdominal ultrasound is to the transplanted liver as a chest radiograph is to the chest. Obtain an ultrasound with Doppler flow assessment to rule out hepatic artery thrombosis in the following situations:
- AST/ALT > 5000 within 12–24 hours of reperfusion.
- A rise in the AST/ALT values when previously they had been slowly declining.
- To assess for portal vein thrombosis or perihepatic fluid collections.
■ In a transplanted graft, the biliary tree typically does not dilate in the face of obstruction.
- Ultrasound is not a good test to evaluate for biliary obstruction.
- MR cholangiopancreatography is only useful if the patient can hold his or her breath, which most patients cannot do in the early postoperative period.
- Most patients require an endoscopic retrograde cholangiopancreatogram if a duct-to-duct anastomosis was performed or a percutaneous transhepatic cholangiogram if a choledochojejunostomy was performed.
■ Suspect bile leak if the patient's general clinical condition declines.
- The serum bilirubin value does not have to be elevated for a bile leak to be present.
- Similarly, sampled ascites may not demonstrate an elevated bilirubin value as the bile leak or collection can be localized and loculated.

REFERENCES

Blumgart LH, Fong Y, eds. *Surgery of the Liver and Biliary Tract*, 3rd ed. Philadelphia, PA: WB Saunders; 2000.

Busuttil RW, Klintmalm GB, eds. *Transplantation of the Liver*, 2nd ed. Philadelphia, PA: Elsevier Saunders; 2005.

Lucey MR, Brown KA, Everson GT, et al. Minimal criteria for placement of adults on the liver transplant waiting list. *Liver Transplant*. 1997;3:628–637.

Mazzaferro V, Regalia E, Doci R, et al. Liver transplantation for the treatment of small hepatocellular carcinomas in patients with cirrhosis. *N Engl J Med*. 1996;334:693–699.

CHAPTER 33

Vascular Access for Dialysis

Frank C. Vandy, MD, and Peter K. Henke, MD

INDICATIONS

- End-stage renal disease; recommendations from the Kidney Dialysis Outcomes Quality Initiative:
  - Creatinine clearance < 25 mL/min.
  - Serum creatinine > 4.0 mg/dL.
  - Dialysis anticipated within 1 year.
- Long-term plasmapheresis.

CONTRAINDICATIONS

- Ipsilateral proximal venous and arterial occlusion or stenosis.
- Systemic or local infection.
- Multiple comorbidities precluding safe intervention.

INFORMED CONSENT

Expected Benefits
- Provides access for dialysis.

Potential Risks
- Clotting, narrowing, or scarring of the graft requiring surgical or radiologic revision.
- Infection of the graft requiring surgical excision and replacement.
- Wound infection.
- Injury to the neurovascular structures of the arm.
- Bleeding.
- Failure of the fistula to mature for adequate dialysis access.
- Pain or numbness.
- Development of arterial "steal," resulting in decreased blood flow to the hand.

EQUIPMENT

- No. 10 or 15 blade scalpel for skin incision.
- Electrocautery unit.

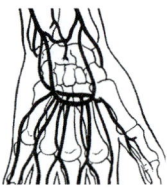
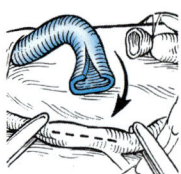
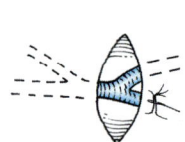
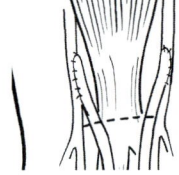

- Heparinized saline solution.
- Prosthetic expanded polytetrafluoroethylene (ePTFE) graft (frequently tapered 4–7 mm) for forearm loop grafts or brachial artery to axillary vein arteriovenous grafts if arteriovenous fistula is not possible.
- Tunneling device if needed.
- Small vascular clamps or vessel loops.
- No. 11 blade scalpel and Micro-Potts scissors.
- Double-armed polypropylene suture.
- Doppler ultrasound unit.

PATIENT PREPARATION

Preoperative History
- Specific focus on history of indwelling catheters, pacemaker, internal automatic cardiac defibrillator, or extremity trauma.
- Dominant extremity should be documented.
- Patients with severe congestive heart failure may not tolerate the additional cardiac output required to circulate blood through the fistula.

Physical Examination
- All pulses should be palpated.
- The Allen test should be performed to evaluate perfusion to the hand.
- Blood pressure should be obtained in both arms to evaluate proximal arterial disease.
- Veins of the wrist, forearm, elbow, and upper arm should be evaluated with or without a tourniquet.
  - Repetitive hand squeeze may make veins more prominent.
  - Visible veins can be considered for access.

Ultrasonography
- Doppler: to assess arterial flow.
- B-mode: to image and size potential veins.
  - Vein segments < 2.5 mm may be technically difficult to use for anastomosis and are associated with higher rates of failure.

Indications for Venography
- Edema in the extremity in which access is planned.
- Collateral vein development in the planned access site.
- Differential extremity size of the considered limb.
- Current or previous central access or transvenous catheter in the ipsilateral limb.
- Previous arm, neck, or chest trauma on the same side as the planned access site.
- Prior failed attempts to establish access in the ipsilateral extremity.

PATIENT POSITIONING

- The patient should be supine with the operative arm extended on an arm board and supinated.
- The arm should be prepared circumferentially from the fingers to the axilla, and the hand covered with a sterile towel.

PROCEDURE

- **Figure 33–1:** Vascular anatomy of the upper extremity.
  - The basilic vein courses medially down the arm and is found in the deeper subcutaneous tissues.

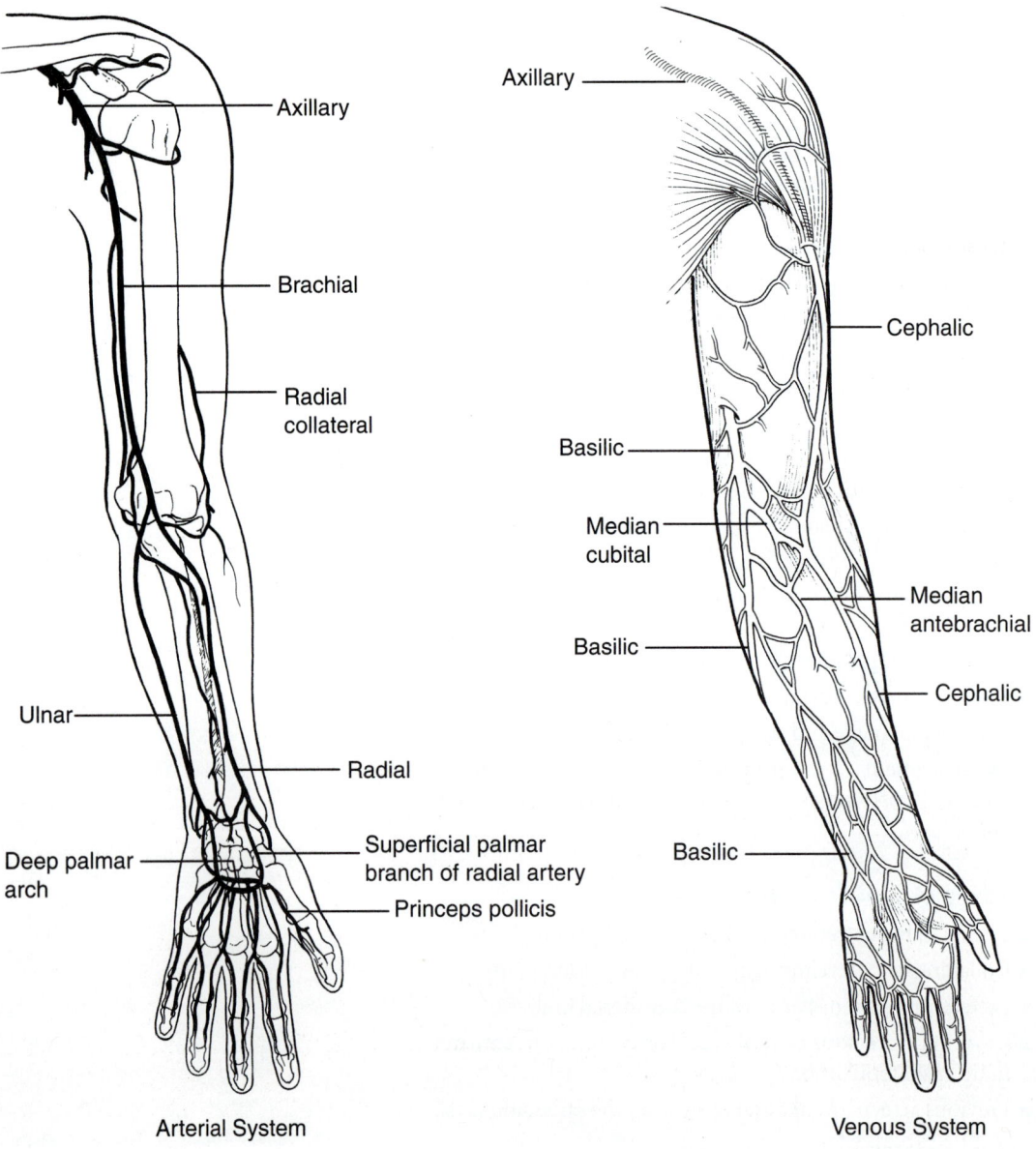

Figure 33–1

- The cephalic vein courses laterally and is very superficial, running under the skin layer.
- The cephalic vein runs posteriorly and laterally, proximal to the antecubital fossa.

Location of Access

- The goal is to provide the greatest surface area available for cannulation while allowing for the highest flow rates.
- The nondominant arm is preferred over the dominant arm.
- A distal location is preferred over a proximal location.

Types of Access

A. AUTOGENOUS RADIAL-CEPHALIC DIRECT WRIST ACCESS

- **Figure 33–2A-D:** Autogenous radial-cephalic direct wrist access is the gold standard in access.
  - The 3-year patency rate is 64%, with most failures occurring in the first 12 months.
  - Approximately 24% of radial-cephalic fistulas do not mature, failing in the first month.
- The procedure may be done with local, regional, or general anesthesia.
- Preoperatively the artery and the vein are located and marked using ultrasound for guidance.
- A single incision may be made between the marked artery and vein (Figure 33–2A).
- The cephalic vein and radial artery are gently dissected away from the surrounding tissues, ligating and dividing any small branches.
- Proximal and distal control of the radial artery is obtained with vessel loops in a Potts fashion.
  - The vessel should not be occluded at this stage (Figure 33–2B).
- The thenar branch of the radial artery, which comes off laterally, is identified and controlled.
- Using ink or a marking pen, the anterior surface of the vein is marked to avoid kinking or twisting.
- The vein is ligated and divided at its most distal aspect. The vein can later be trimmed to avoid redundancy.
- The vein is gently distended with heparinized saline to evaluate for leaks and assess caliber.
- A 3000-unit dose of systemic heparin is administered before occluding the artery with vessel loops.
- Using a No. 11 blade, a small arteriotomy is made on the anterior surface of the artery.
  - Care should be taken not to incise the back wall of the artery with the knife (Figure 33–2C).
- Micro-Potts scissors are used to extend the arteriotomy 5–6 mm, in a slightly angled fashion.

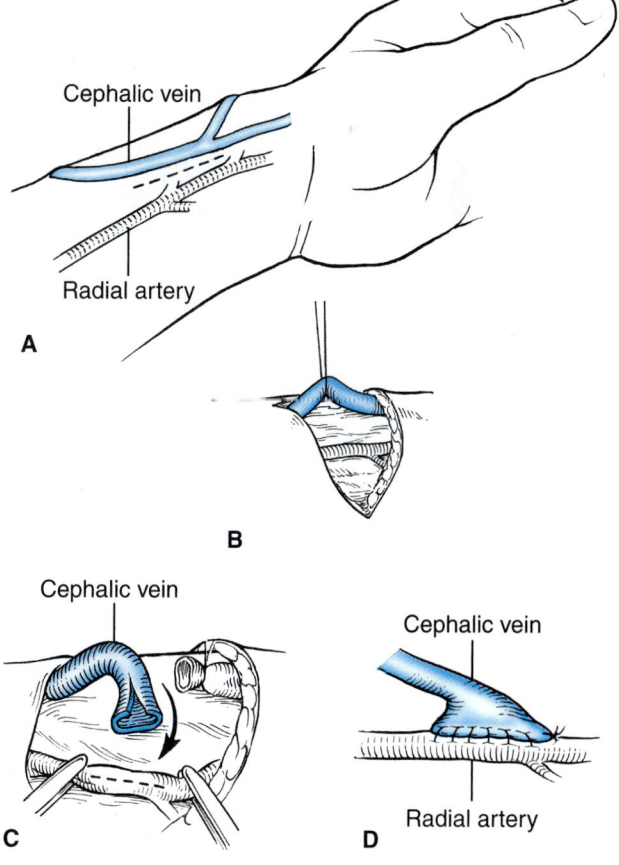

Figure 33–2A–D

- The vein is trimmed so that the anastomosis will be tension free but not redundant.
- The anastomosis is completed with a 6-0 polypropylene suture in an end-to-side fashion.
- Following completion of the anastomosis, a palpable thrill should be felt in the vein.
- The wound may be closed with deep dermal interrupted sutures followed by a running subcuticular absorbable stitch (Figure 33–2D).

B. Autogenous Brachial-Cephalic Access
- Provides superior flow and higher maturation rates than radial-cephalic access.
- Preferable in women, the elderly, and diabetic patients in whom a radiocephalic fistula may fail to mature.
- Associated with a higher incidence of arterial steal than more distal fistulas.

C. Basilic Vein Transpositions
- **Figure 33–3A, B:** Basilic vein transposition is preferred in patients with a sclerotic or small-caliber cephalic vein.
- The basilic vein is a deeper vein and thus less amenable to repeated venipunctures.

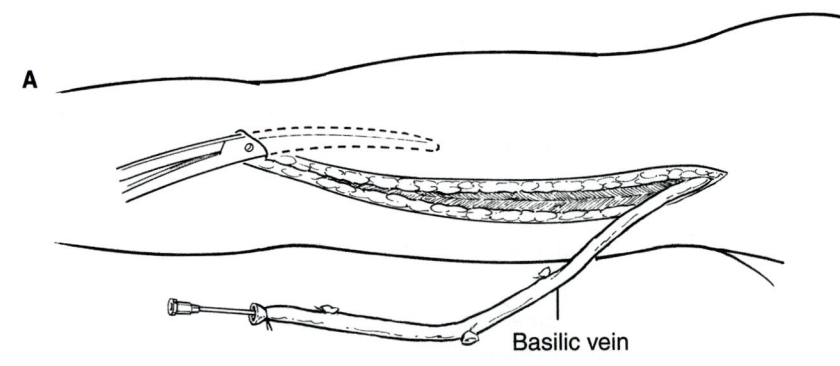

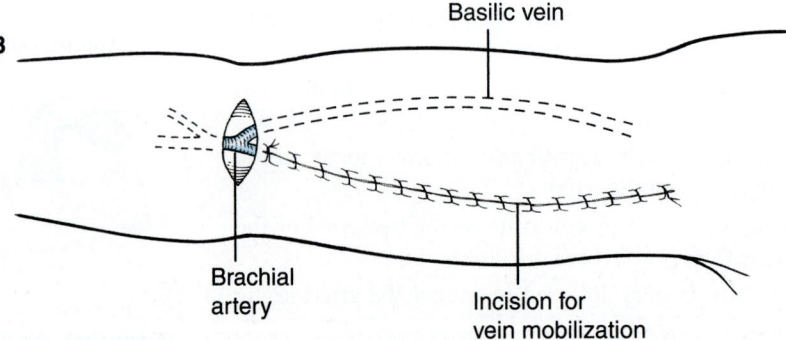

Figure 33–3A–B

- Transposition of the basilic vein to an anterior and superficial location allows for:
  - Easier dialysis cannulation.
  - Elimination of the awkward positioning required during dialysis using posterior arm access.
- Brachial-basilic transposition has a 92% maturation rate with 66% primary patency at 1 year.
- Basilic-forearm transposition has a 91% maturation rate with 84% primary patency at year.
- The procedure may be done with regional or general anesthesia.
- Using ultrasound, the basilic vein can be identified preoperatively anterior to the medial epicondyle of the humerus.
- A longitudinal incision is made along the medial aspect of the upper arm to the axilla for adequate exposure.
- The median cutaneous nerve should be preserved if possible.
- The basilic vein should be gently dissected away from surrounding tissues and mobilized proximally to the brachial vein, with small tributaries ligated and divided.
- The brachial artery can be exposed though the same incision.
- Distal and proximal control is obtained with vessel loops, but the vessel should not be occluded at this stage.
- Using ink or a marking pen, the anterior surface of the vein is marked to avoid kinking or twisting.
- The vein is ligated and divided at its most distal aspect, near the antecubital fossa.
  - The vein can later be trimmed to avoid redundancy.
  - A small Heifitz clamp can be placed on the proximal vein to avoid bleeding.
- The vein is gently distended with heparinized saline to evaluate for leaks and to assess the caliber of the vessel.
- Using a large Kelly clamp or Bainbridge clamp, a superficial tunnel is made through the subcutaneous tissues on the anterior aspect of the upper arm between the axilla and the antecubital fossa.
- The distended vein is pulled gently through the tunnel.
- A 3000-unit dose of systemic heparin is administered before occluding the artery with vessel loops.
- Using a No. 11 blade, a small arteriotomy is made on the anterior surface of the artery.
  - Care should be taken not to incise the back wall of the artery with the knife.
- Micro-Potts scissors are used to extend the arteriotomy 5–6 mm, in a slightly angled fashion.
- The vein is trimmed so that the anastomosis will be tension free but not redundant.
- The anastomosis is completed with a 6-0 polypropylene suture in an end-to-side fashion.

- Following completion of the anastomosis, a palpable thrill should be felt in the vein.
- The wound may be closed in two layers with Vicryl sutures for the subcutaneous tissues followed by a running subcuticular absorbable stitch.
- Care should be taken not to occlude or impinge flow through the graft with a tight or strangulated wound closure.

D. Prosthetic Graft Access

- **Figure 33–4:** PTFE is preferred over Dacron for prosthetic grafts.
  - Prosthetic grafts have lower patency rates than those using autogenous vein, with higher rates of infection; however, grafts can be accessed within 4 weeks of creation, eliminating the wait for maturation, and there are multiple options for sites of insertions.
- Inflow can be obtained from the radial artery, antecubital brachial artery, proximal brachial artery, or axillary artery.
- The procedure may be done with regional or general anesthesia; an interscalene nerve block is also an option.
- A curvilinear incision is made over the antecubital fossa.
- Careful dissection is performed to isolate and gain control of the following venous structures in the fossa using vessel loops:
  - Cephalic vein.
  - Basilic vein.
  - Antecubital vein.
  - Median antecubital vein.
- The median antecubital vein may take off posteriorly and run deep.
- The brachial artery is dissected out, and proximal and distal control is obtained with vessel loops.
  - The artery should not be occluded at this stage.
- A small horizontal counterincision is made distally on the anterior surface of the forearm.
- Using either a commercial tunneling device or a large Kelly clamp, a subcutaneous tunnel is made from the antecubital fossa to the counterincision in a curvilinear fashion.
- The prosthetic graft is gently pulled through the tunnel.
- A similar curvilinear-like tunnel is made from the counterincision back to the antecubital fossa.
- The graft is then gently pulled though the tunnel.
- The tunneled graft should resemble an oval loop, with the apex at the counterincision.
  - The site should be inspected to ensure there are no kinks.
- A 3000-unit dose of systemic heparin is administered before occluding the artery with vessel loops.

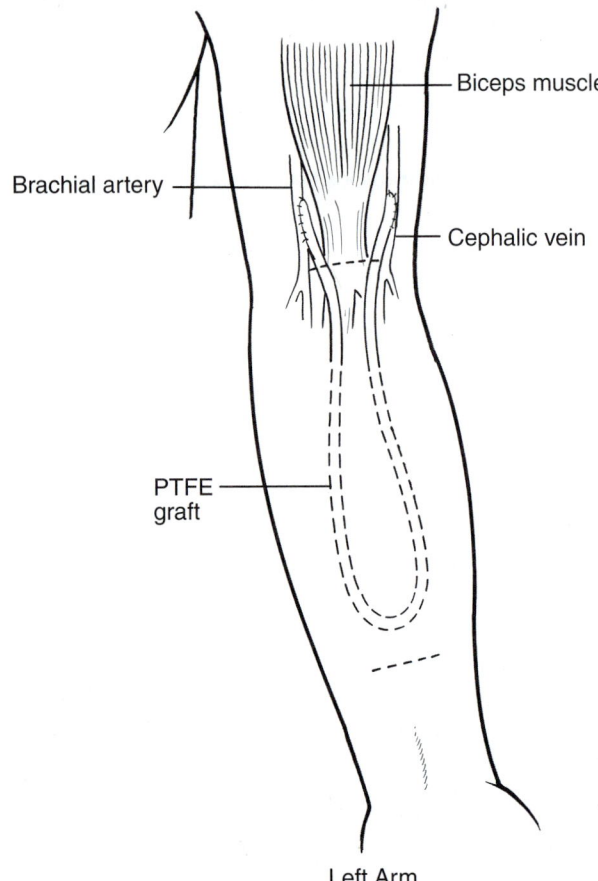

Figure 33–4

- Using a No. 11 blade, a small arteriotomy is made on the anterior surface of the artery.
  - Care should be taken not to incise the back wall of the artery with the knife.
- Micro-Potts scissors are used to extend the arteriotomy 5–6 mm in a slightly angled fashion.
- The graft is anastomosed to the artery using a 5-0 ePTFE suture.
- Following the anastomosis, tension is gently released on the proximal vessel loop to assess arterial flow.
- The vessel loops placed earlier around the venous structures are gently occluded.
- The caliber of the laterally running cephalic vein is often large enough for the venous anastomosis.
- A No. 11 blade is used to make a small venotomy, being careful not to incise the back wall of the vein with the knife.
- Micro-Potts scissors are used to extend the venotomy, usually to approximately 1.5 cm, depending on the graft size.
- The graft is then anastomosed to the vein using a 6-0 ePTFE suture.
- Following completion of the anastomosis, a palpable thrill should be felt in the graft and in the proximal vein.
- The wounds may be closed with deep dermal interrupted sutures followed by a running subcuticular absorbable stitch.

Additional Access Strategies

- Autogenous posterior radial branch-cephalic access.
- Lower extremity venous transposition with the great saphenous vein.
- Lower extremity prosthetic graft insertion.
- Axillary artery prosthetic graft insertion.

POSTOPERATIVE CARE

- The operation should be performed as an outpatient procedure.
- The patient may remove the dressing after 48 hours.
- A sling may be offered for the patient's comfort, although it is not necessary.
- The patient should return for follow-up examination in 4 weeks.
  - The wound is checked for signs of infection or poor healing.
  - The vein is palpated for a thrill.
  - Distal radial and ulnar pulses are palpated.
- Most autogenous fistulas will be ready for use in 8–12 weeks.
  - The vein is assessed to determine if the caliber is large enough to accommodate dialysis access.
- Prosthetic grafts are usually ready for use in 4 weeks.

POTENTIAL COMPLICATIONS

- Early thrombosis.
  - Technical error.
  - Hypercoagulable state.
  - Low cardiac output.
  - Poor inflow.
  - Poor outflow.
- Late thrombosis.
  - Intimal hyperplasia causing progressive outflow venous stenosis.
  - Hypotension during hemodialysis.
  - Worsening inflow stenosis.
  - Poor puncture technique with excessive pressure.
- Arteriovenous access steal syndrome.
  - Diagnosed by clinical examination and history.
  - Cool hand.
  - Diminished distal pulses.
  - Hand pain.
  - Confirmed by Doppler finger waveforms and pressures.
- Ischemic monomelic neuropathy.
  - Acute and potentially irreversible dysfunction of the radial, median, and ulnar nerves.
  - Pain, paresthesia, and diminished motor function of the wrist and hand.
  - Absence of tissue ischemia.
  - Preserved distal palpable radial pulse or Doppler signal.
  - Presumably caused by alteration in blood flow to the vasa vasorum of the above-mentioned nerves.
- Venous hypertension.
  - Hand and upper extremity swelling with pain.
  - Usually secondary to undiagnosed or recently formed central venous stenosis or occlusion; however, severe valvular incompetence with retrograde flow can also produce these symptoms.

PEARLS AND TIPS

- Wear surgical loupes while operating.
- When inserting a prosthetic graft, perform the arterial anastomosis first. The arterial graft is more likely to ooze from needle holes. Place a hemostatic agent around your suture line and perform the venous anastomosis. This allows time for hemostasis to be achieved by the completion of the operation.
- When dissecting out the vein, be cognizant of small venous tributaries that will need to be ligated and divided. Limit tearing of such veins by careful sharp dissection with Metzenbaum scissors rather than using electrocautery for the dissection.

- Sewing the back wall of the arterial venous anastomosis first enables the surgeon to use a forehand approach and quickly finish the anastomosis on the front wall.
- Always dissect out and mobilize more vein than you think will be needed.
- When dissecting out the venous structures in the antecubital fossa, be mindful of posterior perforating veins. These will have to be controlled with a vessel loop in order to perform the anastomosis in a bloodless field.
- Before performing the anastomosis, arterial and venous (although to a lesser degree) spasm can be relieved with topical application of papaverine. Application of papaverine can cause vasodilation, allowing for easier completion of the anastomosis.

REFERENCES

Bohannon WT, Silva MB. Venous Transpositions in the Creation of Arteriovenous Access. In: Rutherford R, ed. *Rutherford Vascular Surgery*, 6th ed. Philadelphia, PA: Elsevier Saunders; 2005:1677–1683.

NKF-K/DOQI Clinical practice guidelines for vascular access: Update 2000. *Am J Kidney Dis.* 2001;37:S137–S181.

Stoney RJ, Effeney DJ. *Comprehensive Vascular Exposures.* Philadelphia, PA: Lippincott; 1998:131–144.

Weiswasser JM, Sidawy AN. Strategies of Arteriovenous Dialysis Access. In: Rutherford R, ed. *Rutherford Vascular Surgery*, 6th ed. Philadelphia, PA: Elsevier Saunders; 2005:1669–1676.

CHAPTER 34

Management of Infrarenal Abdominal Aortic Aneurysm

Michael S. Shillingford, MD, Loay S. Kabbani, MD, and Gilbert R. Upchurch, Jr, MD

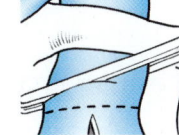
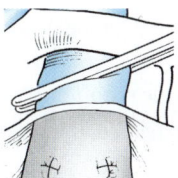
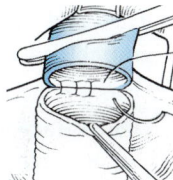
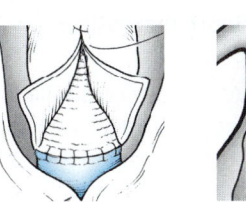
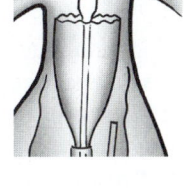

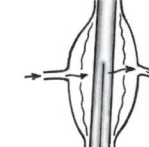

INDICATIONS

- Symptomatic or ruptured abdominal aortic aneurysm (AAA) of any size.
- Asymptomatic AAA ≥ 5.5 cm or > 0.8-cm growth in 12 months.

CONTRAINDICATIONS

Absolute
- None.

Relative
- Malignancy with limited life expectancy.
- Prohibitive medical comorbidities.

INFORMED CONSENT

- Infrarenal AAA may be treated by open or endovascular repair.
- Perioperative mortality:
  - Open repair: 2–5%.
  - Endovascular repair: 1.2–1.6%.
  - Repair of ruptured AAA: 50–75%.

Expected Benefits
- Exclusion of the aneurysm wall from the systemic circulation and associated pressure, thereby preventing its rupture.

Potential Risks
A. OPEN REPAIR
- The established treatment option for AAA for > 50 years.
  - Associated with excellent long-term outcomes and fewer subsequent aneurysm-related procedures than endovascular repair.

- Limited by comorbidities.
- Can treat all aneurysms with no anatomic restraints.
- Involves longer hospital and ICU stays, results in more postoperative pain, and is associated with a higher 30-day mortality rate than endovascular repair.
■ Complications include but are not limited to:
  - Surgical site infections and incisional hernias.
  - Myocardial infarction.
  - Renal or respiratory failure.
  - Retrograde ejaculation.
  - Colonic ischemia.
  - Embolization of clot to the legs.

B. Endovascular Repair
■ Well established for patients who are not surgical candidates and increasingly being used for all anatomically favorable aneurysms.
  - Has specific anatomic requirements.
  - Rate of aneurysm-related reintervention is higher than for open repair.
  - Patients require lifelong follow-up with serial imaging.
  - Is associated with a lower 30-day mortality rate than open repair.
■ Complications following endovascular repair are similar to those for open repair, excluding retrograde ejaculation and incisional hernia. In addition, approximately 15% of patients treated with an endovascular approach will need at least one additional procedure to better seal the aneurysm from an endoleak or to fix a complication (eg, graft migration, stent fracture, graft material fatigue).

EQUIPMENT
Open Repair
■ Vascular surgery instrument tray.
■ Bookwalter or Omni retractor for abdominal exposure.
■ Graft material (Dacron or polytetrafluoroethylene [PTFE]) of various sizes, 12–36 mm).

Endovascular Repair
■ Vascular surgery instrument tray.
■ Sterile angiographic capabilities with a full compliment of catheters and wires.
  - A portable C-arm may be used, but a fixed fluoroscopic unit gives better images.
■ The procedure should be done in a room with operative capabilities (eg, suction, electrocautery, good lighting, etc).
■ An angiogram table that permits fluoroscopic imaging of the abdomen is required.

PATIENT PREPARATION
■ The arterial anatomy needs to be defined clearly.
  - CT angiogram or MR angiogram may provide sufficient detail for operative planning.
■ Preoperative stratification with a full history and physical examination is required.
  - Eagle criteria or another cardiac risk stratification algorithm can be used to calculate the patient's perioperative risk for coronary events and need for further workup.
■ All patients should receive optimal medical therapy in the perioperative period, including:
  - β-Blockers.
  - Statin therapy, with a goal low-density lipoprotein (LDL) cholesterol of < 100 mg/dL.
  - Tight blood glucose control, with a target level < 140 mg/dL (for at least the first 3 days postoperatively).
■ Appropriate prophylactic antibiotics are delivered within 30 minutes of skin incision and are redosed as needed for prolonged procedures (eg, intravenous cefazolin, 1 g preoperatively, then 1 g every 8 hours intraoperatively).
■ Invasive hemodynamic monitoring with at least an arterial line.

Endovascular Repair
■ Preprocedural imaging (CT or MRI) to determine the size of the aneurysm.
  - Aneurysm measurements must be determined precisely in advance of the operation and the appropriate size grafts must be available.
■ Important measurements used to determine the graft sizes are:
  - Location and diameter of the aortic aneurysm neck.
  - Distance between the lowest renal artery and the start of the aneurysm (must be > 10–15 mm).
  - Shape of the neck (a conical-shaped neck is less desirable for endovascular repair).
  - Angulation of the neck (> 60 degrees is less desirable for endovascular repair).
  - Aneurysm lengths (measured from the lowest renal artery to the aortic bifurcation [L1], and from the renal artery to both distal landing zones [L2 and L3]).
  - Diameter of the iliac arteries and their suitability as a landing zone (amount of thrombus and calcium).
  - Diameter of the femoral arteries and external iliac arteries for access (> 7 mm is usually required for most endografts).

PATIENT POSITIONING
Open Repair
■ Anterior approach: the patient should be supine, with a lumbar roll placed to allow for better aortic exposure and arms extended on arm boards.

- Retroperitoneal approach: the patient should be in left lateral decubitus position.

Endovascular Repair
- The patient should be supine on the angiotable, with both arms tucked or extended.

Both Procedures
- A nasogastric tube is inserted.
- A Foley catheter is placed.
- Distal pulses are marked.
- Two large-bore intravenous lines are placed to provide for rapid infusion.
- A radial arterial line is placed for hemodynamic monitoring.

PROCEDURE

Open Repair
- Epidural anesthesia is administered for intraoperative and postoperative pain control.
- **Figure 34–1:** Incision and exposure.
  - A midline incision is made from the xiphoid to below the umbilicus. Transverse or left lateral retroperitoneal incisions can also be made.
  - The abdomen is explored for any additional pathology. The position of the nasogastric tube in the stomach is noted.
  - The small bowel can be packed in the right flank or eviscerated into a plastic bag to help maximize exposure of the retroperitoneum. The transverse colon is reflected cephalad.
  - The retroperitoneum is exposed from the ligament of Treitz to the aortic bifurcation using electrocautery.
  - Care must be taken to ligate or clip all lymphatics.
  - Once the aneurysm is exposed, the aortic neck should be carefully dissected up to the left renal vein. If the aneurysm is pararenal, both renal arteries may need to be dissected out and controlled.
  - The distal anastomosis site depends on the extent of the aneurysm (terminal aorta, common iliac, external iliac, or femoral arteries).
  - Heparin (100 units × wt [kg]) is administered, followed by mannitol, 12.5 g. At least 3 minutes are allowed for appropriate heparin circulation before clamping the aorta. An activated clotting time (ACT) > 250 is maintained throughout the procedure.
  - Vascular clamps are applied distally first (common or external iliac or femoral arteries) and then proximally (aortic neck) to achieve vascular control.
  - The aorta is opened longitudinally, using electrocautery initially followed by surgical scissors.
- **Figure 34–2:** Control of bleeding vessels.

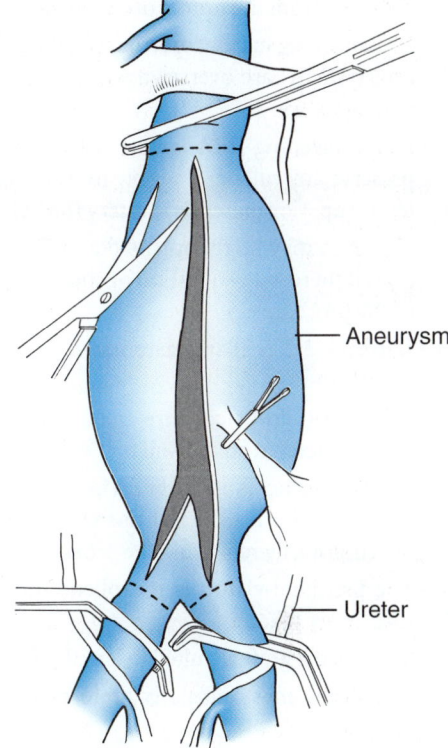

Figure 34–1

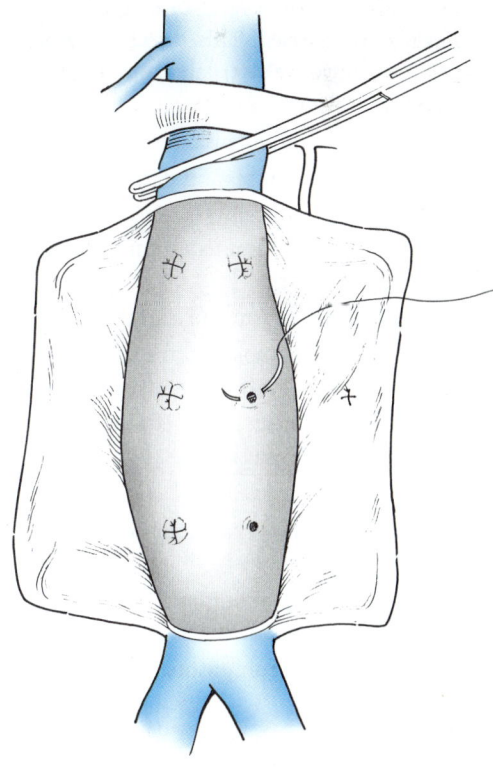

Figure 34–2

- Aneurysm thrombus and atherosclerotic debris are removed from the lumen of the aorta.
- Backbleeding lumbar arteries and the inferior mesenteric artery (IMA) are oversewn with 2-0 silk or 3-0 polypropylene suture.
- A backbleeding IMA is ligated from inside the aorta to preserve any collateral supply from the hypogastric arteries or superior mesenteric artery (SMA).
- The IMA may be reimplanted as a Carrel patch onto the graft if there is any question of colonic ischemia at the end of the procedure.

■ **Figure 34–3:** Vascular anastomosis.
- Proximally, an end-to-end anastomosis is performed using a 3-0 Prolene suture and a strip of felt to reinforce the degenerated aortic wall.
- The anastomosis is checked for leaks first by injecting saline into the distal graft lumen using a bulb syringe, then by temporarily removing the proximal clamp.
- The proximal clamp is reapplied and, if needed, repair sutures are placed.
- Distally, the graft is pulled to length, then cut.
- The distal anastomosis is preformed using 3-0 or 4-0 Prolene.
- The proximal clamp is removed thereby testing the integrity of the distal anastomosis. Any necessary repair sutures are placed.
- The femoral arteries are occluded with manual pressure in each groin for several cardiac cycles while the distal clamps are released. This directs atheroemboli into the pelvis through the internal iliac vessels and not down the legs.
- Sigmoid colon viability is assessed.
- Lower extremity pulses and signals are checked.
- Once all surgical bleeding is controlled, heparin is reversed with intravenous administration of protamine (1 mg per 100 units of heparin).

■ **Figure 34–4:** Aneurysm and abdominal wall closure.
- After adequate hemostasis, the aortic wall is closed over the newly placed graft using 3-0 Prolene sutures.
- The retroperitoneal tissue is reapproximated over the aorta using 2-0 Vicryl sutures.
- Retractors are removed.
- Small and large bowel are replaced into normal anatomic position.
- Standard running abdominal closure of the fascia is performed using looped PDS or Prolene suture.
- Skin closure is accomplished with Monocryl sutures or skin staples.

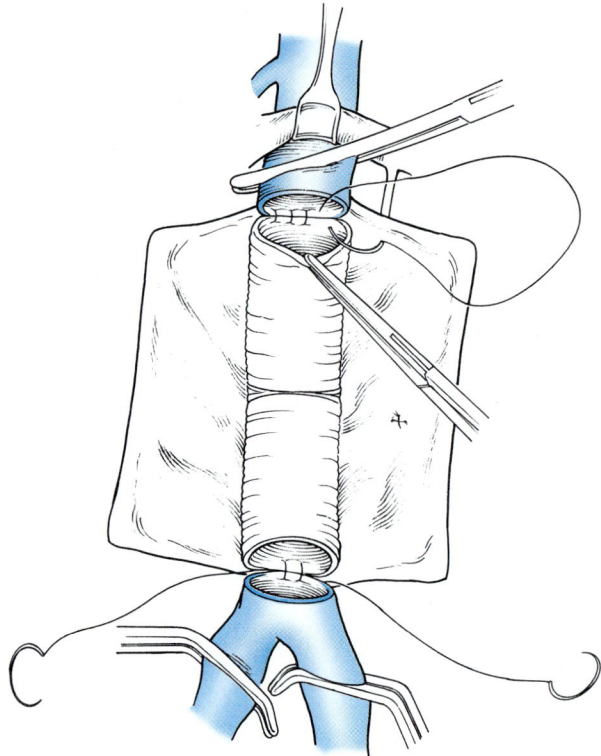

Figure 34–3

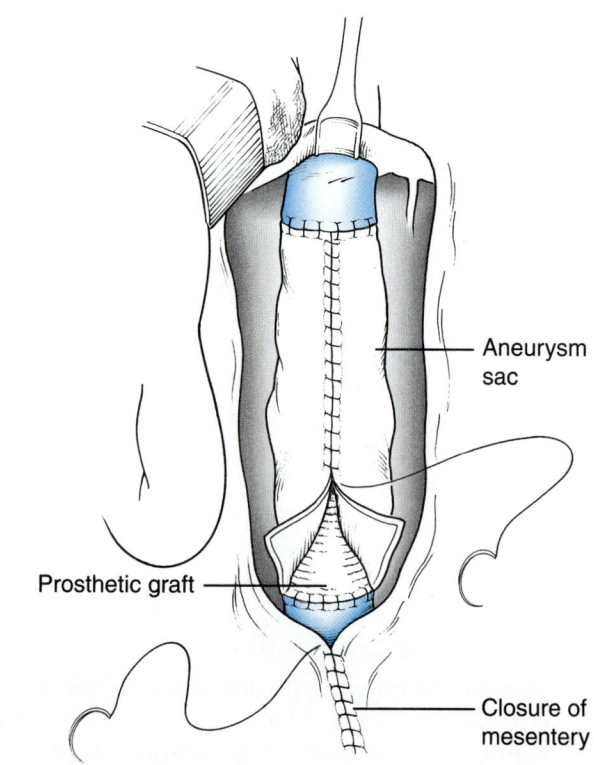

Figure 34–4

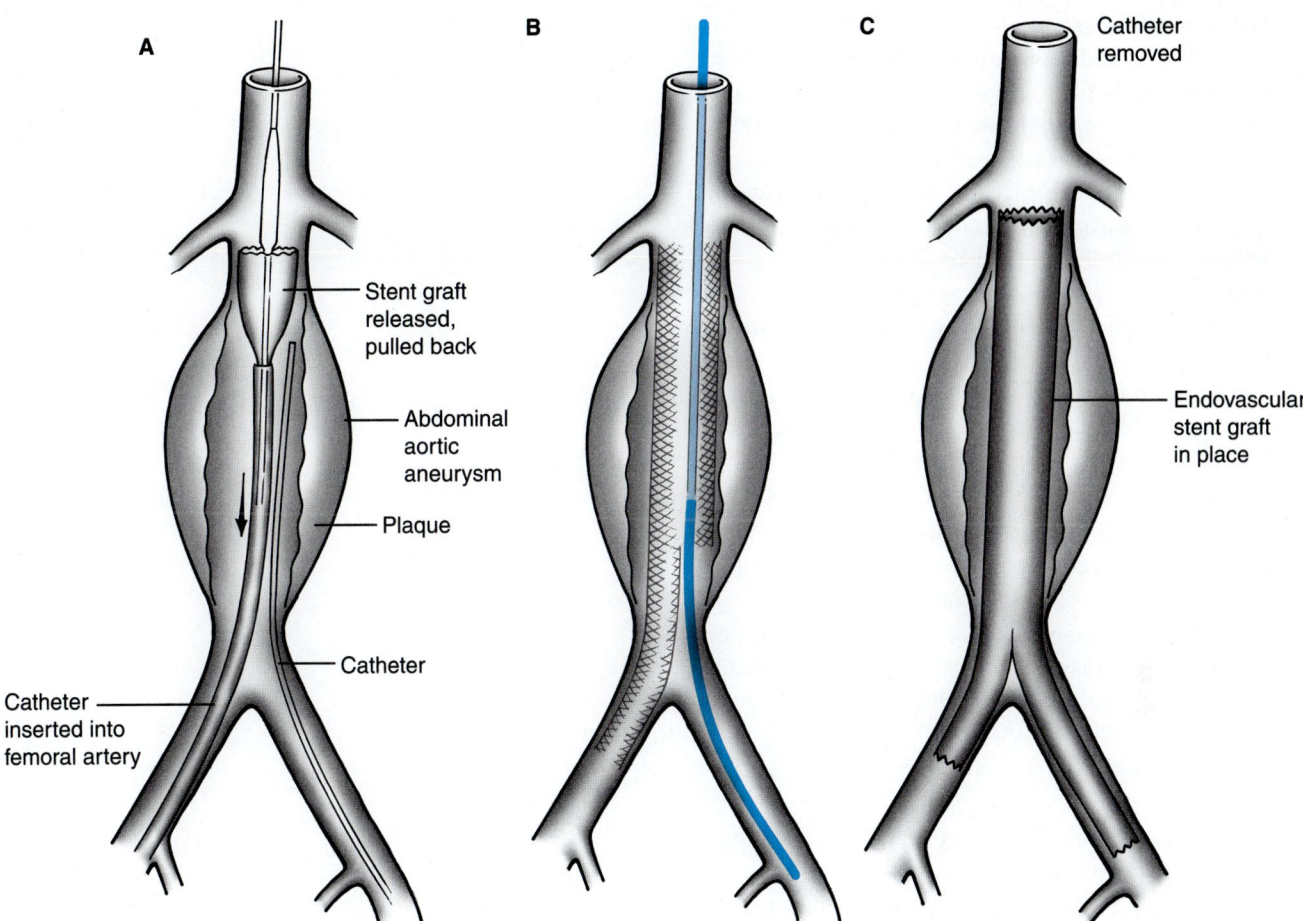

Figure 34–5A–C

Endovascular Repair

- General anesthesia is preferable, but endovascular repair may be attempted under epidural, spinal, or even local anesthesia.
- **Figures 34–5A-C:** Stent graft insertion.
  - The abdomen and each groin are prepared.
  - Exposure of both common femoral arteries is performed with proximal and distal control using vessel loops in a Potts fashion (double looping the artery for hemostatic control).
  - The patient is heparinized with 100 units/kg, and ACT > 250 is maintained throughout the procedure.
  - The ipsilateral (IL) femoral artery (the artery through which the main body of the graft will be inserted) is selected preoperatively based on suitable anatomy.
  - Both the IL femoral and contralateral (CL) femoral arteries are cannulated.
  - Using an 18-gauge needle, the artery is punctured and a 0.035-inch flexible J guidewire is passed under fluoroscopic control into the thoracic aorta.
  - The needle is removed and a 7 French sheath is placed.

- On the IL side, a catheter is inserted over the wire into the thoracic aorta, and the wire is removed. Next, a super-stiff guidewire (eg, Lunderquist wire) is inserted into the catheter and positioned just below the left subclavian artery.
- Using the CL femoral artery, an angio-scaled catheter (eg, pigtail) is inserted to the level of the renal arteries (around L1–2) and an aortogram is preformed. Usually 15 mL/s of iodinated contrast is injected over 2 seconds (for a total of 30 mL).
- The renal arteries and the aortic bifurcation are marked out.
- The main body of the aortic endograft that has already been selected based on preoperative sizing is opened on the field.
- The graft is prepared on the back table.
- Most grafts need to be oriented prior to insertion so that the radiopaque markers on the CL limb of the graft are oriented toward the contralateral artery.
- The graft is inserted into the aorta through the IL femoral artery over the stiff guidewire and positioned so that the covered portion of the graft deploys just below the lowest renal artery (Figure 34–5A).
- The main body of the graft is deployed and the CL limb is released.
- The CL limb is cannulated from the CL groin. An angled guide catheter over a glide wire is used.
- To make absolutely sure the CL limb is cannulated, the angle guide catheter is advanced into the main body of the graft and spun around.
- Injection of a small amount of contrast through the angle guide catheter into the main body of the graft may also document proper cannulation. Alternatively, insertion of a balloon catheter over the wire into the CL limb, and inflation of the balloon, can confirm proper cannulation.
- A stiff guidewire is then inserted into the CL limb and positioned just under the subclavian artery (Figure 34–5B).
- In the pelvis, the location of the CL hypogastric artery is marked after injecting contrast through the CL sheath.
- The CL limb of the graft is then inserted and deployed.
- We use a compliant balloon to seat and seal the graft proximally just below the renal arteries, at the overlapping segments, and at the distal attachment sites (Figure 34–5C).
- A final angiogram is performed to document proper placement and the occurrence of endoleaks, some of which need attention at the time of primary graft placement (type I and III endoleaks), while others may be observed (type II endoleaks).

■ **Figure 34–6:** The four types of endoleaks.
- Type I: leak from the proximal or distal landing zones.
- Type II: leak from a back-bleeding lumbar or inferior mesenteric artery into the aneurysm sac (the most common endoleak).

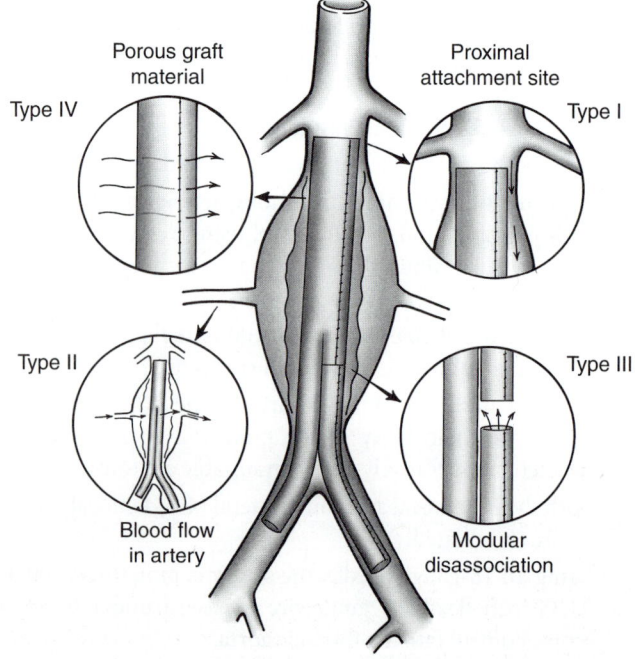

Figure 34–6

- Type III: leak caused by inadequate graft-to-graft overlap at the junctions.
- Type IV: porosity leak through the graft material (rare with the current grafts).
- The sheaths are pulled followed by the wires.
- The femoral arteries are closed with Prolene suture.
- The groins are closed in several layers.
- Distal pulses and signals are documented.

POSTOPERATIVE CARE

Open Repair

- Patients usually are extubated in the operating room or within the first 12 hours and out of bed by postoperative day (POD) 1.
- The typical patient requires up to 2 days in the ICU.
- During the first 24–48 hours, patients require adequate fluid resuscitation.
- We recommend aggressive diuresis of uncomplicated patients starting on POD 3 to prevent cardiac and pulmonary complications.
- All central venous lines and arterial catheters should be removed as early as possible to decrease the risks of catheter-related infections.
- The nasogastric tube may be removed on POD 1 or according to physician preference.
- Most patients who have uncomplicated procedures are ready for discharge home by POD 7.

Endovascular Repair

- Patients are extubated in the operating room.
- Patients should be assigned to a telemetry floor bed.
- Most patients with uncomplicated procedures are ready for discharge by POD 1 or 2.

POTENTIAL COMPLICATIONS

Open Repair

A. Intraoperative Complications
- Injury to the small bowel, colon, ureter, or major venous structures.

B. Postoperative Complications
- Myocardial infarction.
- Bleeding.
- Infections, including urinary tract or wound complications.
- Pneumonia.
- Bowel ischemia (particularly of the descending and sigmoid colon).
- Lower extremity ischemia from distal embolization, thrombosis, or clamp injuries.
- Renal failure.

Endovascular Repair

A. Intraoperative Complications
- Malposition of the graft.
- Arterial dissection or rupture.
- Avulsion of iliac arteries.
- Endoleaks.

B. Postoperative Complications
- Myocardial infarction.
- Infections, including urinary tract or wound complications.
- Pneumonia.
- Bowel ischemia (particularly of the descending and sigmoid colon).
- Lower extremity ischemia from distal embolization, thrombosis, or clamp injuries.
- Renal failure.

PEARLS AND TIPS

- In 5% of patients, the renal vein is retroaortic and can be injured during open para-aortic dissection.
- Use care during dissection around the aortic bifurcation and IMA to prevent sympathetic nerve injuries (the left side of the aorta), which may result in retrograde ejaculation in men. Care must also be taken not to injure the iliac veins (posterior and to the right of the aorta).
- Abdominal pain and loose stools with or without bloody bowel movements in the initial postoperative period may indicate ischemic colitis.
  - Diagnosis is with flexible sigmoidoscopy.
  - Treatment depends on the degree of ischemia and can range from broad-spectrum antibiotics to colectomy with ostomy.
- Treat wound cellulitis early to prevent bacterial seeding of graft.

REFERENCES

Huber T, Lee A, Ozaki K, Seeger J. Abdominal Aortic Aneurysms. In: Mulholland MW, Lillemoe KD, Doherty GM, et al, eds. *Greenfield's Surgery: Scientific Principles & Practice,* 4th ed. Philadelphia, PA: Lippincott Williams & Wilkins; 2006:1711–1747.

Upchurch GR, et al. Complications of Arterial Surgery. In: Mulholland MW, Doherty GM, eds. *Complications in Surgery.* Philadelphia, PA: Lippincott Williams & Wilkins; 2006:317–335.

CHAPTER 35

Carotid Endarterectomy

Christopher Longo, MD, and Ramon Berguer, MD, PhD

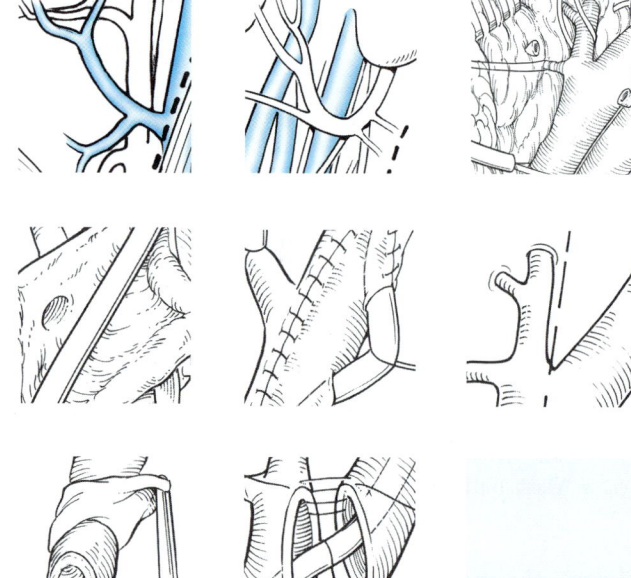

INDICATIONS

- Asymptomatic carotid stenosis > 60% by angiography or 70% by duplex ultrasound.
- Symptomatic carotid stenosis (cerebrovascular accident, transient ischemic attack, or amaurosis fugax) > 50%.
- Carotid endarterectomy can be performed safely under regional anesthesia in patients with severe chronic obstructive pulmonary disease, coronary artery disease (CAD), and other comorbidities.
- Carotid stenting can be considered in patients with a history of neck irradiation, modified radical neck dissection, or reoperative carotid endarterectomy.
- Only patients with concurrent *symptomatic* carotid stenosis and *symptomatic* CAD should be considered for combined carotid endarterectomy and coronary artery bypass grafting.

CONTRAINDICATIONS

- There are no absolute contraindications other than distal internal artery occlusion.

INFORMED CONSENT

Expected Benefits

- Long-term stroke prevention.

Potential Risks

- The risk of perioperative stroke is ≤ 1.5% in expert series.
- The risk of a clinically significant cranial nerve injury is similarly small in experienced hands and includes:
  - Injury to the hypoglossal nerve with tongue deviation toward the operative side.
  - Injury to the vagus nerve or a nonrecurrent laryngeal nerve (which may result in ipsilateral vocal cord paralysis).
  - Superior laryngeal nerve injury (which may result in difficulty speaking at high pitch).

- A retraction injury to the marginal mandibular branch of the facial nerve (which may result in a lower facial droop).
■ Glossopharyngeal nerve injury (a concern in exposures approaching the skull base).
  - Spinal accessory nerve injury (a risk only if dissection is not conducted anterior to the internal jugular vein).
  - Other complications include myocardial infarction, postoperative bleeding requiring reexploration, wound infection, local sensory loss, and restenosis.
■ It should be emphasized that regular postoperative surveillance by duplex ultrasound is required to monitor for restenosis.

EQUIPMENT

■ No special equipment is required.
■ A small, self-retaining retractor such as the "mini" Omnitract may be helpful, particularly if high exposure is necessary.
■ We prefer to control the distal internal carotid artery with an atraumatic clip (eg, Schwartz, Yasargil, or Heifetz).

PATIENT PREPARATION

■ Duplex ultrasound is highly sensitive and specific and is the only preoperative imaging required in most cases.
■ Arteriography (conventional or CT) is generally reserved for cases involving restenosis, a history of radiation or prior neck dissection, or atypical findings on duplex ultrasonography.

PATIENT POSITIONING

■ The patient should be in a semi-seated position with a small roll across the shoulder blades.
  - This allows for gentle extension and external rotation of the head to the contralateral side.
■ The ipsilateral arm is tucked, padding the elbow and wrist.
■ Care should be taken not to over-rotate or extend the head to avoid kinking of the vertebral arteries or contralateral carotid artery.
■ Landmarks such as the ear lobe, angle of the mandible, mastoid process, sternal notch, and clavicle must be included in the prepared area.

PROCEDURE

■ Carotid endarterectomy can be performed under regional anesthesia, general anesthesia with routine shunting, or general anesthesia with selective shunting based on adjuncts such as intraoperative EEG monitoring or stump pressures.

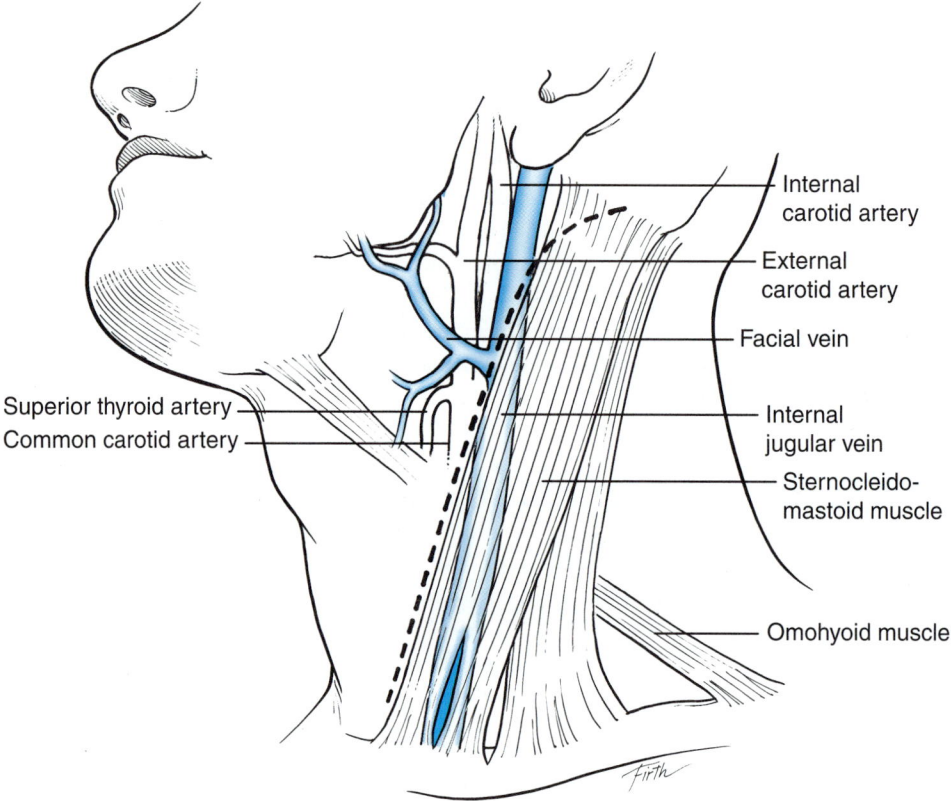

Figure 35–1

- **Figure 35–1:** Most surgeons prefer an oblique incision along the anterior border of the sternocleidomastoid (SCM) muscle.
  - A transverse incision is cosmetically superior and technically feasible for all patients except those with the highest lesions.
  - Electrocautery is used to divide the platysma and dissect along the medial border of the SCM muscle from its tendon superiorly to the level of the omohyoid muscle inferiorly.
  - The medial edge of the internal jugular vein (IJV) is identified by sharp dissection.
  - Ligation and division of the common facial and the middle thyroid vein inferiorly and any hypoglossal veins superiorly, allows for lateral retraction of the SCM and IJV.
- **Figure 35–2:** Great care must be taken to identify the cranial nerves of interest.
  - The vagus nerve usually lies posterolateral to the carotid arteries but can be located anteriorly, placing it at risk of injury early in the dissection.
  - The ansa cervicalis can be divided near its origin and followed in a cephalad direction to the hypoglossal nerve.
  - Dissection of the superior thyroid artery should be kept to its origin to avoid injury to the external branch of the superior laryngeal nerve.

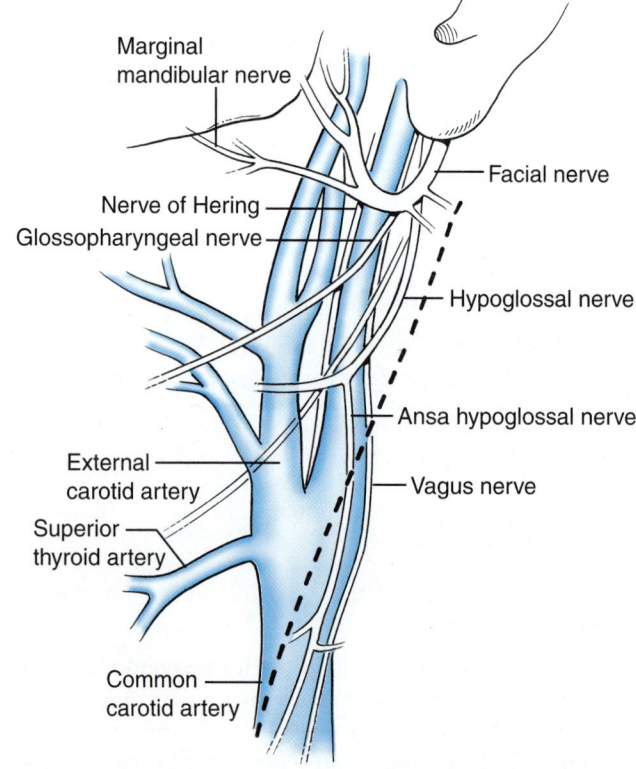

Figure 35–2

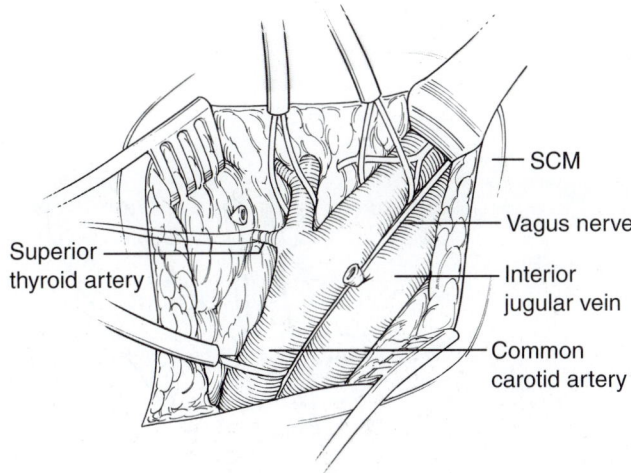

Figure 35–3

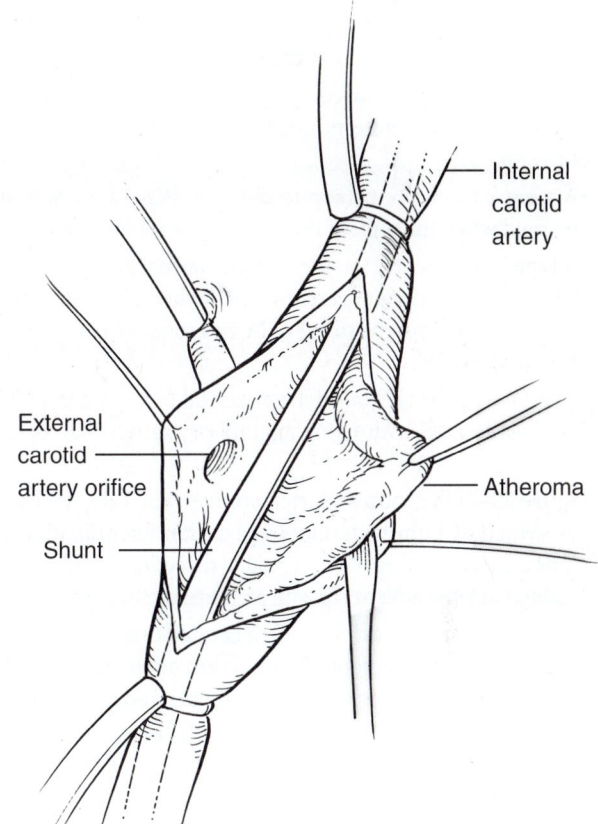

Figure 35–4

- **Figure 35–3:** The common (CCA), external (ECA), and internal carotid (ICA) arteries are circumferentially dissected and encircled with vascular loops.
  - The superior thyroid artery can be looped with a 2-0 silk ligature.
  - The distal ICA can be controlled with a Schwartz clip.
  - A long plaque or high carotid bifurcation necessitates additional distal exposure of the ICA; this requires division of the digastric muscle and any underlying crossing veins.
  - Cephalad mobilization of the hypoglossal nerve is achieved through ligation and division of the occipital artery and the sternocleidomastoid artery.
- **Figure 35–4:** A longitudinal arteriotomy is made and a shunt of the surgeon's choice is used, if indicated.
  - The atheroma is bluntly dissected and elevated in a medial plane.
  - The proximal plaque in a relatively healthy portion of the CCA is sharply cut and the plaque dissected in a cephalad direction toward a finely feathered endpoint.
  - Eversion endarterectomy of the ECA is required.
  - The bed should be irrigated vigorously with heparinized saline and any remaining loose bits of media removed with fine forceps.
  - If a satisfactory endpoint is not found, the remaining distal plaque can be secured to the vessel with interrupted, full-thickness 7-0 sutures tied on the adventitial surface.
- **Figure 35–5:** Once the endarterectomy is complete, a patch of the desired material (Dacron or bovine pericardium) is cut to fit the length and shape of the arteriotomy.
  - Prior to completion of the patch angioplasty the shunt is removed, the ICA is allowed to back-bleed, and the atheroma bed is irrigated with heparinized saline.

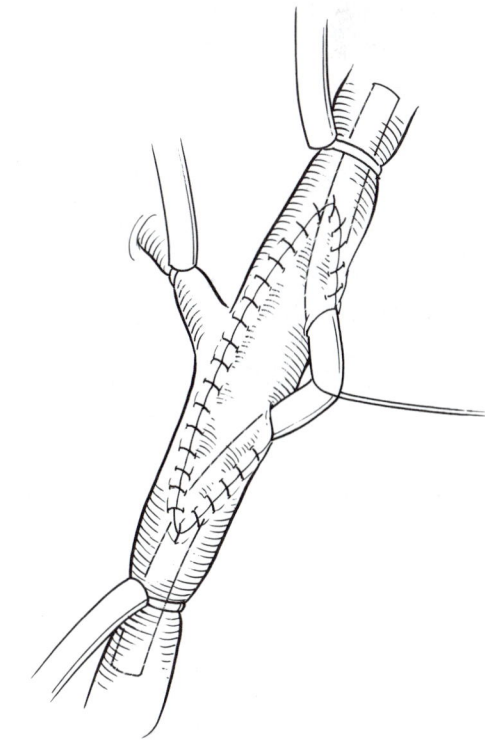

Figure 35–5

- Upon completion of the circumferential and continuous suture line, flow is established into the ECA prior to establishing antegrade flow into the ICA.
- **Figure 35–6:** The transection plane for eversion carotid endarterectomy is determined by the location of the bulk of the plaque.
  - A type I transection (severe oblique, ICA only) is performed when the bulk of the lesion is located in the ICA.
  - A type II transection (gentle oblique, across the CCA 3 mm below the flow divider) is performed when the bulk of the disease lies within the distal CCA and most proximal portion of the ICA.
  - Lesions extending beyond the proximal 2–3 cm of the ICA are best treated with patch angioplasty rather than eversion.
- **Figure 35–7:** Eversion endarterectomy (type I depicted) is performed by bluntly developing a circumferential medial plane and continuing it in a cephalad direction while gently pulling back the adventitia with atraumatic forceps.
  - The arteriotomy is extended in a caudad direction on the lateral CCA and in a cephalad direction on the medial ICA to allow for an even wider, circumferential anastomosis.
- **Figure 35–8:** Once the ICA portion of the eversion endarterectomy is complete a shunt may be placed, as indicated.
  - The primary anastomosis is quite wide, necessitating use of synthetic patch material.
  - If the ICA is redundant in length it may be cut shorter or implanted more proximally on the CCA, making eversion endarterectomy ideal for patients with ICA stenosis in the setting of concurrent ICA elongation.

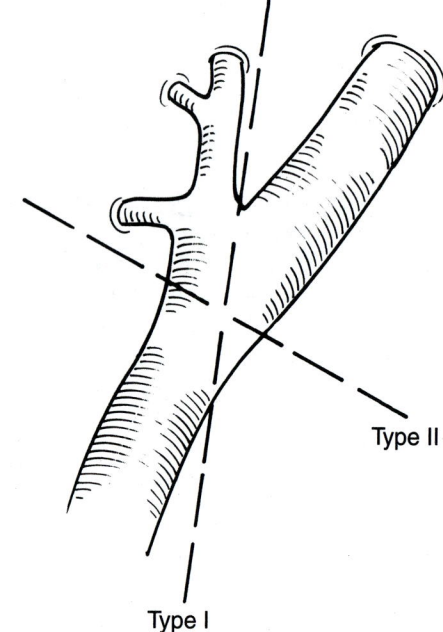

Figure 35–6

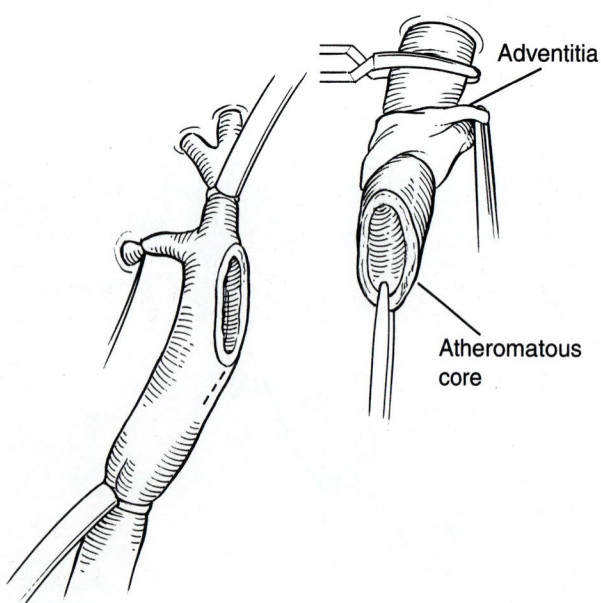

Figure 35–7

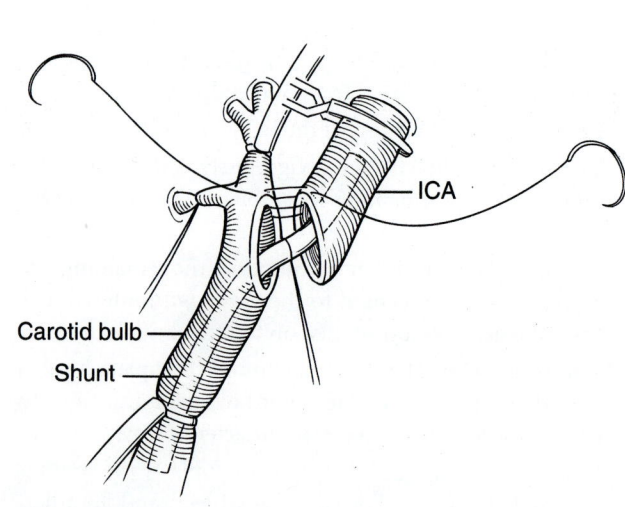

Figure 35–8

POSTOPERATIVE CARE

- Closed suction drain overnight, depending on surgeon preference.
- Strict postoperative management of blood pressure, avoiding hypertension to reduce the risk of hyperperfusion syndrome.
- Discharge following overnight observation and monitoring (possibly 8 hours postoperatively if uncomplicated and with satisfactory blood pressure).

POTENTIAL COMPLICATIONS

- Cranial nerve injury.
- Stroke.
- Myocardial infarction.
- Carotid restenosis.

PEARLS AND TIPS

- Do not hesitate to expose the distal ICA early in the procedure by the techniques discussed.
  - This is much more difficult to do once the ICA is clipped and an arteriotomy has been made.
  - In eversion cases, the ICA can be transposed anterior to the hypoglossal nerve to facilitate distal exposure and anastomosis.
- In rare cases when the ICA must be exposed at the level of C1 or above, a retrojugular approach is preferable.
  - This is more likely in reoperative surgery or if preoperative imaging reveals an extremely long lesion or unusually high bifurcation.
  - Nasotracheal intubation and mandibular subluxation are useful adjuncts for this approach.
- A "nonrecurrent" laryngeal nerve may cross the carotid artery as it courses from the vagus nerve. If not recognized, it can be mistaken for a branch of the ansa cervicalis and damaged or ligated, resulting in ipsilateral vocal cord paralysis.

REFERENCES

Ballotta E, Da Giau G, Baracchini C, Manara R. Carotid eversion endarterectomy: perioperative outcome and restenosis incidence. *Ann Vasc Surg*. 2002;16:422–429.

Chiesa R, Melissano G, Castellano R, et al. Carotid endarterectomy: experience in 5425 cases. *Ann Vasc Surg*. 2004;18:527–534.

Green RM, Greenberg R, Illig K, et al. Eversion endarterectomy of the carotid artery: technical considerations and recurrent stenosis. *J Vasc Surg*. 2000;32:1052–1061.

[CHAPTER 36]

Operative Management of Aortoiliac Occlusive Disease

Gorav Ailawadi, MD

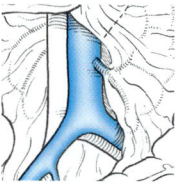 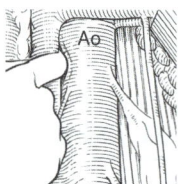 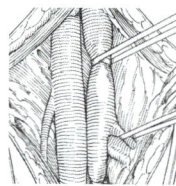
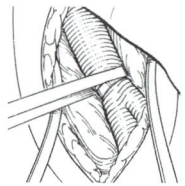 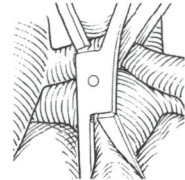 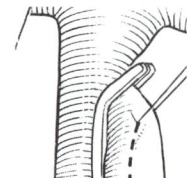
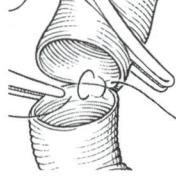 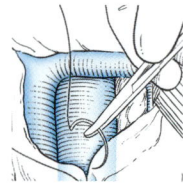 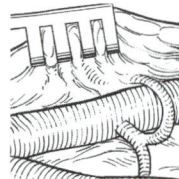

INDICATIONS

- Significant chronic lower extremity ischemia.
  - Lifestyle-limiting claudication, tissue loss, and rest pain.
  - Risk factor modification partially helpful.
- Acute lower extremity ischemia.
  - Thrombosed aortoiliac system.
- Infected aortic graft (prior abdominal aortic graft for aneurysmal or occlusive disease).
- Abdominal aortic aneurysm with iliac disease (occlusive or aneurysmal).

CONTRAINDICATIONS

Absolute
- Chronic ischemia: none.
- Acute ischemia: nonsurvivable acidosis.

Relative
- Cardiopulmonary comorbidities.
- Prior abdominal surgery.
- If significant comorbidities exist, extra-anatomic bypass (axillary-femoral bypass) is preferred.

INFORMED CONSENT

Expected Benefits
- Restoration of adequate blood flow to the pelvis and lower extremities to prevent tissue loss and improve claudication symptoms.

Potential Risks
- Cardiac compromise is common, as more than one third of patients have significant coronary artery disease.
- Respiratory compromise can occur with abdominal approaches.

- Renal dysfunction can occur due to perioperative hemodynamic variation, preoperative intravenous contrast dye administration, and suprarenal aortic cross-clamping.
- Although rare, significant morbidity can occur with graft infections, which can appear late (months to years postoperatively).

EQUIPMENT

- An Omni rectractor is preferred.
- Polytetrafluoroethylene (PTFE) or Dacron bifurcated aortic grafts for aortobifemoral bypass or a ringed PTFE graft for axillary (bi)femoral bypass.
- Vascular clamps and instruments.
- Tunneling device if axillary-femoral bypass is to be performed.
- Doppler ultrasonography is useful to document lower extremity pulses before and after bypass.

PATIENT PREPARATION

- Thorough preoperative workup is essential before recommending aortic surgery.
  - Claudication or rest pain symptoms need to be distinguished from other causes of lower extremity pain.
  - Likewise, tissue loss must be attributable to ischemia, at least in part.
- Screening for peripheral occlusive disease should include ankle-brachial indices (ABIs).
  - Diabetic patients may have calcified vessels, resulting in inaccurate ABIs.
- The gold standard for diagnosis is aortography with evaluation of runoff vessels in the lower extremities.
- CT angiography of the aorta and lower extremity arteries is now frequently used to evaluate aortic and iliac occlusive and aneurysmal disease.
- MR angiography is preferred in patients with renal dysfunction but can overestimate occlusive disease.
- Patient selection is based on preoperative cardiopulmonary testing.
  - Significant cardiac disease can be present in up to 50% of patients.
  - Appropriate cardiac testing, including stress testing, echocardiography, and cardiac catheterization, should be considered in appropriate patients.

PATIENT POSITIONING

- The patient should be supine and prepared from mid chest to the feet.
- The abdomen is entered through a midline incision.
- Groin incisions can be transverse but more often are longitudinal.

PROCEDURE

Aortobifemoral Bypass

- **Figure 36–1:** Exposure of the retroperitoneum and aorta.
  - After a midline laparotomy, the small bowel is retracted to the patient's right side and the transverse colon is lifted superiorly, exposing the ligament of Treitz.
  - The ligament of Treitz is taken down sharply and the duodenum retracted to the right.
  - The retroperitoneum is opened over the aorta, taking care to avoid injuring the duodenum and preserving enough retroperitoneum for later closure.
- **Figure 36–2:** Control of the proximal aorta.
  - The left renal vein is identified crossing the aorta.
  - A noncalcified, minimally diseased region of the aorta suitable for clamping is identified.
  - The infrarenal aorta is dissected free from the surrounding structures.
  - Large lumbar vessels are controlled, preserving collateral vessels, while smaller lumbar vessels can be ligated.
  - The types of vascular clamps used will determine the length of aorta needed; generally this is 3–4 cm.
- **Figure 36–3:** Bilateral femoral artery exposure.
  - Vertical incisions are made over the femoral pulse (artery) at the level of the inguinal ligament.
  - Subcutaneous fat is opened vertically.
  - The femoral sheath is opened sharply, exposing the underlying femoral artery lateral to the femoral vein.
  - The common, superficial, and deep (profunda) femoral arteries are isolated with vessel loops.
  - Circumflex branches are controlled and preserved.
- **Figure 36–4:** Creation of the retroperitoneal tunnel.
  - The proximal common femoral artery is bluntly dissected from the posterior inguinal ligament, taking care to avoid injuring a commonly crossing circumflex vein, and continued onto the anterior external iliac artery.
  - From the abdomen, blunt dissection along the anterior common iliac artery is performed with the contralateral hand lifting the colon and ureter away from the iliac vessels.
  - The dissection is continued bluntly until the contralateral fingers meet.
  - Moving both fingers in a continuous circular motion aids in completion of this tunnel.
  - The tunnel is maintained with a ringed forceps or umbilical tape.
- **Figure 36–5A, B:** Aortic cross-clamping and aortotomy.
  - After adequate heparinization (typically 100 units/kg), the proximal and distal aorta are clamped.
  - Before opening the aorta, the surgeon must ensure that no pulse is present in the clamped aorta and that the clamp is secure.

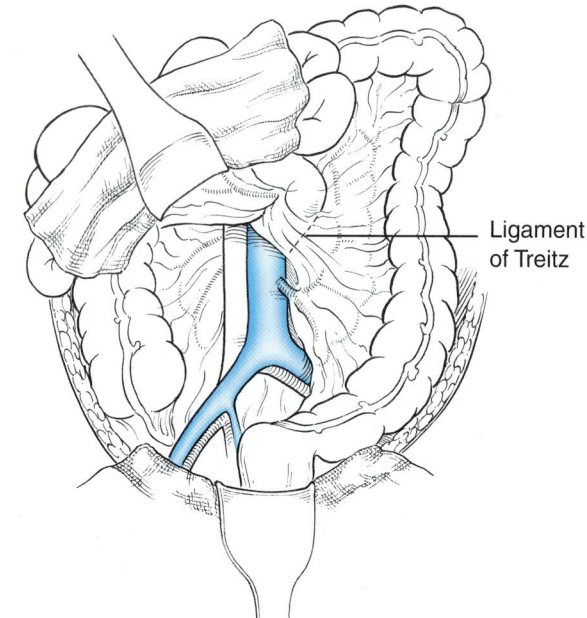

Figure 36–1

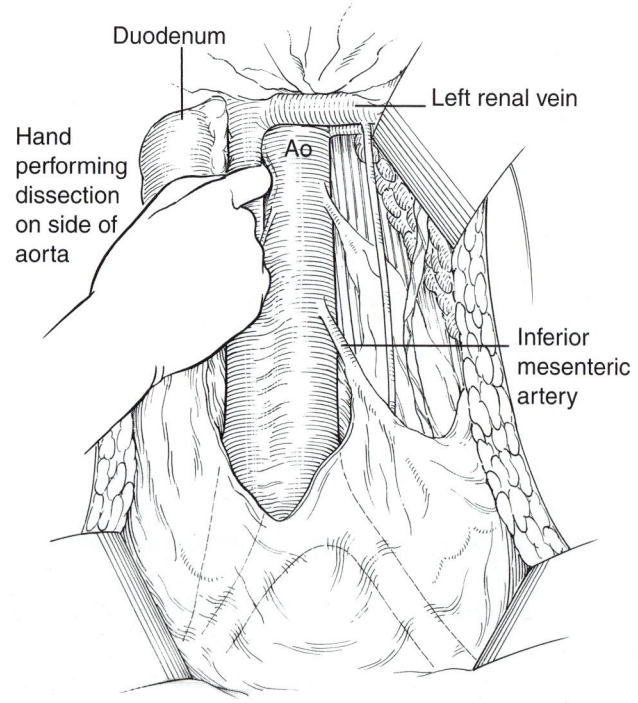

Figure 36–2

Chapter 36 : Operative Management of Aortoiliac Occlusive Disease • 295

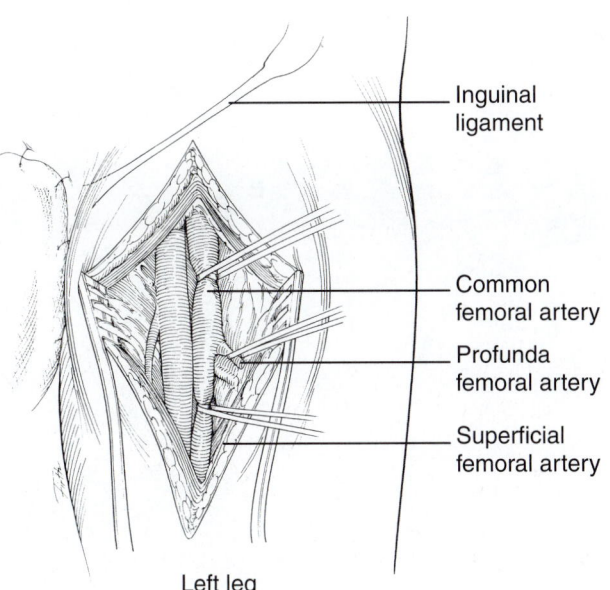

Figure 36–3

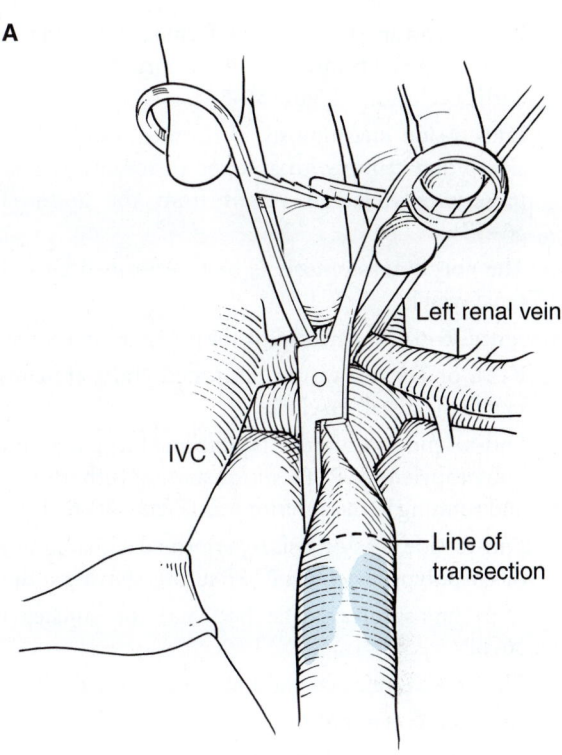

Figure 36–5A–B

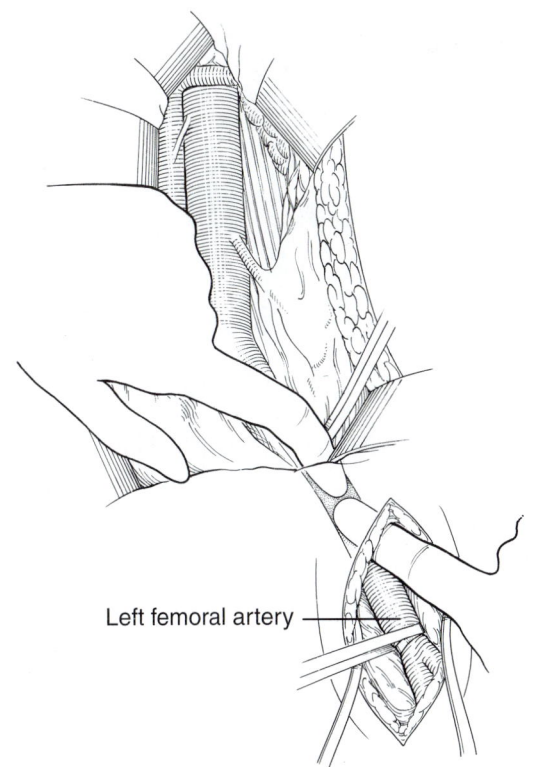

Figure 36–4

- End-to-end anastomosis is performed with a single proximal clamp and transection of the aorta for cases of distal aortic occlusions (Figure 36–5A).
- End-to-side anastomosis, performed using a Satinsky side-biting clamp with anterior aortotomy, is useful for preserving collateral vessels from the aorta (Figure 36–5B).
- The aortic anastomosis is best performed close to the renal vessels.

■ **Figure 36–6A, B:** Performing the proximal anastomosis.
- PTFE or Dacron-woven bifurcated grafts are chosen to match the distal vessel size.
- End-to-end anastomosis is performed with a running 3-0 polypropylene or PTFE suture starting with the back wall and running to the anterior wall (Figure 36–6A).
- End-to-side anastomosis is performed with a running 3-0 or 4-0 polypropylene or PTFE suture, starting at the heel.
- Important sutures are the "heel" and "toe" stitches (Figure 36–6B).
- The clamp is released and anastomosis tested.

■ **Figure 36–7:** Femoral anastomosis.
- The graft limbs are tunneled into the femoral wounds.
- In general, spatulation of the anastomosis onto the profunda femoris is preferred.
- An arteriotomy is preformed with a No. 11 blade after the common, superficial, and deep femoral arteries are clamped.
- The graft is fashioned to length.
- An end-to-side anastomosis is performed, starting at the heel with a running 5-0 polypropylene suture.
- The femoral vessels and graft are flushed to remove debris.
- The anastomosis is completed and flow reestablished.

■ **Figure 36–8:** Closure of the retroperitoneum.
- After ensuring improved distal flow, heparinization is reversed with protamine.
- The retroperitoneum is closed with 2-0 or 3-0 absorbable suture covering the graft from the abdomen.
- The abdominal contents are replaced and the fascia and skin closed.
- The femoral incisions are closed with a deep 2-0 absorbable suture covering the graft and femoral artery.
- Superficial tissue is closed with a running 3-0 absorbable suture.
- Skin is closed in a subcuticular fashion.

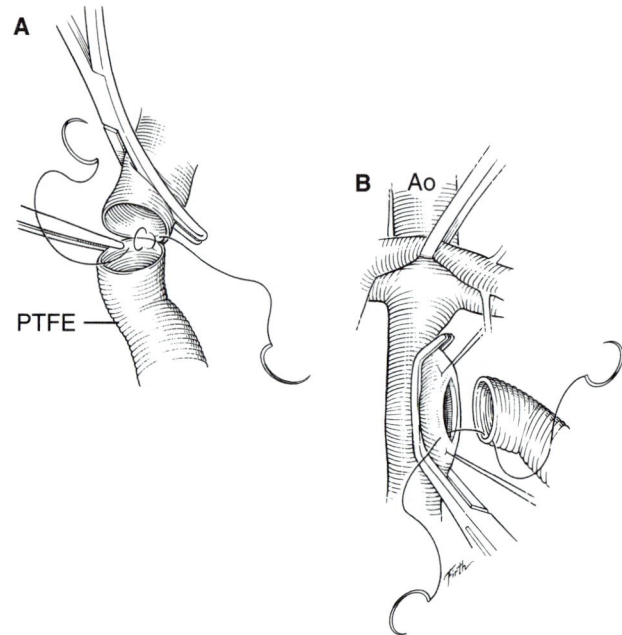

Figure 36–6A–B

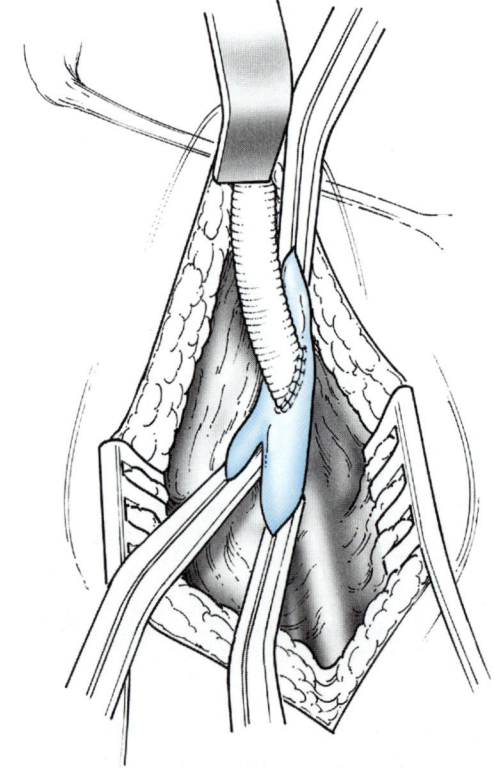

Figure 36–7

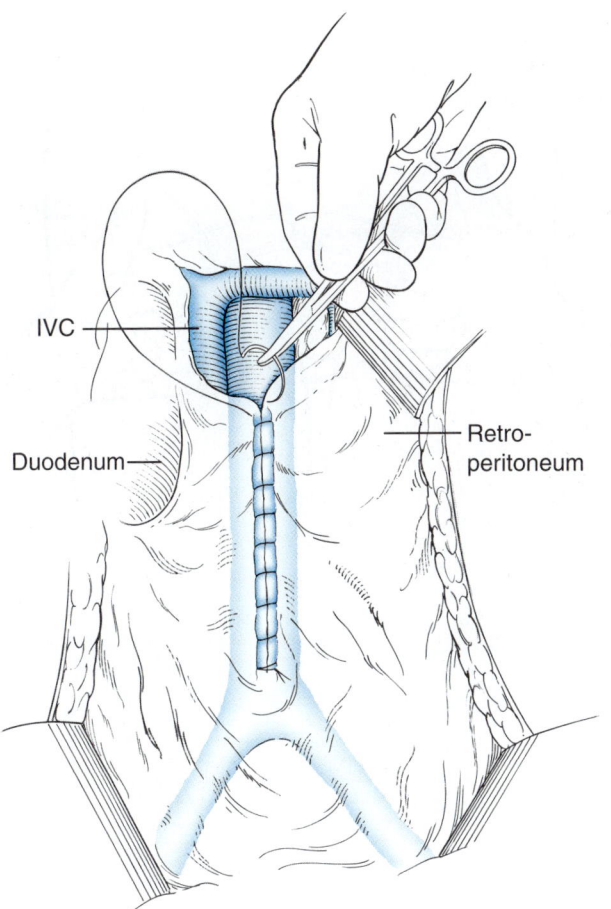

Figure 36–8

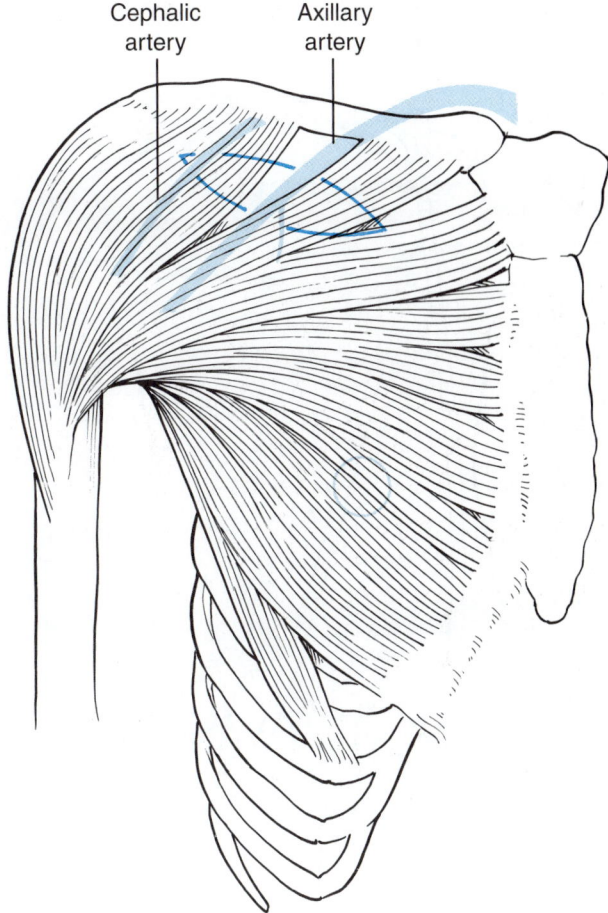

Figure 36–9

Axillary-femoral Bypass

- **Figure 36–9:** Infraclavicular incision.
  - The side of inflow is chosen (if the thoracic aorta needs to be accessed in future, axillary-femoral bypass should be performed on the right side).
  - The incision is made 2 fingerbreadths below the clavicle.
  - The pectoralis major muscle is split and the pectoralis minor insertion is divided.
  - The axillary fat pad is dissected.
- **Figure 36–10:** Exposure of the axillary artery.
  - The axillary vein lies anterior to the artery from this exposure, requiring isolation of the vein and inferior (or occasionally superior) retraction to allow access to the axillary artery.
  - Branch vessels are isolated and controlled.
  - A 3–4-cm length of artery is isolated with vessels loops.

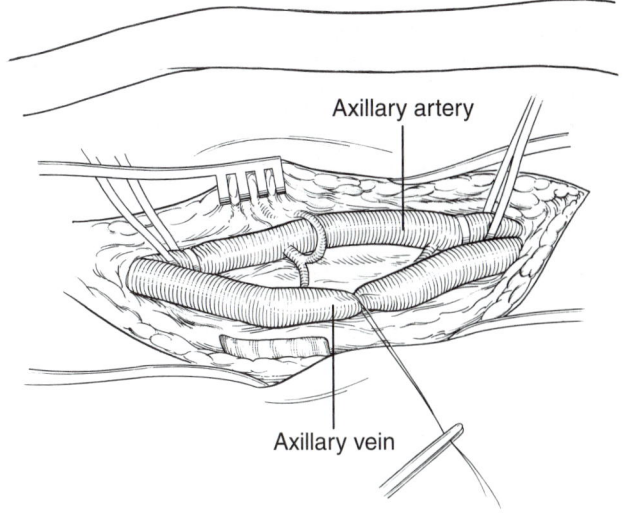

Figure 36–10

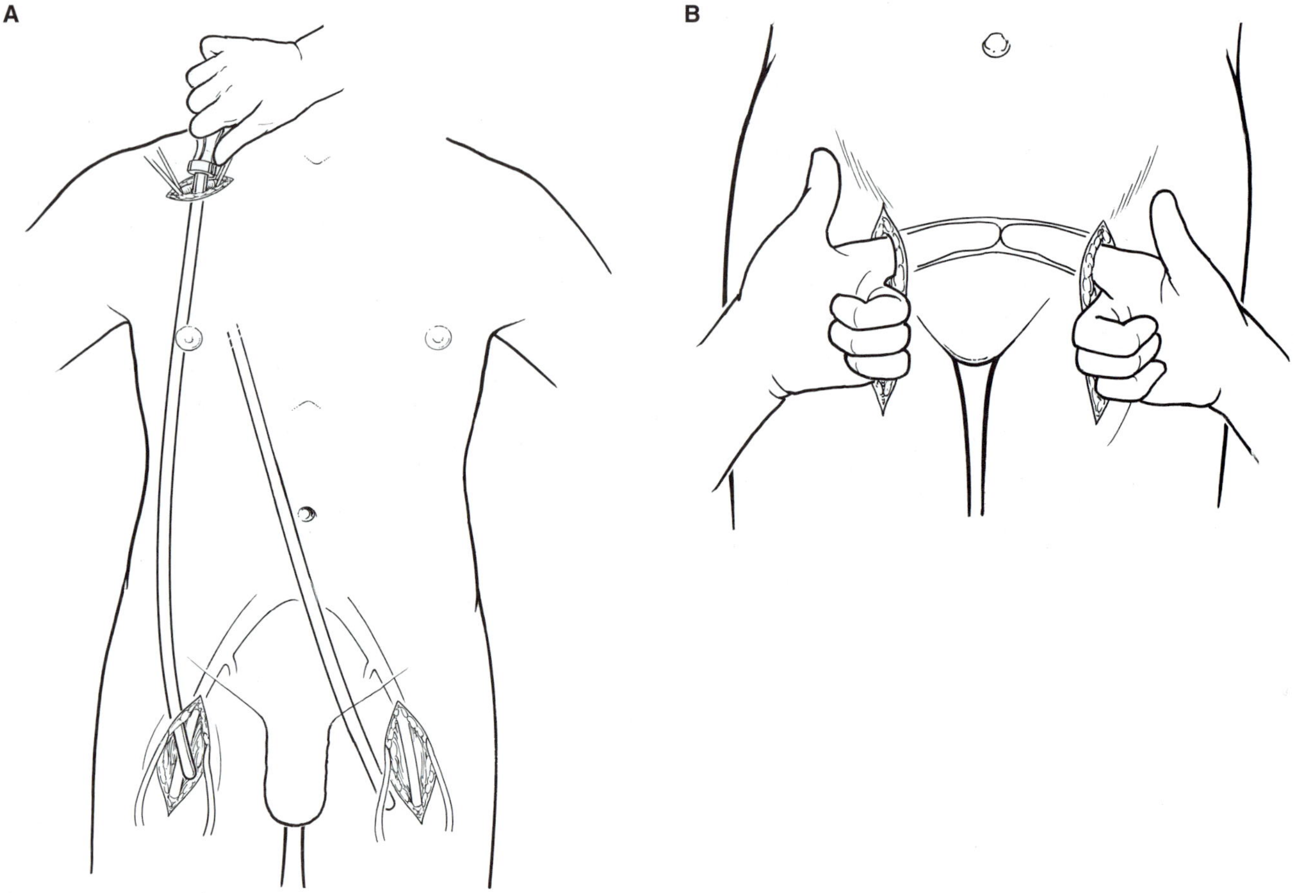

A

B

Figure 36–11A–B

- **Figure 36–11A, B:** Axillary and femoral tunneling.
  - After femoral exposure is performed (see Figure 36–3), a Gore tunneler is used to create a subcutaneous tunnel anterior to the midaxillary line, lateral to the nipple, and above the abdominal fascia from the axillary incision to the femoral incision (Figure 36–11A).
  - A femoral-femoral tunnel is created superior to the pubic bone (Figure 36–11B).
  - The bifurcated ringed PTFE graft is passed from the ipsilateral groin incision to the axillary incision and contralateral femoral incision.
  - Tunneling is preferred prior to heparinization to minimize bleeding.
- **Figure 36–12:** Axillary anastomosis.
  - After heparinization, the axillary artery is clamped proximally and distally with angled ductus clamps.
  - A longitudinal arteriotomy is performed.

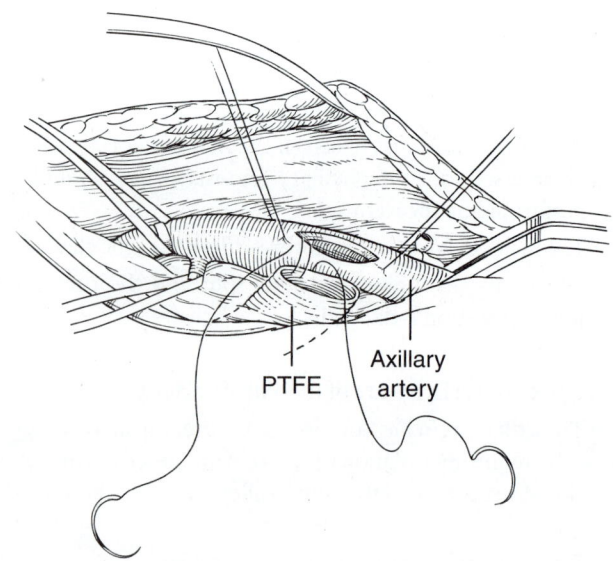

Figure 36–12

- The graft is fashioned and a running end-to-side anastomosis is performed.
- The femoral anastomoses are performed (see Figure 36–7).
- Prior to completion of the anastomoses, femoral arteries and grafts are flushed.
- Flow is reestablished.
- After ensuring improved distal flow, heparinization is reversed.
- The axillary incision is closed with a deep 2-0 absorbable suture, a superficial 3-0 absorbable suture, and subcuticular layer.

POSTOPERATIVE CARE

- Arterial line, central line, and pulmonary artery catheter for hemodynamic monitoring.
- Nothing by mouth.
- A nasogastric tube is needed for decompression for 12–24 hours in cases of abdominal entry.

POTENTIAL COMPLICATIONS

- Respiratory failure.
- Renal failure.
- Myocardial infarction.

PEARLS AND TIPS

- Perioperative hemodynamic monitoring is essential to good outcomes.
- Communication between surgeon and anesthesiologist during aortic clamping and unclamping will minimize hemodynamic fluctuations.
- Early graft thrombosis or pseudoaneurysm is a sign of early graft infection.

REFERENCES

Ernst C, Stanley JC, eds. *Current Vascular Surgery*. St Louis, MO: Mosby; 2001.

Rutherford RB, ed. *Vascular Surgery*. Philadelphia, PA: WB Saunders; 2005.

CHAPTER 37

Surgical Revascularization of Infrainguinal Arterial Occlusive Disease

Loay S. Kabbani, MD, and Peter K. Henke, MD

INDICATIONS
- Disabling claudication.
- Critical limb ischemia, defined as rest pain or tissue loss.

CONTRAINDICATIONS

Absolute
- Debilitated patient with severe comorbidities.
- Unaddressed inflow disease.
- Lack of an appropriate distal target for revascularization.

Relative
- Nondisabling claudication.
- Nonambulatory patient.
- Severe joint contractures.

INFORMED CONSENT

Expected Benefits
- Restoration of adequate blood flow to the lower extremity, thereby relieving ischemic pain, preventing gangrene, and maintaining ambulation.

Potential Risks
- The 30-day mortality and morbidity rates are 2% and 26%, respectively. Morbidity includes:
  - Surgical site infection.
  - Myocardial infarction.
  - Renal and respiratory failure.
- Vein graft patency overall is reported to be 73% at 5 years versus 49% for a polytetrafluoroethylene (PTFE) graft.
  - Primary and secondary vein graft patency at 5 years is reported to be 50% and 70%, respectively, with a limb salvage rate of 73%.

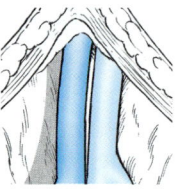
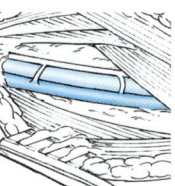
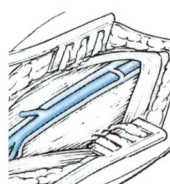
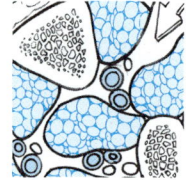
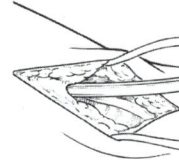
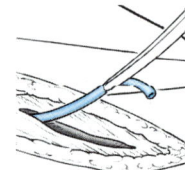
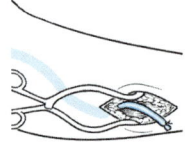
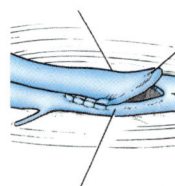

EQUIPMENT
- No special equipment is needed other than a standard vascular instrument tray.

PATIENT PREPARATION
- Ankle-brachial indices (ABIs) or segmental pressures.
- The arterial anatomy must be defined clearly.
  - A lower extremity angiogram, CT angiogram, or MR angiogram may provide sufficient detail for operative planning.
- Preoperative stratification with a full history and physical examination.
  - Eagle criteria, American Heart Association guidelines for perioperative cardiovascular evaluation for noncardiac surgery, or another cardiac risk stratification algorithm can be used to calculate the patient's perioperative risk for coronary events and need for further workup.
- All patients should receive optimal medical therapy in the perioperative period, including:
  - Daily aspirin.
  - β-Blockers to titrate the heart rate to < 70 beats/min.
  - Statin therapy to achieve a goal low-density lipoprotein level < 100 mg/dL.
  - Tight blood glucose control with a target level < 140 mg/dL (for at least the first 3 days postoperatively).
- Appropriate prophylactic antibiotics are delivered within 30 minutes of skin incision and are redosed as needed for prolonged cases (eg, intravenous cefazolin, 1 g preoperatively, then 1 g every 8 hours intraoperatively).

PATIENT POSITIONING
- The patient should be supine with both arms extended; procedure-specific positioning is indicated later.
- A Foley catheter is inserted.
- A radial arterial line is placed.

PROCEDURE

Principles of Open Infrainguinal Revascularization

A. INFLOW
- The artery from which the bypass will originate must have an adequate pressure and allow suturing. Significant vascular calcification can present challenges.

B. OUTFLOW
- The vessel should be the least diseased vessel with dominant blood flow to the foot.

C. Conduit

- The great saphenous vein (GSV) has superior long-term patency rates for all infrainguinal bypasses.
- In the absence of an ipsilateral GSV, the contralateral vein may be used.
- Alternatively basilic, cephalic, or lesser saphenous veins may be used as a composite graft.
- The GSV may be used in situ, reversed, or nonreversed transposed with equivalent long-term patency results, depending on the surgeon's experience.
- Although prosthetic grafts have mediocre long-term patency rates in infrainguinal bypasses, they can be used if no other conduit is available.

Anatomy, Exposure, and Preparation of Proximal and Distal Targets

- **Figure 37–1:** Anatomy of the target site.
  - The mnemonic NAVEL aids in recollection of the anatomy; from lateral to medial, the **N**erve, **A**rtery, **V**ein, **E**mpty space, and **L**ymphatics will be encountered—the latter is where a femoral hernia may occur.

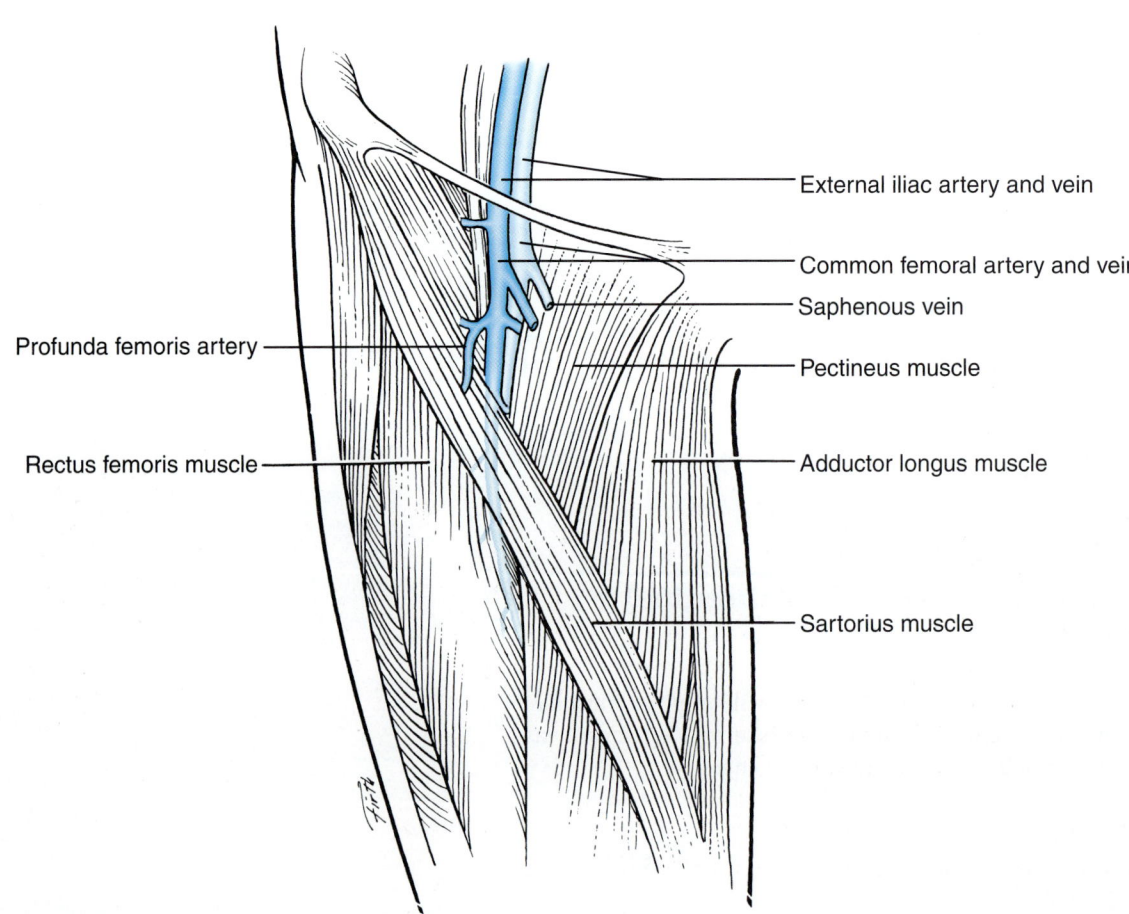

Figure 37–1

- The GSV joins the femoral vein at the saphenofemoral junction.
- The common femoral artery (CFA) begins at the inguinal ligament as a continuation of the external iliac artery.
- The femoral artery bifurcates approximately 5 cm distal to the inguinal ligament into the superficial femoral artery (SFA) and the deep femoral artery, also known as the profunda femoris (PF), the latter traveling laterally and posteriorly.

A. Common Femoral Artery

- **Figure 37–2:** Exposure and preparation for bypass.
  - A vertical incision 3–5 cm in length is made proximal to the inguinal ligament and continued for about 3–4 cm distally over the femoral pulse.
  - If the pulse is absent, the incision should be made 1–2 cm lateral to the pubic tubercle where the femoral artery is usually located.
  - A calcified artery may be pulseless but is easily palpated.
  - The femoral artery should be exposed longitudinally to avoid lymphatic disruption and the lymphatics dissected laterally; we ligate or clip larger lymphatics when present.
  - A Weitlaner or cerebellar retractor is used to help expose the vessel.
  - The CFA, SFA, and PF artery are dissected and isolated with vessel loops.
  - The lateral circumflex femoral vein is located between the origins of the SFA and PF. During dissection of the femoral artery bifurcation, this vein tends to be injured and bleed if not sought out and carefully mobilized.
  - We have found that the proximal CFA is best clamped using a Satinsky or a Dara clamp. The external iliac artery may be mobilized, instead, if it is a better vessel to clamp; this sometimes entails dividing the inguinal ligament, which is repaired at the end of the operation.
  - A severely diseased CFA may require an endarterectomy with patch angioplasty in order to make it suitable for bypass grafting.
  - Caution must be undertaken with this maneuver as suitable end points after endarterectomy are rare.

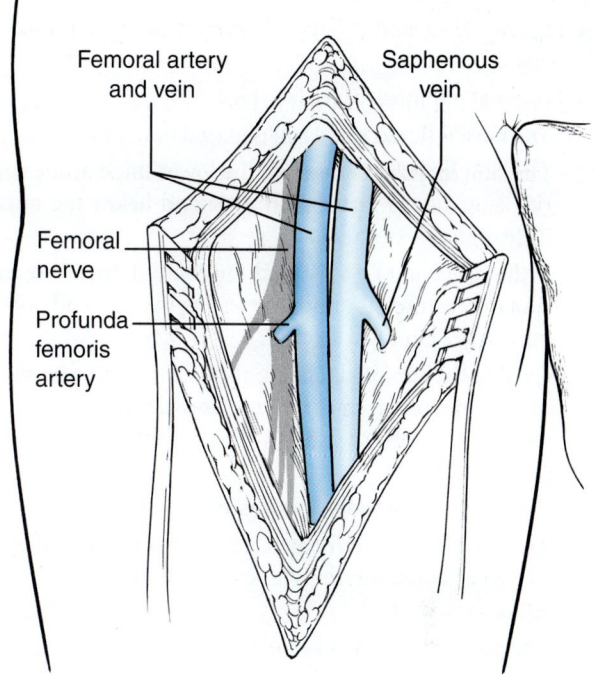

Figure 37–2

B. Popliteal Artery

- **Figures 37–3 and 37–4:** Exposure and preparation for bypass.
- Proximal popliteal artery (see Figure 37–3).
  - The knee is flexed and a roll is placed under the thigh.
  - The skin incision is made in the lower thigh at the superior edge of the sartorius muscle and below the muscle belly of the vastus medialis.
  - If the ipsilateral GSV is used for conduit, then one incision may be used for both harvesting the vein and dissecting out the popliteal artery.
  - Cutting the superficial fascia allows entry into the sheath of the sartorius muscle; this muscle is isolated and reflected posteriorly along with the semitendinosus and gracilis muscles.
  - The popliteal fat space is exposed.
  - The dissection is performed close to the femur, retracting the great adductor muscle anteriorly and exposing the adductor hiatus.
  - The popliteal artery is found by palpation.
  - Doppler localization is helpful in patients with larger legs and small nonpalpable arteries.
- Distal popliteal artery (see Figure 37–4).
  - A roll is placed under the distal thigh.
  - The incision starts 1 cm behind the medial tibial condyle, runs for 1–2 cm behind the posterior edge of the tibia, and then courses down the upper third of the leg; we extend it proximally or distally as needed.
  - The medial head of the gastrocnemius is retracted posteriorly using a Weitlaner or an Adson retractor.
  - A Beckman retractor is placed, lifting the soleus muscle up and the gastrocnemius muscle down.
  - The popliteal artery is surrounded by two veins, and the tibial nerve lies posterior to it.
  - Careful sharp dissection is carried out using Metzenbaum scissors.
  - The popliteal artery gives off the anterior tibial artery and the tibioperoneal trunk 2–7 cm before diving into the soleus muscle.
  - To expose the tibioperoneal trunk, follow the popliteal artery caudally, dividing the soleus muscle with cautery.
  - The anterior tibial artery is isolated with vessel loops at its origin at the proximal end of the soleus muscle.

C. Posterior Tibial and Peroneal Arteries

- Patient positioning.
  - The patient should be supine with the thigh rotated 30–50 degrees.
  - A bump is placed below the thigh to help exposure.
  - A tourniquet or microvascular Heifitz clips may be used for homeostasis at the time of bypass.

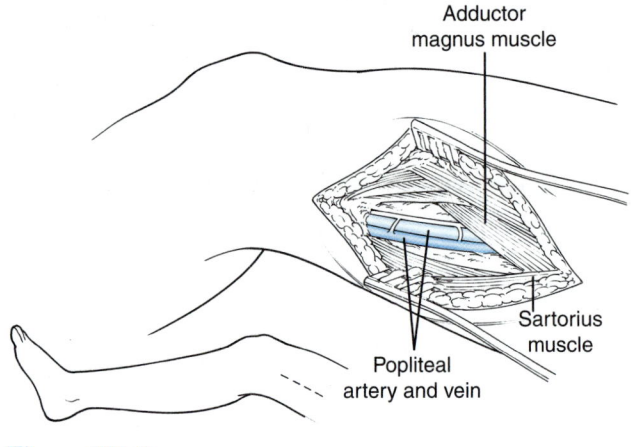

Figure 37–3

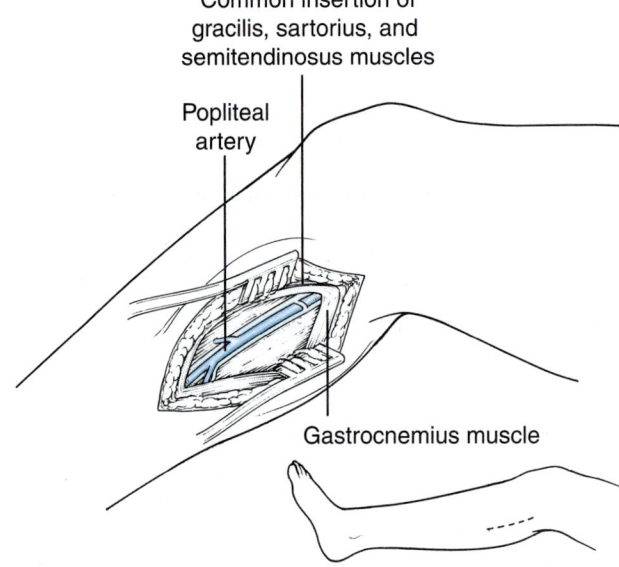

Figure 37–4

- **Figures 37–5 and 37–6:** Exposure and preparation for bypass.
  - Upper and middle leg: the incision is placed 1–2 cm behind the posterior edge of the tibia midway in the leg. This incision usually overlies the GSV.
  - The fascia is cut and the gastrocnemius muscle is freed and retracted posteriorly while the insertion of the soleus muscle is taken down from the posterior aspect of the tibial bone, exposing the deep posterior compartment of the calf.
  - Both the posterior tibial artery and, a little deeper to it, the peroneal artery lie inside this compartment.
  - With the use of a tourniquet, only the anterior and lateral aspects of the vessels need to be exposed, and there is no need for circumferential exposure or vessel loops.

D. Anterior Tibial Artery
- Patient positioning.
  - The leg is maintained at 30 degrees of flexion and a roll is placed under the thigh.
- Exposure and preparation for bypass.
  - The skin and fascia are incised over the space between the anterior tibial muscle and the long extensor of the toes.

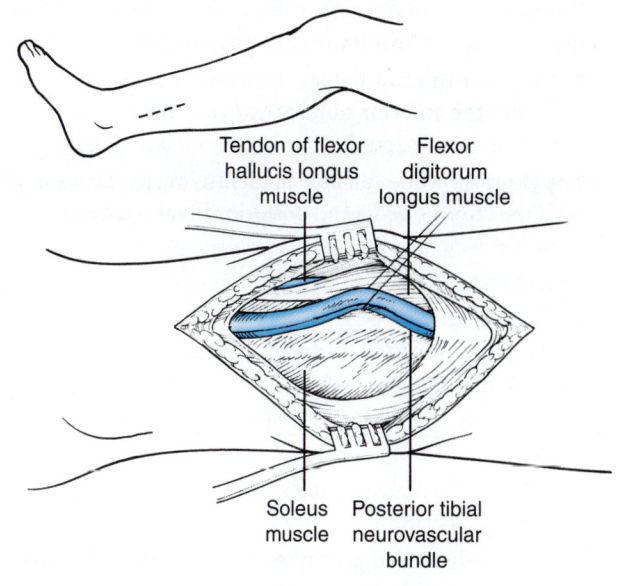

Figure 37–5

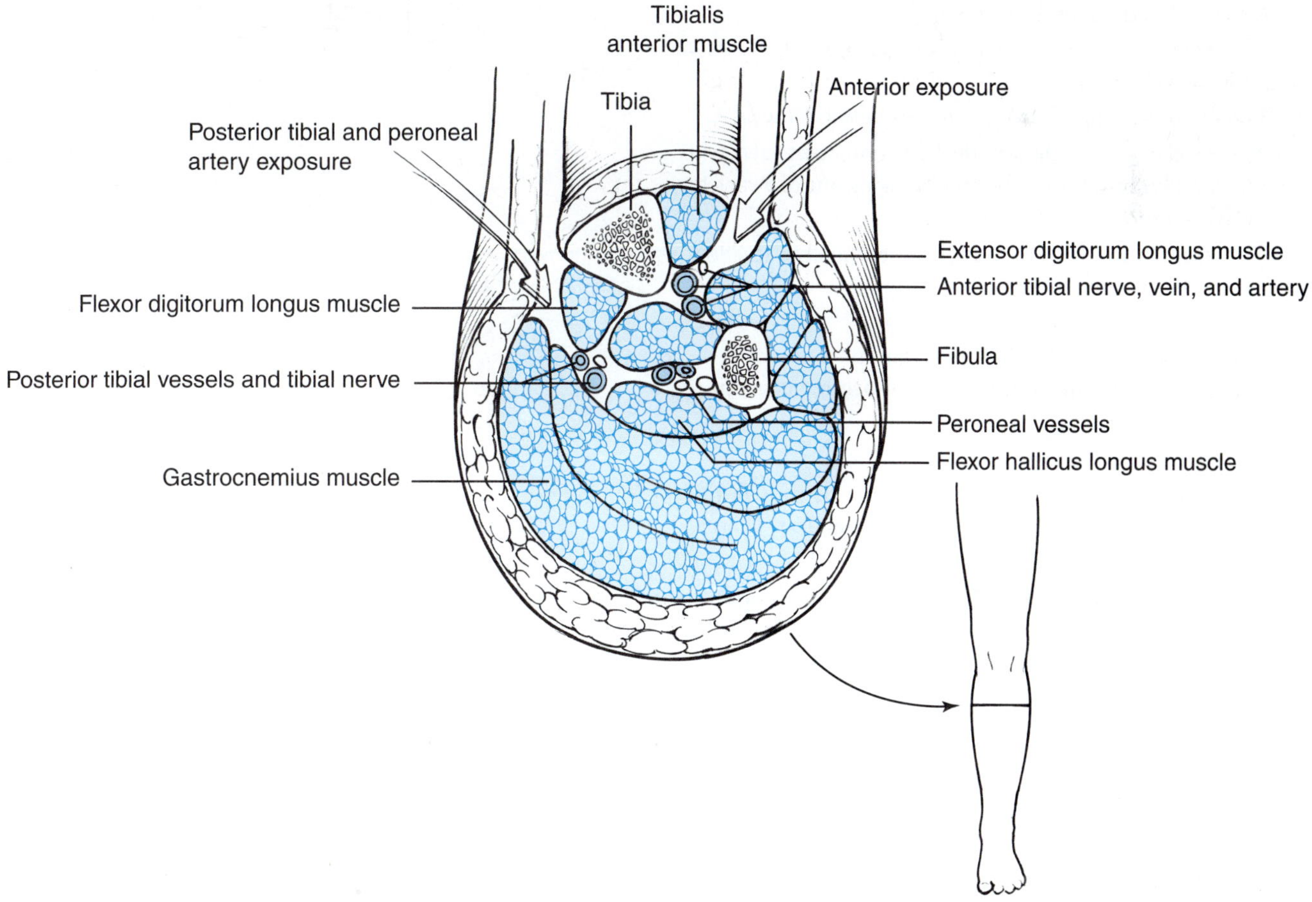

Figure 37–6

- The anterior tibial artery runs with the deep peroneal nerve on top of the interosseous membrane.
- In the lower third of the leg the muscles are more tendinous and the anterior tibial artery runs behind the anterior tibial muscle and the extensor hallucis longus.
- The Doppler probe can aide in identifying the location of both the dorsalis pedis and posterior tibial arteries.

Preparing the Conduit

A. Vein Harvest
- The GSV is harvested through a separate skin incision medial to the CFA incision.
  - Cephalic, basilic, or lesser saphenous veins may also be harvested.
- Once the vein is removed, it should be placed in a solution containing heparin.
  - The vein is distended gently and any leaks are addressed.
  - Tributaries are ligated with 4-0 silk ties.

B. In-Situ Bypass
- Here the vein is not mobilized from its bed except at the proximal and distal ends.
  - As the vein is exposed, tributaries are tied off with silk ties.
  - The proximal GSV is mobilized, excising the first valve under direct vision.
- Then the GSV is spatulated and anastomosed to the CFA.
- Once the clamps are released, the first competent valve will hold up; valve lysis is then performed using one of a variety of valvulotomes.
  - It is essential to preserve the vein side branches to allow passage of the valvulotome.

C. Routes for Bypass and Creating the Tunnel
- **Figure 37–7A, B:** The graft is tunneled before heparinization.
- Popliteal route.
  - The graft is tunneled beneath the sartorius muscle but superficial to the adductor magnus tendon (Figure 37–7A).
  - If the distal anastomosis target is the below-knee popliteal artery, then the graft should be further tunneled in an anatomic position (Figure 37–7B).
- Posterior tibial artery route.
  - The GSV is mobilized for approximately 10 cm.
  - The aponeurosis of the leg should be incised high enough to avoid angulation of the vein.
  - In reversed bypasses, either a subcutaneous or an anatomic route may be used.

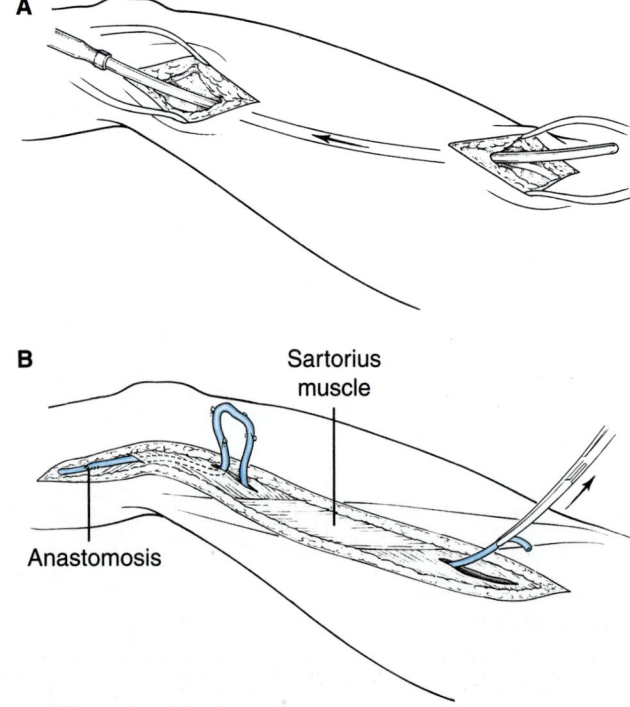

Figure 37–7A–B

- The anatomic route follows the posterior edge of the sartorius, enters the popliteal fossa between the two heads of the gastrocnemius, and passes anterior to the soleus muscle to the posterior tibial artery.
- This route is used preferentially for reversed saphenous vein graft and prosthetics; it is less susceptible to the risk of superficial infections and is not subject to kinking when the knee is flexed.
- When using a subcutaneous route, a tunnel is made that runs along the anterior medial surface of the thigh and continues on the medial side of the knee and leg.
- The diameter of the tunneling instrument must be sufficient to create a tunnel wide enough to prevent compression.
■ Peroneal artery route.
- When accessed through the medial approach, the trajectory is the same as for the posterior tibial artery.
■ Anterior tibial artery route.
- In-situ bypasses: the lower part of the popliteal fossa is divided, and the interosseous membrane is freed and then incised longitudinally for 2–3 cm.
- A blunt instrument is passed from the anterior compartment to the popliteal fossa.
- The distal anastomosis should be performed far enough from the point where the vein graft crosses the interosseous space so that the vein is parallel to the artery.
- The path for a reversed GSV may follow the anatomic route behind the sartorius, between the heads of the gastrocnemius, before joining the anterior compartment.

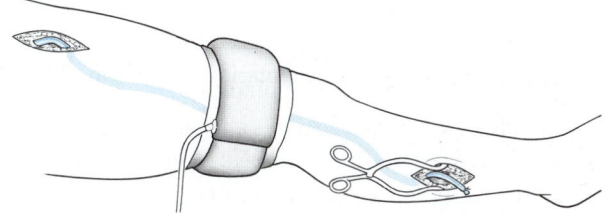

Figure 37–8

D. Performing the Bypass
■ Before occluding the inflow, the patient is given an initial heparin bolus of 100 units/kg; the activated clotting time (ACT) is kept above 250 seconds.
■ **Figures 37–8 and 37–9:** The arteriography is made using a No. 11 blade and then extended with Potts scissors.
■ The graft is spatulated and a polypropylene suture (eg, Prolene) is used to create the proximal anastomosis.
- We usually use 5-0 Prolene suture for the CFA and 6-0 Prolene suture for the distal target vessels.
■ After completing the proximal anastomosis, the inflow is released and the graft is distended and then marked for orientation.
- The graft is passed through the tunnel carefully making sure there are no twists.
■ For the leg vessels a tourniquet may be used to ensure a bloodless field (see Figure 37–8).
■ An arteriotomy is made in the distal vessels with a No. 11 blade, and a 1.5–2.5-mm coronary dilator is carefully passed to ensure patency.

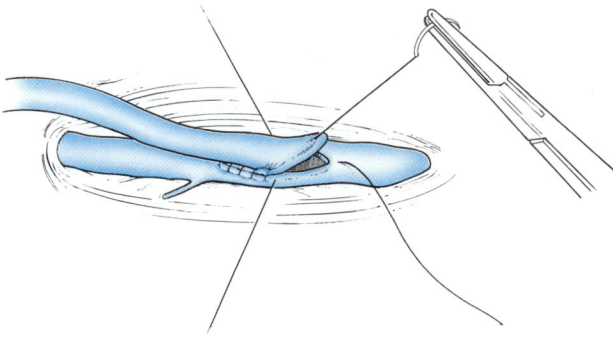

Figure 37–9

- The graft is cut to size with the leg extended, and the end is spatulated. The anastomosis is created (see Figure 37–9).
- Before completion of the anastomosis the artery is back-bled and the graft is flushed.
- Some centers perform completion angiograms; we use intraoperative duplex ultrasonography to scan the inflow anastomosis, the outflow anastomosis, and the graft for any abnormalities.
  - In cases of a threefold increase in flow velocities or a velocity above 300 cm/s, close evaluation is needed to identify technical errors, flaps, or retained valves.
- The groin wound is closed in at least three layers of 3-0 Vicryl, obliterating all the potential space.
- The leg wounds are closed by approximating the fascia only.
- The skin is closed with staples, interrupted nylon, or subcuticular stitches.

POSTOPERATIVE CARE

- Doppler ultrasound signals should be checked frequently to monitor graft patency.
- Patients are maintained on a β-blocker, an antiplatelet agent, and a statin unless contraindicated.
- Antibiotics are stopped 24 hours after surgery unless there is an active infection (eg, an infected ulcer or toe).
- Epidural injection or patient-controlled analgesia may be used for postoperative pain management.
- Venous thromboembolic prophylaxis is started on postoperative day 1 using unfractionated heparin administered subcutaneously.
- Patients with significant edema and pedal wounds are treated with an Ace wrap and leg elevation.
- Sutures in the foot are removed only when the wounds are solidly healed, and not before 4 weeks.

POTENTIAL COMPLICATIONS

- Local wound infections.
- Hematoma.
- Lymph leaks.
- Graft thrombosis.

PEARLS AND TIPS

- Vessel exposure in previously operated groins requires patience and care.
  - Doppler insonation is useful for locating difficult-to-palpate arteries and grafts.
  - Sharp knife dissection is also helpful in groins that are very scarred.
- Patients should continue to take aspirin preoperatively as this improves graft patency. However, clopidogrel is associated with excessive bleeding, and we recommend stopping this drug 7 days before the operation.
- Perioperative antibiotics, excellent homeostasis, and good incision closure technique are essential to decrease postoperative problems.
- If there are no distal targets, amputation may be required.
  - The level of amputation may be determined based on segmental pressures and the angiogram.
  - A below-the-knee amputation should heal if the popliteal pressure is > 50 mm Hg or there is a patent PF artery.

REFERENCES

Branchereau A, Berguer R. *Vascular Surgical Approaches.* New York, NY: Futura; 1999.

Zelenock G. *Mastery of Vascular and Endovascular Surgery.* Philadelphia, PA: Lippincott Williams & Wilkins; 2006.

CHAPTER 38

Management of Lower Extremity Venous Insufficiency

K. Barrett Deatrick, MD, and Thomas W. Wakefield, MD

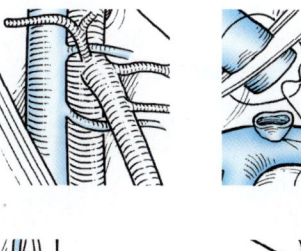
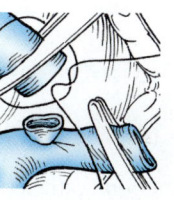
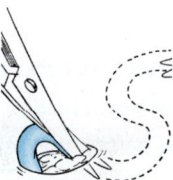
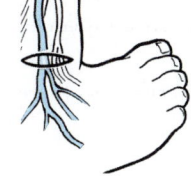
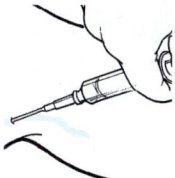
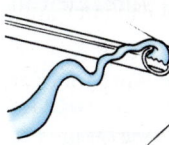

INDICATIONS

- Swelling.
- Leg heaviness.
- Aching.
- Cramping.
- Skin discoloration.
- Venous ulcers.

CONTRAINDICATIONS

- Acute deep venous thrombosis.
- Malformation of the deep venous system.
- Active infection.
- Symptomatic peripheral arterial disease.
- Cardiopulmonary comorbidities (relative).

INFORMED CONSENT

Expected Benefits

- Removal of varicose veins of the lower extremity.

Potential Risks

- Phlebectomy.
  - Bleeding or hematoma formation at the operative site.
  - Superficial surgical site infection.
  - Paresthesias.
  - Recurrent varicose veins.
- Endovenous laser or radiofrequency ablation.
  - Recanalization.
  - Thromboembolism.
  - Burning pain.
  - Swelling.
  - Bruising.
  - Scarring.

EQUIPMENT

Stab Phlebectomy
- No. 11 blade scalpel.
- Mosquito clamps.
- Vein hooks of several sizes.

Endovenous Laser Ablation
- No. 11 blade scalpel.
- Micropuncture kit.
- Endovenous laser generator, laser catheter.
- Ultrasonographic equipment.
- Tumescent anesthesia (infused by hand or Klein pump): lidocaine 1% with epinephrine, 50 mL; sodium bicarbonate 1 mEq/mL, 30 mL; saline 0.9%, 1000 mL.

Endovenous Radiofrequency Ablation
- No. 11 blade scalpel.
- Micropuncture kit.
- Radiofrequency generator, catheter.
- Ultrasonographic equipment.
- Tumescent anesthesia (as discussed earlier).

TriVex Transilluminated Power Phlebectomy
- No. 11 blade scalpel.
- Power phlebectomy unit and handpiece.
- Tumescent anesthesia.

PATIENT PREPARATION

- Nothing by mouth after midnight on the evening before the procedure.
- Ultrasound mapping.
- Veins should be marked in the preoperative area while the patient is standing upright to distend affected veins.
- Antimicrobial prophylaxis: cefazolin, 1 g intravenous, if phlebectomy is indicated (not needed for ablation only) or if skin changes indicative of chronic venous insufficiency are present.
- Deep vein thrombosis prophylaxis as appropriate for risk factors, using unfractionated or low-molecular-weight heparin.

PATIENT POSITIONING

- The patient is usually placed in the supine position initially, with exposure of the entire affected extremity.
- The leg should be prepared circumferentially from the inguinal ligament to the foot.

- If necessary, the patient may be repositioned prone.
  - This is especially helpful when access to posterior perforators or the small saphenous vein is necessary.

PROCEDURE

- The patient may receive either general or regional (spinal) anesthesia.
- **Figure 38–1A:** The anatomy of the superficial veins of the lower extremity, showing the location of the great saphenous vein (GSV) and small saphenous vein (SSV) as well as the tributaries to the GSV near the saphenofemoral junction.
  - Ablation of the GSV and SSV reduces venous hypertension transmitted to the varicose veins.
- **Figure 38–1B:** The saphenofemoral junction.
  - The tributaries that join the GSV near the saphenofemoral junction are shown in greater detail.

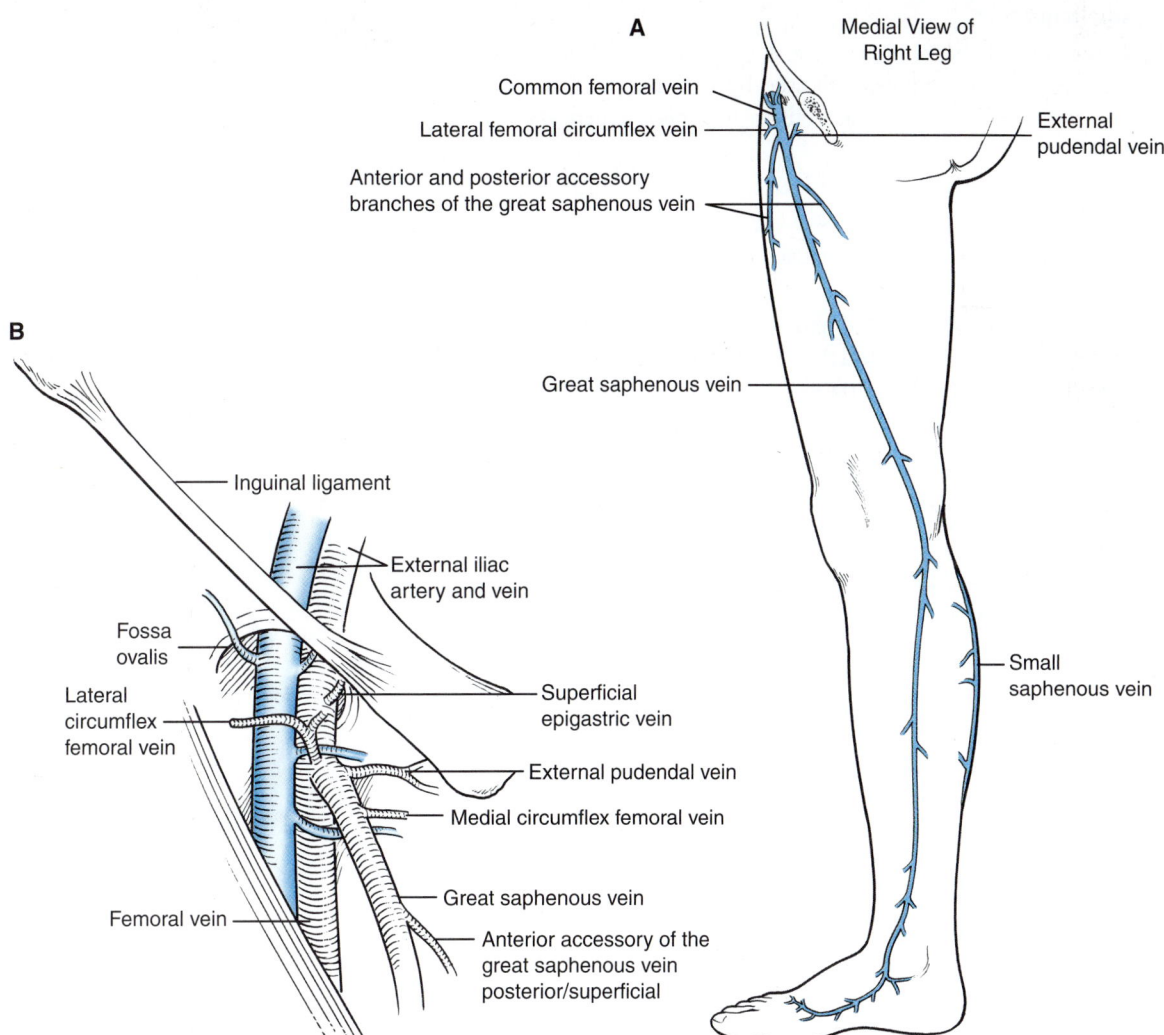

Figure 38–1A–B

- Formal stripping requires identification and division of these branches.
- **Figure 38–2A:** A 3-cm incision is made in the medial thigh, below the inguinal ligament, lateral to the femoral arterial pulse.
- **Figure 38–2B:** The tributaries to the saphenofemoral junction are identified, ligated, and divided.
  - The GSV is traced distally from the saphenofemoral junction, then doubly ligated and divided 1 cm distal to the junction.
- **Figure 38–3A-D:** Stab avulsion.
  - Small (< 1 cm) incisions are made directly over the varicosities marked preoperatively.
  - The vein segments are then pulled to the surface using small hemostatic clamps or small specially modified crochet hooks.
- **Figure 38–4:** The SSV courses in close proximity to the sural nerve.
- **Figure 38–5:** Essentials of endovenous ablation (laser and radiofrequency).
  - Using ultrasonographic guidance, the GSV is accessed and a guidewire is introduced, followed by a sheath and the catheter containing the laser fiber or radiofrequency probe.
  - With the catheter in place, tumescent anesthesia is introduced into the perivascular space.
  - Placement of the catheter 2 cm distal to the saphenofemoral junction is confirmed.
  - A laser catheter is activated and withdrawn at a rate of 1 mm/s for 100 seconds, and then 2.5 mm/s until the laser tip is 1 cm from the skin surface.

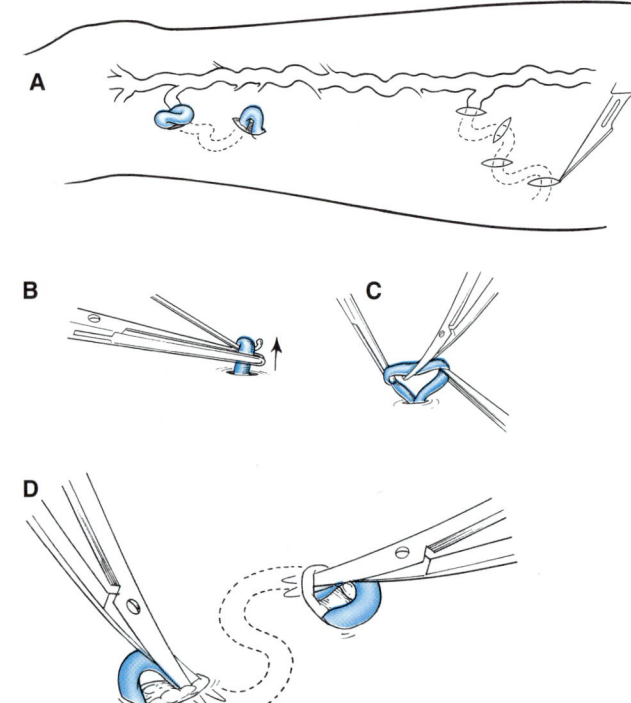

Figure 38–3A–D

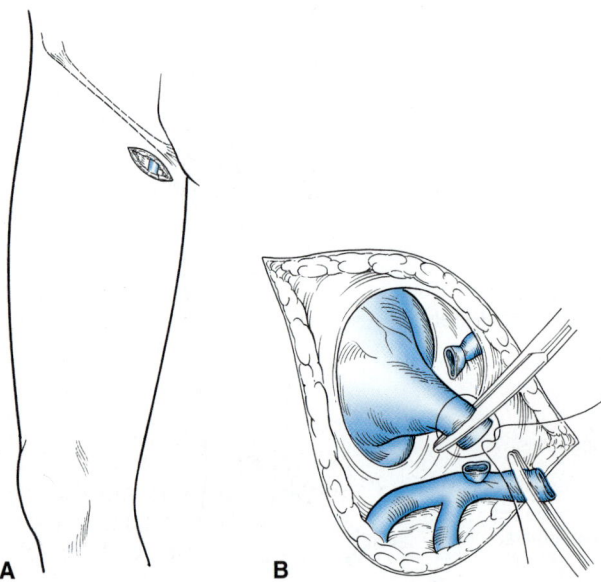

Figure 38–2A–B

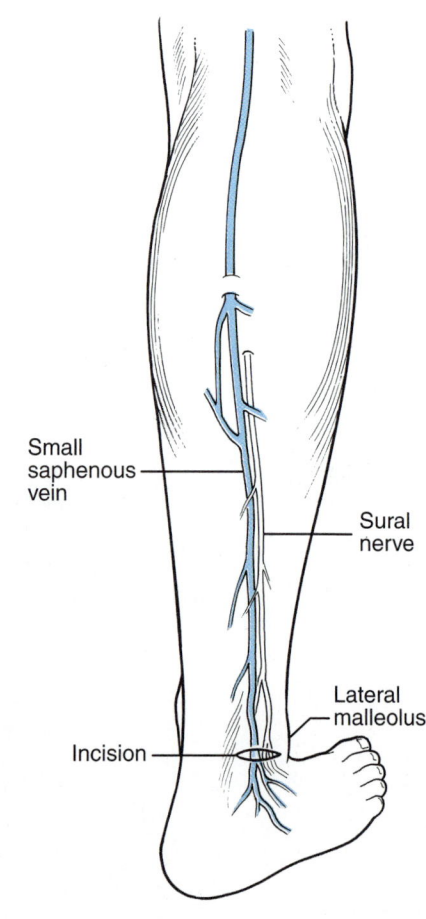

Figure 38–4

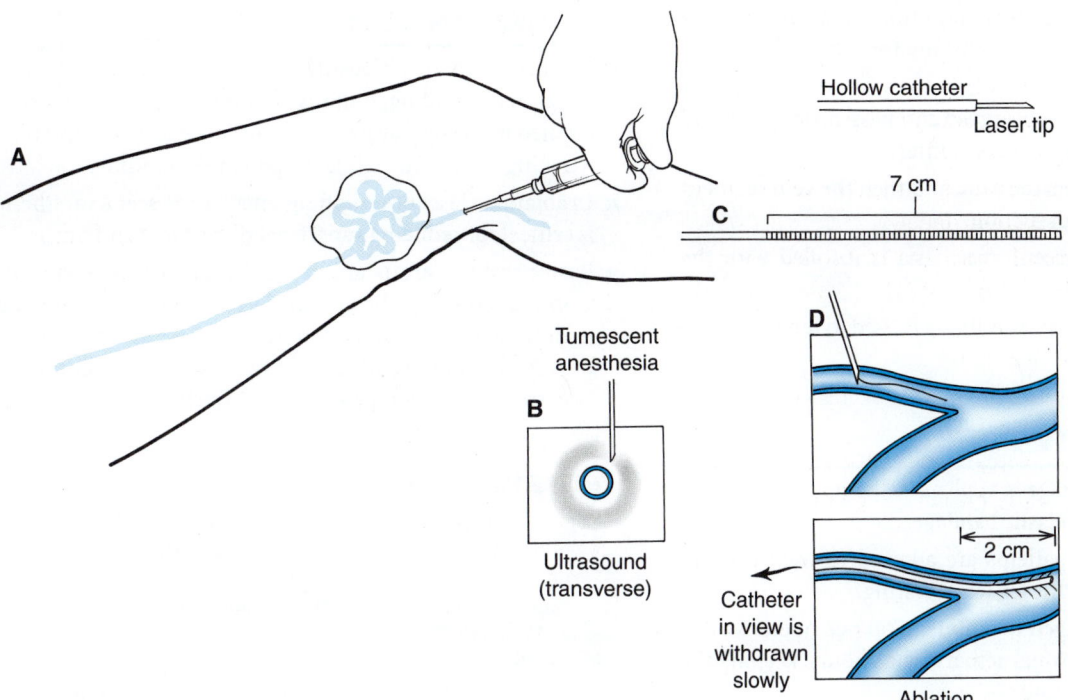

Figure 38–5A–D

- A radiofrequency catheter is heated to a temperature of 120°C and withdrawn in steps.
- The catheter is activated at each 7-cm segment and activated at each station until pulled back to its insertion site.

■ **Figure 38–6:** Transilluminated powered phlebectomy.
- The area of varicosities is marked preoperatively.

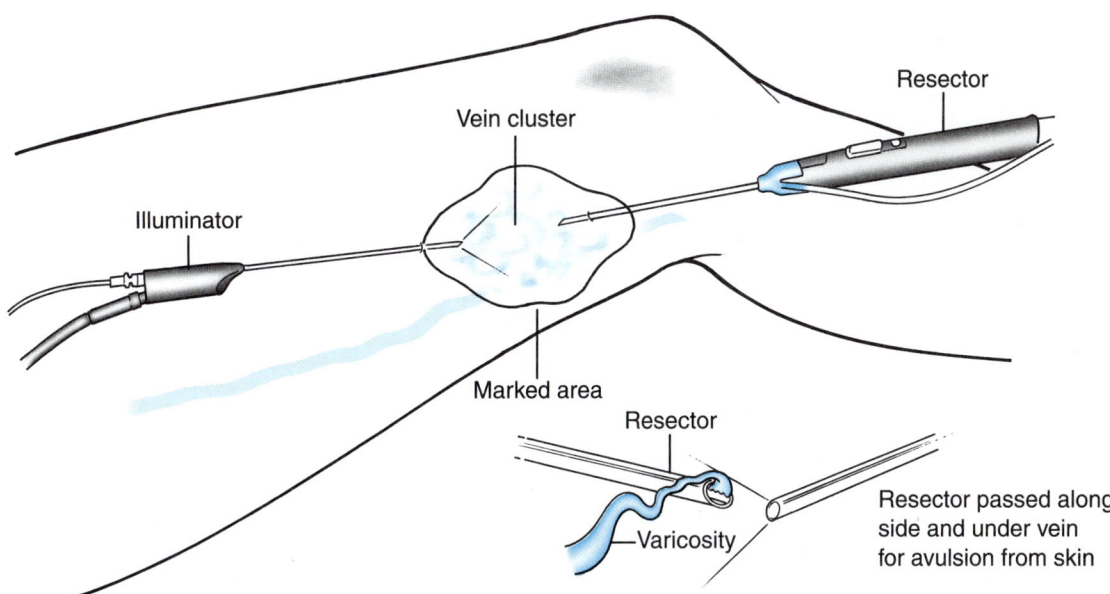

Figure 38–6

- In the operating room, first-stage tumescent anesthesia is instilled using the irrigated illuminator, causing hydrodissection.
- The resector is then introduced and passed alongside and underneath the vein clusters of interest.
- The resector disrupts the vein, and then the vein segment is removed with high suction.
- Second-stage tumescent anesthesia is instilled with the illuminator.
- Third-stage tumescent anesthesia is used to remove blood from the incisions.

POSTOPERATIVE CARE

- A short stretch bandage is applied in the operating room, and covered with an elastic bandage.
- For the first night, patients are allowed to walk and are instructed to elevate the leg when resting.
- Patients are encouraged to ambulate on postoperative day 1 and to return to normal activity by 48 hours, keeping the leg elevated when resting.
- The dressing may be removed after 48 hours; the leg should be kept clean and dry.
- Compression stockings or wraps should be worn thereafter, with the patient continuing to elevate the legs when possible.

POTENTIAL COMPLICATIONS

- Bleeding or hematoma formation.
- Surgical site infection.
- Deep venous thrombosis.
- Leg swelling.

PEARLS AND TIPS

- It is best to mark varicosities in the preoperative area with the patient standing. If this is not done, a tourniquet can be applied in the operating room, but this is less effective than marking varicosities while the patient is standing.
- In ablation (laser or radiofrequency), tumescent anesthesia is critical for reducing superficial discomfort and burns.
- Postoperative care is an essential part of this operation. Compression must be applied in the operating room and maintained for the first 48 hours postoperatively. Following removal of the bandages, patients should use compression stockings or wraps and elevate the legs when possible.

REFERENCES

Caggiati A, Bergan JJ, Gloviczki P, et al. International Interdisciplinary Consensus Committee on Venous Anatomical Terminology. Nomenclature of the veins of the lower limb: extensions, refinements, and clinical application. *J Vasc Surg.* 2005;41:719–724.

Knipp BS, Blackburn SA, Bloom JR, et al. Michigan Venous Study Group. Endovenous laser ablation: venous outcomes and thrombotic complications are independent of the presence of deep venous insufficiency. *J Vasc Surg.* 2008;48:1538–1545.

Pfeifer JR, Engle JS. Surgical Management of Varicose Veins by Saphenous and Perforator Ligation with Sparing of the Saphenous Vein. In: Zelenock GB, Huber TS, Messina LM, et al, eds. *Mastery of Vascular and Endovascular Surgery.* Philadelphia, PA: Lippincott Williams & Wilkins; 2006.

Spitz GA. *Transilluminated Powered Phlebectomy (Trivex):* An Illustrated Guide. Andover, MA: Smith and Nephew; 2000.

CHAPTER 39

Below- and Above-the-Knee Amputation

Jeffrey H. Kozlow, MD, Andrew M. Zwyghuizen, MD,
and Thomas W. Wakefield, MD

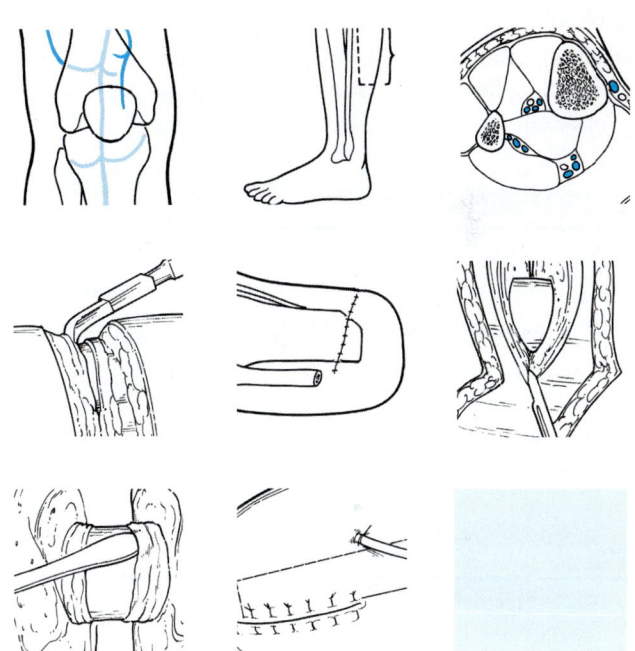

INDICATIONS

Below-the-Knee Amputation (BKA)

- Nonsalvageable lower extremity infection.
- Chronic nonhealing lower extremity wounds.
- Acute lower extremity infection.
- Trauma with vascular or neurologic injury; open tibia fracture with posterior tibial nerve disruption or warm ischemia > 6 hours.

Above-the-Knee Amputation (AKA)

- Severe peripheral vascular disease not amenable to bypass graft with popliteal pressures inadequate to heal BKA.
- Chronic nonhealing BKA wound.
- Nonreconstructible traumatic injury to the lower extremity involving the knee joint or proximal tibia.

CONTRAINDICATIONS

Below-the-Knee Amputation

- Cardiopulmonary disease and inability to tolerate surgery (relative contraindications).
- Fixed knee contracture that would cause pressure on the distal stump after amputation (AKA is indicated in these cases).
- Nonfunctional limbs (an indication for AKA).
- Paraplegia (relative contraindication).
- Infection that extends above the knee.
- Inadequate blood flow to heal a BKA (popliteal artery pressures < 50 mm Hg).

Above-the-Knee Amputation

- Aortoiliac occlusive disease with inadequate femoral artery flow to heal an AKA wound.
- Osteomyelitis of the proximal femur, femoral head, or acetabulum.

- Cardiopulmonary disease and inability to tolerate surgery (relative contraindications).

INFORMED CONSENT

Potential Risks
- Nonhealing wound.
- Phantom pain.
- Chronic pain.
- Neuroma.
- Persistent infection.
- Need for higher amputation.
- Loss of mobility.
- Bleeding requiring transfusion.
- Complications related to general medical condition, including heart attack, stroke, venous thromboembolism, or death.

EQUIPMENT
- Tourniquet.
- Electrocautery and surgical ties for hemostatic control.
- Bone-cutting saw (either a powered oscillating saw or Gigli saw).
- Bone rasp.
- Amputation knife.
- Standard vascular and soft tissue instruments.

PATIENT PREPARATION
- Ankle-brachial index studies (if applicable) and segmental arterial pressures of the lower limb.
  - Popliteal artery pressure of 50 mm Hg is generally considered adequate to heal a BKA.
- Full vascular evaluation for possible salvage procedures, including angioplasty, stenting, or vascular bypass (see Figure 39–1).
- Full medical evaluation (given the high incidence of cardiac disease among patients).
  - Consider cardiac optimization with aspirin, a statin, and a β-blocker as tolerated.
- Preoperative Physical Medicine and Rehabilitation Amputee service consultation.
- Preoperative anesthesia consultation for spinal or regional block.
- Discussion among orthopedic, vascular, and plastic surgery services regarding limb viability in patients with traumatic injury.
- Preoperative type and crossmatch, as appropriate.

PATIENT POSITIONING
- For either BKA or AKA, the patient should be supine.

PROCEDURE
- **Figure 39–1:** Vascular anatomy of the lower extremity, showing locations for skin incision and femoral and tibial transection.

Below-the-Knee Amputation
- General, epidural, or long-acting spinal anesthesia may be used.
- The entire leg is prepared circumferentially to the level of the proximal thigh; open wounds should be prepared with povidone-iodine.
- A sterile thigh tourniquet is applied.
  - Caveat: a tourniquet should not be used in patients with severe vascular occlusive disease.
- The distal foot is covered with stockinette or Ioban antimicrobial drape to further exclude it from the operative field.
- Ideally, 10 cm of tibia distal to the tibial tuberosity is maintained; this can be measured with a ruler or using the width of the surgeon's hand.
- The planned skin incision is marked 1–2 cm distal to the planned site of tibial transection to allow for soft tissue coverage.

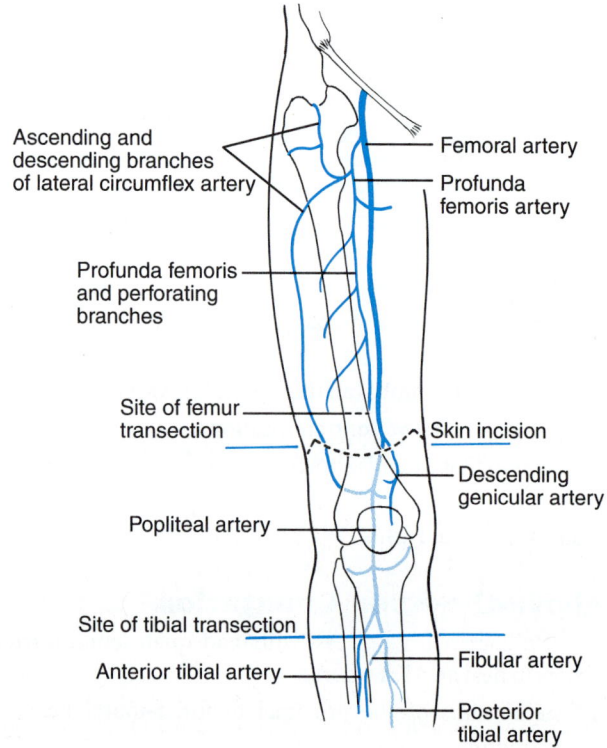

Figure 39–1

- **Figure 39–2:** Marking of the incision site.
  - The planned incision is marked to proceed around the anterior two thirds of the lower extremity circumference.
  - The posterior flap is then marked by measuring one third of the lower extremity circumference with slight tapering at the distal end; this measurement can be made with a suture or umbilical tape cut to the circumference of the lower extremity at the site of amputation.
  - A slight beveling of the incision proximally at the corner can allow for better closure at the end of the case.
  - The marked incisions are then made and carried down through the skin, subcutaneous fat, and fascia.
  - Care is taken to identify and ligate the great saphenous vein.
- **Figure 39–3:** Cross-sectional anatomy of the calf.
  - With electrocautery, the musculature of the anterior and lateral compartments is divided down to the periosteum of the tibia and fibula.
  - Special care is taken when dissecting through the muscle bellies to achieve hemostasis.
  - The anterior tibial vessels are identified and ligated.

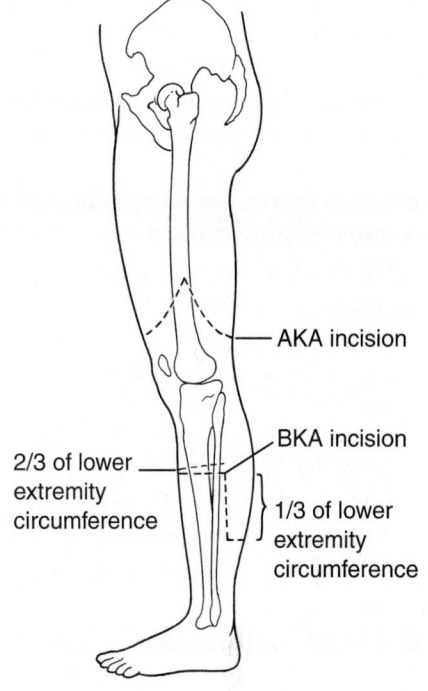

Figure 39–2

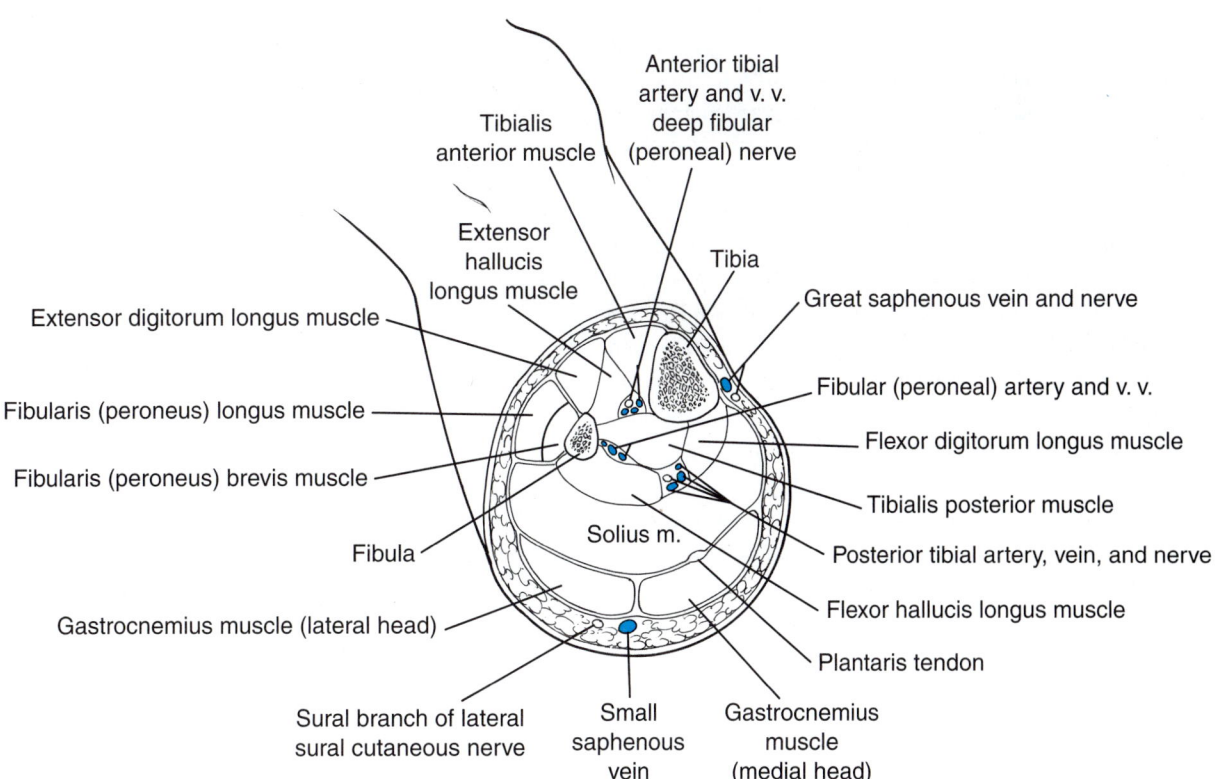

Figure 39–3

- **Figure 39–4A:** Using a rake retractor, the subcutaneous tissues are retracted proximally over the tibia to expose the planned site of transection.
  - The periosteum is divided around the tibia and a periosteal elevator is used to separate the proximal periosteum from the tibia.
- **Figure 39–4B:** Either a reciprocating saw or a Gigli saw is used to transect the tibia.
  - To avoid causing a pressure point under the prosthesis, the anterior edge of the tibia is then beveled at a 45-degree angle using either the reciprocating saw or a bone rasp.
  - Attention is next turned to the fibula; the periosteum is again divided and a periosteal elevator is used to strip the proximal periosteum from the fibula.
- **Figure 39–4C:** The fibula is then transected 1 cm proximal to the location of the tibial transection in order to prevent the fibula from becoming a pressure point.
  - This can be done with a reciprocating saw, Gigli saw, or bone cutter.
- Next, an amputation knife is used to transect the posterior soft tissues.
  - The initial knife cut is perpendicular to the limb axis in a posterior direction to divide the deep posterior compartment.
  - The knife is then turned in a coronal plane to develop a posterior flap consisting of skin, subcutaneous fat, and the muscles of the superficial posterior compartment.
  - Care must be taken to keep the knife within the previous lateral incisions made at the start of the operation to maintain an adequate skin for flap closure.
- At the distal aspect of the incisions, the gastrocnemius and soleus tendons are cut and the amputated specimen is handed off for pathologic examination.
- If a tourniquet is not used, pressure is held on the remaining tissue to control hemorrhage mainly from the transected popliteal trunk.
- Hemostasis is achieved with specific attention paid to identification and ligation of the posterior vasculature using electrocautery or suture ligatures.
- The transected nerves are sharply cut as proximal as possible and allowed to retract up into the soft tissue.
- Rough edges of bone are rasped smooth.
- After irrigation, the posterior flap is rotated anteriorly.
- **Figure 39–5A-C:** The deep fascia of the superficial posterior compartment may be sutured to the anterior periosteum of the tibia with absorbable sutures to secure muscle coverage over the tibia, although not all surgeons perform this step.
- Deep dermal sutures are then placed followed by skin staples or nylon sutures; the final stump has the appearance of Figure 39–5.

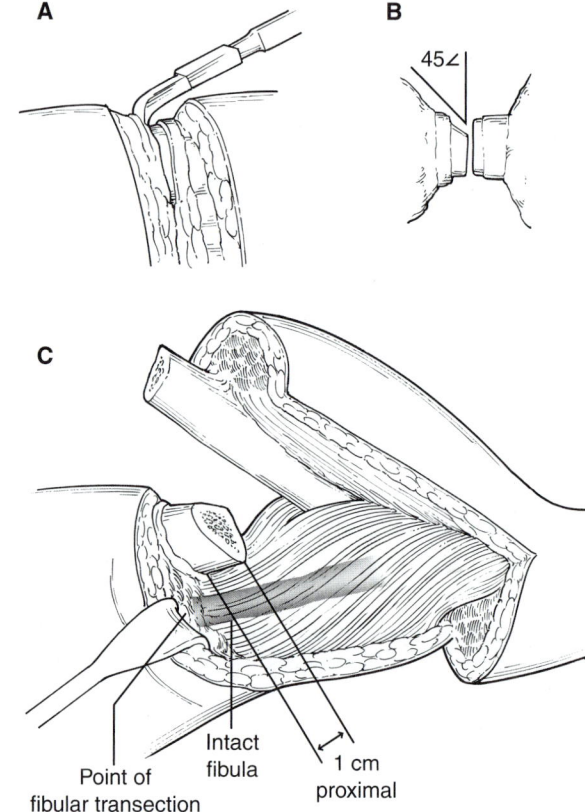

Figure 39–4A–C

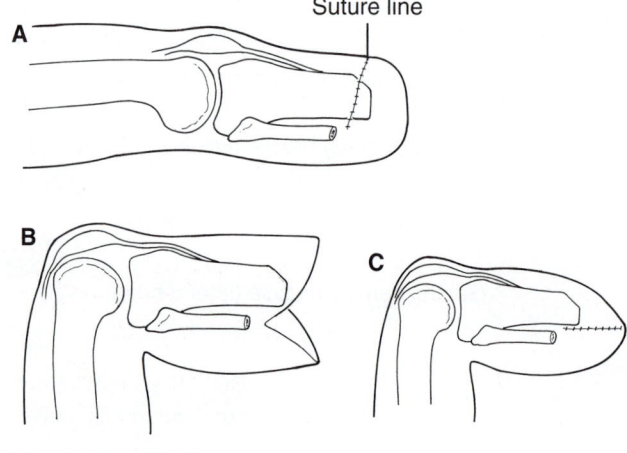

Figure 39–5A–C

- Based on the clinical situation, a Penrose drain may be left under the flap and brought out through a corner of the incision.
- A soft, gently compressive dressing is placed.

Above-the-Knee Amputation

- As in BKA, general, epidural, or a long-acting spinal anesthetic is administered.
- The operative leg is circumferentially prepared and an extremity drape is applied.
- A sterile tourniquet can be placed high on the thigh but may not be necessary in the patient with severe vascular disease.
- A fish-mouth incision is designed with equal anterior and posterior flaps that end just proximal to the knee, maximizing the length of the amputated thigh (see Figure 39–2).
- **Figure 39–6:** Cross-sectional anatomy of the thigh.
  - If a tourniquet is used, the leg should be exsanguinated by either elevation or compression with an Ace or Esmarch bandage.

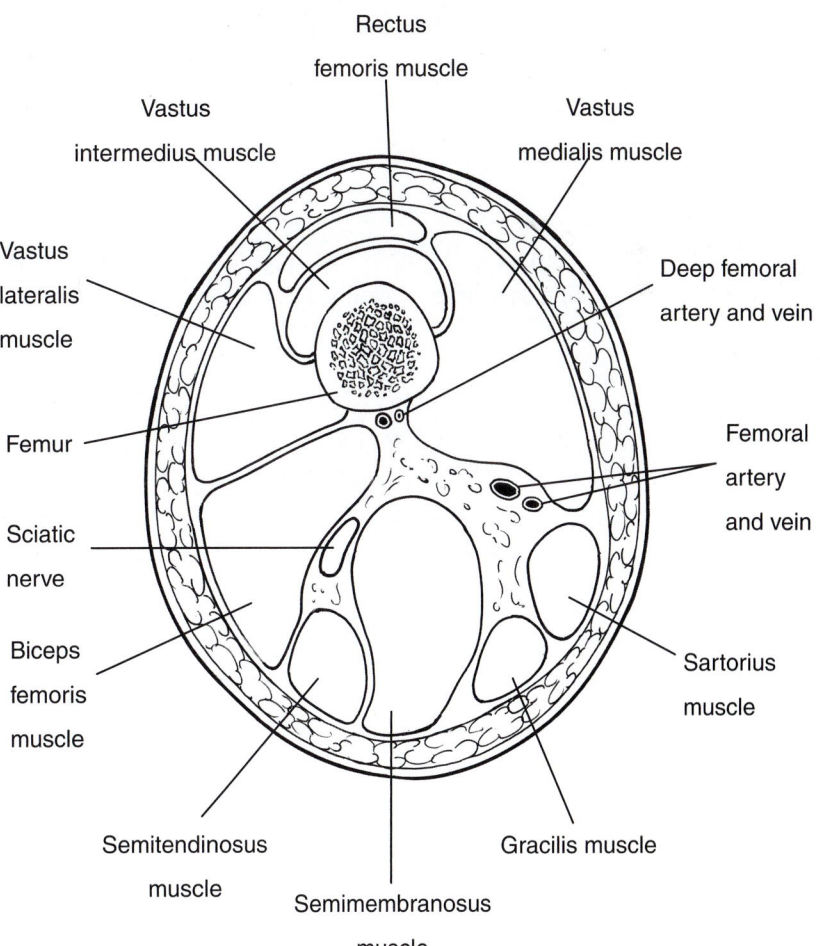

Figure 39–6

- The tourniquet is then insufflated to 250 mm Hg.
- The skin incision is made with a No. 10 blade.
- Dissection is continued straight down to the femur through the subcutaneous fat, rectus femoris, and vastus musculature anteriorly using electrocautery.

■ **Figure 39–7A:** In patients with severe vascular disease, some surgeons prefer the entire dissection to be performed sharply with a No. 10 blade followed by focused hemostasis using suture ligature to minimize thermal tissue trauma.

■ **Figure 39–7B:** On the medial side of the leg, the great saphenous vein is clamped between hemostats, divided sharply, and ligated with 2-0 silk ties.

■ **Figure 39–7C:** Dissection continues through the hamstring and adductor muscles of the medial and posterior thigh until the femoral artery and vein are located.
- The artery and vein are isolated and suture-ligated.
- Near the femoral artery and vein, the sciatic nerve is identified.
- Proximal resection of the nerve is essential to minimize chance of palpable neuroma.
- The nerve is placed on tension and cut sharply to allow the proximal end to retract up the thigh within the posterior musculature.

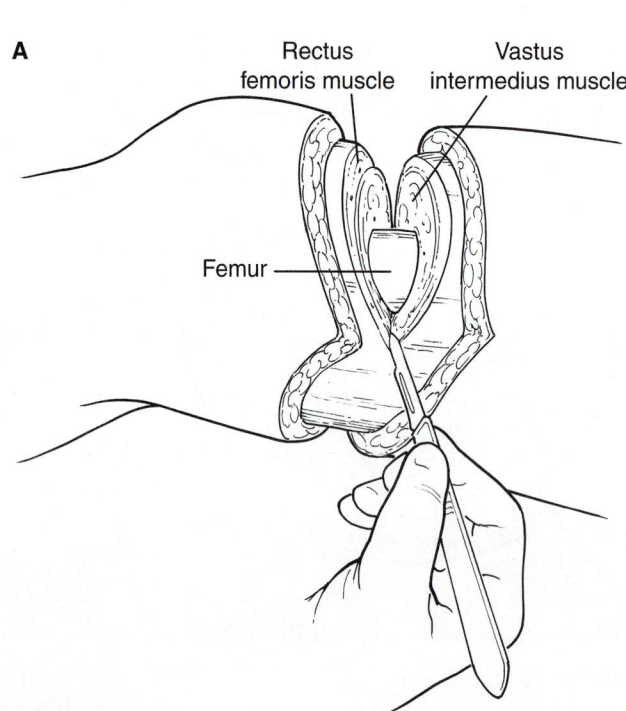
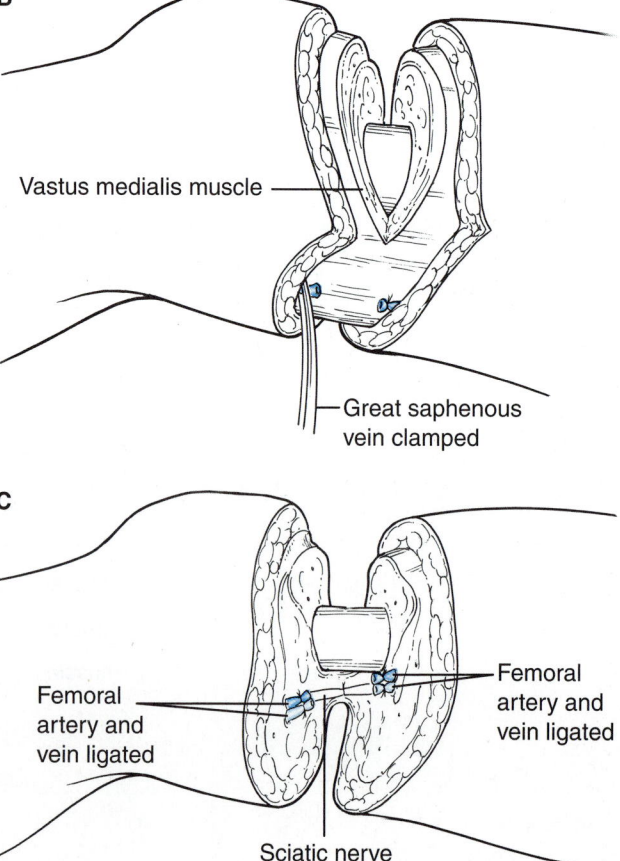

Figure 36–7A–C

- **Figure 39–8A:** Transection of the femur.
  - A periosteal elevator is used to expose the femur 2–3 cm proximal to the deep corner of the fish-mouth incision.
  - Alternatively, the femur can be transected before the posterior musculature and soft tissues are transected.
- **Figure 39–8B:** A powered oscillating saw or Gigli saw is used to cut the bone.
  - No bevel is needed because of the thickness of the muscle bellies in the thigh.
- If a tourniquet was used, the pressure is released and hemostasis is achieved with a combination of electrocautery and suture ligature.
- The wound is copiously irrigated and the viability of the anterior and posterior muscle flaps is assessed.
- A 10 French closed suction drain, if clinically indicated, is placed in the subfascial space through a separate stab incision on the lateral aspect of the leg.
- **Figure 39–8C, D:** The wound is closed in layered fashion.
- First, the fascia is closed with interrupted figure-of-eight 2-0 Vicryl sutures over the drain.

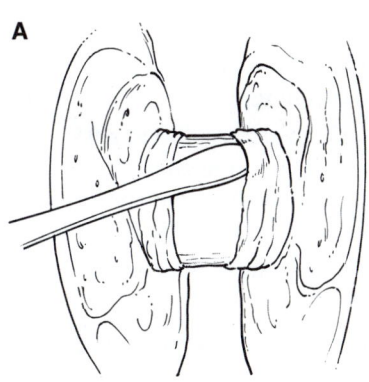
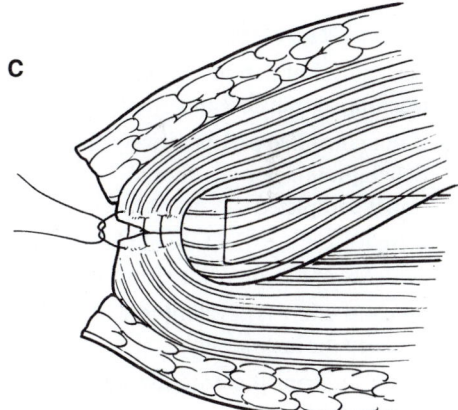
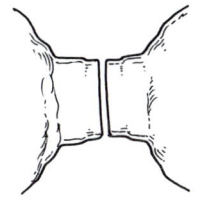
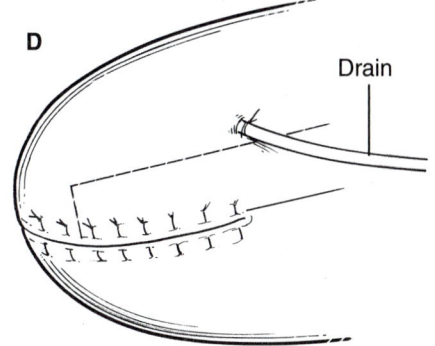

Figure 39–8A–D

- Next, the skin is closed with deep dermal 3-0 Vicryl sutures followed by either staples or vertical mattress 3-0 nylon sutures.
- The wound is dressed with nonadherent iodinated petrolatum gauze dressing and soft gauze wrap.

POSTOPERATIVE CARE

Wound Care
- Most surgeons keep the initial dressing in place for 2 days before examining the wound.
- For both AKA and BKA, the lower extremity stump must be kept strictly elevated at all times to reduce edema.

Medical Management
- A patient-controlled analgesia pump is often used for postoperative pain.
- Perioperative tight glucose control is essential to decrease the risk of wound infection and optimize healing.
- Due to concomitant cardiovascular disease in many patients undergoing amputation, perioperative aspirin, statins, and β-blockers should be continued.
- Patients should be closely monitored for symptoms of cardiac ischemia.

Rehabilitation
- Early physical therapy consultation is required to initiate teaching of transfers and one-legged mobility.
- If not consulted preoperatively, the Physical Medicine and Rehabilitation service should be consulted after amputation is completed.
- With BKA, the patient should be monitored closely for any evidence of flexion contracture at the knee.
  - If contracture is developing, a posterior splint can be used to keep the knee straight.
- Some surgeons prefer to use a rigid removal cast dressing in the initial postoperative period to protect the stump and help prevent flexion contracture.
- The patient should remain non-weight bearing on the amputated extremity for a minimum of 3 months.
- A prosthesis may be fit at 6 weeks but should not be used until all wounds have completely healed.

POTENTIAL COMPLICATIONS
- Delayed wound healing.
  - May occur during the first few postoperative weeks secondary to persistent infection or poor vascular inflow.
  - Often managed with antibiotics when indicated and local wound care but can require surgical debridement, revision, or higher amputation
- Hematomas.
  - Should be drained to prevent future infection.
- Joint contractures of the knee.
  - Contracture after BKA is often difficult to correct; early intervention with physical therapy can be helpful, including splinting of the knee in an extended position.
  - With an AKA, contractures can occur at the hip joint; prevention involves having the patient lie in a prone position and aggressive physical therapy.
- Neuromas.
  - Can occur at sites of transected nerves from overactive axonal regeneration.
  - If close to the skin, these sensitive nodules cause shooting pain with contact and may limit fitting of a prosthetic limb.
  - Occurrence is minimized by dividing the nerve as proximally as possible and then burying the nerve stump under the muscle.
- Phantom limb sensations.
  - Occur in most amputations and can be quite disabling and difficult to treat.
  - Early desensitization therapy and involvement of an amputee specialist can decrease the risk of this disabling complication.
  - Medicines for neuropathic pain (eg, pregabalin or gabapentin) may also be effective to prevent phantom sensations.
- Cardiovascular events, including heart attack, stroke, venous thromboembolism, or death.
  - These are significant risks given the frequent comorbidities in amputation patients and significant physiologic stress of the amputation procedure.
  - Preoperative optimization and close postoperative monitoring are the best interventions to decrease this risk.

PEARLS AND TIPS
- In cases of wet gangrene, uncontrolled lymphedema, or critical illness, a guillotine amputation (either above or below the knee) may be performed to remove the infected tissue. Formal amputation is planned once the patient is physiologically stable and the infection has been controlled with systemic antibiotics and local wound care.
- With any amputation, preoperative optimization is necessary to decrease the risk of morbidity and mortality.
- Thorough knowledge of the cross-sectional anatomy of the thigh or calf will facilitate quick and easy identification of major vessels and nerves.
- In BKA, dissection of the posterior flap with the amputation knife can be tricky; it is best to have too much flap and trim to fit rather than not have enough and be forced to shorten the amputation.

- The posterior flap is most commonly used because the vascular supply to the gastrocnemius musculocutaneous flap is from the sural artery, which arises above the knee; alternatively, sagittally based flaps or anterior-posterior fishmouth flaps can be used if clinically necessary.
- Division of any nerves should be performed on tension to allow the nerve to retract up the leg, minimizing the chance of neuroma development.

REFERENCES

Giglia J, Jarboe MD. Lower Extremity Amputation. In: Mulholland MW, Lillemoe KD, Doherty GM, et al, eds. *Greenfield's Surgery: Scientific Principles & Practice*, 4th ed. Philadelphia, PA: Lippincott Williams & Wilkins; 2006:1310–1334.

Rapp JH, MacTaggart J. Arteries. In: Doherty GM, ed. *Current Diagnosis and Treatment: Surgery.* New York, NY: McGraw-Hill; 2010:753–787.

CHAPTER 40

Inguinal Hernia Repair

Timothy L. Frankel, MD, and Richard E. Burney, MD

INDICATIONS

- Recent literature suggests that patients who are asymptomatic or "minimally symptomatic" may be managed without surgical intervention.
- All symptomatic inguinal hernias (pain, neurologic symptoms) should be repaired unless a specific contraindication exists.
- Inguinal hernias that are incarcerated and are reduced in a timely fashion should be repaired on an urgent basis.
- Hernias that are unable to be reduced should be treated as a surgical emergency and repaired expeditiously.

CONTRAINDICATIONS

- There are no absolute contraindications.
- In the event the patient cannot undergo general or spinal anesthetic, the repair can be performed under local anesthetic with sedation.

INFORMED CONSENT

Potential Risks

- Bleeding.
- Infection (potentially requiring reoperation to remove infected mesh).
- Damage to nerves resulting in loss of inner thigh skin sensation.
- Damage to the vas deferens or testicular vessels potentially leading to decreased fertility.
- Recurrence.
- Neuralgia.

PATIENT PREPARATION

- Nothing by mouth for 6 hours before surgery.
- Blood thinners should be discontinued with adequate time for normalization of coagulation.
- Foley catheter insertion is required for laparoscopic procedures only.

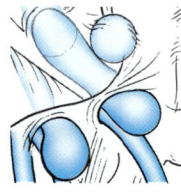
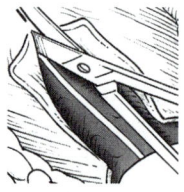
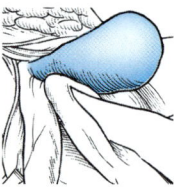
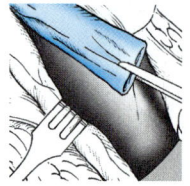
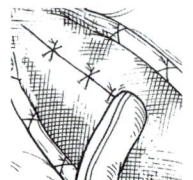
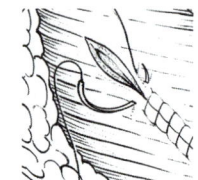
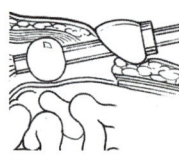
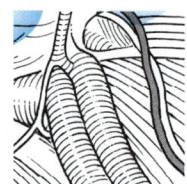
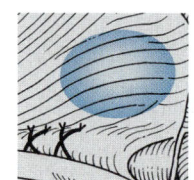

PATIENT POSITIONING

- The patient should be supine.

PROCEDURE

Open Inguinal Hernia Repair

- The operation may be performed under spinal, local, or general anesthesia.
- **Figure 40–1:** Inguinal hernia locations.
- **Figure 40–2A:** Landmarks for skin incision are the anterior superior iliac spine and pubic tubercle.
  - The incision should be superior to the inguinal ligament and, if possible, hidden in a natural skin crease.
- **Figure 40–2B:** The subcutaneous tissue should be divided until the external oblique fascia is encountered.
  - A regional local anesthetic block may be placed at this time (10 mL of 0.5% bupivacaine infiltrated subfascially into the deep muscular layers and retroperitoneum along the iliac fossa region 2 cm medial and cephalad to the anterior superior iliac spine).
  - The external oblique fascia is then divided sharply to expose the underlying cord and hernia.

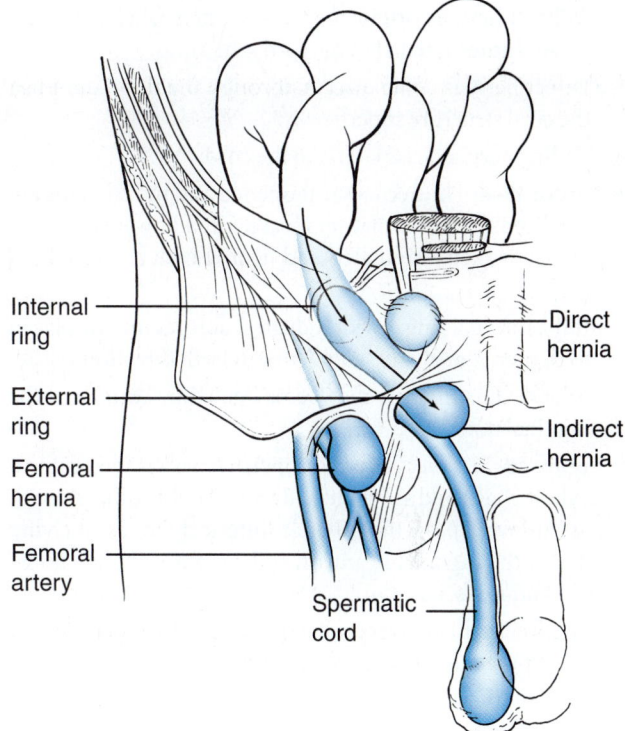

Figure 40–1

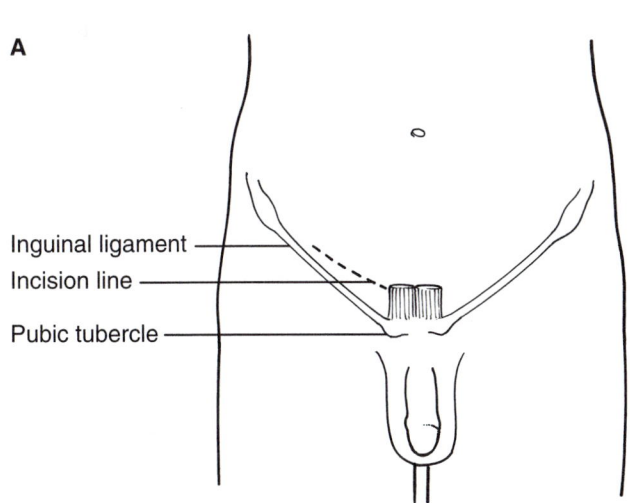

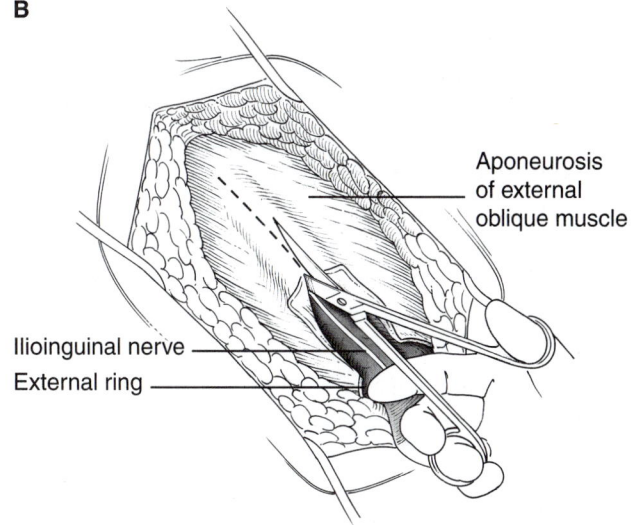

Figure 40–2A–B

- **Figure 40–3:** The hernia sac is dissected free from the associated cord structures.
  - Care should be taken to identify the ilioinguinal nerve and retract it away from the area of dissection to avoid injury.
  - Indirect hernias originate from the internal ring and are located anteromedial to the cord structures.
  - Direct hernias come directly through the floor and push the cord structure superficially.
  - Sliding hernias arise lateral to the cord.
- **Figure 40–4:** The hernia sac is opened and the contents are visualized to ensure that no incarcerated bowel is present. The sac is then amputated and ligated with a suture ligature.
  - If the internal ring is widely dilated, sutures may be placed to tighten it medially, laterally, or in both directions.
  - A large direct hernia may be navigated by sutures in the inguinal floor.
- **Figure 40–5:** A piece of polypropylene mesh is then cut to a keyhole shape and sewn medially to the pubic tubercle with a 2-cm overlap on the tubercle, inferiorly to the shelving edge of the inguinal ligament, and superiorly to the internal oblique fascia.
  - The internal ring is recreated by sewing together the two tails of the mesh lateral to the cord.
  - The tails then extend laterally beneath the external oblique fascia.
- **Figure 40–6:** After the mesh is secured, the external oblique fascia is closed using a running stitch in a medial to lateral direction. The medial closure will form the new external inguinal ring.

Laparoscopic Total Extraperitoneal Inguinal Hernia Repair

- The operation is performed under general anesthesia for laparoscopic hernia repair.
- **Figure 40–7A, B:** A 10-mm port is placed at the umbilicus (Figure 40–7A).
  - Care is taken to insert a balloon dilator between the rectus muscle and posterior sheath fascia.
  - By advancing the dilator toward the pubis, the preperitoneal space is entered.
  - The balloon is inflated and held in place for 5 minutes to ensure hemostasis of small vessels avulsed on entry (Figure 40–7B).
  - The preperitoneal space is then insufflated.
  - Two 5-mm ports are placed in the midline between the umbilicus and pubis into the preperitoneal space (see Figure 40–7A).

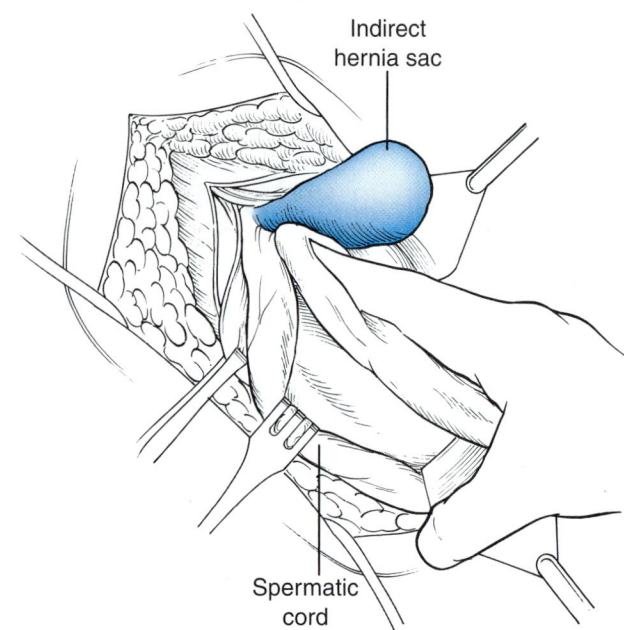

Figure 40–3

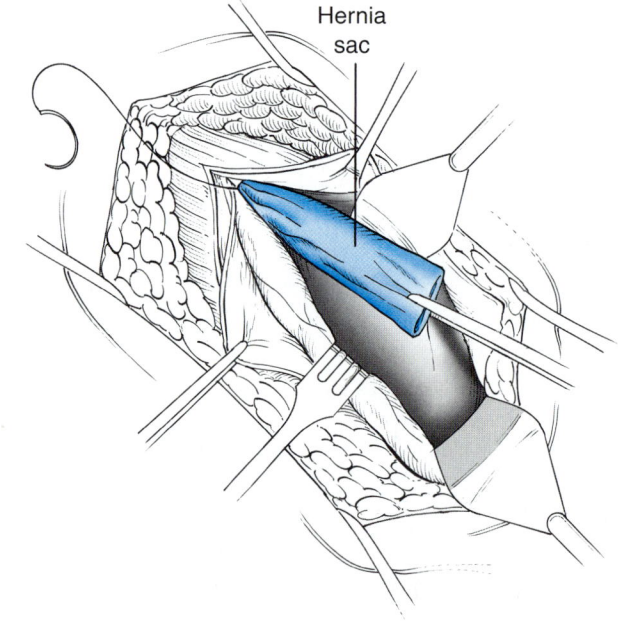

Figure 40–4

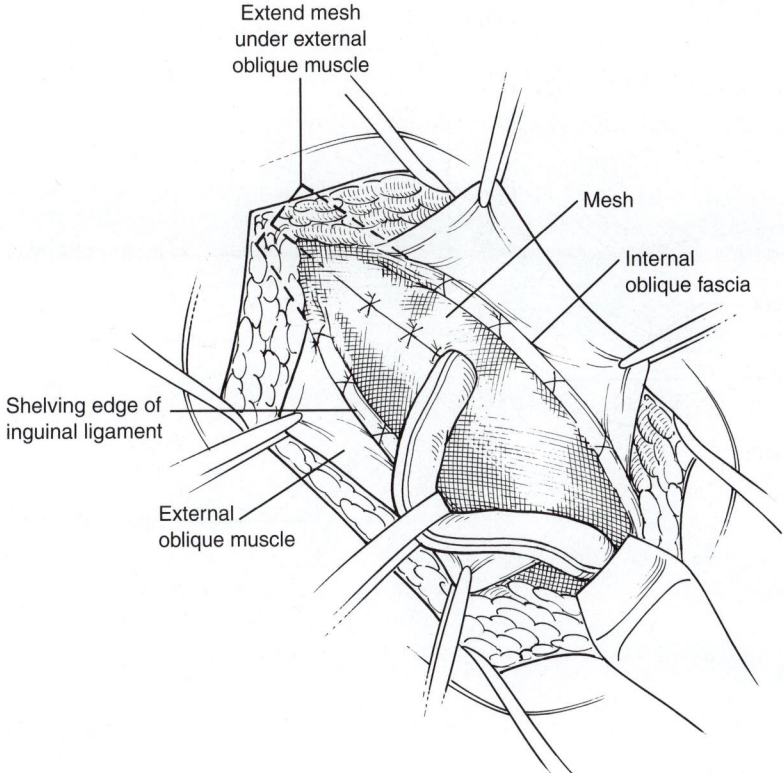

Figure 40–5

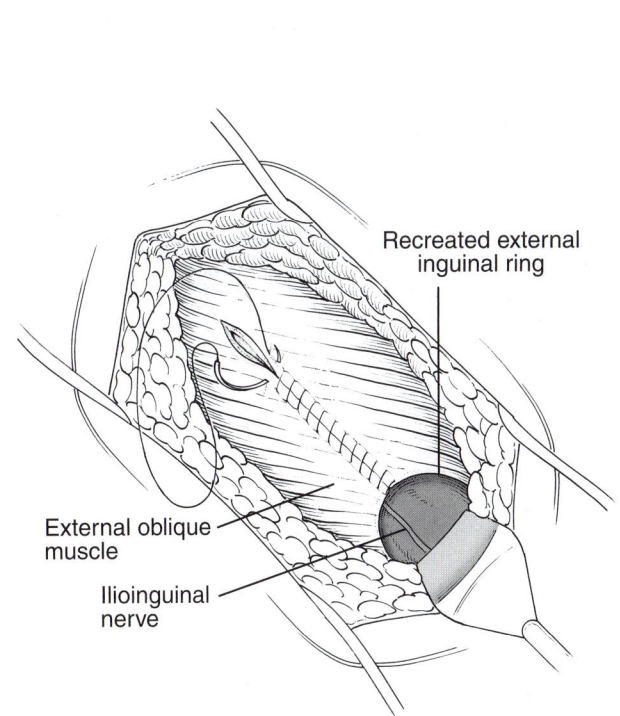

Figure 40–6

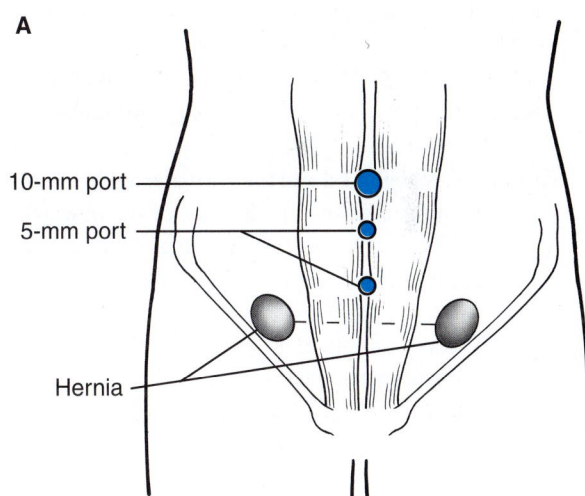

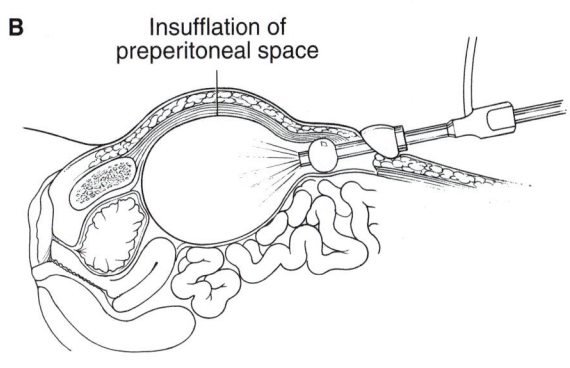

Figure 40–7A–B

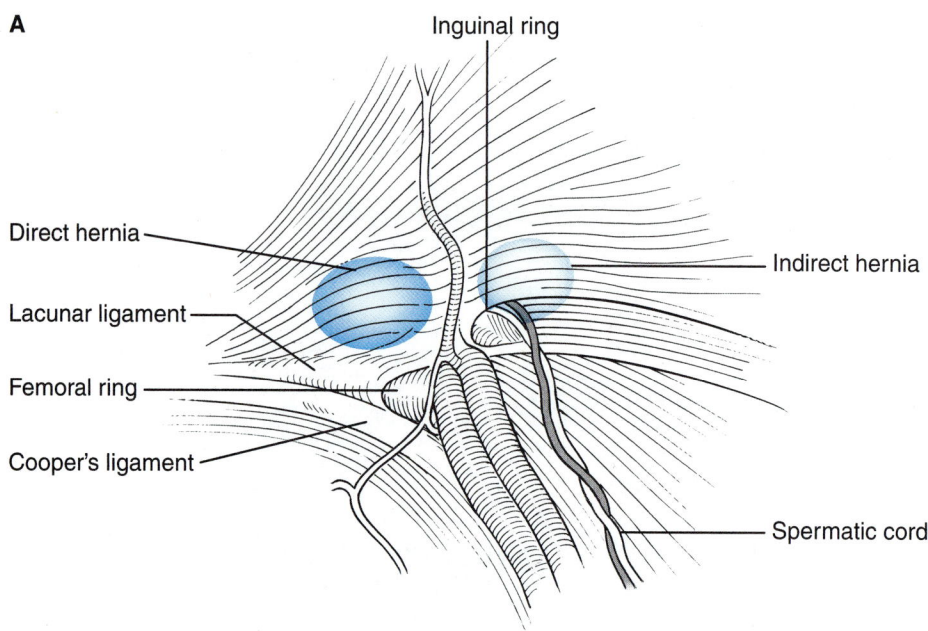

Figure 40–8A

- **Figure 40–8A:** The pubic tubercle and Cooper's ligament are identified medially (this view is of the right groin).
  - The space lateral to the hernia and cord structures is then developed bluntly.
  - The hernia is identified and the sac dissected free from the cord structures. It is then pulled out of the internal ring for an indirect hernia using a hand-over-hand technique.
  - Great care should be taken to avoid creating a hole in the hernia sac or peritoneum during this dissection as this leads to development of a pneumoperitoneum, which collapses the preperitoneal working space.
  - A direct hernia may also be reduced using a hand-over-hand technique if necessary, although often insufflation of the preperitoneal space alone will reduce a direct inguinal hernia.
- **Figure 40–8B:** Once the hernia sac has been swept clear of the cord structures and anterior abdominal wall, a piece of preformed mesh is placed through the 10-mm port and positioned using graspers.
  - The mesh is positioned to cover the entire myopectineal orifice and then tacked medially to the pubis or Cooper's ligament, or both.
  - Direct, indirect, and femoral hernia defects are covered by the mesh, as shown.

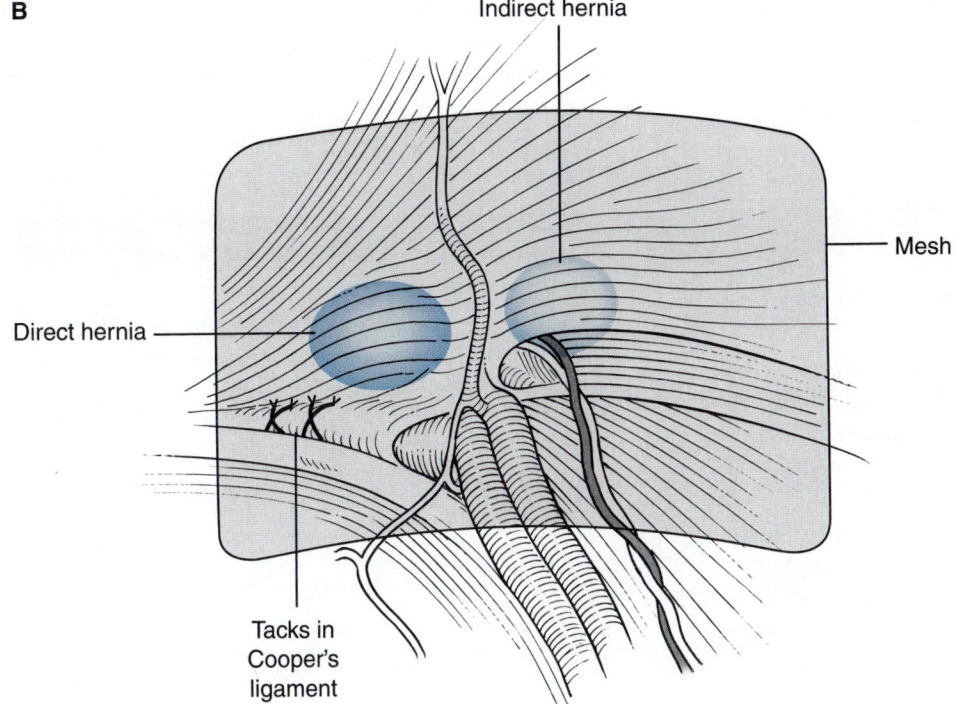

Figure 40–8B

POSTOPERATIVE CARE

- Uncomplicated open or laparoscopic hernia repair is performed on an outpatient basis.
- Postoperative pain control is achieved with anti-inflammatory medications and narcotics for severe pain.

POTENTIAL COMPLICATIONS

- Bleeding can range from a subcutaneous hematoma to hemoscrotum.
  - This rarely requires reoperation, but patients must be informed about potential groin or scrotal bruising.
- Life-threatening hemorrhage is exceedingly rare but may occur if an unrecognized retroperitoneal arterial injury occurs.
  - Typical manifestations are hypotension, decreased urine output, and possibly flank bruising.
- Damage to the ilioinguinal or genitofemoral nerves may result in paraesthesia to the inner thigh or scrotum, or both.
  - This complication is often temporary when caused by traction but may be permanent if caused by transection.
- Chronic groin pain is believed to be caused by nerve entrapment during repair. Occasionally, the pain is debilitating enough to require reexploration.

- Some surgeons electively transect the ilioinguinal nerve when it is encountered to avoid this complication, although this has not been proven to be effective.

PEARLS AND TIPS

- In open repair, take care to identify the ilioinguinal nerve and retract it away from the repair to avoid entrapment. Entrapment most often occurs when sewing the mesh superiorly to the internal oblique fascia and when closing the external oblique fascia.
- During laparoscopic repair, avoid overly aggressive blunt dissection in the region inferior and medial to the hernia and cord to avoid damage to the femoral vessels. To avoid injury to blood vessels and nerves, do not place tacks inferior to the inguinal ring.
- Avoid tearing of the peritoneum during laparoscopic repair as this will cause pneumoperitoneum, decreasing the preperitoneal working space. If this does occur, a Veress needle can be inserted in the periumbilical region to decompress the peritoneum.
- To prevent recurrence after laparoscopic repair, ensure that the mesh used is large enough to cover the entire myopectineal orifice.
- The most common site of recurrence following laparoscopic repair is posteriorly. This is likely the result of failure to adequately reduce the posterior peritoneum (hernia sac) far enough cephalad.

REFERENCES

Fitzgibbons RJ, Giobbie-Hurder A, Gibbs JO, et al. Watchful waiting vs. repair of inguinal hernia in minimally symptomatic men. *JAMA.* 2006;295:285–292.

Franz MG. Complications of Abdominal Wall and Hernia Operations. In: Mulholland MW, Doherty GM, eds. *Complications in Surgery.* Philadelphia, PA: Lippincott Williams & Wilkins; 2006:575–593.

CHAPTER 41

Vental Hernia Repair

Kristoffer B. Sugg, MD, Edwin Y. Chang, MD, and Michael G. Franz, MD

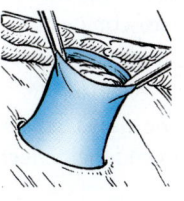 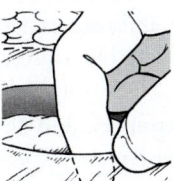 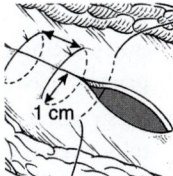
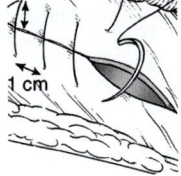 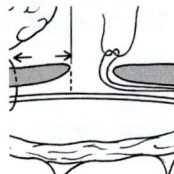 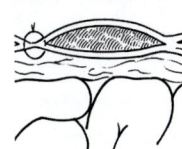
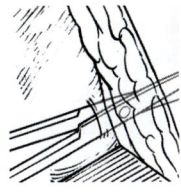  

INDICATIONS

- Incarceration.
- Strangulation.
- Bowel obstruction.
- Functional or cosmetic deformity.
- Threatened overlying skin.
- Pain.

CONTRAINDICATIONS

Absolute

- Inability to tolerate general anesthetic (cardiopulmonary risk).
- Absence of tissue for reconstruction (myofascia or skin).
- Massive loss of peritoneal domain.

Relative

- Infection.
- Moderate loss of peritoneal domain.
- Morbid obesity.
- Malnutrition.
- Tobacco use.
- Bleeding diathesis.
- Ascites.

INFORMED CONSENT

Expected Benefits

- Restoration of the structure and therefore function of the abdominal wall by reestablishing myofascial continuity and preventing evisceration.

Potential Risks

- Recurrence rates are as high as 50% depending on the type of repair (primary vs mesh, open vs laparoscopic).
- Complications include:

- Surgical site infection.
- Mesh-associated infection and fistulization.
- Bleeding.
- Seroma formation.
- Damage to adjacent structures.
- Hernia recurrence.
- Risks related to any major operation (myocardial infarction, pneumonia, and venous thromboembolism).

EQUIPMENT

- No special equipment is required for an open repair.
- Laparoscopic repair utilizes standard laparoscopic equipment, including camera (30 degree), monitor, and appropriately sized ports (5 or 10 mm) with associated trocars.
- Mesh selection is complex and should be based on an understanding of mesh material properties and their effect on wound healing.
  - Meshes may be made of permanent synthetic plastics, rapidly absorbed polymers, or biologic extracellular matrices.

PATIENT PREPARATION

- The number of previous attempts at hernia repair should be elicited, including whether or not mesh was used.
- If the patient smokes or is overweight, lifestyle changes should be recommended prior to the operation.
- Nutrition should be optimized and medications adjusted as necessary (eg, discontinuing methotrexate and steroids) to decrease the likelihood of wound healing problems.
- Visual inspection should include looking for existing abdominal scars that may influence the operative plan.
- The fascial defect should be palpated to determine if the contents of the hernia sac are reducible.
- CT imaging is helpful for outlining the exact size and location of the fascial defect, which is often larger than it may appear on clinical examination.
- CT imaging also reveals the contents of the hernia sac, condition of the abdominal wall musculature for reconstruction, and the presence of other hernias.

PATIENT POSITIONING

- The patient should be supine for the most common midline incisional hernias.
- Modified decubitus positions are used for flank incisional hernia repairs, with appropriate pressure points padded.
- Limited hip flexion can help relax the abdominal wall musculature.

- Tilting the head of the operating table up or down, left or right, aids in gravity-assisted retraction of the abdominal viscera and reduction of the hernia sac contents.

PROCEDURE

- **Figure 41–1:** Sharp dissection is carried down through the skin and subcutaneous tissue to the underlying fascia.
  - The hernia sac (blue) can sometimes be difficult to expose, especially if its contents are already reduced secondary to proper patient positioning.
  - If present, the thin layer of overlying fascia is delicately teased off the hernia sac and dissected back to fascia with sufficient bulk and robust blood supply to hold suture material.
  - The thickened, fibroplastic "hernia ring" should be fully exposed.
  - The hernia sac is opened, being cognizant that loops of bowel may be adherent to the posterior peritoneal surface.
  - Under direct visualization, the contents of the hernia sac are definitively reduced.
  - The excess peritoneum (hernia sac) is then excised.
- **Figure 41–2:** The fascial defect is clearly outlined by removing fat and other devitalized tissue from the fascial edges.
  - It is important to allow at least 5 cm of clearance in all directions before closure is attempted.
  - This is easily accomplished by a careful finger sweep in the subfascial layer to release any further adherent intra-abdominal contents from the posterior peritoneal surface.
- **Figure 41–3A, B:** Primary repair is reserved for small, uncomplicated hernias (<3 cm).

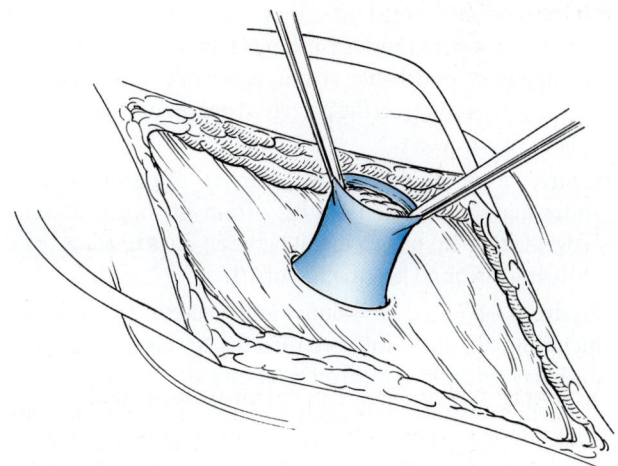

Figure 41–1

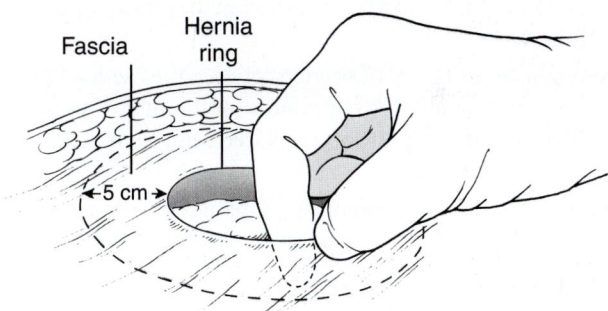

Figure 41–2

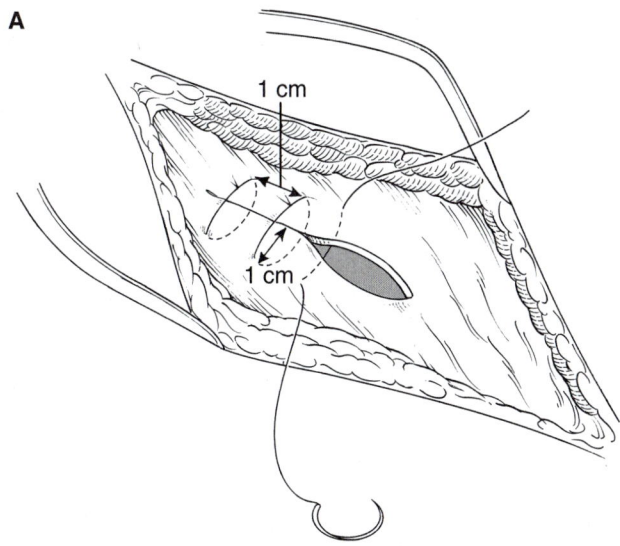

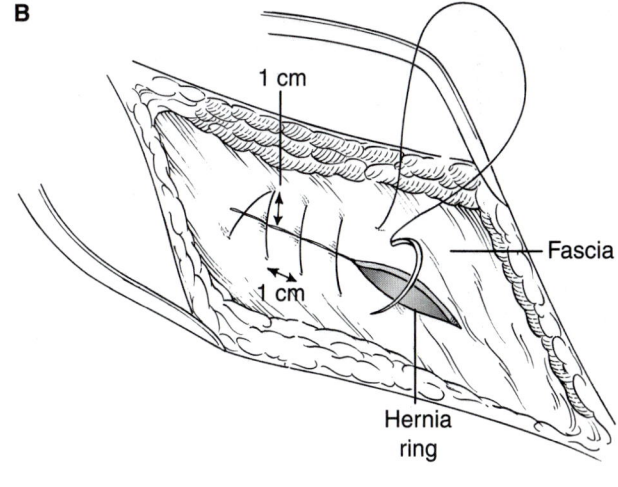

Figure 41–3A–B

- It can be performed in either an interrupted (Figure 41–3A) or a continuous running (Figure 41–3B) fashion using either resorbable or nonresorbable monofilament suture, depending on the perceived degree of wound healing or tissue defect.
- During a continuous suture repair, it is important to take bites that are at least 1 cm back from the normal fascial edge, with 1 cm of spacing in between bites to allow for a suture-to-wound length ratio of 4:1.

■ **Figure 41–4:** There are various mesh placement techniques, including the onlay, inlay, retrorectus, and intraperitoneal underlay (intraperitoneal onlay of mesh).
- The figure shows retrorectus placement, in which the mesh is placed between the rectus abdominis muscle and posterior rectus sheath above the arcuate line and in the preperitoneal space below the arcuate line.
- This technique allows for preservation of the hernia sac and thus maintains a barrier between the mesh and underlying bowel.
- Again, at least 5 cm of overlap between the mesh and fascia should be allowed to promote optimum fibrous tissue ingrowth; tacking sutures are placed 3 cm from the fascial edge.

■ **Figure 41–5:** The components separation technique is a useful alternative for large midline abdominal defects.
- Fibrotic stiffness of the external oblique muscle layer plays a key role in the development of these hernias and hinders successful closure.
- Release of this muscle 1–2 cm lateral to its insertion into the anterior rectus sheath allows medial advancement of the remaining trimuscle complex composed of the rectus abdominis, internal oblique, and transverse abdominis muscles.
- The neurovascular bundle is preserved because it travels in the layer between the internal oblique and transverse abdominis muscles.

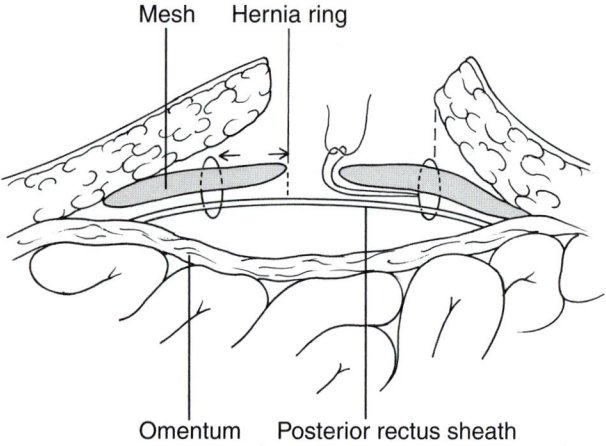

Figure 41–4

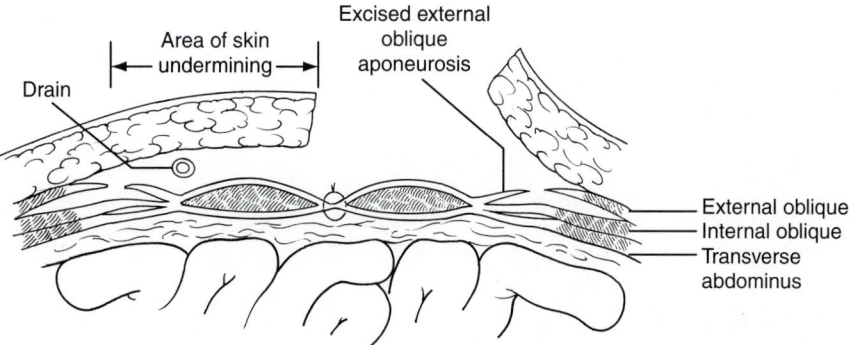

Figure 41–5

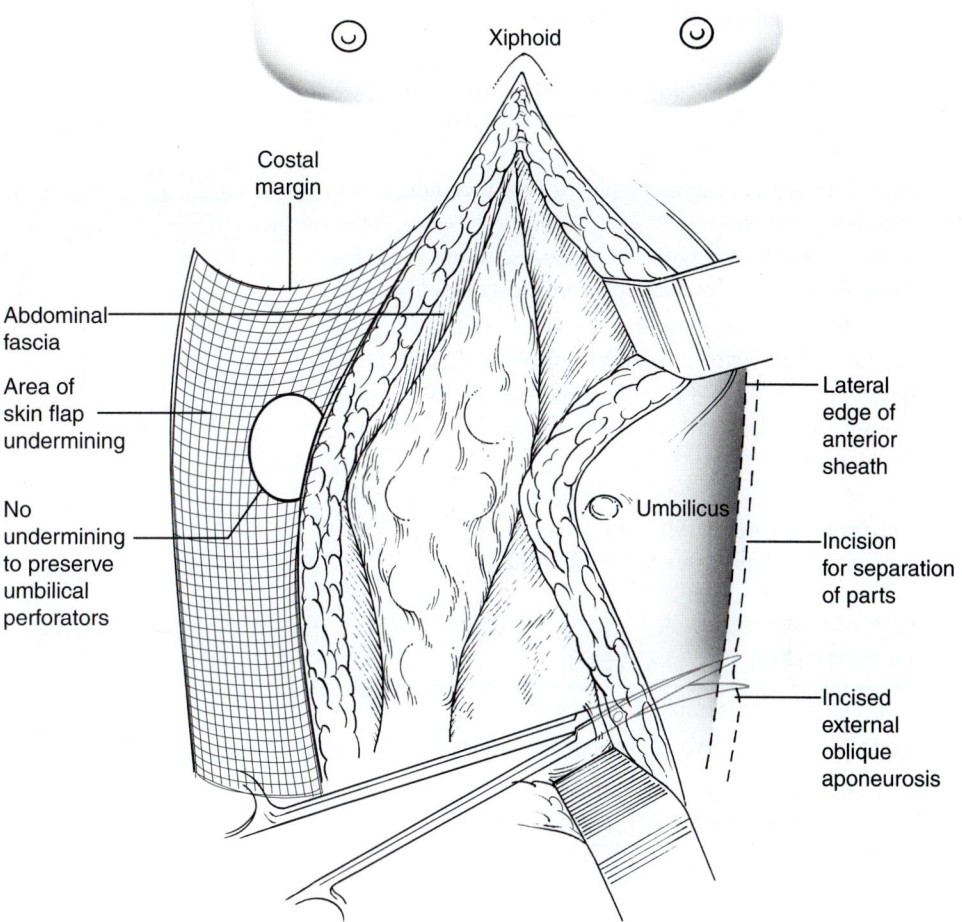

Figure 41–6

- Typical mobility includes 5 cm of unilateral advancement in the epigastric region, 10 cm at the umbilicus, and 3 cm in the suprapubic region.
- This technique minimizes the use of foreign material implants and preserves the innate dynamic nature of the abdominal wall musculature. Fibrotic lateral oblique stiffness is also released.

■ **Figure 41–6:** Newer modifications to the components separation technique include preservation of the umbilical perforators.
- This modification allows for better blood supply to the periumbilical watershed area and can decrease the risk of infection and wound healing problems.

■ **Figure 41–7:** If laparoscopic repair is preferred, the first trocar may be placed in the midline superior or inferior to the hernia defect.

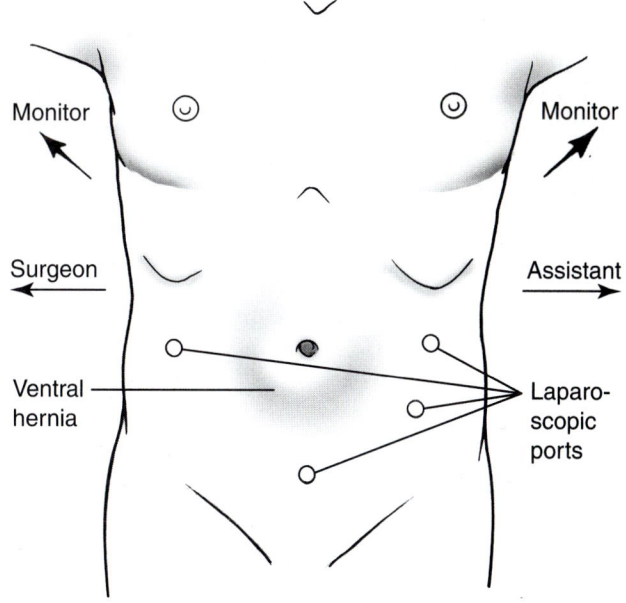

Figure 41–7

- A Veress needle technique can often be safely used in the left upper quadrant, where complicating adhesions are less common.
- Once pneumoperitoneum is established, insertion of the laparoscope (30 degree) aids in proper placement of the remaining trocars.
- Additional trocars should be placed on either side, as far lateral as possible.
- A 10-mm port assists with mesh placement into the peritoneum; otherwise, smaller operating ports are effective.
- An additional 5-mm port can be placed on the patient's opposite side to help with dissection and mesh fixation.
- **Figure 41–8:** At least 5 cm of overlap should be allowed between the fascia and mesh to promote good fibrous tissue ingrowth.
  - The mesh is secured in place by either tacking or through-and-through sutures. Most surgeons prefer a combination of both to optimize early mesh fixation.

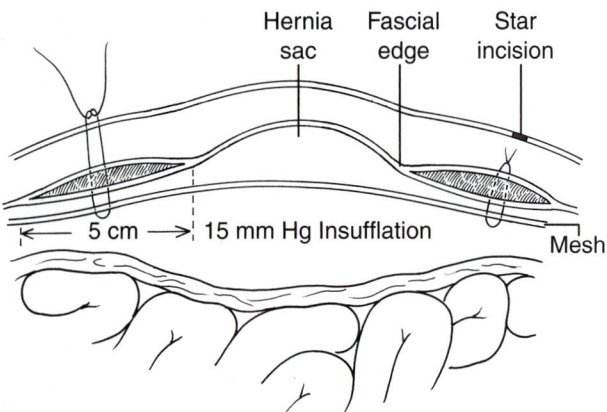

Figure 41–8

POSTOPERATIVE CARE

- Bowel rest until ileus resolves.
- Drains to prevent seroma formation if large flaps are raised.
- Binder for comfort (except after the components separation technique, in which compression may compromise blood flow to the abdominal wall skin flaps).

POTENTIAL COMPLICATIONS

- Recurrence.
  - Early (within 1 month): usually related to technical issues.
  - Late (after 1 year): most often due to patient factors leading to wound healing problems. The best clinical and preclinical evidence now supports the idea that the majority of incisional hernias are the result of very early laparotomy defects.
- Mesh (wound) infection or mesh extrusion.
- Bowel or bladder injury.
- Hematoma and seroma.
- Pain.

PEARLS AND TIPS

- Avoid mesh-on-bowel contact.
- Select the appropriate mesh material based on the surgical circumstances.

- Allow at least 5 cm of overlap between the fascia and mesh to promote good fibrous tissue ingrowth.
- Avoid large gaps between sutures to prevent bowel interposition (Richter's hernia).
- Optimize mesh fixation.
- Repair all questionable deserosalizations to prevent missed enterotomy.

REFERENCES

Burger JW, Luijendijk RW, Hop WC, et al. Long term follow-up of a randomized controlled trial of suture versus mesh repair of incisional hernia. *Ann Surg.* 2004;240:578–585.

Grevious MA, Cohen M, Jean-Pierre F, et al. The use of prosthesis in abdominal wall reconstruction. *Clin Plastic Surg.* 2006;33:181–197.

Korenkov M, Paul A, Sauerland S, et al. Classification and surgical treatment of incisional hernia: Results of an experts' meeting. *Langenbecks Archiv Surg.* 2001;386:65–73.

Nguyen V, Shestak KC. Separation of anatomic components method of abdominal wall reconstruction: clinical outcome analysis and an update of surgical modifications using the technique. *Clin Plastic Surg.* 2006;33:247–257.

Ramirez OM, Ruas E, Dellon L. "Components separation" method for closure of abdominal-wall defects: an anatomic and clinical study. *Plastic Reconstruct Surg.* 1990;86:519–526.

[CHAPTER 42]

Wound Closure Techniques

Brent M. Egeland, MD, and Paul S. Cederna, MD

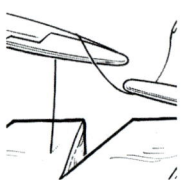 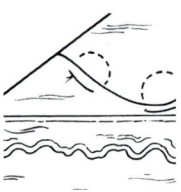 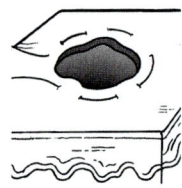
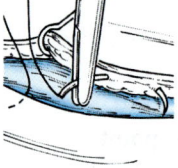 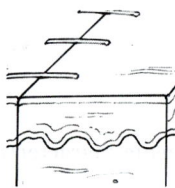 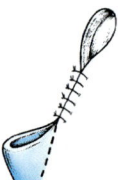

INDICATIONS
- Surgical wounds.
- Traumatic wounds.

CONTRAINDICATIONS

Absolute
- Multiple comorbidities precluding safe intervention.
- Active infection.
- Foreign body (except surgical implants).
- Active bleeding.

Relative
- Impaired healing (corticosteroids, malnutrition, radiation, chronic disease).

INFORMED CONSENT
- Usually implied with consent for major procedure, must obtain consent otherwise.

Potential Risks
- Scarring (normal and abnormal).
- Bleeding (may require reoperation or transfusion).
- Infection (may require antibiotics or reoperation).
- Failure of operation or need for secondary intention healing.
- Need for revision.

EQUIPMENT

Instruments
- Appropriate instruments vary by wound type but include at a minimum a needle driver and tissue handling forceps.

Sutures
- Consist of both a needle and suture material, each with multiple subtypes and characteristics.

- The needle and suture material may vary widely based on different types of wounds in different locations.

Needle

- **Table 42–1:** Point characteristics.
- Swage: the method of attaching the suture material to the needle.
  - Channel swage: a channel is crimped over suture material (swage diameter > body diameter).
  - Drill swage: suture material is placed in the drill hole at the rear of needle, which is then crimped (swage diameter < body diameter).
  - Nonswaged: eyed needle (similar to sewing needle). Closed-eye needles require suture material to be passed through the eye each time it is threaded. French eye needles have a posterior slit allowing suture to be placed in the eye without direct threading; this causes more tissue trauma and reduced suture integrity (eye > body diameter).
  - Pop-off: swage is designed to allow suture material to be gently removed from the needle with traction.

Table 42–1. Needle characteristics—point.

Category	Type	Description	Tissue Use	Diagram
Cutting	Conventional cutting	Triangular point that changes to a flattened body with one cutting edge on the concave surface of the needle (surface seeking)	Skin and tendon	
	Reverse cutting	Cutting edge on convex curvature of the needle (depth-seeking). Stronger than conventional cutting	Dense tissue, including skin, oral mucosa, and tendon	
	Side-cutting (spatula)	Flat with 2 cutting edge to reduce tissue injury and improve depth control	Ocular tissues	
	Taper-point (round needle)	Stretches tissue without direct cutting action to minimize tearing. Sharpness increases with taper ratio (slope) (8–12:1) and decrease with tip angle (20–35 degrees)	Easily penetrated tissues, including abdominal viscera, dura, and peritoneum	
Blunt	Blunt	Dissects through tissue rather than cutting it	Friable tissue, including kidney and liver	

- **Table 42–2:** Needle body characteristics.
  - Designed to transmit the penetrating force to the point.
  - Varied alloy characteristics can make a needle soft or firm (ductility).
  - Diameter: gauge or thickness of needle.

PATIENT PREPARATION

- Nothing by mouth the evening before surgery if the patient will be undergoing general anesthesia.
- Preoperative antibiotics per institutional policy and based on wound characteristics.
- Anesthesiology consultation as needed.

Anesthesia

- Under general anesthesia, no additional preparation is necessary.
- In a conscious patient, local anesthetic (lidocaine, bupivacaine, etc) must be used.

Wound Preparation

- Wound must be clean.
- Clean wounds may need no specific preparation prior to closure.
- Highly contaminated wounds should be irrigated (bulb, pulse-lavage, etc).
- Lacerations.
  - May use a prefabricated syringe-mounted ocular flushing system.
  - A saline bottle with 5–10 needle punctures provides a low-cost, effective irrigator in the acute setting.

Table 42-2. Needle Characteristics—body.

Type	Notes		Diagram
Straight	Used in easily accessible tissue Tissue is manipulated to allow passage of needle (eg, Keith needle)		Needle length
Curved	Most common Needle follows predicable path through tissue with even tension distribution	Chord length: linear distance between tip and swage (bite width)	Chord length
		Needle length: distance between tip and swage along curvature of needle	Needle length
		Radius: distance form center of arc of rotation of needle to needle itself—determines bite depth	
Compound	Compound curved: variable radius Used in ophthalmologic and microsurgical procedures		$r_1 \neq r_2$

- Skin edge.
  - Complex lacerations and damaged skin edges should be resected to healthy tissue where possible.
  - "Freshen" skin edges to allow more accurate apposition of wound margins.
- Hair is generally removed to fully expose wounds and reduce infection.

PATIENT POSITIONING

- The wound should be fully exposed and at comfortable working distance from the surgeon.
- A light source is often necessary in the emergency department setting.

PROCEDURE

Suture Closure Techniques

- **Figure 42–1:** Running continuous stitch.
  - Widely used technique to close many wounds varying from lacerations to midline laparotomy wounds.
  - Depth of bite and layers of tissue incorporated are dependent on site and tissue characteristics.
- Advantages of running technique.
  - Allows expeditious wound closure.
  - Closure is completed with one continuous length of suture material.
  - Achieves approximation of wound margins.
- Disadvantages of running technique.
  - Less reliable than interrupted closure.
  - Wound edge eversion is difficult and there is greater potential for misalignment of wound edges, particularly if the tissue is pliable and the wound is long.
- **Figure 42–2:** Simple interrupted suture.
  - Most common and basic suturing technique.
  - Depth of bite and layers of tissue incorporated are dependent on site and tissue characteristics.
- Advantages of interrupted technique.
  - Closure is completed suture by suture.
  - The depth of bite, layers of tissue incorporated, and tension on the closure can be carefully adjusted for each individual stitch.
  - Achieves accurate approximation of wound margins with optimal control.
  - More reliable closure than continuous stitch.
- Disadvantages of interrupted technique.
  - Time consuming.
  - Multiple knots may contribute to foreign body response and additional scarring.

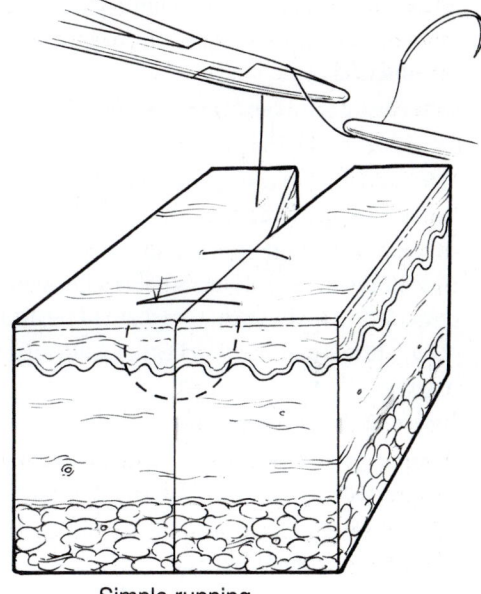

Simple running

Figure 42–1

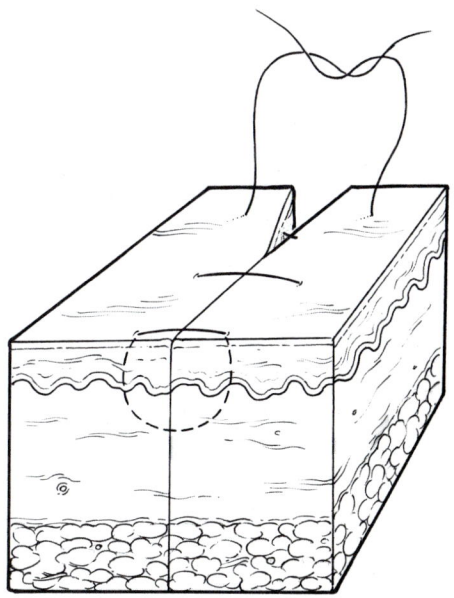

Simple interrupted

Figure 42–2

- Additional suture material may contribute to infections in the wound (suture abscess).
■ Mattress suture: interrupted suturing technique in which the needle is passed through tissue multiple times.
■ **Figure 42–3:** Horizontal mattress technique.
  - The initial simple suture is placed perpendicular to the wound.
  - Instead of tying the suture, the needle is advanced parallel to the wound margin and passed back through the tissue at an equal bite depth to a point on the initial wound edge equidistant to the length of advance on the opposite wound edge.
  - The suture is tied and now lies parallel to the wound edge.
■ **Figure 42–4:** Vertical mattress technique.
  - The initial simple suture is placed perpendicular to the wound using a large bite depth.
  - Instead of tying the suture, the needle is returned to the side of the initial bite at a smaller bite depth and without any advancement down the length of the wound.
  - The suture is tied and now lies perpendicular to the wound edge.
■ **Figure 42–5:** Half-buried horizontal mattress technique.
  - Similar to the horizontal mattress technique, but the suture does not pass out of the tissue on the edge opposite the initial bite.
  - The suture remains buried.
■ Advantages of mattress suture techniques.

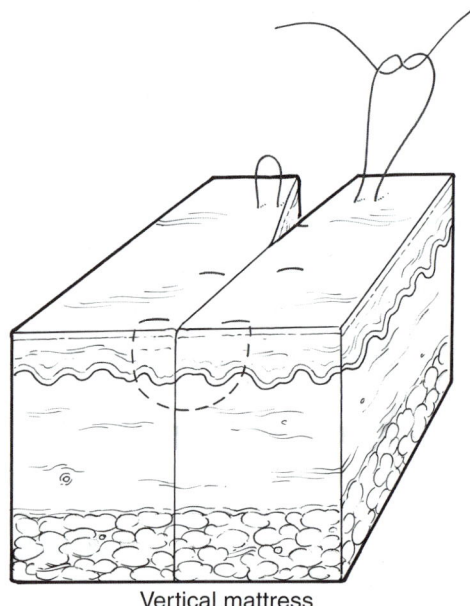
Vertical mattress
Figure 42–4

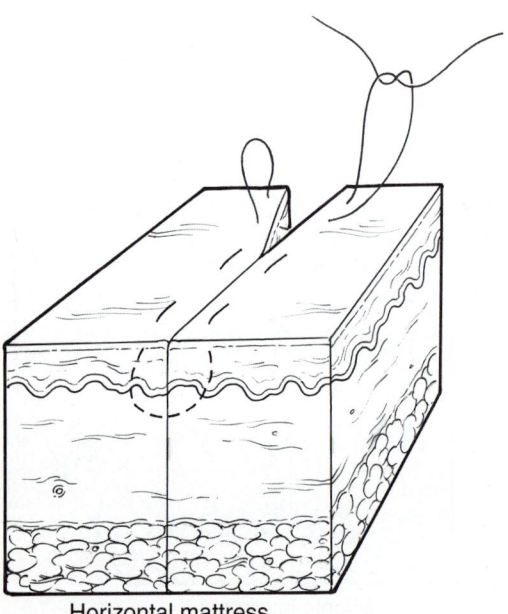
Horizontal mattress
Figure 42–3

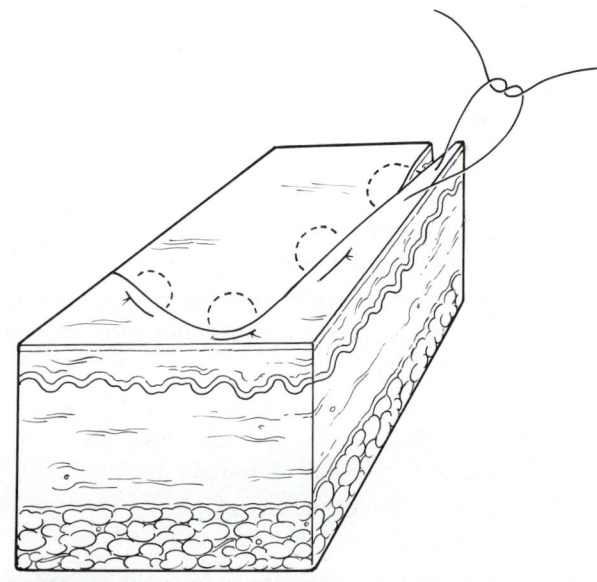
Half-buried horizontal mattress
Figure 42–5

- Tissue eversion is easily controlled.
- Wound tension is distributed in friable tissue to prevent the suture from tearing through the tissue.
- Strong closure.
■ Disadvantages of mattress suture techniques.
- Can create ischemic tissue either directly under the suture (vertical mattress) or constrict tissue within the confines of each suture leading to tissue ischemia (horizontal mattress).
■ Figure 42–6: Purse-string suture.
- Used to close wounds by circumferential constriction of the wound edge.
- Commonly used in closing the end of a hollow viscus such as bowel or appendiceal stumps, around a catheter, or in reconstructive and cosmetic surgery.
- Uses a running suture technique.
- The suture is passed in and out of tissue around the circumference of the wound without entering the lumen of the viscera.
- As the suture reaches the origin, it can be tightened to reduce the circumference of the initial wound in a manner similar to the leather strings on a pliable "purse."
- If the technique is executed properly, the viscera can be reduced into the wound as the suture is tightened, creating a seal.
■ Advantages of purse-string technique.
- Provides equal wound tension distribution around the circumference of the wound.
- Rapid closure.
■ Disadvantages of purse-string technique.
- Creates pleating, which may lead to a poor seal, unfavorable scarring, or both.
- When used on skin, may lead to scar-widening as tissue stretches.
■ Figure 42–7: Subcuticular suture.
- Used to close superficial skin edges to achieve accurate wound margin approximation.
- Sutures are not placed through the epidermis, thus avoiding potential scarring related to suture placement.
- The suture is introduced through normal skin and brought out of the deep tissue into the epidermal-dermal junction.
- The suture is then passed back into tissue and out of tissue at this same level, alternating edges of the wound (the suture should not penetrate epidermis).
- The suture exits deep tissue through the epidermis just distal to the wound.
- The tails are trimmed so they may be accessed to pull the suture out after several days (some prefer to tie or bury the suture).

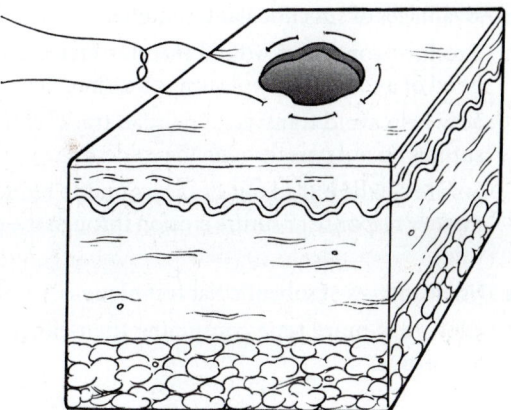

Figure 42–6

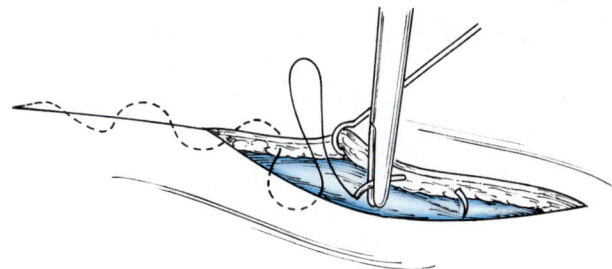

Figure 42–7

- Advantages of subcuticular technique.
  - Excellent control of wound margins increases the likelihood of a cosmetically pleasing outcome.
  - May help avoid transverse "railroad track" scarring since sutures do not pass through the epidermis.
  - Suture can be pulled out of the wound to reduce inflammatory response or suture erosion through the skin (spitting).
- Disadvantages of subcuticular technique.
  - Closure is more time consuming than either staples or tissue glue.

Nonsuture Closure Techniques

- **Figure 42–8:** Stapled closure.
  - Used to close superficial skin edges.
  - Skin edges are held up and everted using tissue forceps.
  - A staple is deployed at this site.
  - The process is repeated down the length of the wound.
- Advantages of stapled closure.
  - Rapid skin edge closure.
  - Individual staples can be removed in the event of wound infection.
- Disadvantages of stapled closure.
  - May contribute to transverse hatching of the scar in a "railroad track" pattern.
  - Staple removal can be uncomfortable.
- Tissue glue.
  - Used to close superficial skin edges to achieve close edge approximation.
  - Skin edges are approximated manually or with pull-out sutures.
  - The wound is cleaned of necrotic debris, foreign material, and dried blood.
  - A bed of glue is applied down the length of the wound, typically in one pass.
- Advantages of tissue glue.
  - Rapid skin edge closure.
  - Minimal tissue handling.
- Disadvantages of tissue glue.
  - Glue cannot be removed easily if need be (eg, opening an infected wound).
  - Expensive.

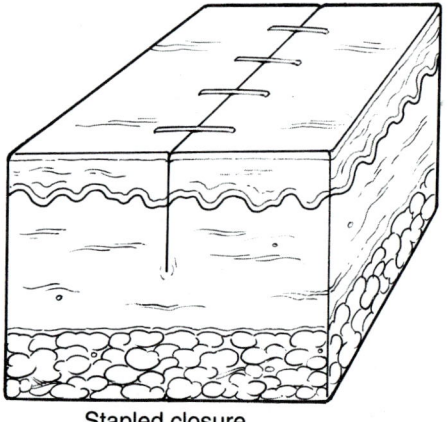

Stapled closure

Figure 42–8

POSTOPERATIVE CARE

- Wound edges should remain clean.
- Sutures should be removed several days (typical in face) or weeks following repair, depending on the location of the wound and characteristics of the tissue.

- Pain control with analgesics is appropriate.
- Antibiotics are not necessary for most wounds but may be recommended in contaminated wounds following closure.

POTENTIAL COMPLICATIONS

- Wound infection.
  - Infected wounds, particularly those involving deep spaces, are typically opened to prevent systemic spread.
- Unfavorable scarring.
  - Some scarring is expected, but hypertrophic scars, keloids, or wound contraction leading to functional limitation may occur, often without a known cause.
  - Some wounds with unfavorable scarring may require scar revision.
- **Figure 42–9:** Standing cutaneous deformities ("dog ears") may be a result of individual wound length differences leading to excess tissue on one side of the wound, or occur in cases in which tissue rearrangement is necessary to achieve closure.
  - These cutaneous deformities may persist and can often be addressed at primary closure.
  - To remove a standing cutaneous deformity, the tissue leading to the deformity can be lifted away from the plane of tissue and resected in an elliptical fashion.
  - If executed properly, the dimensions of the newly created ellipse will allow primary closure without a standing cutaneous deformity.

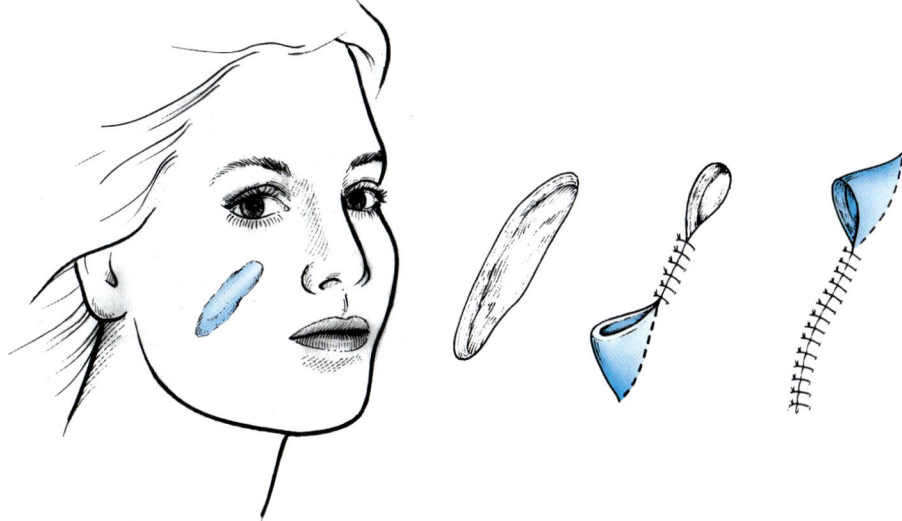

Figure 42–9

PEARLS AND TIPS

- Remember that not all wounds require or are well-managed by primary closure.
- To prevent injury to yourself and others, never handle needles directly.
- Returning suture by grasping the suture material instead of the needle will reduce the risk of the needle ejecting out of the needle holder.
- Use instruments appropriate for both the needle and the tissue you are suturing.

REFERENCES

Aston SJ, Beasley RW, Thorne CH, et al. *Grabb and Smith's Plastic Surgery,* 5th ed. Philadelphia, PA: Lippincott-Raven Publishers; 1997.

Baker SR, Swanson NA. *Local Flaps in Facial Reconstruction.* St Louis, MO: Mosby-Year Book; 1995.

Evans GRD. *Operative Plastic Surgery.* Stamford, CT: Appleton & Lange; 2000.

Johnson & Johnson. *Ethicon Wound Closure Manual,* 2001. Available at: http://www.orthonurse.org/portals/0/wound%20closure%20manual.pdf. Accessed August 12, 2008.

McGregor IA. *Fundamental Techniques of Plastic Surgery and Their Surgical Applications,* 10th ed. Edinburgh, New York: Churchill Livingstone; 2000.

Sanders RJ. Subcuticular skin closure–description of technique. *J Dermatol Surg.* 1975;1:61–64.

CHAPTER 43

Central Venous Access

Laura A. Monson, MD, and Melissa E. Brunsvold, MD

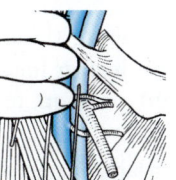 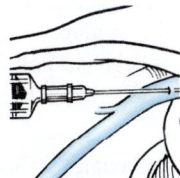 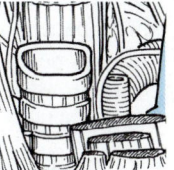
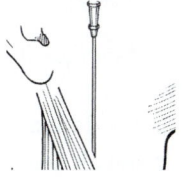 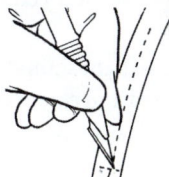 

INDICATIONS
- Intravenous hemodynamic monitoring.
- Central venous sampling.
- Parenteral nutrition.
- Hemodialysis.
- Transvenous pacing.
- Placement of pulmonary artery catheters.

CONTRAINDICATIONS
- Significant coagulopathy, especially with platelet counts < 50,000/μL.

INFORMED CONSENT
Potential Risks
- Infection.
- Pneumothorax.
- Dysrhythmia.
- Arterial puncture.
- Guidewire loss.
- Pseudoaneurysm.
- Thrombosis.
- Retroperitoneal dissection.
- Arteriovenous fistula.

EQUIPMENT
- Chlorhexidine skin preparation solution.
- Sterile gown, gloves, and drapes.
- Hat and mask.
- 1% lidocaine.
- Sterile gauze pads.
- 22-gauge finder needle.
- 18-gauge introducer needle.
- J-tip guidewire.
- Transduction tubing.

348 • Current Procedures: Surgery

- Tissue dilator.
- Sterile saline for flushing the line.
- Catheter.
- 2-0 silk sutures.
- Sterile dressing.

PATIENT PREPARATION
- Short-acting antianxiety or pain medications as needed in consultation with the patient's nurse.

PATIENT POSITIONING
- The patient should be supine, in Trendelenburg (head-down) position for subclavian and internal jugular lines, and in reverse Trendelenburg (head-up) position for femoral lines.
- For infraclavicular subclavian vein access in larger patients, and those in whom the clavicle is difficult to palpate, a rolled towel can be placed between the shoulder blades to facilitate access.
- For femoral lines the patient should be placed supine with the leg slightly abducted and externally rotated.
- The patient should be placed on continuous monitoring.
- The area chosen should be widely exposed and all necessary hair trimmed.
- The area is prepared with a chlorhexidine-based skin solution and sterile drapes are applied.

PROCEDURE

Femoral Vein Access
- **Figure 43–1:** Landmarks used for placement are the anterior iliac spine and the symphysis pubis.
  - The vein is found halfway between these landmarks just below the inguinal ligament, lateral to the artery and medial to the nerve.
- One hand is placed over the femoral pulse, and the syringe is held in the other with the needle at a 30–40-degree angle to the skin and the bevel up.
- The needle typically encounters the vein within 2–4 cm but may be hubbed before encountering the vein in an obese patient.
- If there is no return of blood, the needle should be withdrawn slowly as the vein may be entered on withdrawal.
- The needle should be moved medially to laterally in a systematic manner until the vein is encountered.

Subclavian Vein Access
- **Figure 43–2A, B:** The axillary vein continues as the subclavian vein at the lateral border of the first rib.

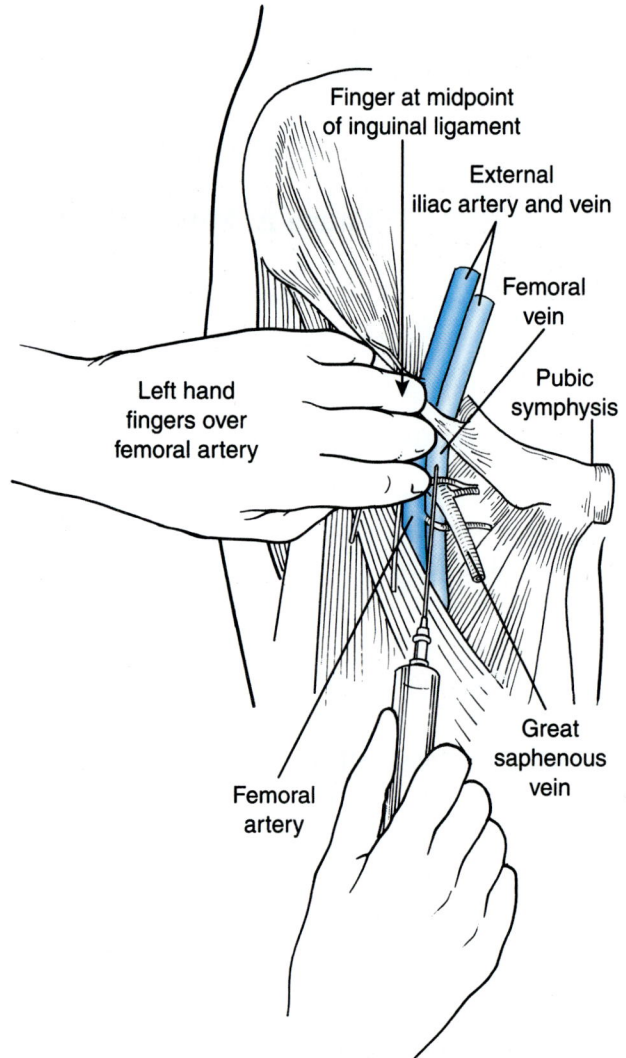

Figure 43–1

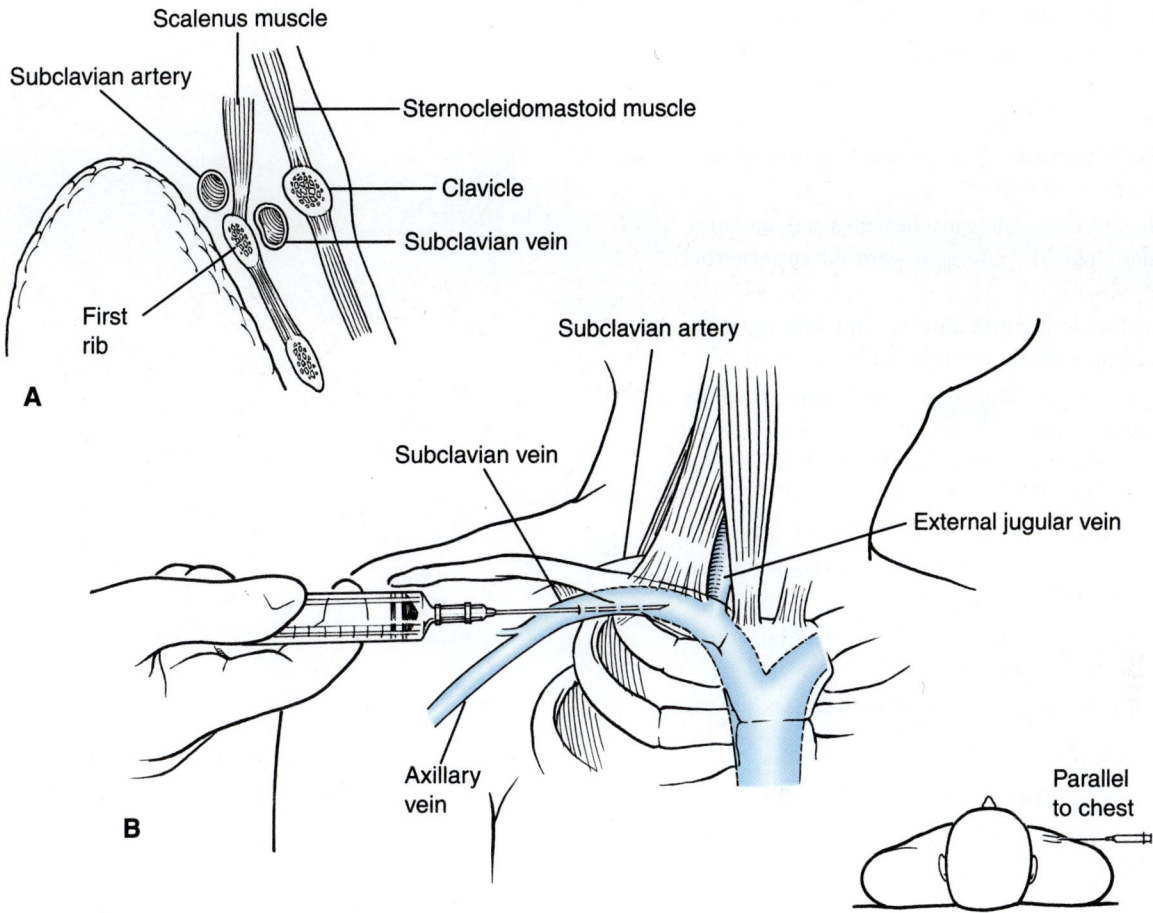

Figure 43-2A-B

- It arches superiorly behind the medial clavicle and then joins the internal jugular vein to become the brachiocephalic vein posterior to the sternoclavicular joint.
- The subclavian artery runs with the vein, separated by the anterior scalene muscle, in a superior and posterior position (Figure 43-2A).
- The apex of the lung can rise above the level of the first rib on the left but is usually situated more inferiorly on the right. It lies deep and inferior to the subclavian vein.
- The subclavian vein can be accessed along the length of the clavicle, but the midpoint approach is the most common (Figure 43-2B).
  - The needle is inserted at the midpoint, approximately 1 cm lateral to the bend and 2-3 cm inferior to the clavicle.
  - The needle is held at an angle that would allow it to skim just beneath the clavicle and is aimed toward the suprasternal notch.
  - If the clavicle is encountered, the needle should be marched down until it skims just beneath.

- Alternatively, a more lateral approach can be used.
  - The clavicle is thinner lateral to the midclavicular line, so the needle is held parallel to the floor, still aiming toward the suprasternal notch (Figure 43–2B, inset).
- The subclavian vein can also be approached more medially at the convergence of the great veins.
  - To access this site, the needle must be held at a much more perpendicular angle, still aiming toward the suprasternal notch.
  - The medial clavicle is much thicker, and this approach also must pass through the costoclavicular ligament.
- The subclavian vein can also be accessed from above the clavicle, although this is much less commonly done.
  - This approach enters the vein near its junction with the internal jugular vein.
  - The most important surface landmark for this approach is the posterior (clavicular) head of the sternocleidomastoid (SCM) muscle.
  - The patient's head is turned to the contralateral side in order to delineate the muscle.
  - The needle is inserted approximately 1 cm superior to the clavicle and 1 cm posterior to the clavicular head of the SCM muscle.
  - The needle is oriented at an angle to slip just behind the medial clavicle and toward the contralateral nipple.
  - The vein is encountered within 1–2 cm.

Internal Jugular Vein Access

- **Figures 43–3 and 43–4:** The internal jugular vein runs within the carotid sheath along with the internal and common carotid arteries.
  - The vein becomes anterolateral to the artery as they pass beneath the SCM.
  - The vein runs just beneath the SCM before it emerges between the sternal and clavicular heads; at this point it lies 1–1.5 cm beneath the skin.
- Internal jugular localization is initially done with a finder needle to minimize damage to the carotid artery in case of an inadvertent puncture.
- The finder needle is left in place and the introducer needle is inserted alongside it, following the same trajectory.
- There are three main approaches to catheterization of the internal jugular vein: central, posterior, and anterior.
- The central approach is most commonly used, and utilizes the triangle made by the two bellies of the SCM and the clavicle as the external landmark.
  - The needle is inserted at the apex of the triangle, approximately 5 cm superior to the clavicle, just lateral to the carotid pulsation at an angle of 30–45 degrees.
  - The needle is directed toward the ipsilateral nipple and should enter the vein within 2.5 cm.

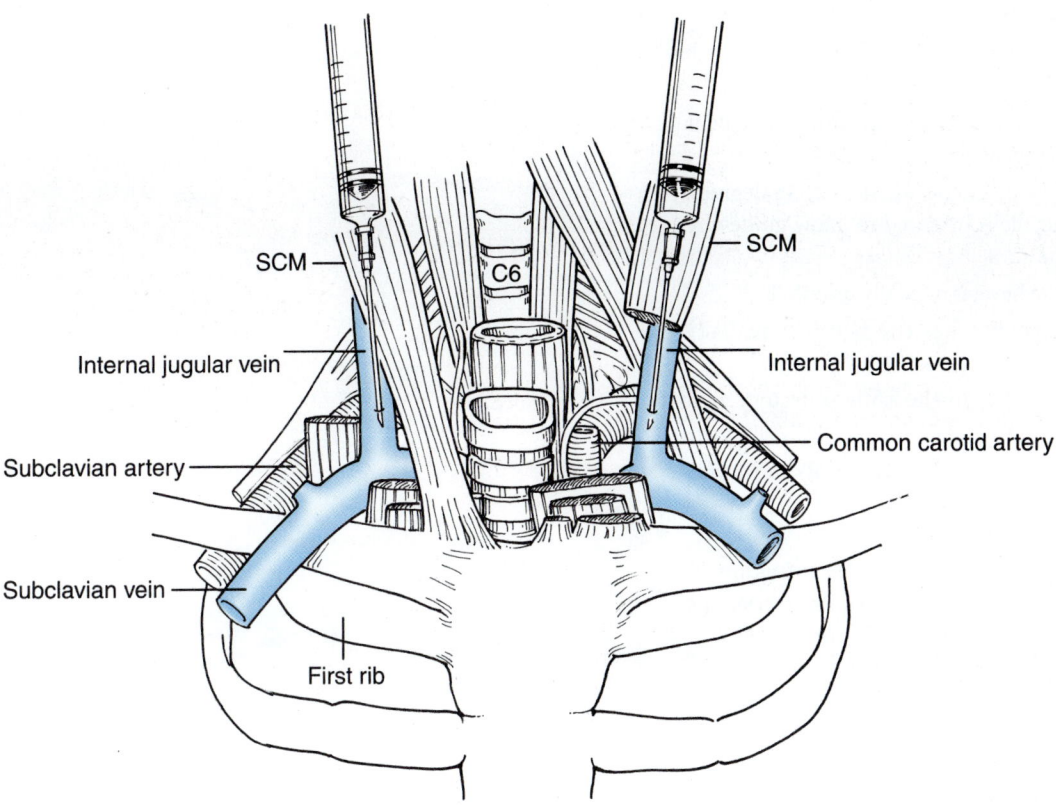

Figure 43-3

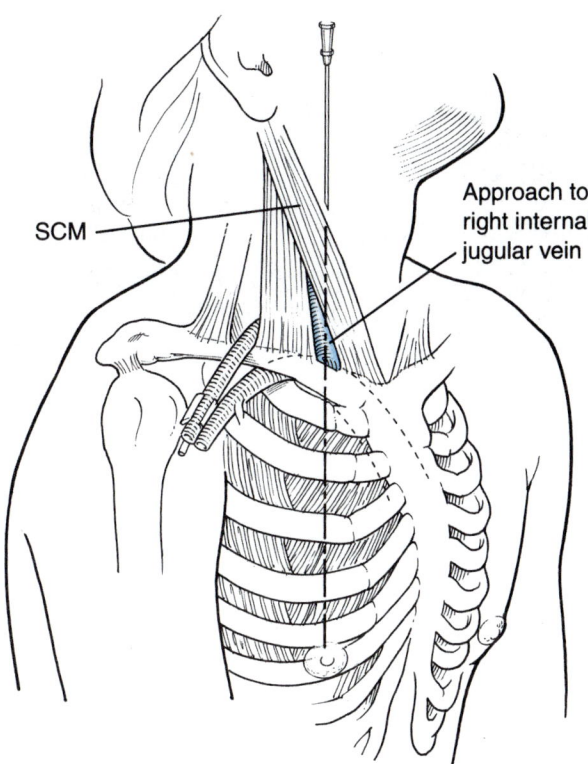

- To access the internal jugular vein from the posterior approach, the patient's head is turned to the contralateral side to accentuate the landmarks of the SCM.
  - The needle is inserted between the middle and lower thirds of the SCM, along the posterior border.
  - This point can also be identified by the external jugular vein, which often crosses at this point.
  - The needle is directed toward the sternal notch and held at an angle to slide just beneath the SCM.
- The internal jugular vein can also be accessed anterior to the sternal head of the SCM.
  - The carotid pulsations are palpated with one hand, and the needle is inserted at the midpoint of the anterior border of the SCM, about 5 cm above the clavicle.
  - The needle should follow a trajectory aimed at the ipsilateral nipple.

Figure 43-4

Seldinger Technique

- **Figure 43–5A–E:** The vein is first accessed using a small needle, typically 21 or 22 gauge.
- Once the vein is located, an 18-gauge introducer needle is used for guidewire placement.
- The skin is punctured with the needle held at 45 degrees, and the bevel of the needle is oriented to allow guidewire placement into the vena cava.
  - For subclavian lines the bevel is caudally oriented.
  - For internal jugular approaches the bevel is medially oriented.
- The needle is inserted slowly in the same trajectory as it entered the skin, while aspirating continuously.
- Once beneath the skin, the needle should only move forward and backward, never side to side as this can lacerate the vein.
- Dark, nonpulsatile blood return indicates intraluminal venous position, but a blood gas sample or an arterial line transducer can be used to confirm the position as well.

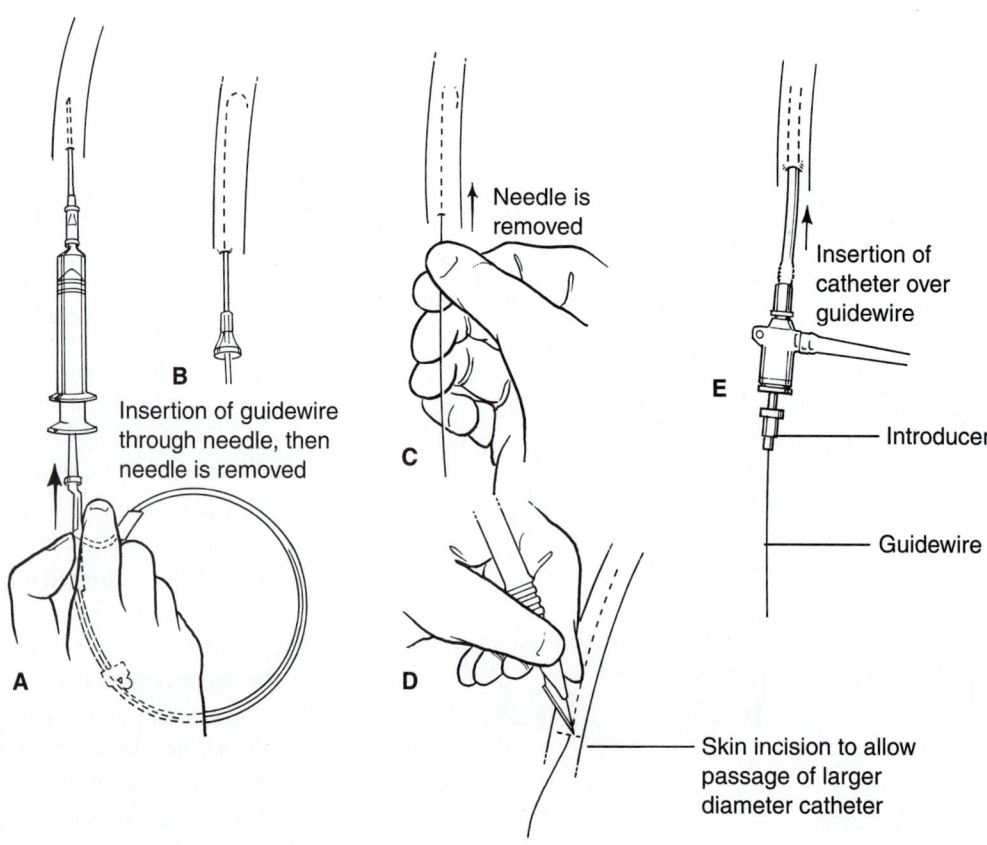

Figure 43–5A–E

- When intraluminal position is confirmed, the syringe is removed and a guidewire is inserted through the needle.
- Once the wire is advanced, the needle is removed.
- A scalpel is used to make a small incision over the wire to allow passage of the dilator.
- The dilator is inserted over the wire to the depth of the vessel with a steady twisting motion, and then removed leaving the wire in place.
- The catheter is advanced over the wire to the desired depth.
- The wire is removed through the distal port.
- Blood is then back through all ports to confirm all are in working order and the catheter is then sutured into place.
- A sterile dressing is applied.

POSTOPERATIVE CARE

- Placement of internal jugular and subclavian central venous catheters is confirmed with a chest radiograph; no radiographs are required for femoral line placement.
- In general, it is recommended that the catheter tip lie within the superior vena cava, outside of the right atrium and above the pericardial reflection. On chest radiographs, therefore, the tip should lie above the level of the carina.
- A sterile dressing is applied to the central line, which is changed weekly.
- Current guidelines indicate that catheters should only be replaced if there is evidence of sepsis or localized infection, and that routine replacement is not indicated.
- Topical antibiotic ointment at the insertion site does not reduce infection rates and should not be used.
- Central venous catheters should be removed as soon as possible.

POTENTIAL COMPLICATIONS

- Each year 250,000 central venous catheter-related infections occur in the United States, with an associated mortality of 12–25% and a cost of $25,000 per infection.
- Femoral venous catheters have higher rates of infection and iliofemoral thrombosis in comparison with subclavian and internal jugular sites.
- When the femoral technique is used in patients during cardiac arrest, misplacement in the retroperitoneum, femoral artery, or elsewhere occurs in up to 30% of cases.
- Pneumothorax may occur with both internal jugular and subclavian vein access approaches.
- Review of the literature reveals no difference in the rates of major complications, including pneumothorax, between subclavian and internal jugular vein catheters.
- If a patient might require dialysis in the future, an internal jugular approach is preferred to a subclavian approach to prevent the possible complication of subclavian vein stenosis, which would limit arteriovenous dialysis access options.
- Malposition of the catheter.
- Dysrhythmia, often caused by advancing the wire into the right atrium.
- Arterial puncture.
- Guidewire loss.
- Venous thrombosis and stenosis.
- Retroperitoneal dissection.
- Arteriovenous fistula, a late complication.

PEARLS AND TIPS

- If an internal jugular or subclavian approach has been chosen, prepare the area widely enough so that the other ipsilateral site may be used without changing drapes if placement at the first site is unsuccessful.
- If unsuccessful in placing either an internal jugular or subclavian line on one side, obtain a chest radiograph to rule out the presence of a pneumothorax before attempting line placement on the contralateral side.
- To ascertain intravenous position, a pressure transducer or manometer tubing can be used. The needle can be connected directly to a pressure line and transduced as would be done with an arterial line. The pressure and waveform can then be visualized on the monitor.
- Alternatively, a saline-filled length of single-lumen tubing can be connected to the needle. The tubing is then raised to a vertical position; variation with respirations will be seen with venous blood, and pulsations will be seen with arterial placement.
- For subclavian lines, orienting the J-tip of the guidewire caudally facilitates placement into the superior vena cava. Manually occluding the ipsilateral jugular vein will also decrease the chance of malposition of the guidewire into the internal jugular vein.
- Having the patient turn his or her head to the contralateral side against resistance can help identify the triangle formed by the sternal and clavicular heads of the SCM.
- For most patients, the right internal jugular vein is chosen as an access site over the left. This is due to its larger caliber, the lower apex of the right lung, and the technical ease for the right-handed surgeon. The left internal jugular vein is significantly smaller than the right in about one third of patients.

- Placing downward traction on the arm during subclavian line placement increases the amount of overlap between the artery and vein and improves cannulation success; 5 cm below neutral has been shown to be the optimal position.
- The clavicular periosteum should be included in the local anesthetic field when placing a subclavian line.

REFERENCES

Ambesh SP, Dubey PK, Matreja P, et al. Manual occlusion of the internal jugular vein during subclavian vein catheterization: a maneuver to prevent misplacement of catheter into internal jugular vein. *Anesthesiology.* 2002;97:528–529.

Emerman CL, Bellon EM, Lukens TW, et al. A prospective study of femoral versus subclavian vein catheterization during cardiac arrest. *Ann Emerg Med.* 1990;19:26–30.

Fortune JB, Feustel P. Effect of patient position on size and location of the subclavian vein for percutaneous puncture. *Arch Surg.* 2003;138:996–1000.

McGee DC, Gould MK. Preventing complications of central venous catheterization. *N Engl J Med.* 2003;348:1123–1133.

Mumtaz H, Williams V, Hauer-Jensen M, et al. Central venous catheter placement in patients with disorders of hemostasis. *Am J Surg.* 2000;180:503–505.

Polderman KH, Girbes AJ. Central venous catheter use. Part 1: mechanical complications. *Intensive Care Med.* 2002;28:1–17.

Ruesch S, Walder B, Tramer MR. Complications of central venous catheters: internal jugular versus subclavian access—a systematic review. *Crit Care Med.* 2002;30:454–460.

Sanchez R, Halck S, Walther-Larsen S, et al. Misplacement of subclavian venous catheters: importance of head position and choice of puncture site. *Br J Anaesth.* 1990;64:632–633.

Schuster M, Nave H, Piepenbrock S, et al. The carina as a landmark in central venous catheter placement. *Br J Anaesth.* 2000;85:192–194.

Stone MB, Price DD, Anderson BS. Ultrasonographic investigation of the effect of reverse Trendelenburg on the cross-sectional area of the femoral vein. *J Emerg Med.* 2006;30:211–213.

Tanner J, Khan D. Surgical site infection, preoperative body washing and hair removal. *J Perioper Pract.* 2008;18:232,237–243.

Tripathi M, Dubey PK, Ambesh SP. Direction of the J-tip of the guidewire, in Seldinger technique, is a significant factor in misplacement of subclavian vein catheter: a randomized, controlled study. *Anesth Analg.* 2005;100:21–24.

CHAPTER 44

Tube Thoracostomy

Peter Sassalos, MD, and Melissa E. Brunsvold, MD

INDICATIONS
- Pneumothorax.
- Hemothorax.
- Chylothorax.
- Empyema.
- Pleural effusion (persistent).
- Thoracic trauma or surgery.

CONTRAINDICATIONS
Absolute
- None.

Relative
- Coagulopathy.
- Overlying skin infection.
- Overlying chest wall malignancy.
- Intrapleural adhesions.
- Loculated pleural collection.

INFORMED CONSENT
Potential Risks
- Bleeding.
- Infection.
  - Skin and subcutaneous infection.
  - Empyema.
- Risk of anesthetic if used.
- Death.
- Possible injury and need for repair of surrounding structures.
  - Intercostal neurovascular injury.
  - Great vessel injury.
  - Pulmonary parenchymal injury.

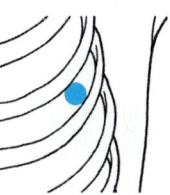 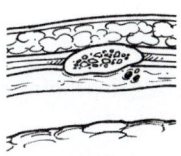 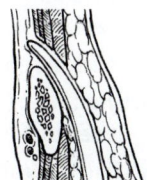
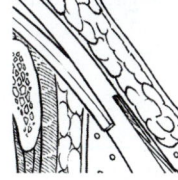 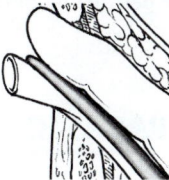 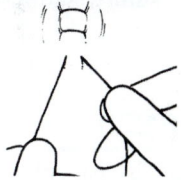

- Diaphragmatic injury.
- Cardiac injury.
- Splenic injury on left side.
- Hepatic injury on right side.
■ Persistent air leak.
■ Need for emergent thoracotomy or future additional procedures.

EQUIPMENT

■ Sterile gown and gloves, cap, mask, eye protection.
■ Povidone-iodine or chlorhexidine preparation, sterile towels.
■ Local anesthesia.
■ Chest tube (varied sizes, depending on indication and size of patient).
■ Chest tube management system.
■ Scalpel, Kelly clamp, needle driver, scissors, nonabsorbable suture, Xeroform or petroleum gauze, sterile gauze, foam tape.

PATIENT PREPARATION

■ The patient does not need to have an empty stomach although this is preferable if conscious sedation is used in the nonemergent setting.
■ Preoperative antibiotics are not required.

PATIENT POSITIONING

■ The patient should be supine with the ipsilateral arm positioned over the head to facilitate adequate exposure of the anterolateral thoracic wall.

PROCEDURE

■ Local anesthesia with or without conscious sedation may be used.
  - When local anesthesia is used, infiltration of the skin, subcutaneous tissue, muscle, and parietal pleura provides the best anesthesia.
■ **Figure 44–1:** A transverse skin incision parallel to the intercostal space is planned, usually at approximately the fourth or fifth intercostal space at the midaxillary or anterior axillary line.
  - The goal of this placement is to avoid the diaphragm, intra-abdominal organs, and breast tissue (in women), and to allow for placement anterior enough that the patient does not lie on the tube after placement.

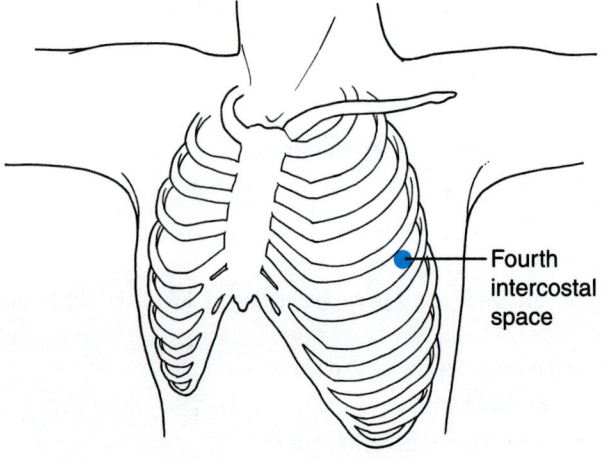

Figure 44–1

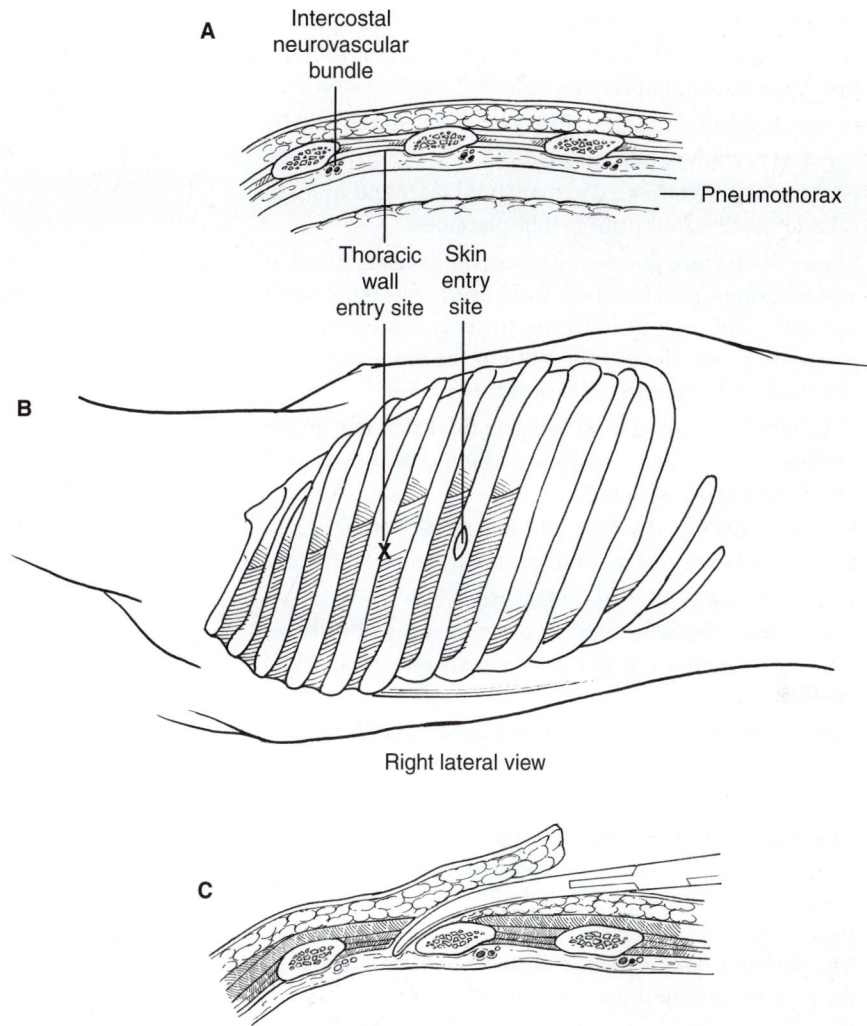

Figure 44–2A–C

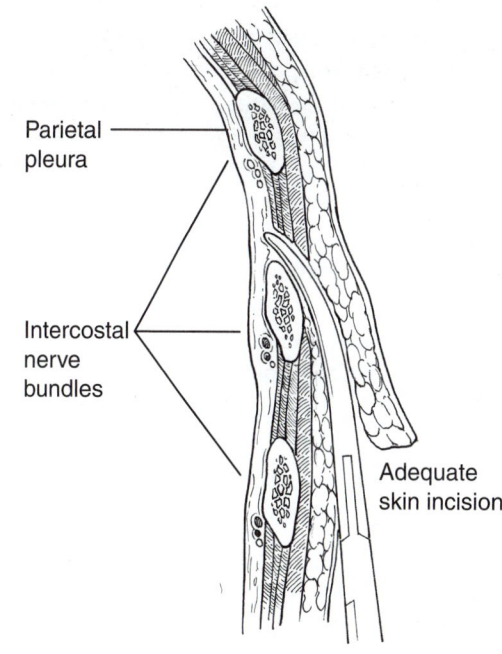

Figure 44–3

- **Figure 44–2A–C:** The skin incision is made using a scalpel at one intercostal level below the planned entry site of the chest tube into the pleural space.
  - The subcutaneous tissue and intercostal muscles are dissected bluntly in a transverse direction using a hemostat or Kelly clamp until the parietal pleura is reached.
- **Figure 44–3:** During dissection of the subcutaneous tissue and muscles, the Kelly clamp should be directed cranially toward the rib above and the tips should be pointed toward the superior aspect of this rib to avoid the course of the intercostal neurovascular bundle inferior to each rib.

- **Figure 44–4:** Using a Kelly clamp, the pleural space is entered parallel to the ribs in a controlled fashion with the tips of the instrument closed.
  - Once the pleural space is penetrated, the clamp should be opened to allow egress of air or fluid.
  - A finger should be placed in the pleural space and swept to check for adhesions prior to tube placement.
- **Figure 44–5:** Once the pleural space is entered and freed of any adhesions, the chest tube is clamped at its fenestrated end with a Kelly clamp and, using finger guidance, the tube is advanced into the pleural space in the posterosuperior direction of the apex to the desired tip location.
  - The tube is advanced to various lengths depending on the patient; however, all fenestrations should be intrapleural to create a closed system.
- **Figure 44–6:** Once the chest tube is in place, it is connected and secured to a chest tube management system and placed on suction, typically at 20 cm H_2O negative pressure.
  - The chest tube is secured in place by a nonabsorbable U-stitch through the skin with ends wrapped and tied around the tube.
  - Xeroform or petroleum gauze is placed around the tube opening and gauze and foam tape are applied.

POSTOPERATIVE CARE

- A chest radiograph should be obtained at the conclusion of the procedure to assess placement.
- The patient's hemodynamic status should be monitored for signs of cardiopulmonary distress.
- The chest tube output should be recorded; if there is considerable blood loss a thoracotomy should be considered.
- Each time the patient is evaluated, assessment of the nature of the output and presence of an air leak should be noted.
- Typically, when the patient has clinically improved, the output is decreased (values vary based on surgeon preference), and an air leak has resolved the chest tube is transitioned from suction to water seal in anticipation of removal.
- To remove a chest tube, great care must be taken to prevent introduction of air into the pleural space.
  - An assistant should hold pressure with petroleum gauze and dry gauze over the tract as the tube is rapidly removed at the end of an inspiration.
  - The previously placed U-stitch may be tied to close the skin opening (see Figure 44–6); however, this is optional.
- A chest radiograph should be obtained to assess for interval development of a pneumothorax.

POTENTIAL COMPLICATIONS

- Bleeding: intercostal neurovascular or great vessel injury.
  - May present with hemorrhage.

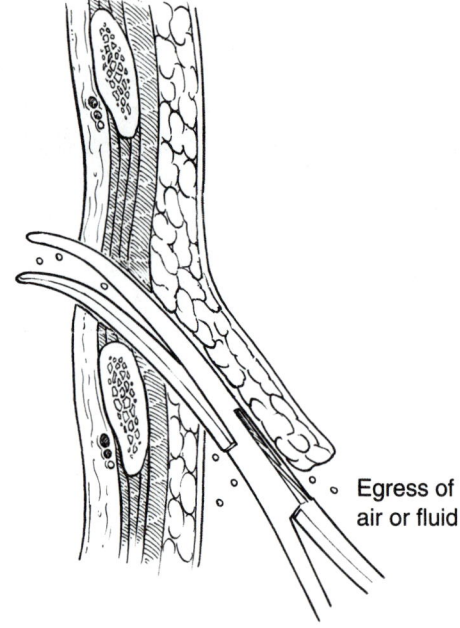

Figure 44–4

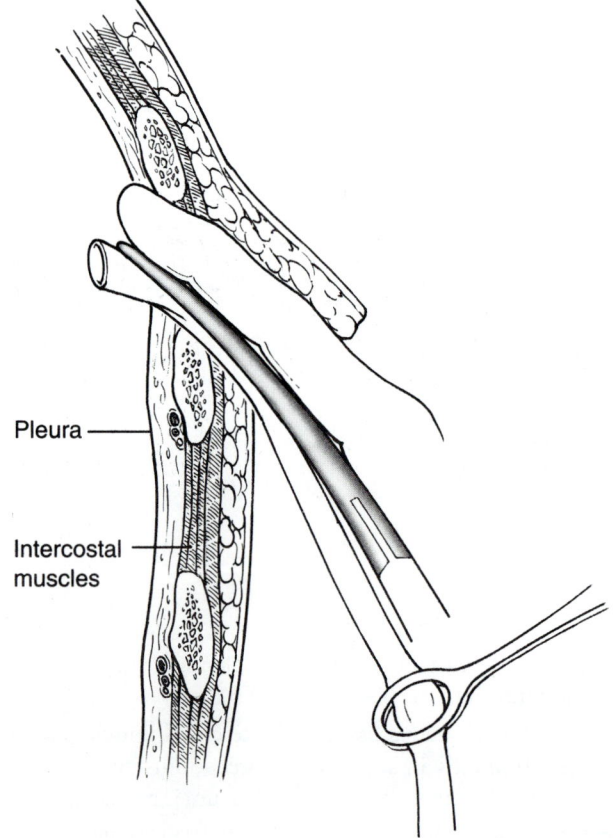

Figure 44–5

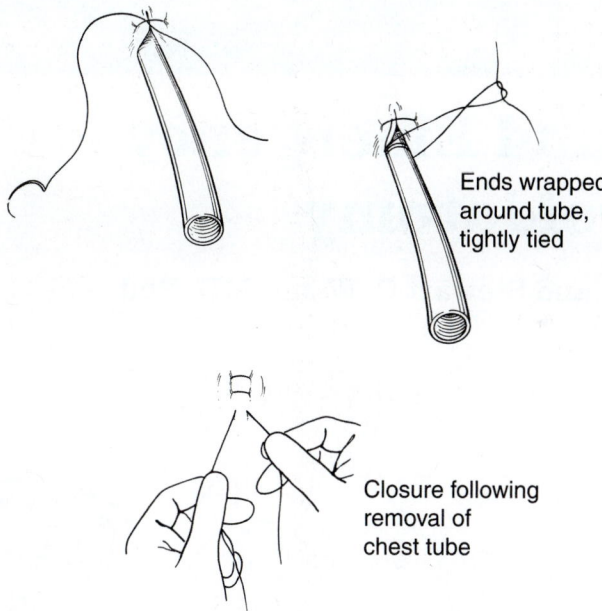

Figure 44-6

- Treatment includes resuscitation, hemostatic control through possible thoracotomy, and consultation with a cardiovascular surgeon.
- Solid organ injury: pulmonary parenchymal injury, diaphragmatic injury, cardiac injury, splenic injury on the left side, or hepatic injury on the right side.
  - May present with bleeding or dysfunction of the involved organ.
  - Treatment is directed at the affected organ system.
- Persistent air leak.
  - May manifest if a bronchopleural fistula is present or pulmonary parenchymal injury has occurred.
  - Treatment would require surgical management by a thoracic surgeon.

PEARLS AND TIPS

- Infiltration of the parietal pleura prior to the procedure provides the best anesthesia.
- Although the fourth or fifth intercostal space is typically used for tube thoracostomy, any variety of intercostal locations can be used if pathologic findings preclude standard placement.
- To avoid loss of the pleural opening, spread the Kelly clamp widely after entering the pleural space and do not remove the clamp before a finger is placed into the pleural space.
- Sweep a finger in the pleural space before placing the chest tube to avoid parenchymal injury.
- Use nonabsorbable suture to secure the chest tube; the area is often moist from chest tube output and bleeding and an absorbable suture might dissolve.

REFERENCES

Rozycki GS, McNeil J, Thal ER. Diagnostic Procedures Used to Establish Priorities. In: Thal ER, Weigelt JA, Carrico J, eds. *Operative Trauma Management: An Atlas.* New York, NY: McGraw-Hill; 2002:20–34.

CHAPTER 45

Tracheostomy and Emergency Cricothyroidotomy

Michael L. Bernstein, MD, PhD, and Stewart C. Wang, MD, Phd

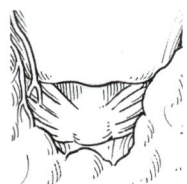 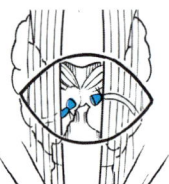 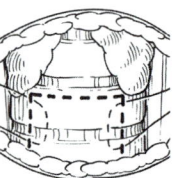
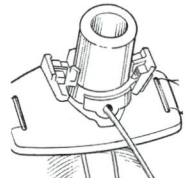 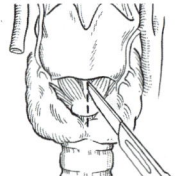 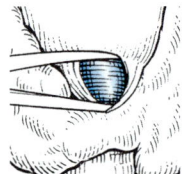
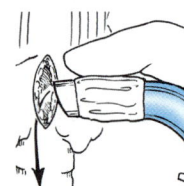  

INDICATIONS

Tracheostomy
- Supralaryngeal obstruction.
- Secure airway access.
- Prolonged intubation and mechanical ventilation.
- Inability to control secretions.

Emergency Cricothyroidotomy
- Inability to obtain an oral or nasopharyngeal airway in a patient who requires emergent intubation.
- Severe facial or head and neck trauma.
- Acute loss of the airway due to supralaryngeal obstruction secondary to tumor, anaphylaxis, foreign body, trauma, or burn injury.

CONTRAINDICATIONS

Tracheostomy
- Significant coagulopathy can be considered a relative contraindication because bleeding into the airway can be catastrophic.

Emergency Cricothyroidotomy
- There are few contraindications to cricothyroidotomy in the emergent setting with a patient in extremis.

INFORMED CONSENT
- The emergent circumstances under which cricothyroidotomy are considered typically preclude informed consent.

Expected Benefits (Tracheostomy)
- Provision of a secure airway and prevention of complications of prolonged oral or nasal intubation.

Potential Risks (Both Procedures)
- Surgical site infection.
- Bleeding.

- Tracheal stenosis (1.6–6%).
- Vocal cord injury.
- Subglottic stenosis.
- Tracheoesophageal fistula formation.
- Rates of complications and vocal cord injury are higher for emergent cricothyroidotomy as compared with elective tracheostomy.

EQUIPMENT

- No special equipment is required, although a bronchoscope can be useful in some instances.
- Small self-retaining retractors are useful for exposing the operative field.

PATIENT PREPARATION AND POSITIONING

- If possible, patient preparation should include the use of a folded sheet, sandbag, or other supporting device placed transversely under the shoulders; this helps in extending the neck and exposing the operative area.
- Endotracheal intubation is also extremely useful to maintain the airway during the procedure.
- In emergent situations when the patient is in respiratory distress, there may not be any time for such preparations.

PROCEDURE

Anatomic Landmarks

- **Figure 45–1:** The anatomy of the neck with pertinent landmarks.

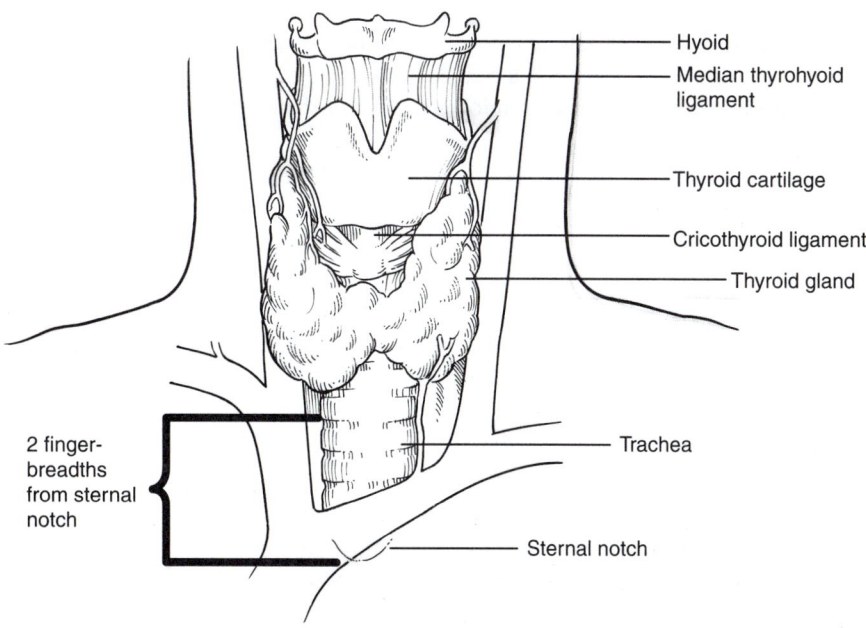

Figure 45–1

- The location of the thyroid cartilage in relation to the cricoid cartilage and the trachea is shown.
- Incision for the tracheostomy is made either transversely or vertically, approximately 2 fingerbreadths above the sternal notch.
- An emergency cricothyroidotomy is performed between the thyroid cartilage and the cricoid cartilage.
- A vertical incision is preferred for emergency cricothyroidotomy to minimize bleeding secondary to venous laceration. Additionally, if the initial incision is off target, it is easier to extend a vertical incision rather than make another transverse incision.

Open Tracheostomy

- **Figure 45–2:** After incision (shown here as a transverse incision), dissection is carried down through the subcutaneous tissues.
  - Often there is an anterior jugular vein crossing the field which may be tied off and divided.
- A small self-retaining retractor is useful to hold the incision open.
- Once the strap muscles are identified, they are divided vertically in the midline to expose the trachea.
- Often, the thyroid isthmus can be seen in the superior portion of the dissection; it may need to be divided for exposure.
  - It is preferable to ligate the lateral aspects of the thyroid isthmus prior to division in the midline.
  - Bleeding from thyroid tissue can be troublesome to control once initiated.
- **Figure 45–3A–C:** Once the trachea is exposed, two polypropylene sutures are placed around the third or fourth tracheal ring.
  - These are placed well laterally so as not to be divided when the trachea is opened, and care should be taken not to suture the balloon of the endotracheal tube if it is present.
  - The balloon on the endotracheal tube can be deflated temporarily during suture placement to avoid inadvertent puncture.
  - If the patient is intubated and oxygenation permits, the inspired Fio_2 should be decreased to 50% to minimize the possibility of endotracheal fire should cautery be required to control bleeding after tracheal opening.
  - The trachea is then typically entered with a vertical incision through the third and fourth rings.
  - Care must be taken not to cut the posterior wall of the trachea so as to avoid injury to the underlying esophagus.
  - Several different methods exist for creation of lateral tracheal flaps to facilitate insertion of the endotracheal tube: T-shaped incision (Figure 45–3A), H-shaped incision (Figure 45–3B), and trapdoor-type incision (Figure 45–3C).

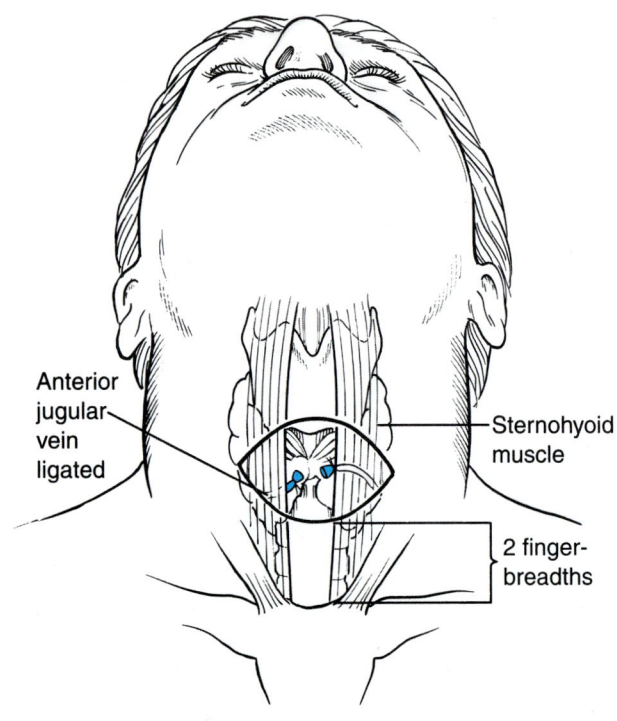

Figure 45–2

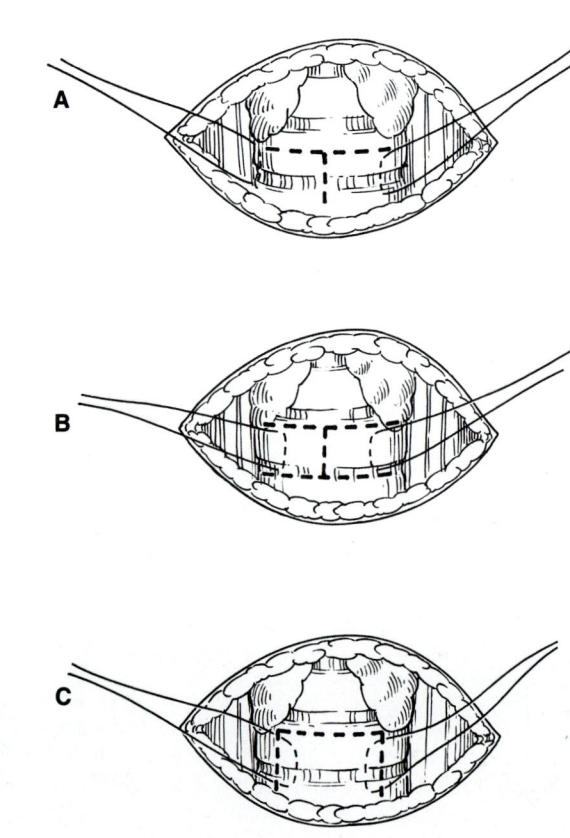

Figure 45–3A–C

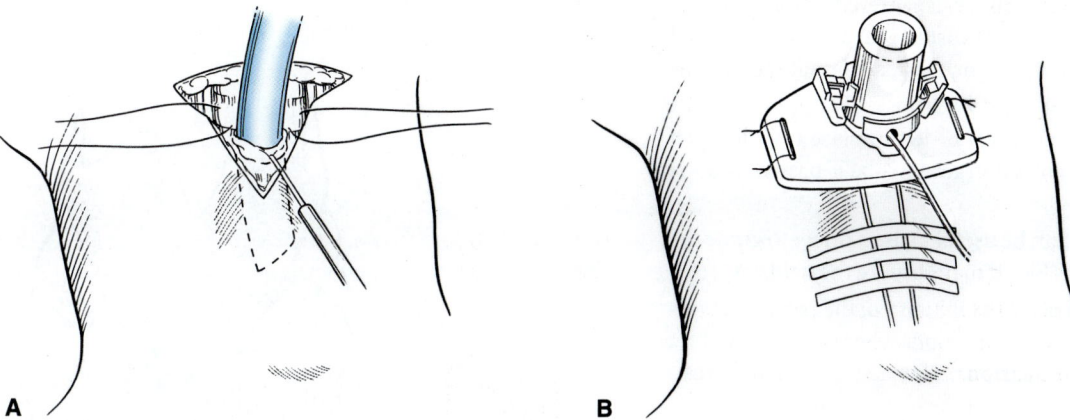

Figure 45–4A–B

- **Figure 45–4A, B:** Once the tracheal flaps have been created, a tracheal spreader is used to dilate the opening in preparation for tube placement.
  - The polypropylene sutures can be used to help retract the tracheal flaps laterally to facilitate placement of the tracheostomy tube into the trachea, but care must be taken not to pull the sutures through the delicate tracheal tissues (Figure 45–4A).
  - Once in place, the balloon is inflated and the tracheostomy tube is connected to the ventilator.
  - At this point, confirmation of proper placement of the tube into the trachea is of paramount importance. The detection of end-tidal CO_2 confirms appropriate tube placement in the trachea.
  - Once the ability to ventilate the patient is confirmed, the incision is closed loosely with nylon sutures and the cuff of the tracheostomy tube is sutured in place with four nylon sutures (Figure 45–4B).
  - The tracheostomy tube should also be secured with straps around the neck.
  - The polypropylene sutures in the tracheal flaps are left in place for several days in case replacement of the tracheostomy tube is needed.

Emergent Cricothyroidotomy

- **Figure 45–5:** Emergency cricothyroidotomy is performed using a vertical skin or stab incision to reduce bleeding.
  - The scalpel is stabbed through the skin and cricoid membrane between the thyroid cartilage and cricoid cartilage.

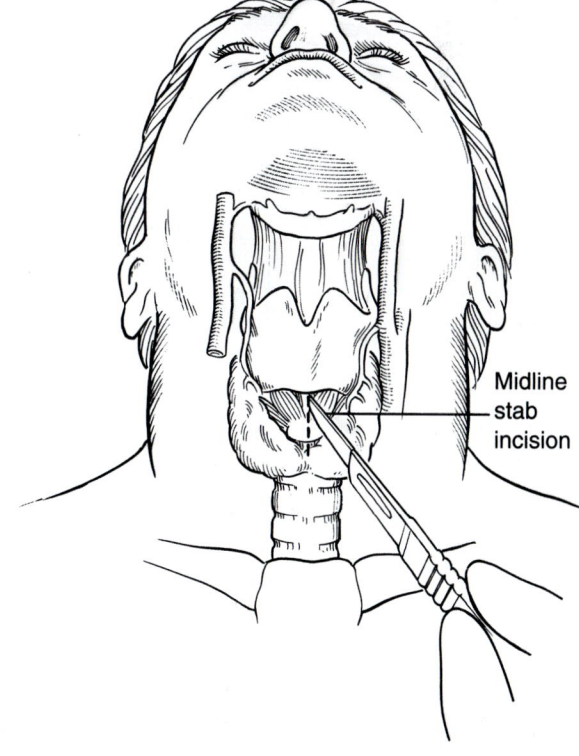

Figure 45–5

- **Figure 45–6:** Once the airway is entered, a hemostat or the knife handle (if no hemostat is available) is passed into the airway and spread or twisted to dilate the opening in the cricothyroid membrane.
  - If a hemostat is used, it can be left in place to hold open the incision while an endotracheal tube is passed into the airway.
- **Figure 45–7A, B:** It can be useful to use a finger to guide the endotracheal tube as blood may obscure the field.
  - Once the emergency airway is secured, the patient is typically taken to the operating room where conversion to a formal tracheostomy can be performed, although this can be delayed for several days if the patient is unstable.

POSTOPERATIVE CARE

- A replacement tracheostomy tube should be available at the patient's bedside at all times, and close monitoring is necessary in the first several days after tracheostomy.
- The inhaled air should be humidified since the upper airway is bypassed.
- Frequent endotracheal suctioning is often required to clear secretions.
- In the comatose patient, continuous pulse oximetry and frequent arterial blood gas monitoring may be needed.
- Delayed bleeding in the wound can often be difficult to visualize because the tracheostomy tube hinders exposure.

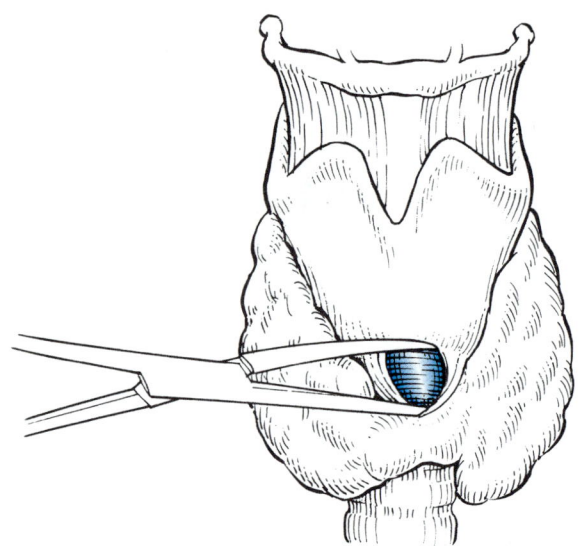

Figure 45–6

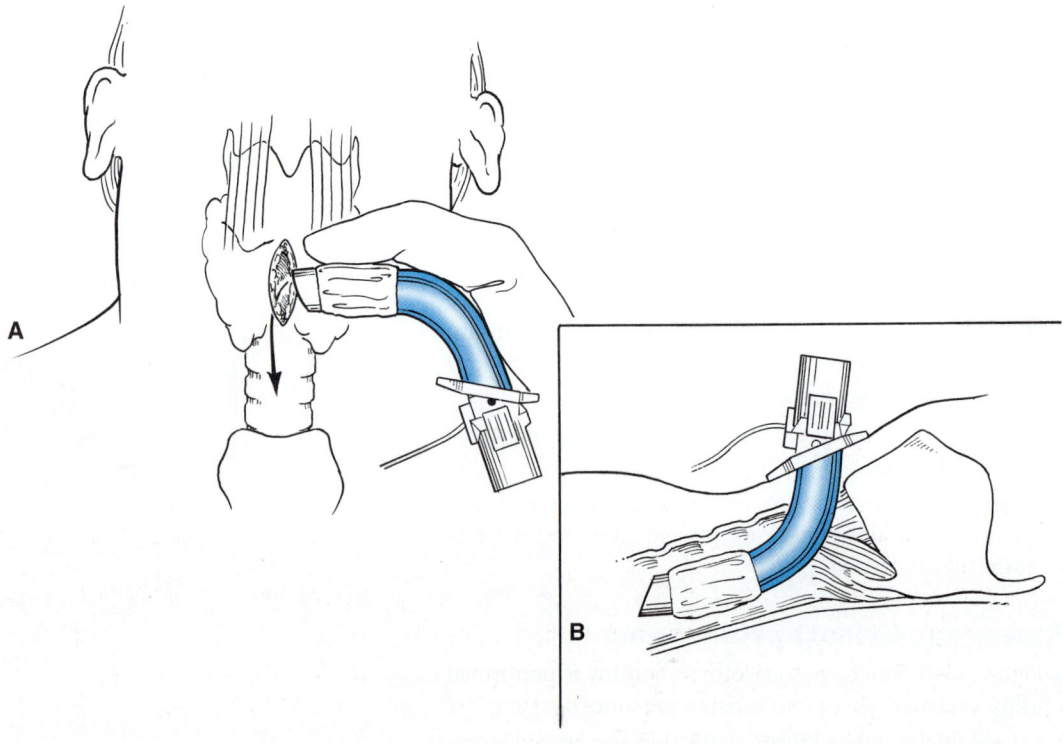

Figure 45–7A–B

- In such situations, packing of the wound with a long piece of hemostatic material (eg, Surgicel) may control the bleeding.
- Packing with small pieces should be avoided to prevent aspiration into the airway.
■ The initial tracheostomy tube is usually left in place for a minimum of 5–7 days, after which it may be removed and replaced.
■ The polypropylene sutures in the tracheal flaps can be cut and removed at the time of the first tracheostomy tube change if the change goes smoothly.

POTENTIAL COMPLICATIONS

■ Tracheal stenosis.
■ Subglottic stenosis.
■ Tracheoesophageal fistula.
■ Bleeding.

PEARLS AND TIPS

■ Staying in the midline will facilitate a more bloodless dissection.
■ A bronchoscope can be used to visualize the airway from inside the trachea if needed.

REFERENCES

Hemmila M, Wahl W. Management of the Injured Patient. In: Doherty GM, ed. *Current Diagnosis and Treatment: Surgery*, 13th ed. New York, NY: McGraw-Hill; 2010:176–209.

CHAPTER 46

Operative Management of Pyloric Stenosis: Pyloromyotomy

Benjamin Levi, MD, and George B. Mychaliska, MD

INDICATIONS

- Projectile nonbilious emesis in an infant.
- Palpable "olive" on physical examination.
- "String sign" on an upper gastrointestinal series.
- Pyloric muscle wall thickness ≥ 4 mm and pyloric channel length ≥ 16 mm on ultrasound examination.

CONTRAINDICATIONS

- Severe hypochloremic, hypokalemic metabolic alkalosis.
- Severe dehydration.

INFORMED CONSENT

- The procedure is successful in nearly 100% of cases.

Expected Benefits

- Elimination of the mechanical gastric outlet obstruction caused by a hypertrophic pylorus.

Potential Risks

- Incomplete myotomy (usually gastric).
- Mucosal perforation (usually duodenal).
- Wound infection.
- Postoperative bleeding.
- Fascial dehiscence.

EQUIPMENT

- Open pyloromyotomy: pyloric spreader (Benson).
- Laparoscopic pyloromyotomy.
  - Veress needle and sheath.
  - 5-mm umbilical port.
  - 3-mm instruments, including laparoscopic pyloric spreader.

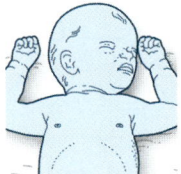
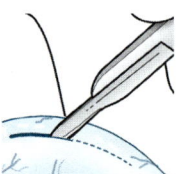
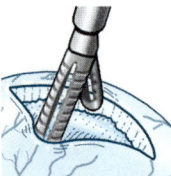
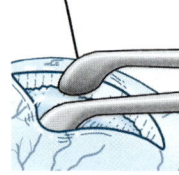

PATIENT PREPARATION

- Pyloric stenosis is not a surgical emergency; the goal of preoperative evaluation is to confirm the diagnosis and to correct metabolic derangements caused by persistent vomiting.
- Diagnosis is based on a thorough history and physical examination and is usually confirmed by radiographic findings.
  - A history of projectile nonbilious vomiting between ages 4 and 6 weeks and a palpable "olive" is sufficient for diagnosis.
  - If the diagnosis is unclear, ultrasound examination of the pylorus is the radiologic procedure of choice.
- Criteria for ultrasound diagnosis are pyloric muscle wall thickness ≥ 4 mm and pyloric channel length ≥ 16 mm.
- Once the diagnosis is suspected, the patient should not ingest anything orally.
- Preoperative nasogastric decompression is not required and may exacerbate the metabolic alkalosis.
- The most common metabolic abnormality is hypochloremic, hypokalemic metabolic alkalosis ($HCO_3 \geq 30$ mEq/L) and overall volume deficit.
- The patient should be rehydrated with 20 mL/kg boluses of normal saline until urinating and then given D5½ normal saline (10–20 mEq KCl/L if indicated) at a maintenance rate of 1.5. Lactated Ringer solution is contraindicated because it may exacerbate the metabolic alkalosis.

PATIENT POSITIONING

- **Figure 46–1A:** For both open and laparoscopic procedures, the infant should be supine on the operating table.
- Laparoscopic procedure.
  - The infant is positioned supine at the end of the operating table with appropriate padding.
  - The lower extremities are secured to the operating table in a frog leg position.

PROCEDURE

- Before induction of anesthesia, nasogastric decompression should be performed.
- **Figure 46–1B:** A longitudinal incision is made in the umbilicus and a Veress needle and trocar sheath are inserted.
  - A CO_2 pneumoperitoneum is established to a level of 10–12 mm Hg, and a 5-mm port is inserted.
  - Under direct vision, a No. 11 blade is used to make two 3-mm stab incisions in the upper abdominal wall.
- **Figure 46–1C:** An open pyloromyotomy is performed using a right upper quadrant or umbilical skin incision.

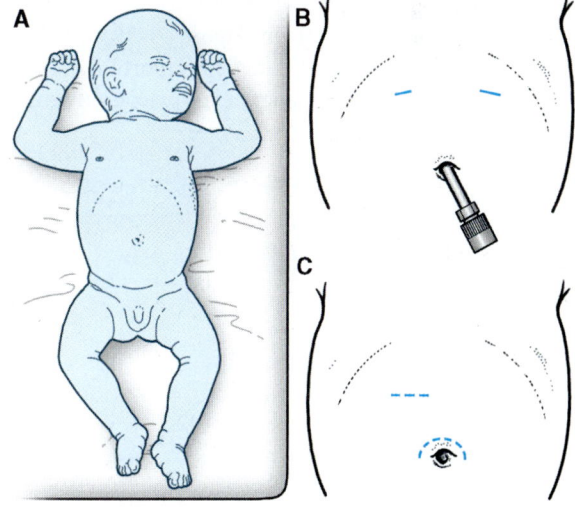

Figure 46–1A–C

- Right upper quadrant incision: a transverse incision is made directly over the right rectus muscle midway between the xiphoid and umbilicus. The rectus muscle may be divided transversely or the rectus fascia divided longitudinally to facilitate splitting of the rectus muscle.
- Umbilical incision: a supraumbilical curvilinear skin incision is made. The subcutaneous tissue is dissected until the midline fascia is exposed. The fascia is incised longitudinally and extended as far cephalad as required to locate the pylorus.

■ **Figure 46–2:** Cross-sectional view through a hypertrophic pylorus. The hypertrophic pylorus is readily apparent laparoscopically.

■ In the open procedure, mobilization of the pylorus out of the wound requires grasping the greater curvature of the stomach with a gauze sponge and gently "rocking" the pylorus outside the abdominal wall.

■ **Figure 46–3A, B:** Pyloromyotomy.
- Laparoscopic procedure: 3-mm instruments are used to grasp the duodenum and elevate the pylorus into view. Using a guarded Bovie tip, the serosa is cauterized in a linear fashion in an avascular area 2 mm proximal to the pyloroduodenal junction (noted by color and texture change and the Mayo vein) and extending to the antrum (Figure 46–3A). The cold "guarded" Bovie tip is used to extend the incision through the muscular layer. In the midportion of the incision, the Bovie tip is twisted to separate the pyloric musculature.
- Open procedure: cautery is not typically used. Using a scalpel, an incision is made in an avascular region of the pylorus, 2 mm proximal to the pyloroduodenal junction and extending to the antrum (Figure 46–3B). The back of the scalpel handle is placed in the midportion of the incision and then twisted to separate the pyloric musculature.

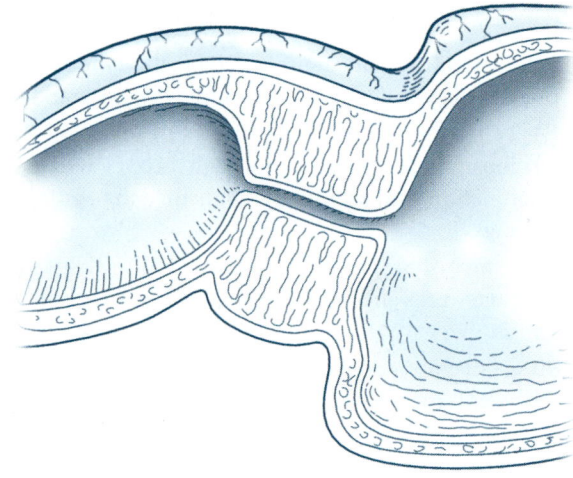

Figure 46-2

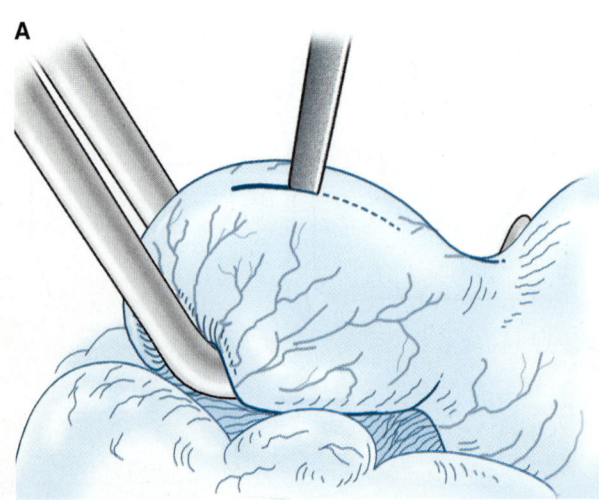
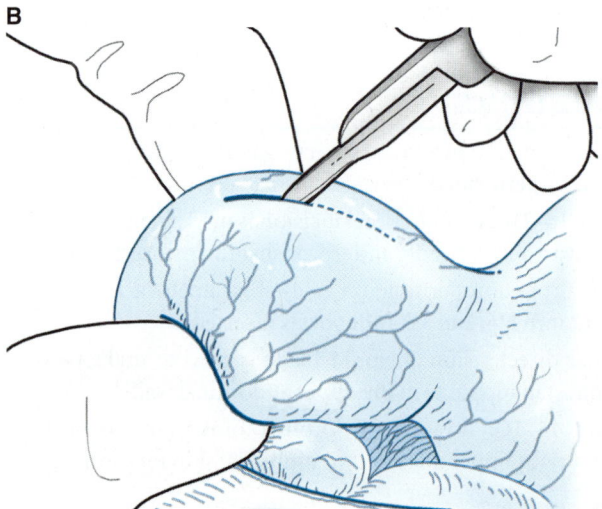

Figure 46-3A-B

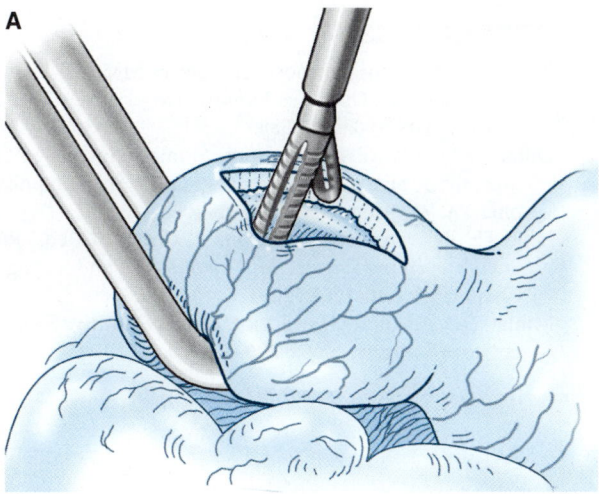
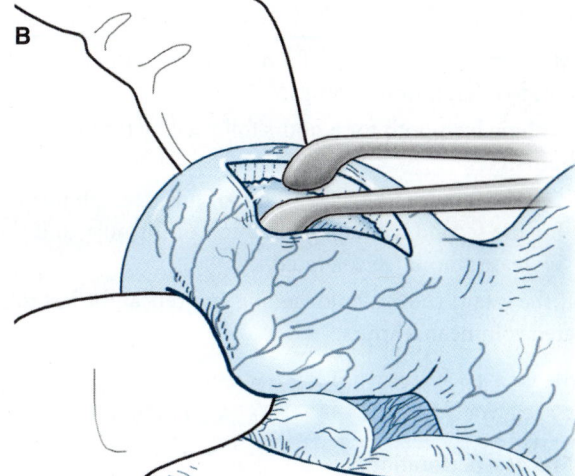

Figure 46–4A–B

- **Figure 46–4A, B:** Splitting the pyloric musculature.
  - Laparoscopic procedure: a laparoscopic spreader is used to slowly spread the hypertrophied muscle fibers until the submucosa bulges out (Figure 46–4A).
  - Open procedure: a Benson spreader is placed in the incision and used to slowly spread the hypertrophied muscle until the submucosa bulges out (Figure 46–4B).
- **Figure 46–5A, B:** Laparoscopic or open pyloromyotomy is complete when the two halves of the pyloric muscle appear askew, move independently, and normal antral muscle fibers are visualized proximally.
- Bleeding is venous and self-limited and should never be cauterized due to potential mucosal injury.
- At the conclusion of the procedure, the proximal duodenum is gently compressed and 60 mL of air is injected through a nasogastric tube to rule out mucosal perforation.

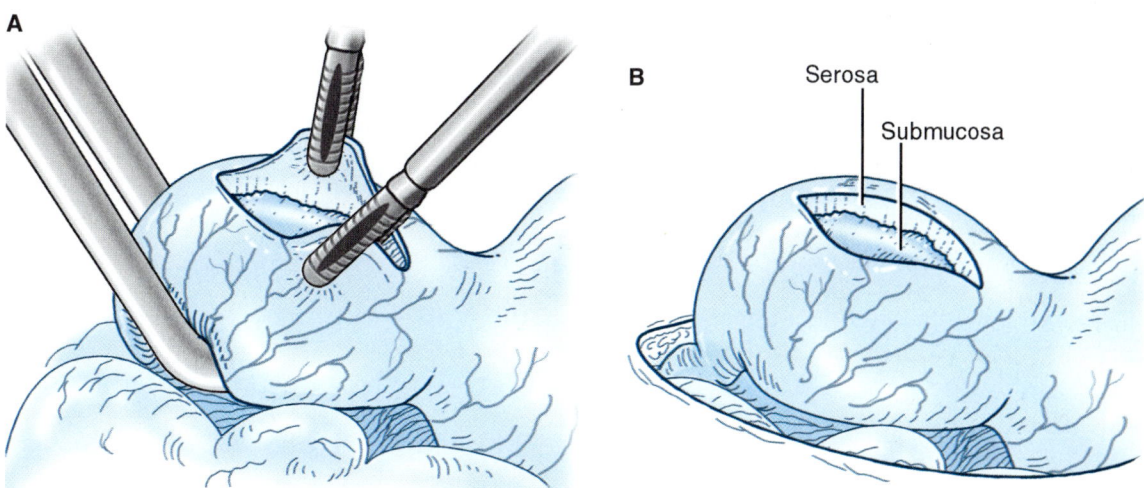

Figure 46–5A–B

POSTOPERATIVE CARE

- Maintenance intravenous fluids are given until the infant is able to tolerate oral feedings.
- Nothing by mouth for 6 hours followed by feeding every 3 hours:
  - For the first feeding, give 30 mL of full-strength formula; for the second feeding, give 60 mL of formula, and then increase amount as tolerated.
- If the infant vomits, hold feeding and repeat the last tolerated volume in 3 hours.

POTENTIAL COMPLICATIONS

- Mucosal perforation.
- Incomplete myotomy.
- Wound infection.

PEARLS AND TIPS

- Preoperatively, ensure correction of electrolyte abnormalities, adequate hydration, and $HCO_3 \leq 30$ mEq/L.
- Preoperative nasogastric decompression is contraindicated because gastric secretions are tolerated and metabolic alkalosis may be exacerbated with persistent loss of gastric acid.
- Intraoperatively, test for intestinal perforation by administering 60 mL of air via the nasogastric tube and looking for bubbles or bile staining.

REFERENCES

Barksdale EM. Pyloric Stenosis. In: Ziegler MM, Azizkhan RG, Weber TR, eds. *Operative Pediatric Surgery.* New York, NY: McGraw-Hill; 2003:583–588.

Dillon PW, Cilley RE. Lesions of the Stomach. In: Ashcraft KW, Murphy JP, Sharp RJ, et al, eds. *Pediatric Surgery.* Philadelphia, PA: WB Saunders; 2000:391–406.

Lobe TE. Pyloromyotomy. In: Spitz L, Coran AG, eds. *Rob & Smith's Operative Surgery: Pediatric Surgery.* London, England: Chapman & Hall; 1995:320–328.

Miniati DN, Albanese CT. Pyloric Stenosis. *Operative Techniques in General Surgery.* 2004;6:296–306.

CHAPTER 47

Pediatric Vascular Access

Kimberly McCrudden Erickson, MD

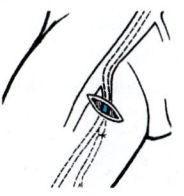 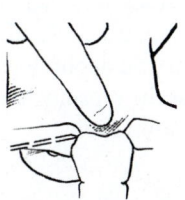 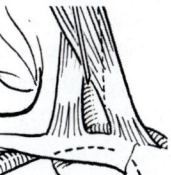
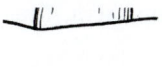 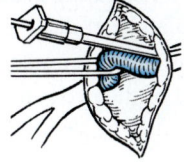 
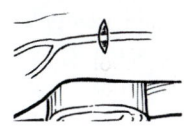

INDICATIONS

- Need for acute resuscitation.
  - Trauma.
  - Critical care monitoring.
- Need for long-term central venous access.
  - Total parenteral nutrition.
  - Chemotherapy.
  - Hemodialysis.
  - Long-term antibiotic therapy.
  - Limited peripheral access in ill child.

CONTRAINDICATIONS

Absolute
- None.

Relative
- Coagulopathy.
- Severe thrombocytopenia.

INFORMED CONSENT

Expected Benefits
- Stable vascular access in infants and children to aid a variety of therapeutic interventions.

Potential Risks
- Bleeding.
- Pneumothorax.
- Hemothorax.
- Catheter infection.
- Line sepsis.
- Catheter malfunction or thrombosis.
- Venous thrombosis.

EQUIPMENT

- Cutdown central venous lines in premature infants and neonates require very fine vascular pickups and small right-angle clamps. It is best to assemble a sterile neonatal cutdown tray to have available at all times.
- A portable ultrasound machine is helpful for internal jugular venous punctures.
- All lines inserted in the operating room should be placed using live fluoroscopy on an appropriate radiolucent table.
- A wide range of catheter types and sizes should be available at all times.
  - For both acute and long-term hemodialysis catheters, it is best to develop a weight-based catheter size chart in conjunction with pediatric nephrologists to ensure that the catheter placed has the capacity to provide adequate flow for dialysis or hemofiltration.

PATIENT PREPARATION

- Preoperative blood work should include hematocrit, platelet count, and coagulation studies.
- If the child has had previous central lines, a duplex Doppler vascular ultrasound of the neck and upper extremity vessels should be performed to identify potential preoperative thromboses.
  - If multiple thromboses are seen, a magnetic resonance venogram is useful for preoperative planning.

PATIENT POSITIONING

- The patient is most often positioned supine with a shoulder roll in place.
- If a saphenous vein cutdown or femoral vein catheterization is planned, the leg should be straight and abducted away from the midline.

PROCEDURE

- **Figure 47–1:** Saphenous vein cutdown.
  - This procedure is used most often for premature infants and neonates and can be performed at the bedside.
  - The location of the femoral artery is identified by palpation.
  - After infiltration of the area with local anesthesia, a short transverse incision is made 1 cm below the groin crease and medial to the femoral artery.
  - The saphenous vein is identified, ligated distally, and encircled proximally.
  - A 5-mm stab wound is made on the medial thigh just above the knee.

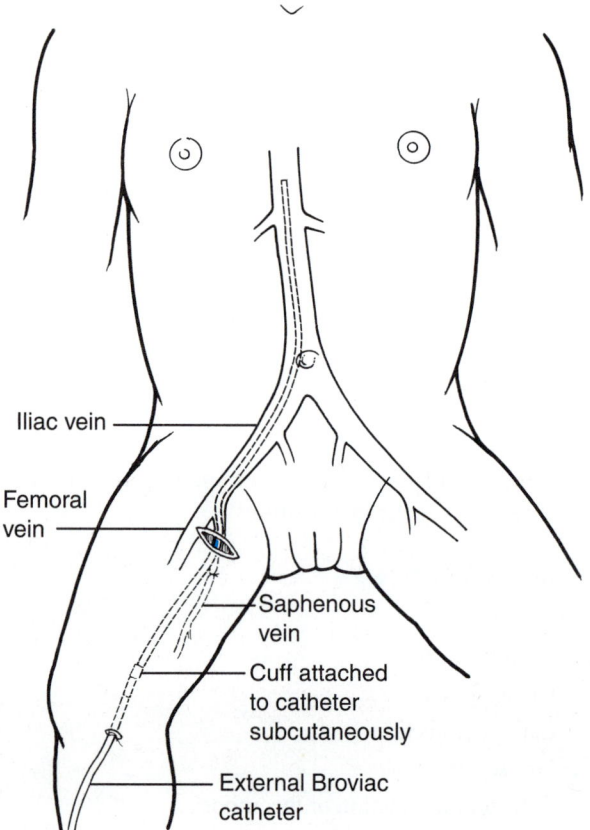

Figure 47–1

- A Broviac catheter is tunneled from the distal incision to the venous cutdown site until the Dacron cuff is midway between the two incisions.
- The catheter is measured to lie in the subdiaphragmatic superior vena cava (SVC) and is cut on a very acute angle to the appropriate length.
- Using a No. 11 blade, an anterior venotomy is performed and the catheter placed *bevel down* into the vein.
- Once in place, the catheter is secured in the vein with the previously placed suture.
- The catheter is then checked to ensure that blood can be withdrawn and the catheter flushes easily.
- The catheter is secured at the skin exit site with a nylon suture and the wound closed with either a running nylon or absorbable suture.

■ **Figure 47–2A, B:** Subclavian vein puncture.
- This procedure is safe and effective in both infants and children.
- The patient should be in Trendelenburg position with a small horizontal shoulder roll.
- The needle is attached to an empty 5-mL syringe and inserted just lateral to the midportion of the clavicle, at a depth of approximately 5 mm below the clavicle.
- The needle is advanced medially toward the suprasternal notch while aspirating continuously.
- Placing a finger in the suprasternal notch may help guide the angle of advancement (Figure 47–2A).
- In smaller children and infants, the needle should be angled more superiorly to a spot 1 cm above the suprasternal notch (Figure 47–2B).

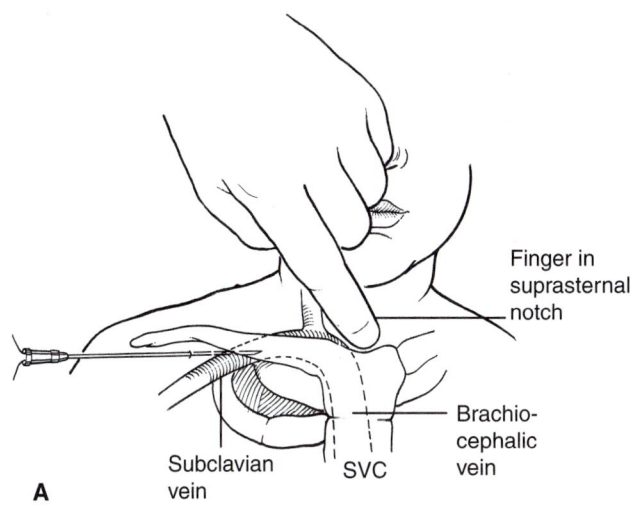
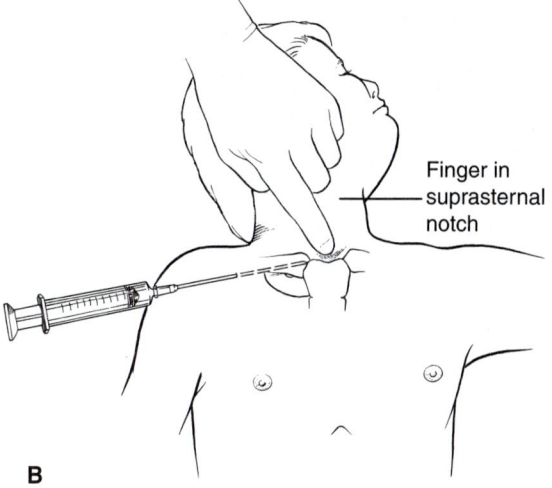

Figure 47–2A–B

- Free return of venous blood during aspiration signals successful venipuncture.
- The needle is then carefully stabilized as the syringe is removed and a flexible J-tipped guidewire passed through the needle and into the vein.
- Fluoroscopy is essential at this point to confirm proper position of the wire in the right atrium.
- This wire will then be used to place either a temporary central venous catheter or the introducer and sheath required for a tunneled catheter.

■ **Figure 47–3:** Internal jugular vein puncture.
- This procedure is also safe and effective in both infants and children and can be facilitated by the use of intraoperative portable ultrasound.
- The right internal jugular vein provides direct access to the right atrium and is the preferred route for placing dialysis catheters.
- The patient should be in Trendelenburg position with a shoulder roll in place and the head turned to the left.
- The needle is attached to an empty 5-mL syringe and inserted between the two heads of the sternocleidomastoid muscle at the level of the cricoid cartilage.
- This puncture site is just above the apex of the triangle formed by the two muscle heads and lateral to the carotid artery.
- The needle is directed inferiorly and laterally toward the ipsilateral nipple at an angle of 15–30 degrees to the skin.
- Free return of venous blood during aspiration signals successful venipuncture.
- If the artery is accidentally punctured, the needle is removed and direct pressure applied for 5 minutes.
- The needle is then carefully stabilized as the syringe is removed and a flexible J-tipped guidewire passed through the needle and into the vein.
- Fluoroscopy is essential at this point to confirm proper position of the wire in the right atrium.
- This wire is then used to place either a temporary central venous catheter or the introducer and sheath required for a tunneled catheter.

■ **Figure 47–4A–C:** Radial artery cutdown.
- This technique is most commonly used in neonates when the percutaneous route is unsuccessful.
- The hand is taped to an armboard and a small gauze roll is placed under the supinated, extended wrist (Figure 47–4A).
- A 1-cm transverse incision is made over the area of the radial artery just proximal to the wrist.
- The artery is often deeper than expected and usually located directly over the head of the radius.
- A suture is placed distally around the artery for traction.

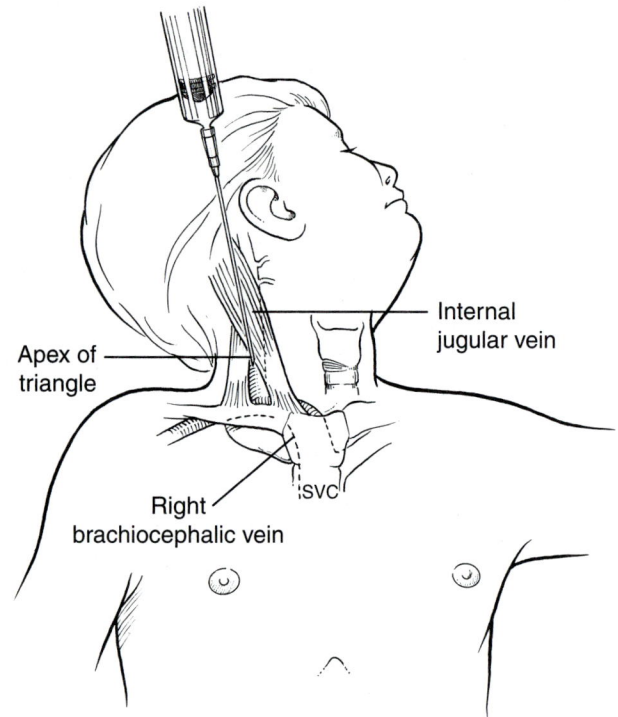

Figure 47–3

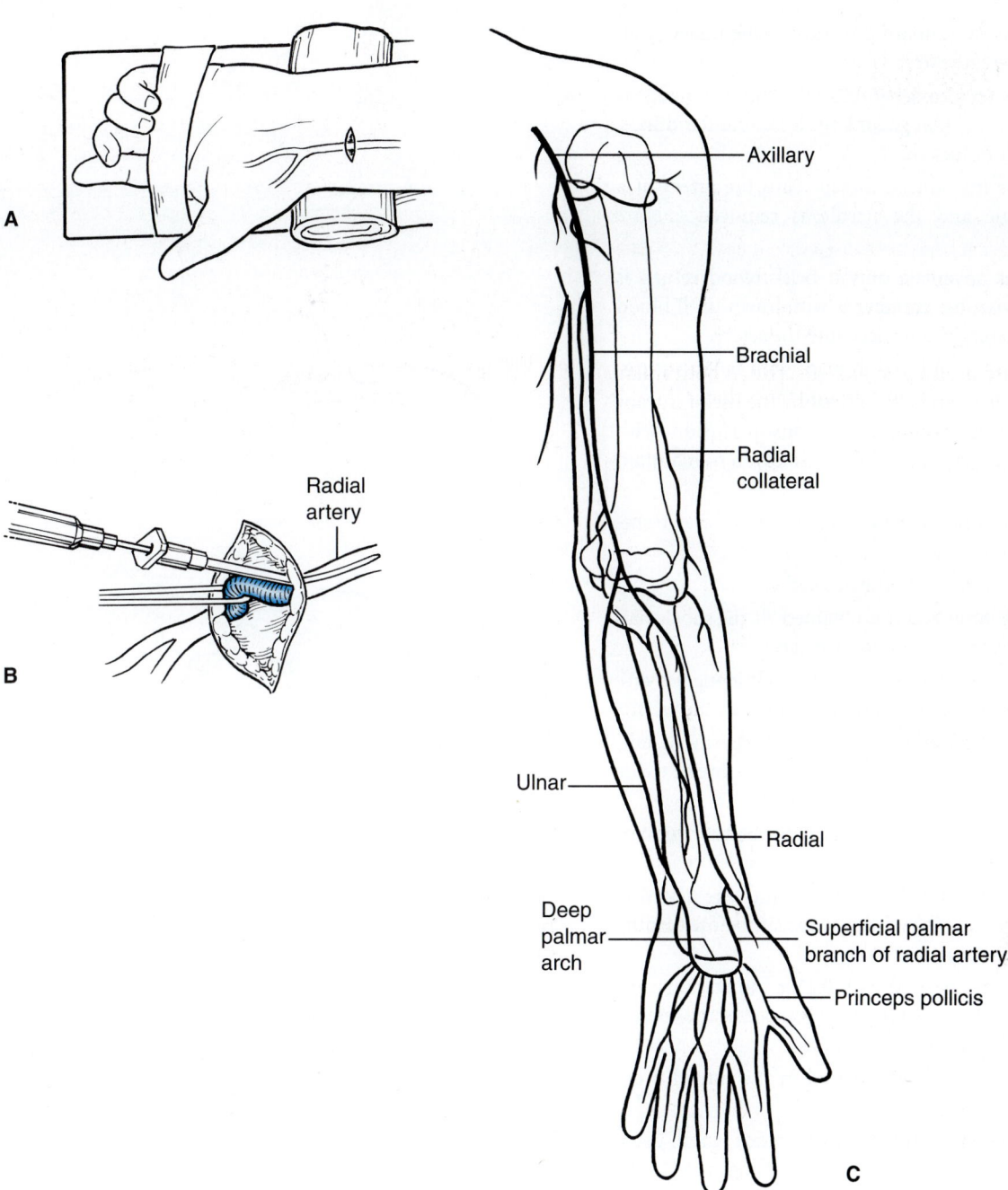

Figure 47-4A-C

- Cannulation is via standard puncture of the vessel by an over-the-needle catheter device.
- Choice of catheter size depends on the child: 24-gauge is best for neonates, 22-gauge for large infants and toddlers, and 20-gauge for older children.
- The catheter is introduced directly into the artery at a 30-degree angle and the needle is removed (Figure 47–4B).
- The catheter is advanced only if brisk blood return is noted. Otherwise, the catheter is withdrawn until blood returns, then carefully advanced into the artery.
- The catheter hub is sutured in place with nylon sutures and the skin incision is closed around the catheter.
- Arterial catheters require continuous perfusion with 0.5–1.0 mL/h of heparinized saline solution to maintain patency.
- Figure 47–4C outlines the anatomy of the upper extremity arterial system.

■ **Figure 47–5:** Placement of tunneled catheters.
  - Initial central venous access is obtained via the subclavian or internal jugular route as outlined earlier.
  - A small 5-mm incision is made transversely along the wire at the wire insertion site using a No. 11 blade.
  - A second incision is made on the anterior chest wall, taking into consideration the presence of future breast tissue in girls.
  - This incision can be made superior to the breast region or in the midline over the sternum.
  - A tendon passer is then tunneled from the wire insertion site, passing lateral to the venous access site before turning and traveling to the skin exit site.
  - The tunnel is anesthetized with 0.25% bupivacaine; the proximal end of the catheter is then grasped by the tendon passer and pulled through the tunnel.
  - The Dacron cuff should be placed in the tunnel 2 cm proximal to the exit site.
  - The catheter is measured to the appropriate length using fluoroscopic guidance and cut on a slight angle.
  - The dilator and associated peel-away sheath are placed over the wire and advanced under fluoroscopic guidance only as far as the SVC.
  - The wire and dilator are then removed together, the tunneled catheter is inserted into the sheath, and the sheath is peeled away.
  - Catheter position is confirmed by fluoroscopy, and catheter function is assured by easy bidirectional flow of blood and saline.
  - The venous access site is closed with a single 5-0 absorbable subcuticular suture and the catheter secured in place at the skin exit site with a nylon suture.

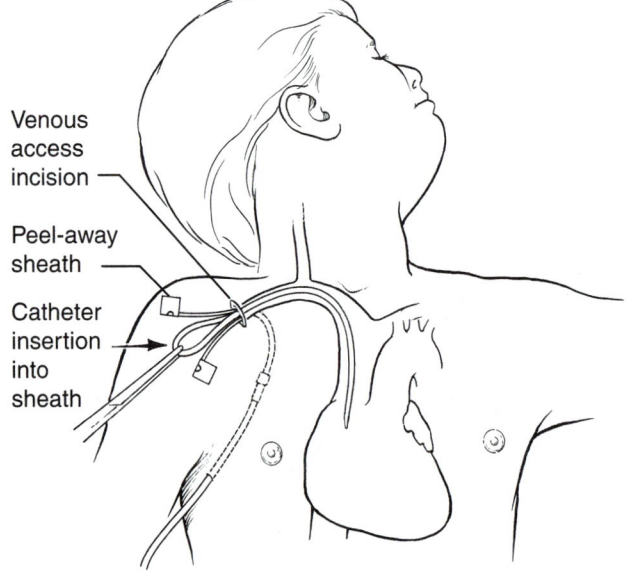

Figure 47–5

- The catheter is then flushed with heparinized saline (10 units/mL concentration) unless it is a hemodialysis catheter.

POSTOPERATIVE CARE

- All lines except radial arterial lines require a post-procedure radiograph to confirm catheter position and look for complications.
  - These films may pick up a subtle pneumothorax not seen by fluoroscopy during catheter placement.
- Meticulous aseptic technique must be used for routine catheter care and every time the catheter is accessed for infusion or blood draw.

POTENTIAL COMPLICATIONS

Acute
- Pneumothorax.
- Hemothorax.
- Catheter malposition.
- Pericardial tamponade.

Chronic
- Catheter infection.
- Bacteremia and line sepsis.
- Catheter thrombosis.
- Vessel thrombosis.
- Septic emboli.
- SVC syndrome.

PEARLS AND TIPS

- For standard central venous access indications, premature infants usually require a 2.7 French catheter, while full-term infants will tolerate a 4.2 French line. Larger catheters (ie, 7 French) required in urgent settings should be placed in the right internal jugular vein.
- Percutaneous access in infants and smaller children is best obtained using a 21-gauge needle. Older children may be accessed using the standard 18-gauge needle.
- After securing any Broviac catheter in place and closing the venous access site, always flush the catheter again and ensure easy blood withdrawal as sometimes the securing sutures are placed too tightly and partially occlude the catheter.
- It is best to use a concentration of 10 units of heparin per milliliter of saline as the standard solution for line flushes in children in the pediatric operating room.
  - Small accidental flushes of a more concentrated solution can fully heparinize an infant and increase bleeding complications.
  - Higher concentrations of heparinized saline (100–1000 units/mL) required for hemodialysis catheters should be specifically requested during those cases.

REFERENCES

Coran AG, Hirschl RB. Cardiovascular Considerations. In: O'Neill JA, Grosfeld JL, Fonkalsrud EW, et al, eds. *Principles of Pediatric Surgery*, 2nd ed. St Louis, MO: Mosby; 2004:437–442.

Janik JE, Conlon SJ, Janik JS. Percutaneous central access in patients younger than 5 years: size does matter. *J Pediatr Surg*. 2004;39:1252–1256.

Johnson EM, Saltzman DA, Suh G, et al. Complications and risks of central venous catheter placement in children. *Surgery*. 1998;124:911–916.

CHAPTER 48

Pediatric Inguinal Hernia

Kimberly McCrudden Erickson, MD

INDICATIONS

- Presence of a hernia (elective).
- Incarceration or strangulation (emergent).

CONTRAINDICATIONS

Absolute
- Coagulopathy.
- Thrombocytopenia.

Relative
- Extreme prematurity.
- Cardiopulmonary comorbidities.
- Immunosuppression.

INFORMED CONSENT

Expected Benefits
- The most important goal is to eliminate the risk of incarceration and strangulation.
- Repair can also provide relief from discomfort associated with the hernia.

Potential Risks
- Risks include:
  - Bleeding.
  - Wound infection.
  - Injury to the vas deferens.
  - Injury to the testicular vessels.
  - Injury to the ilioinguinal nerve.
- Parents should also be informed that the procedure is performed under general anesthesia.

EQUIPMENT

- A basic pediatric soft tissue tray should provide the various small retractors (Davis, U.S. Army retractors) needed for the surgery.

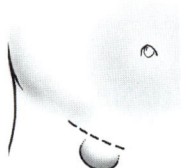
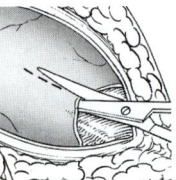
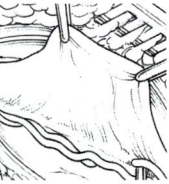
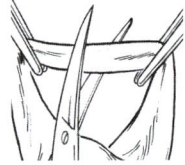
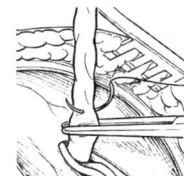
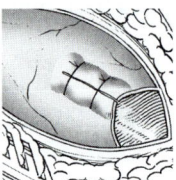

- Peritoneoscopy equipment.
  - 2.7-mm, 70-degree angled laparoscope.
  - Small, blunt-tipped metal 3-mm trocar.
  - Laparoscopy equipment (light cord, camera cord, and a single video monitor).

PATIENT PREPARATION

- No special preparation is required other than a thorough preoperative examination with attention to both inguinal regions.
- The side of the symptomatic hernia should be marked by the surgeon on the patient on the day of surgery with the parent or guardian present.

PATIENT POSITIONING

- The patient should be supine on the operating table.
- Following induction of general anesthesia, the patient may be turned on his or her side for placement of a caudal block if appropriate.

PROCEDURE

- The following steps describe the procedure for a male patient. The procedure is performed under general anesthesia with or without the addition of a caudal block.
- The entire lower abdomen, perineum, and upper thighs are scrubbed, prepared with povidone-iodine, and draped in the standard sterile fashion.
- **Figure 48–1:** A 1–2-cm transverse skin incision is made along the lowest inguinal skin crease approximately 1 cm superior and lateral to the pubic tubercle.
  - The subcutaneous fat is separated to expose Scarpa's fascia, which is incised with either Metzenbaum scissors or electrocautery.
- **Figure 48–2:** The opening in Scarpa's fascia is then explored using a hemostat to expose the external oblique aponeurosis below. This allows for placement of small Davis retractors into the wound.
  - A key maneuver at this point is to dissect laterally to fully expose the groove between the abdominal wall and the lateral border of the external oblique fascia.
  - This groove is then followed inferiorly to the external ring, where the spermatic cord and associated hernia sac exit the inguinal canal.
  - A hemostat is placed in the external ring and a small nick is made in the ring using a knife.
  - The hemostat is briefly removed to allow the ilioinguinal nerve to fall away and is then replaced in the external ring.

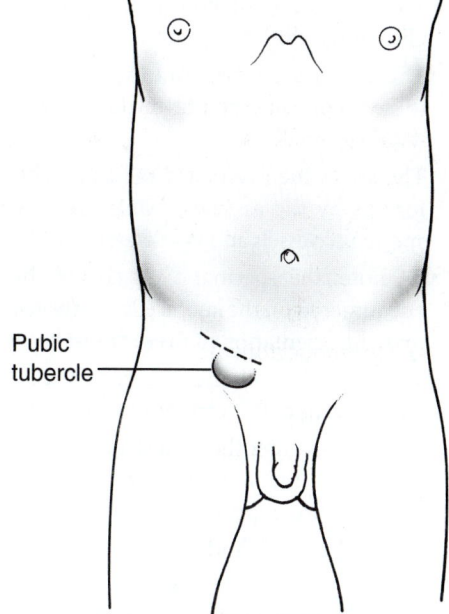

Figure 48–1

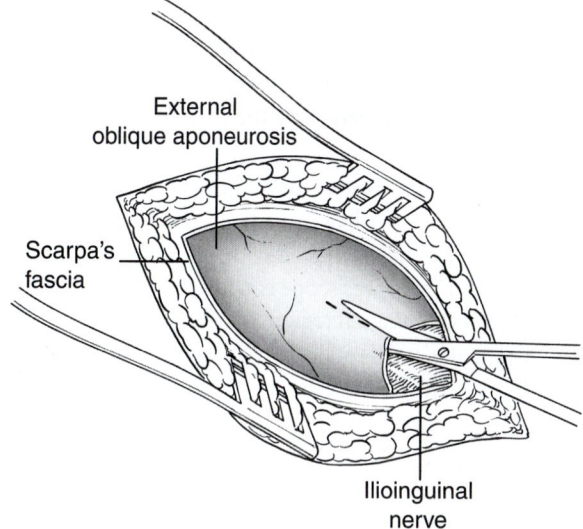

Figure 48–2

- The external oblique fascia is incised from along its fibers for a distance of 1–2 cm.
- The edges of the opened external oblique fascia are grasped with atraumatic forceps and the undersurface of each leaf is gently brushed clear of the underlying cord structures to protect the nerve and facilitate later closure.
- The ilioinguinal nerve should then be visualized and gently dissected free.
- **Figure 48–3:** Using atraumatic tissue forceps, the cremasteric fibers are grasped and separated to identify the underlying hernia sac.
  - The sac lies anteromedial to the cord structures and has a glistening, whitish appearance.
  - The sac is grasped with one forceps while the other is used to sweep the muscular fibers down toward the floor of the inguinal canal.
  - The sac is then retracted medially with two atraumatic forceps by the assistant, while the surgeon dissects the spermatic vessels and vas deferens off the sac.
  - Of note, the spermatic vessels are the first structures encountered on the lateral edge of the sac. If the vas is seen first, the orientation of the sac must be evaluated.
  - The vas and vessels must never be directly grasped or held with forceps as this can cause significant damage.
- **Figure 48–4:** After the cord structures have been separated from the sac, the sac is inspected to ensure that no abdominal viscera are trapped within.
  - Unless the sac is blind-ending, it is divided between hemostats.
  - The proximal end of the sac is lifted vertically and the cord structures are dissected free down to the level of the internal ring, where properitoneal fat is identified.
  - To facilitate this dissection, the assistant should place gentle downward traction on the spermatic cord structures.
- At this point, peritoneoscopy may be performed if the clinical situation warrants and the sac appears sturdy.
  - To perform peritoneoscopy, the sac is opened and secured with hemostats.
  - A 3-mm blunt metal trocar is inserted directly into the sac and secured with a heavy silk tie.
  - The abdomen is insufflated with CO_2 (8–12 mm Hg), and a 2.7-mm, 70-degree scope is inserted with the lens facing the opposite inguinal region.
  - The vas deferens and spermatic vessels on the opposite side are identified and the region is inspected for a patent processus vaginalis on the contralateral side.
  - The scope and trocar are removed, and desufflation is ensured by placing a tissue forceps into the sac and observing for release of air and abdominal decompression.

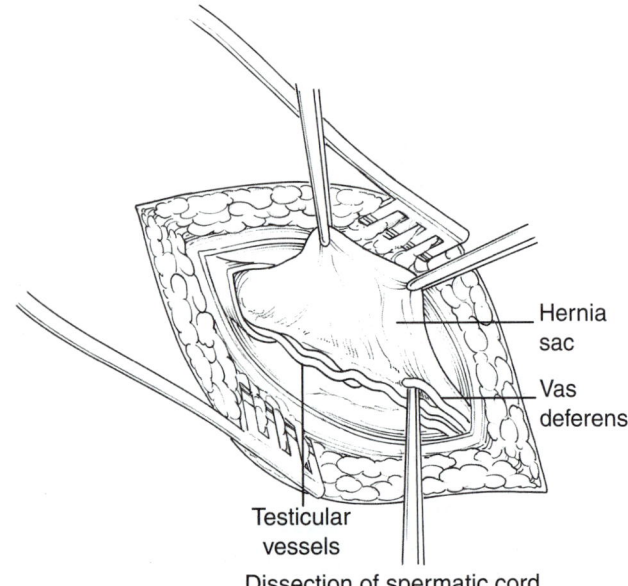

Dissection of spermatic cord

Figure 48–3

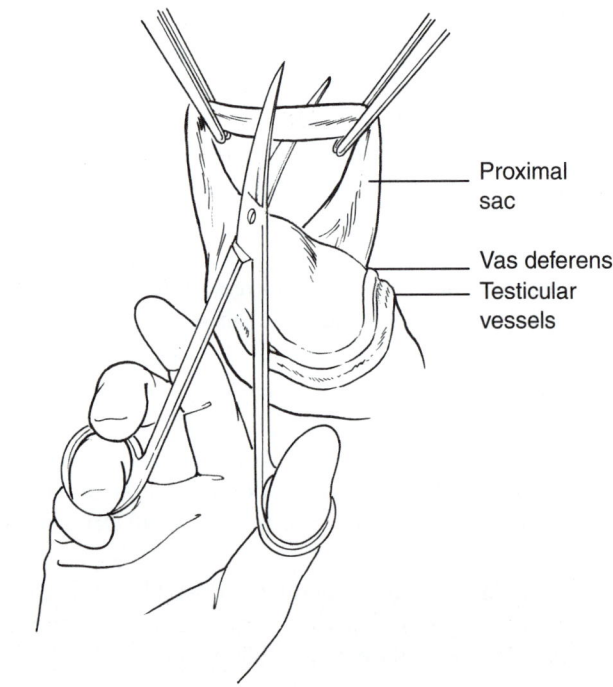

Figure 48–4

- **Figure 48–5:** High ligation of the proximal sac is then performed by twisting the sac and placing two 3-0 or 4-0 Vicryl suture ligatures at the base.
  - Care must be taken to avoid incorporating the cord structures in these sutures as twisting the sac may alter the anatomy at the internal ring.
  - Following ligation, the excess sac is removed with scissors.
  - The distal end of the sac heading toward the scrotum may be opened widely along its anterior surface.
  - If a noncommunicating hydrocele also exists, it should be opened widely and a portion of this sac excised.
  - If the testicle is visualized, any associated appendix testes should be excised or cauterized. The testicle must be placed back in the scrotum prior to closure.
- **Figure 48–6:** Once hemostasis is ensured, the external oblique fascia is closed using interrupted Vicryl sutures, taking care to identify and protect the ilioinguinal nerve.
  - If a preoperative caudal block was not used, an ilioinguinal nerve block can be placed under direct visualization at this juncture.
  - Scarpa's fascia is then reapproximated using buried, interrupted Vicryl sutures.
  - The skin is closed with a running 5-0 Monocryl suture. The wound may be dressed using an adhesive (Collodion, Dermabond, Indermil) in children who are still in diapers, or Steri-Strips with Benzoin in older children.

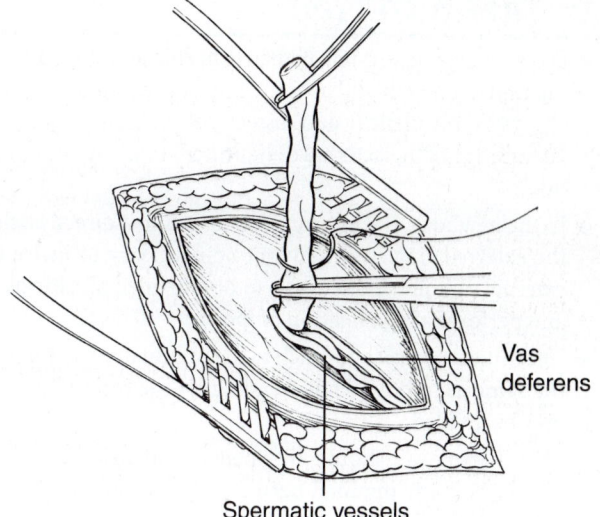

Figure 48–5

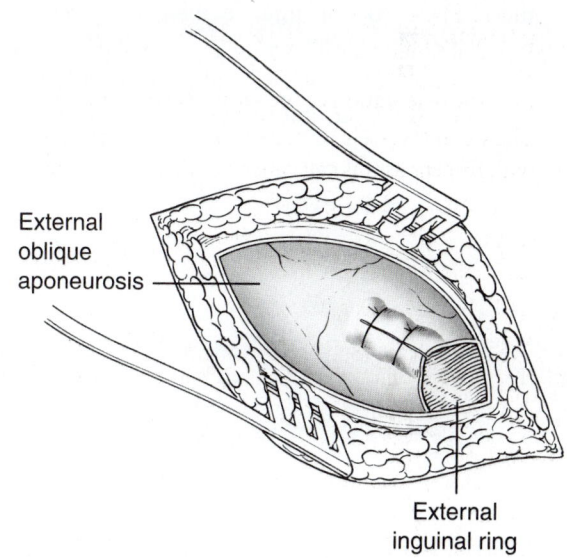

Figure 48–6

POSTOPERATIVE CARE

- Analgesia using acetaminophen, ibuprofen, and narcotics as needed.
- Heavy lifting and high-contact sports in older children and adolescents should be limited for 4–6 weeks postoperatively.

POTENTIAL COMPLICATIONS

Acute
- Bleeding.
- Wound infection.
- Injury to spermatic vessels.
- Injury to vas deferens.
- Postoperative hydrocele.
- Damage or entrapment of ilioinguinal nerve.

Chronic
- Testicular atrophy.
- Recurrence.
- Iatrogenic undescended testicle.

PEARLS AND TIPS

- To avoid getting lost in a pediatric hernia and thereby risking injury to the bladder or the floor of the inguinal canal, always clearly identify and dissect out the groove along the lateral edge of the external oblique fascia early in the operation.
- In the newborn, the internal ring lies almost directly below the external ring so it may not be necessary to incise the external oblique aponeurosis to obtain adequate exposure and perform a high ligation of the sac.
- The initial surgical approach to the inguinal canal in girls is the same as in boys. However, in girls the round ligament may be divided.
  - The hernia sac should be opened and inspected in all cases, as many inguinal hernias in girls contain a sliding component.
  - The ovary, fallopian tube, and mesosalpinx can be present either in the hernia sac or within the wall of the sac. Care must be taken to avoid injury to these structures.
  - If the fallopian tube lies within the wall of the sac, a purse-string closure of the sac may be performed followed by inversion of the sac and separate closure of the internal ring.

REFERENCES

Ein SH, Njere I, Ein A. Six thousand three hundred sixty-one pediatric inguinal hernias: a 35-year review. *J Pediatr Surg.* 2006;41:980–986.

Fonkalsrud EW, Stolar CJ. Disorders of the Inguinal Canal. In: O'Neill JA, Grosfeld JL, Fonkalsrud EW, et al, eds. *Principles of Pediatric Surgery,* 2nd ed. St Louis, MO: Mosby; 2004:437–442.

Manoharan S, Samarakkody U, Kulkarni M, et al. Evidence-based change of practice in the management of unilateral inguinal hernia. *J Pediatr Surg.* 2006;40:1163–1166.

Index

Note: Page numbers followed by *f* and *t* indicate figures and tables, respectively.

A

abdominal aortic aneurysm, infrarenal, management, 279-285, 279*f*, 281*f*-284*f*. *See also* infrarenal abdominal aortic aneurysm, management
abdominoperineal resection (APR), with total mesorectal excision, in rectal tumor management, 192-202
above-the-knee amputation (AKA), 315-323, 315*f*, 316*f*, 319*f*-321*f*
abscess(es)
   anorectal, management of. *See* anorectal abscess and fistula, management
   hemorrhoidal, simple drainage of, 214, 215*f*, 216
adrenalectomy, 14-21, 14*f*, 16*f*-19*f*
   disease states associated with, 14
      postoperative care, 20
   laparoscopic, 14-18
   open, 15, 16
   open anterior, 18-20
AKA. *See* above-the-knee amputation (AKA)
Altemeier procedure, for rectal prolapse. *See* perineal rectosigmoidectomy, for rectal prolapse
amputation(s)
   above-the-knee, 315-323, 315*f*, 316*f*, 319*f*-321*f*. *See also* above-the-knee amputation (AKA)
   below-the-knee, 315-323, 315*f*-318*f*, 322-323. *See also* below-the-knee amputation (BKA)
anastomosis(es)
   Billroth I, 72-73, 72*f*
   Billroth II, 73, 73*f*
   cervical esophagogastric, in transhiatal esophagectomy, 39-40, 39*f*-40*f*
   hand-sewn, in small bowel resection, procedure, 151-152, 151*f*-153*f*
   ileal pouch anal. *See* Ileal pouch anal anastomosis
   stapled, in small bowel resection, 154, 154*f*
aneurysm(s), abdominal aortic, infrarenal, management. *See* infrarenal abdominal aortic aneurysm, management
anorectal abscess and fistula, management, 210-216
anorectal procedures, benign, 210-216, 210*f*, 212*f*-215*f*. *See also* specific procedures *and* benign anorectal procedures
antibiotic(s), in bile duct injury management, postoperative care, 113
antrectomy, truncal vagotomy and, for gastric ulcers, 72-74
aortic aneurysm, abdominal, infrarenal, management. *See* infrarenal abdominal aortic aneurysm, management
aortoiliac occlusive disease, operative management, 292-299, 292*f*, 294*f*-298*f*
appendectomy, 156-160, 156*f*-159*f*
   procedures, 158-160, 158*f*-159*f*
      laparoscopic appendectomy, 157*f*, 158*f*, 159-160
      open appendectomy, 158, 158*f*-159*f*
APR. *See* abdominoperineal resection (APR)
areolar duct excision, in breast cancer management, 218-227
arterial occlusive disease, infrainguinal, surgical revascularization, 300-308, 300*f*, 302*f*-307*f*. *See also* infrainguinal arterial occlusive disease, surgical revascularization

B

below-the-knee amputation (BKA), 315-323, 315*f*-318*f*
benign anorectal procedures, 210-216, 210*f*, 212*f*-215*f*. *See also* specific procedures
   types, 212-215, 212*f*-215*f*
      anorectal fistula management, 214-215, 215*f*
      circular stapled hemorrhoidopexy, 213-214, 213*f*
      hemorrhoidectomy, 212-213, 212*f*-213*f*
      pilonidal cyst excision and marsupialization, 214, 214*f*
      simple abscess drainage, 214, 215*f*
bile duct injuries
   classification, procedure, 110-111, 110*f*
   evaluation, equipment, 107
   at index operation, procedure, 111
   management, 106-114, 106*f*, 108*f*, 109*t*, 110*f*-113*f*
      procedures, 110-113, 110*f*-113*f*
         delayed reconstruction, 111-113, 111*f*-113*f*
         Roux-en-Y hepaticojejunostomy, 113, 113*f*
biliary decompression, contraindications, 106-107
biliary duct catheters, in bile duct injury management, postoperative care, 113

biliary stone disease, complex management. *See also* complex biliary stone disease, management
   management of, 97-105, 97f, 99f-104f
biliary strictures
   extrahepatic, causes of, 109, 109t
   management, 106-114, 106f, 108f, 109t, 110f-113f. *See also* bile duct injuries, management
Billroth I anastomosis, 72-73, 72f
Billroth II anastomosis, 73, 73f
biopsy(ies), sentinel lymph node, in breast cancer management. *See* sentinel lymph node biopsy, in breast cancer management
BKA. *See* below-the-knee amputation (BKA)
bleeding, from duodenal ulcer. *See* duodenal ulcer, bleeding
breast cancer, operative management, 217-228, 217f, 220f-226f
   procedures, 220-226, 220f-226f
      breast lumpectomy, 220-221, 220f-221f
      modified radical mastectomy, 221-224, 221f-224f
breast lumpectomy, in breast cancer management

C

cancer(s)
   breast, operative management of, 217-228, 217f, 220f-226f. *See also* breast cancer, operative management
   gastric, lymph node distribution for, procedure, 55, 55f
carotid endarterectomy, 286-291, 286f, 288f-291f
catheter(s), biliary duct, in bile duct injury management, postoperative care, 113
central venous access, 347-354, 347f-349f, 351f-352f
   procedures, 348-353, 348f-352f
      femoral vein access, 348, 348f
      internal jugular vein access, 350-351, 351f
      Seldinger technique, 352-353, 352f
      subclavian vein access, 348-350, 349f
   risks, 347
cervical esophagogastric anastomosis, in transhiatal esophagectomy, 39-40, 39f-40f
children
   inguinal hernia in, repair of, 378-382, 378f-381f. *See also* inguinal hernia repair, in children
   vascular access in, 371-377, 371f-376f. *See also* vascular access, in children
cholecystectomy, laparoscopic, 89-96, 89f, 91f-95f. *See also* laparoscopic cholecystectomy
choledochoduodenostomy, in complex biliary stone disease management, 98-105, 102f-104f
chronic pancreatitis, operative management, 137-144, 137f, 139f-144f
circular stapled hemorrhoidopexy, 213-214, 213f
colectomy, 180-191, 180f, 182f-189f
   with ileostomy, in inflammatory bowel disease management, 167-176, 167f, 169f-174f, 176f
      procedures, 169-174, 169f-174f

colectomy, with ileostomy, in inflammatory bowel disease management, procedures (*Cont.*):
      ileal pouch anal anastomosis, 171-174, 172f-174f
      total abdominal colectomy with end ileostomy, 169-170, 169f-170f
      total proctocolectomy with end ileostomy, 170, 171f
   procedures, 182-190, 182f-189f
      laparoscopic colectomy, 189-190, 189f
      left hemicolectomy, 186-188, 186f-187f
      right colectomy, 184-185, 184f-185f
      sigmoid colectomy, 188, 188f
      transverse colectomy, 186
   right, procedure, 184-185, 184f-185f
   sigmoid, procedure, 188, 188f
   total abdominal, with end ileostomy, in inflammatory bowel disease management, 169-170, 169f-170f
   transverse, procedure, 185
colitis, ulcerative, operative management of
   colectomy with ileostomy, 167
   ileal pouch anal anastomosis, 167
colostomy, loop. *See* loop colostomy
common bile duct, open exploration
common femoral artery, surgical revascularization of infrainguinal arterial occlusive disease and, 303, 303f
complex biliary stone disease, management, 97-105, 97f, 99f-104f
   procedures, 99-104, 99f-104f
      choledochoduodenostomy, 102-104, 102f-104f
      open common bile duct exploration, 99-100, 99f-100f
      transduodenal sphincteroplasty, 100-101, 100f-101f
cricothyroidotomy, emergency, 360-365, 360f-364f. *See also* emergency cricothyroidotomy
Crohn's disease, operative management
   colectomy with ileostomy, 167
   ileal pouch anal anastomosis, 167
   stricturoplasty, 176-179, 178f. *See also* stricturoplasty, in Crohn's disease management
Csendes procedure, for gastric ulcers, 73, 73f

D

deep vein thrombosis, after bile duct injury management, prevention, 113
dialysis, vascular access for, 270-278, 270f, 272f-274f, 276f
   procedure, 272-277, 272f-274f, 276f
distal pancreatectomy, 131-136, 131f, 133f-135f
donor nephrectomy
   laparoscopic transperitoneal donor nephrectomy, 246-248, 247f-248f
   open donor nephrectomy, 245-246, 245f-246f
donor pancreatectomy, procedure, 254-256, 254f-255f
drain(s), management, in bile duct injury management, postoperative care, 113

duodenal ulcer
  emergency operations, 70-71, 70*f*
    pyloroplasty, 70
    truncal vagotomy, 70-71
  oversewing of, 70, 70*f*, 74
  perforated, emergency operations for, procedure, 69-70, 69*f*
  vagotomy for, indications, 67

E

emergency cricothyroidotomy, 360-365, 360*f*-364*f*
  procedure, 363-364, 363*f*-364*f*
end ileostomy 161-166, 164*f*
  procedure, 163-164, 164*f*
  with total abdominal colectomy, in inflammatory bowel disease management, 169-170, 169*f*-170*f*
  with total proctocolectomy, in inflammatory bowel disease management, 170, 171*f*
endarterectomy, carotid, 286-291, 286*f*, 288*f*-291*f*. *See also* carotid endarterectomy
endocrine pancreas, surgery of, 22-28, 22*f*-27*f*
  procedure, 23-26, 23*f*-27*f*
endovenous laser ablation, in lower extremity venous insufficiency management, 310
endovenous radiofrequency ablation, in lower extremity venous insufficiency management, 310
esophagectomy, transhiatal, 29-41, 29*f*, 31*f*, 33*f*-40*f*. *See also* transhiatal esophagectomy

F

femoral artery, common, surgical revascularization of infrainguinal arterial occlusive disease and, 303, 303*f*
femoral vein access, 348, 348*f*
Finney stricturoplasty, in Crohn's disease management, 178-179, 178*f*
fistula(s), anorectal, management of. *See* anorectal abscess and fistula, management
full-thickness skin graft, in melanoma management, 235-237, 236*f*
fundoplication
  laparoscopic, hiatal. *See* laparoscopic fundoplication, hiatal
  open Nissen, hiatal

G

gastrectomy
  distal, procedure, 45-50, 45*f*-49*f*
  subtotal, procedure, 45-50, 45*f*-49*f*
  total, procedure, 50-54, 50*f*-54*f*
gastric band, laparoscopic adjustable. *See* laparoscopic adjustable gastric band
gastric bypass, Roux-en-Y. *See* Roux-en-Y gastric bypass
gastric cancer, lymph node distribution for, procedure, 55, 55*f*

gastric lesions, operative management, 42-56, 42*f*-47*f*, 49*f*-55*f*
  procedures, 43-55, 43*f*-47*f*, 49*f*-55*f*
    anatomy related to, 43-44, 43*f*-44*f*
    distal and subtotal gastrectomy, 45-50, 45*f*-49*f*
    lymph node distribution for gastric cancer, 55, 55*f*
    overview, 43-44, 43*f*-44*f*
    total gastrectomy, 50-54, 50*f*-54*f*
gastric ulcers
  classification, 71-73, 71*f*-73*f*
  emergency operations, procedures, 71-73, 71*f*-73*f*
gastrostomy
  in enteral access
    percutaneous endoscopic. *See* percutaneous endoscopic gastrostomy
    Stamm. *See* Stamm gastroscopy
Graham patch
  for gastric ulcers, pearls/tips, 74
  laparoscopic, for perforated duodenal ulcer, 69-70
  open, for perforated duodenal ulcer, 69, 69*f*

H

hand-sewn anastomosis, in small bowel resection, procedure, 151-152, 151*f*-153*f*
Heineke-Mikulicz stricturoplasty, in Crohn's disease management, 178, 178*f*
hemicolectomy, left, procedure, 186-188, 186*f*-187*f*
hemorrhoidectomy, 211-216, 212*f*-213*f*
  procedure, 212-213, 212*f*-213*f*
hemorrhoidopexy, circular stapled, 213-214, 213*f*
hepatectomy, 115-120, 115*f*-119*f*
  procedure, 116-118, 116*f*-119*f*
hepaticojejunostomy, Roux-en-Y, in bile duct injury management, procedure, 113, 113*f*
hernia(s)
  hiatal, repair of, laparoscopic. *See* laparoscopic hernia repair, hiatal
  inguinal, repair of, 324-330, 324*f*-329*f*. *See also* inguinal hernia repair
    in children, 378-382, 378*f*-381*f*. *See also* inguinal hernia repair, in children
  ventral, repair of, 331-337, 331*f*, 333*f*-336*f*. *See also* ventral hernia repair
hiatus, surgery of, 57-66, 57*f*, 59*f*-65*f*
  indications, 57
    open Nissen fundoplication, 57
    open paraesophageal hernia repair, 57
  procedures, 59-65, 59*f*-65*f*
    laparoscopic hernia repair, 63-65, 63*f*-65*f*
    open Nissen fundoplication, 59-62, 59*f*-62*f*
    open paraesophageal hernia repair, 63-65, 63*f*-65*f*
hyperaldosteronism, adrenalectomy in patients with, postoperative care, 20
hypercortisolism, after adrenalectomy, postoperative care, 20

I

ileal pouch anal anastomosis, in inflammatory bowel disease management, 171-174, 172f-174f
ileostomy
   end, 161-166, 161f, 164f. See end ileostomy
   loop. See loop ileostomy
inflammatory bowel disease, operative management, 167-179, 167f, 169f-174f, 176f, 178f
   colectomy with ileostomy, 167-176, 167f, 169f-174f, 176f
   Crohn's disease, 167, 176-179, 178f. See also Crohn's disease
   ileal pouch anal anastomosis, 167-176, 167f, 172f-174f, 176f
infrainguinal arterial occlusive disease, surgical revascularization, 300-308, 300f, 302f-307f
infrarenal abdominal aortic aneurysm, management, 279-285, 279f, 281f-284f
inguinal hernia repair, 324-330, 324f-329f
   in children, 378-382, 378f-381f
   procedures, 325-328, 325f-329f
      laparoscopic total extraperitoneal repair, 326, 327f-329f, 328
      open repair, 325-326, 325f-327f
inguinal lymph node dissection, in melanoma management, 232-235, 232f-235f
internal jugular vein access, 350-351, 351f

J

jejunostomy, Witzel. See Witzel jejunostomy

L

laparoscopic adjustable gastric band, for morbid obesity, 79-80, 79f
laparoscopic appendectomy, procedure, 157-160, 157f-158f
laparoscopic cholecystectomy, 89-96, 89f, 91f-95f
laparoscopic colectomy, procedure, 188-190, 189f
laparoscopic fundoplication, hiatal, 59-62, 59f-62f
laparoscopic Graham patch, for perforated duodenal ulcer, 69-70
laparoscopic hernia repair, hiatal. 57, 58, 63-65, 63f-65f
laparoscopic splenectomy, procedure, 146-147, 146f-147f
laparoscopic total extraperitoneal inguinal hernia repair, 326, 327f-329f, 328
laparoscopic transperitoneal donor nephrectomy, procedure, 246-248, 247f-248f
LAR. See low anterior resection (LAR)
laser ablation, endovenous, in lower extremity venous insufficiency management, 310
left hemicolectomy, procedure, 186-188, 186f-187f
lesion(s), gastric, operative management of, 42-56, 42f-47f, 49f-55f. See also gastric lesions, operative management
liver transplantation, 261-269, 261f, 263f-268f
lobectomy, thyroid, indications, 1
longitudinal pancreaticojejunostomy, in chronic pancreatitis management, 137-142, 139f-142f
loop colostomy, 161-166, 162f-163f
loop ileostomy, 161-166, 165f
low anterior resection (LAR), with total mesorectal excision, in rectal tumor management, 192-202, 195f-198f
lower extremity venous insufficiency, management, 309-314, 309f, 311f-313f
lumpectomy, breast, in breast cancer management. See breast lumpectomy, in breast cancer management

M

marsupialization, pilonidal cyst excision and. See pilonidal cyst excision, marsupialization and
mastectomy, radical, modified. See modified radical mastectomy
melanoma, operative management, 229-237, 229f, 231f-236f
   full-thickness skin graft, 235-237, 236f
   inguinal lymph node dissection, 232-235, 232f-235f
   wide local excision, 231-232, 231f
modified radical mastectomy, 218-224, 221f-224f
morbid obesity, surgeries for, 75-80, 75f-79f
   laparoscopic adjustable gastric band, 79, 79f
   Roux-en-Y gastric bypass, 76-78, 76f-78f

N

neck dissection, 1-7, 1f, 4f-6f
needle(s), in wound closure, 339-340, 339f, 340t
nephrectomy, donor, 242-251, 242f, 245f-251f. See also donor nephrectomy
Nissen fundoplication, open, hiatal

O

obesity, morbid, surgeries for, 75-80, 75f-79f. See also morbid obesity, surgeries for

P

pancreas, endocrine, surgery of, 22-28, 22f-27f. See also endocrine pancreas, surgery of
pancreas transplantation, 252-260, 252f, 254f, 255f, 257f-259f
   donor pancreatectomy, 254-256, 254f-255f
pancreatectomy
   distal, 131-136, 131f, 133f-135f. See also distal pancreatectomy
   donor, procedure, 254-256, 254f-255f
pancreatic pseudocyst-gastrostomy, pseudocyst-jejunostomy with, in chronic pancreatitis management, 137-144, 142f-144f
pancreaticoduodenectomy, 121-130, 121f, 123f-129f
pancreaticojejunostomy, longitudinal, in chronic pancreatitis management. See longitudinal pancreaticojejunostomy, in chronic pancreatitis management
pancreatitis, chronic, operative management of, 137-144, 137f, 139f-144f. See also chronic pancreatitis, operative management
paraesophageal hernia repair, open, hiatal
parathyroidectomy, 8-13, 8f-12f
pediatric inguinal hernia repair. See inguinal hernia repair, in children
pediatric vascular access. See vascular access, in children
peptic ulcer disease, emergency operations, 67-74, 67f, 69f-73f
   bleeding duodenal ulcer, 70-71, 70f
   Csendes procedure, 73, 73f

peptic ulcer disease, emergency operations (*Cont.*):
    gastric ulcers, 71-73, 71*f*-73*f*
    perforated duodenal ulcer, 69-70, 69*f*
percutaneous endoscopic gastrostomy, in enteral access, 82-87, 83*f*
perineal rectosigmoidectomy, for rectal prolapse, 203-209
peroneal artery, posterior, surgical revascularization of infrainguinal arterial occlusive disease and, 304-305, 305*f*
pheochromocytoma, adrenalectomy in patients with, postoperative care, 20
phlebectomy, TriVex transilluminated power, in lower extremity venous insufficiency management, 310
phlebotomy, stab, in lower extremity venous insufficiency management, 310
pilonidal cyst excision, marsupialization and, 210-216, 214*f*
popliteal artery, surgical revascularization of infrainguinal arterial occlusive disease and, 304, 304*f*
proctocolectomy, total, with end ileostomy, in inflammatory bowel disease management, 170, 171*f*
prolapse, rectal, operative management, 203-209, 203*f*-208*f*. *See also* rectal prolapse, operative management
pseudocyst-gastrostomy, pancreatic, pseudocyst-jejunostomy with, in chronic pancreatitis management. *See* pancreatic pseudocyst-gastrostomy, pseudocyst-jejunostomy with, in chronic pancreatitis management
pseudocyst-jejunostomy, pancreatic pseudocyst-gastrostomy with, in chronic pancreatitis management. *See* pancreatic pseudocyst-gastrostomy, pseudocyst-jejunostomy with, in chronic pancreatitis management
pyloric stenosis, operative management, 366-370, 366*f*-369*f*
pyloromyotomy, 366-370, 366*f*-369*f*
pyloroplasty, truncal vagotomy and
  for bleeding duodenal ulcer, procedure, 70
  for gastric ulcers, 72-74, 72*f*-73*f*

R

radical mastectomy, modified. *See* modified radical mastectomy
radiofrequency ablation, endovenous, in lower extremity venous insufficiency management, 310
rectal prolapse, operative management, 203-209, 203*f*-208*f*
    perineal rectosigmoidectomy, 206-208, 206*f*-208*f*
    resection rectopexy, 204-205, 204*f*-205*f*
rectal tumors, operative management, 192-202, 192*f*, 194*f*-201*f*. *See also specific procedures*, 192-202, 194*f*-201*f*
    APR with total mesorectal excision. *See* abdominoperineal resection (APR), with total mesorectal excision, in rectal tumor management
    LAR with total mesorectal excision. *See* low anterior resection (LAR), with total mesorectal excision, operative management
    transanal resection. *See* transanal resection, in rectal tumor management

rectopexy, resection, for rectal prolapse. *See* resection rectopexy, for rectal prolapse
rectosigmoidectomy, perineal, for rectal prolapse. *See* perineal rectosigmoidectomy, for rectal prolapse
renal transplantation, 242-251, 242*f*, 245*f*-251*f*
    donor nephrectomy, 242-251, 242*f*, 245*f*-251*f*. *See also* donor nephrectomy
resection rectopexy, for rectal prolapse, 203-208, 204*f*-205*f*
right colectomy, procedure, 184-185, 184*f*-185*f*
Roux-en-Y gastric bypass, for morbid obesity, 76-80, 76*f*-78*f*
Roux-en-Y hepaticojejunostomy, in bile duct injury management, procedure, 113, 113*f*

S

sarcoma(s), soft tissue, operative management, 238-241, 238*f*-241*f*. *See also* soft tissue sarcoma, operative management
Seldinger technique, 352-353, 352*f*
sentinel lymph node biopsy, in breast cancer management, 217-228, 224*f*-225*f*
sigmoid colectomy, procedure, 188, 188*f*
small bowel resection, 149-155, 149*f*, 151*f*-154*f*
    hand-sewn anastomosis, 151-152, 151*f*-153*f*
    stapled anastomosis, 154, 154*f*
soft tissue sarcoma, operative management, 238-241, 238*f*-241*f*
sphincteroplasty, transduodenal. *See* transduodenal sphincteroplasty
splenectomy, 145-148, 145*f*-148*f*
    laparoscopic, 146-147, 146*f*-147*f*
    open, 147-148, 147*f*-148*f*
stab phlebotomy, in lower extremity venous insufficiency management, 310
Stamm gastrostomy, in enteral access, 82-88, 84*f*-86*f*
stapled anastomosis, in small bowel resection, 154, 154*f*
stenosis(es), pyloric, operative management, 366-370, 366*f*-369*f*. *See also* pyloromyotomy
stricturoplasty
  in Crohn's disease management, 176-179, 178*f*
    Finney stricturoplasty, 178-179, 178*f*
    Heineke-Mikulicz stricturoplasty, 178, 178*f*
subclavian vein access, 348-350, 349*f*
suppression status, uncertain, after adrenalectomy, postoperative care, 20
suture(s), in wound closure, 338-339

T

thoracostomy, tube, 355-359, 355*f*-359*f*. *See also* tube thoracostomy
thrombosis(es), deep vein, prevention, in bile duct injury management, 113
thyroid lobectomy, indications, 1
thyroidectomy, 1-7, 1*f*-6*f*
tibial artery
  anterior, surgical revascularization of infrainguinal arterial occlusive disease and, 305-306

tibial artery (*Cont.*):
   posterior, surgical revascularization of infrainguinal arterial occlusive disease and, 304-305, 305*f*
total abdominal colectomy with end ileostomy, in inflammatory bowel disease management, 169-170, 169*f*-170*f*
total mesorectal excision
   APR with, in rectal tumor management. *See* abdominoperineal resection (APR), with total mesorectal excision, in rectal tumor management
   LAR with, in rectal tumor management. *See also* low anterior resection (LAR), with total mesorectal excision, in rectal tumor management
total proctocolectomy, with end ileostomy, in inflammatory bowel disease management, 170, 171*f*
tracheostomy, 360-365, 360*f*-364*f*
   anatomic landmarks, 361-362, 361*f*
transanal excision of tumor, in rectal tumor management, 192-201
transduodenal sphincteroplasty, in complex biliary stone disease management, 97-104, 100*f*-101*f*
transhiatal esophagectomy, 29-41, 29*f*, 31*f*, 33*f*-40*f*
   abdominal phase, 32-34, 33*f*
   cervical esophagogastric anastomosis, 39-40, 39*f*-40*f*
   cervical phase, 34-35, 34*f*
   gastric conduit creation, 37-39, 37*f*-38*f*
   mediastinal dissection, 35-37, 35*f*-36*f*
transplantation(s)
   liver, 261-269, 261*f*, 263*f*-268*f*. *See also* liver transplantation
   pancreas, 252-260, 252*f*, 254*f*, 255*f*, 257*f*-259*f*. *See also* pancreas transplantation
   renal, 242-251, 242*f*, 245*f*-251*f*. *See also* renal transplantation
transverse colectomy, procedure, 185

TriVex transilluminated power phlebectomy, in lower extremity venous insufficiency management, 310
truncal vagotomy, pyloroplasty and
   for bleeding duodenal ulcer, procedure, 70-71
   for gastric ulcers, 72-74, 72*f*-73*f*
tube thoracostomy, 355-359, 355*f*-359*f*
tumor(s), rectal. *See* rectal tumors

# U
ulcer(s)
   duodenal. *See* duodenal ulcer
   gastric, 71-73, 71*f*-73*f*
   peptic, 67-74, 67*f*, 69*f*-73*f*
ulcerative colitis, operative management
   colectomy with ileostomy, 167
   ileal pouch anal anastomosis, 167

V
vagotomy
   for bleeding duodenal ulcer, indications, 67
   truncal. *See* truncal vagotomy
vascular access
   in children, 371-377, 371*f*-376*f*
   for dialysis, 270-278, 270*f*, 272*f*-274*f*, 276*f*. *See also* dialysis, vascular access for
venous access, subclavian, 348-350, 349*f*
venous insufficiency, lower extremity, management, 309-314, 309*f*, 311*f*-313*f*. *See also* lower extremity venous insufficiency, management
ventral hernia repair, 331-337, 331*f*, 333*f*-336*f*

W
Witzel jejunostomy, in enteral access